THIRD EDITION

INTRODUCTION TO Veterinary Anatomy AND Physiology TEXTBOOK

Victoria Aspinall BVSc MRCVS
Senior Lecturer in Veterinary Nursing, Hartpury College, Gloucester, UK

Melanie Cappello BSc(Hons) Zoology PGCE VN
East Grinstead, West Sussex, UK

Contribution by

Catherine Phillips RVN REVN CertEd PGDip FHEA
Head of Department, Veterinary Nursing, Hartpury College, Gloucester, UK

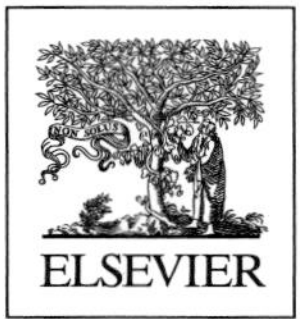

Edinburgh London New York Oxford Philadelphia St Louis Sydney Toronto 2015

ELSEVIER

First edition 2004
Second edition 2009
Reprinted 2009, 2010 (twice), 2011
Third edition 2015
Reprinted 2015

ISBN 978-0-7020-5735-9

Notices

Knowledge and best practice in this field are constantly changing. As new research and experience broaden our understanding, changes in research methods, professional practices, or medical treatment may become necessary.

Practitioners and researchers must always rely on their own experience and knowledge in evaluating and using any information, methods, compounds, or experiments described herein. In using such information or methods they should be mindful of their own safety and the safety of others, including parties for whom they have a professional responsibility.

With respect to any drug or pharmaceutical products identified, readers are advised to check the most current information provided (i) on procedures featured or (ii) by the manufacturer of each product to be administered, to verify the recommended dose or formula, the method and duration of administration, and contraindications. It is the responsibility of practitioners, relying on their own experience and knowledge of their patients, to make diagnoses, to determine dosages and the best treatment for each individual patient, and to take all appropriate safety precautions.

To the fullest extent of the law, neither the Publisher nor the authors, contributors, or editors, assume any liability for any injury and/or damage to persons or property as a matter of products liability, negligence or otherwise, or from any use or operation of any methods, products, instructions, or ideas contained in the material herein.

Printed in China
Last digit is the Print Number: 9 8 7 6 5 4 3 2

Introduction to Veterinary Anatomy and Physiology Textbook

Content Strategist: Robert Edwards
Content Development Specialist: Carole McMurray
Project Manager: Anne Collett
Designer/Design Direction: Miles Hitchen
Illustration Manager: Amy Faith Heyden
Illustrator: Electronic Publishing Services Inc

Contents

Preface

By the time this third edition of *Introduction to Veterinary Anatomy and Physiology* is published, six years will have passed since the second edition, and we decided that it was time to update it. The book is used as a standard text for many animal-based courses in both higher and further education and in particular all veterinary nursing courses. So with this in mind we decided to increase the clinical content and to answer the question 'Why do we have to learn anatomy and physiology?' As lecturers in the subject we are well aware that many students resent time spent away from clinical nursing, both theoretical and practical, and find 'A/P' 'boring', so it is our job to link the theory with what might be seen in practice. In all chapters there are increased numbers of short descriptions of disease conditions that are relevant to the system being described – most of them are common; a few, especially those in exotic species, may only be seen in specialist practices.

We have also included a new chapter on the anatomy and physiology of farm animals. Recently, new courses of study for veterinary nurses have been developed to widen the range of animals to include large animals. This is in response to the demand of mixed veterinary practices, especially those in the country, that require their nurses to be able to work with all types of animal. There are many books written on the subject but these are either very dated or aimed at a higher level of study. Our chapter on large animals provides information at a similar level to the rest of the text and offers a comparison between the anatomy of the dog, cat and especially the horse and pays particular attention to the important differences in the skeletal and digestive systems of the species.

Once again we feel that we have produced a useful, accurate and informative text book that we both hope will continue to be used as the 'bible' of anatomy and physiology for veterinary nurses and all other students in animal-related courses.

Victoria Aspinall
Melanie Cappello

About the authors

Victoria Aspinall, BVSc, MRCVS, qualified from Bristol University in 1974 and went into small animal practice in Kings Lynn, Norfolk, with her husband, Richard, who is also a vet. After five years, including brief spells in practices in Sussex and Swindon, they set up a small animal practice in Gloucester. In 1991 Vicky was employed to help start the new Animal Care department at Hartpury College, Gloucester, and in 1993 was appointed Head of Animal Care and Veterinary Nursing. In 1999 she left the college to start Abbeydale Vetlink Veterinary Training Ltd above her husband's practice and then sold it in 2010 when it moved to Monmouth. While running the business, Vicky also taught vet nurses at Filton College, Bridgwater College and Bridgend College, although not all at the same time! She has recently returned to teach part time at Hartpury College. Vicky has four children, none of whom has followed their parents into the profession!

In the last few years, Vicky has written articles on many veterinary nursing subjects for the *Veterinary Nursing Journal* and the *Veterinary Nursing Times*. She has also been responsible for a series of CD-ROMs on anatomy and physiology and has been a contributor to several major veterinary nursing textbooks, including *BSAVA Textbook of Veterinary Nursing*, 4th edition. Vicky has also acted as editor for *Clinical Procedures in Veterinary Nursing* and *The Complete Textbook of Veterinary Nursing* and has written the companion to this book, *Essentials of Veterinary Anatomy and Physiology*. Recently, with her husband, she produced *Clinical Procedures in Small Animal Veterinary Practice*, designed for veterinary surgeons.

Melanie Cappello, BSc(Hons), Zoology PGCE VN, started out as a veterinary nurse, qualifying in 1990, and working in both mixed and small animal practice, before working at the Royal Veterinary College (RVC) from 1991 to 1993. She then left to undertake a degree in Zoology at University College London, where she graduated with honours in 1996. After taking a break to start a family, Melanie then went into teaching and taught anatomy and physiology to student veterinary nurses from 1998 to 2004, at the College of Animal Welfare's RVC site. During this time she completed a Postgraduate Certificate in Education.

In June 2004 Melanie took up a post as Clinical Skills Tutor in the RVC's new Clinical Skills Centre, which was the first of its kind in a UK veterinary school. She became particularly interested in the educational aspects of clinical skills teaching and this prompted her to pursue a Research Fellowship in the RVC's LIVE Centre. In 2008 Melanie and her family relocated to West Sussex when her husband (who is a specialist in veterinary neurology) took a position in a private referral practice. Since then, Melanie has worked as an Ophthalmology nurse in a referral practice, which allowed her to refresh and update her skills in veterinary nursing. Melanie is currently taking a break from her career while she looks after her four children, two ponies, two dogs and two cats!

Melanie has written a chapter on the evolution of the wolf and the domestication of the dog for the *Ultimate Dog Care Book* and has co-authored (with Victoria Aspinall) the chapter on anatomy and physiology in the *BSAVA Textbook of Veterinary Nursing*, 4th edition.

Acknowledgements

The completion of this book would not have been possible without the continuing support of all the members of our respective families, including Richard, Polly, Charlie, William, Nico, Evelyn, Ken, Sebastian, Elizabeth, Matilda, Alexander and Rodolfo, who put up with starvation and neglect, obsession with hitting deadlines, and our grumpiness!

We would also like to thank Catherine Phillips from Hartpury College in Gloucester, who has updated the chapter on the Horse. As ever, the team at Elsevier have been helpful and supportive, and in particular Robert Edwards, who despite rising up his profession and being ever busier, stills finds time to discuss tactics!

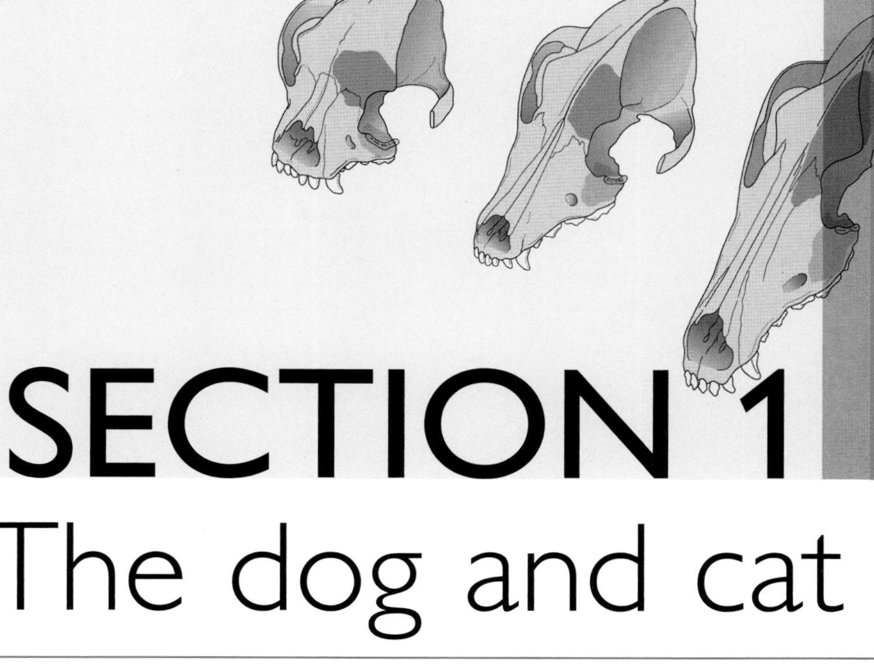

SECTION 1
The dog and cat

This section describes the anatomy and physiology of the two most common species treated in small animal veterinary practice: the dog and cat. Following an introduction to cell biology, each body system is covered separately.

CHAPTER 1

Principles of cell biology

KEY POINTS

- All living organisms can be classified into different orders, classes and families linked by certain common characteristics. These groups can be further divided into a genus and species, which describes an individual type of organism.
- The body is made up of a number of systems, each of which has a specific function. These systems form the structural framework of the body or lie within one of three body cavities.
- Each system consists of a collection of tissues and organs, which are composed of the smallest units of the body – the cells.
- Cells can only be seen under the microscope and all have a basic structure with certain anatomical differences, which adapt them to their specific function.
- Each structure within the cell plays a vital part in the normal function of the cell and therefore in the normal function of the body system.
- Cells grow and divide by means of mitosis. Each mitotic division results in the production of two identical daughter cells containing the diploid (or normal) number of chromosomes.
- The healthy body contains 60–70% water, distributed into two principal fluid compartments – the extracellular fluid (ECF) (surrounding the cells) and the intracellular fluid (ICF) (within the cells).
- Body fluids move between these compartments and this movement is controlled by the chemical constituents of the fluid and the physical processes of diffusion and osmosis.
- Body fluids contain inorganic and organic compounds. The structure and percentage of all of these is fundamental to the balance and normal function of the body. Within the body there are many systems involved in maintaining a state of equilibrium – this is known as homeostasis.

'Anatomy' and 'physiology' are scientific terms used to describe the study of the structure of the body (anatomy) and how the body actually 'works' (physiology). In this section, we will study the anatomy and physiology of the dog and cat. In Section 2, we describe the comparative anatomy and physiology of the horse, the most common farm animals and some of the most commonly kept exotic species. We start by looking at the basic unit of the body – the cell – and then work our way through the tissues, organs and systems until the picture is complete.

Animal classification

When studying any aspect of biology it is important to have a basic understanding of the classification system used to group animals. How the species that one may meet in a veterinary practice fit into this classification system should also be understood. Classification is the way in which we 'sort' species into orderly groups, depending on how closely they are related in terms of their evolution, structure and behaviour. The science of classification is known as *taxonomy*.

If organisms have certain basic features in common they are grouped together into a *kingdom*. For example, if an organism is composed of more than one cell (i.e., it is multicellular) and obtains its food by ingestion, it is placed in the animal kingdom. Other kingdoms include plants and fungi. The animal kingdom is then further subdivided, based upon similarities of organisms, into a hierarchical system (Table 1.1). This narrows the classification down until we eventually reach a particular *genus* and *species*. Most living organisms are identified by a genus and species – a method known as the binomial system, invented by the Swedish scientist Carl Linnaeus.

All the species within the animal kingdom are divided into those with backbones – the vertebrates – and those that do not have backbones – the invertebrates (e.g., insects, worms, etc.). The vertebrates are divided into eight *classes*. The classes that are of the most veterinary importance are:

- Amphibia – approximately 3080 species
- Reptilia – approximately 6600 species
- Aves or birds – approximately 8500 species
- Fish – approximately 30,000 species.
- Mammalia – approximately 4070 species.

These classes are then further divided into *orders*, and so on, until a species is identified, as in Table 1.1.

Most of this section of the book concerns the mammals, because the majority of animals seen in veterinary practice will be from this class. The distinctive features of mammals are the production of milk by the mammary glands and the possession of hair as a body covering. Examples of mammalian orders include:

- Insectivores (e.g., shrews, moles)
- Rodents (e.g., mice, rats)
- Lagomorphs (e.g., rabbits, hares)
- Carnivores (e.g., cats, dogs, bears, seals)
- Ungulates (e.g., cows, sheep, horses)
- Cetaceans (e.g., whales, dolphins)
- Primates (e.g., monkeys, apes)

Table 1.1 Classification of the domestic dog and cat

Taxonomic group	Dog	Cat
Kingdom	Animal	Animal
Phylum	Chordata (vertebrate)	Chordata (vertebrate)
Class	Mammalia (mammal)	Mammalia (mammal)
Order	Carnivora	Carnivora
Family	Canidae	Felidae
Genus	*Canis*	*Felis*
Species	*familiaris*	*catus*
Common name	Domestic dog	Domestic cat

Generally speaking, all mammals have a similar basic structural plan in terms of anatomy and physiology, but each species has been modified to suit its specific lifestyle. In other words, mammals have become specialised for activities such as running, digging, gnawing, jumping and eating specific foods.

Anatomical definitions

When studying anatomy and physiology it is important to understand the terms that are used to describe where structures lie in relation to one another. These are illustrated in Fig. 1.1 and named as follows:

- *Median plane* – divides the body longitudinally into symmetrical right and left halves; can be described as 'the line down the middle of the animal' from nose to tail
- *Superficial* – near to the surface of the body
- *Deep* – closer to the centre of the body
- *Cranial/anterior* – towards the front of the animal (i.e., towards the head)
- *Caudal/posterior* – towards the rear end or tail of the animal (i.e., away from the head)
- *Medial* – structures that lie towards or near the median plane (i.e., closer to the middle of the animal)
- *Lateral* – structures that lie towards the side of the animal (i.e., away from the median plane)
- *Dorsal* – towards or near the back or vertebral column of the animal and the corresponding surfaces of the head, neck and tail
- *Ventral* – towards or near the belly or lowermost surface of the body and the corresponding surfaces of the head, neck and tail
- *Rostral* – towards the nose; used to describe the position of structures on the head
- *Proximal* – structures or part of the structure that lie close to the main mass of the body (e.g., the 'top' of the limb that attaches to the body); also used to describe parts that lie near the origin of a structure
- *Distal* – structures or part of the structure that lie away from the main mass of the body or origin (e.g., the free end of the limb)

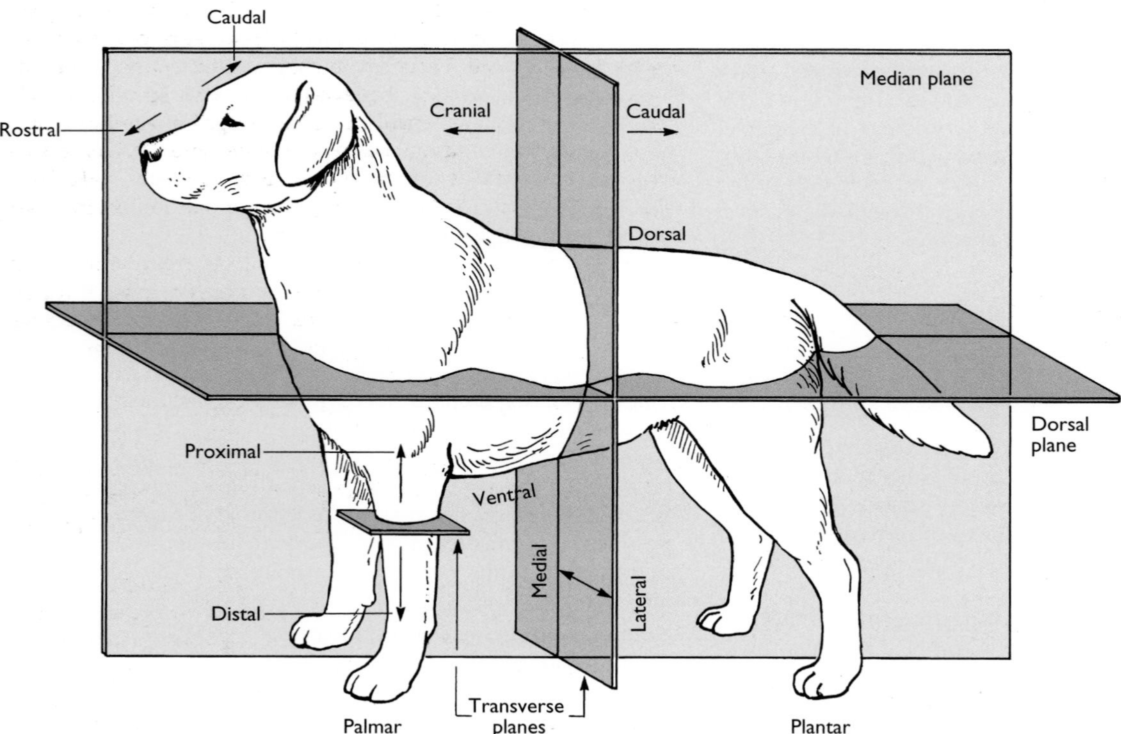

Fig. 1.1 Anatomical planes and directional terms used to describe the relative position of structures in the body. (With permission from T Colville, JM Bassett, 2001. Clinical anatomy and physiology for veterinary technicians. St Louis, MO: Mosby, p. 3.)

- *Palmar* – the rear surface of the fore paw that bears the footpads; the opposite surface (i.e., the front surface of the paw) is the dorsal surface
- *Plantar* – the rear surface of the hind paw that bears the footpads; the opposite surface (as above) is the dorsal surface.

An understanding of anatomical terminology is useful when you are helping the vet in diagnostic imaging. For example, you may be asked to position the patient for a ventrodorsal chest X-ray and knowing the meaning of the words 'ventral' and 'dorsal' will help you position the animal correctly.

The basic plan of the body

The body is made up of a number of systems and each of them has a specific job, enabling the body to function effectively. These systems can be placed in one of three groups depending on their function:

- *Structural systems* – provide the basic 'framework' and transport system for the body
- *Coordinating systems* – the control mechanisms of the body
- *Visceral systems* – includes all the basic functional systems that do the general duties for the body; found within one of the three body cavities: thoracic, abdominal and pelvic

Structural systems

- *Skeletal system* – the supporting frame upon which the body is built (i.e., the bones and joints)
- *Muscular system* – the mechanism by which the bones are moved to bring about locomotion (this relates to skeletal muscle only, the other categories of muscle are considered separately)
- *Integument* – the covering of the body (i.e., skin and hair)
- *Cardiovascular system* – transports the blood around the body

Coordinating systems

- *Nervous system* – carries information to and from the central 'control station' of the body (i.e., the brain); controls and monitors the internal and external environment of the body
- *Endocrine system* – controls the body's functions via a communication system of chemical messengers or hormones

Visceral systems

- *Digestive system* – responsible for taking in food and breaking it down to its basic components so that the body can utilise them
- *Respiratory system* – responsible for taking in oxygen and removing carbon dioxide
- *Urinary system* – responsible for eliminating waste and toxic substances from the body
- *Reproductive system* – responsible for producing offspring

Each system of the body is made up of a collection of specific types of *tissue* arranged as *organs*. Each tissue is composed of a specialised type of *cell* (the smallest unit of the body).

The mammalian cell

Cells are the minute units of a tissue that can only be seen under a microscope. Cells can be considered to be the basic structural and functional unit of an organism. In fact they are like 'little bodies' themselves because they carry out a number of basic functions such as taking in nutrients and excreting waste, respiring or 'breathing', and reproducing. These and other functions are carried out by various structures that make up the cell – mainly by the organelles, or 'little organs', that float within the cytoplasm of the cell.

Cell structure and function

The components of a cell are shown in Figs. 1.2 and 1.3 and are as follows:

- Cell membrane
- Nucleus
- Organelles:
  - Mitochondria
  - Ribosomes
  - Rough endoplasmic reticulum
  - Smooth endoplasmic reticulum
  - Golgi apparatus
  - Lysosomes
  - Centrosome

Cell membrane

The cell membrane covers the surface of the cell and may also be called the plasma membrane. It is responsible for separating the cell from its environment and controls the passage of substances in and out of the cell. Carbohydrates are found on the surface of the cell membrane and it is believed that these help cell recognition, meaning that they enable a cell to recognise whether or not it is in contact with another cell of the same type. The cell membrane of a mammalian cell is composed of a *phospholipid bilayer* (Fig. 1.4). This is a double layer of phospholipid molecules with protein molecules embedded within it.

The nature of its structure means that the cell membrane is *selectively permeable*, allowing some substances to pass through it while others may either be excluded or must travel across the membrane by means of specialised transport systems. These include:

- *Pores in the cell membrane* – small molecules can pass through these pores
- *Simple diffusion* – molecules that are soluble in lipids (or fats) will passively dissolve in the lipid part of the cell membrane and diffuse across it; oxygen and water enter the cell in this way
- *Facilitated diffusion* – another type of passive diffusion, where the substance is moving down a concentration gradient, but the substance enlists the help of a carrier protein to help it across the membrane; glucose uses this method to enter the cell
- *Active transport mechanisms* – substances are usually being moved from a region of low concentration to one of higher concentration (i.e., they are travelling against a concentration gradient). This is like going up a steep hill – it is hard work and therefore requires energy. Substances that require active

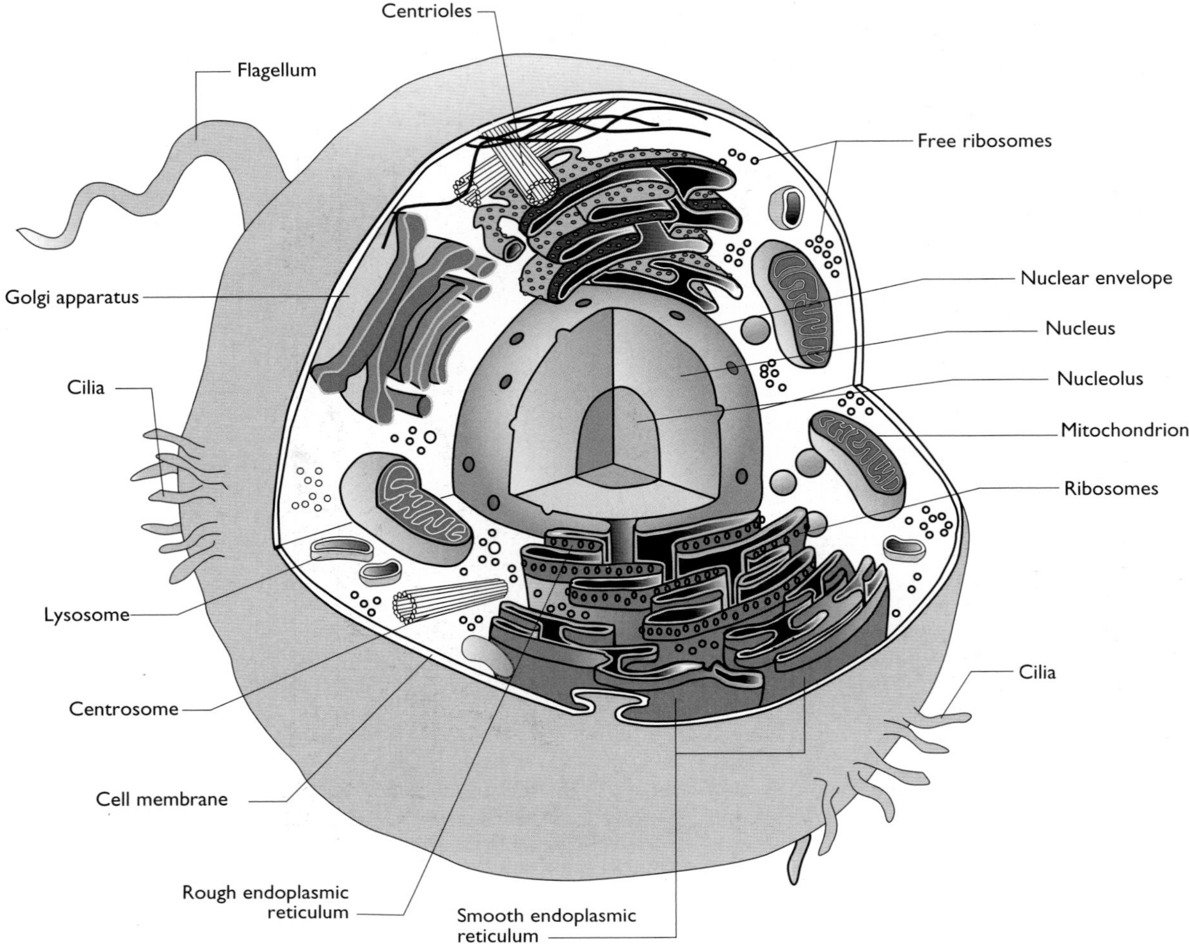

Fig. 1.2 Components of the mammalian cell. (With permission from T Colville, JM Bassett, 2001. Clinical anatomy and physiology for veterinary technicians. St Louis, MO: Mosby, p. 11.)

transport mechanisms to cross the cell membrane use a carrier protein to transport them across. The 'cost' for this service is that energy is required, and is supplied by the cell's 'energy currency' – molecules of adenosine triphosphate (ATP). Sodium enters the cell this way.

Cytoplasm

This is the fluid that fills the interior of the cell, providing it with support. The nucleus and organelles are found within the cytoplasm, along with solutes such as glucose, proteins and ions.

Nucleus

The nucleus is the information centre of the cell. It is surrounded by a nuclear membrane and contains the *chromosomes*. Chromosomes are the bearers of the hereditary material, DNA, which carries the information for protein synthesis. DNA is the 'set of instructions' that tells the cell how to function, and these instructions are then passed on to the cell's descendants. The nucleus also contains several nucleoli, where the ribosomes (see below) are manufactured.

Organelles

- *Mitochondria* – these are responsible for cellular respiration and are the site where energy is extracted from food substances and stored in a form that the cell can use: ATP. Mitochondria have a smooth outer membrane and a highly folded inner membrane, which increases the surface area on which ATP production can take place (Figs. 1.2 and 1.3). Mitochondria are found in abundance in cells that are very active in terms of energy consumption (e.g., skeletal muscle). When a cell requires energy it uses its store of ATP molecules. The energy itself is stored in the bond that connects the phosphate group to the rest of the molecule (Fig. 1.5). If one of these phosphate groups is 'snapped off' the molecule, the bond is broken and energy is released. The remaining molecule is now called adenosine *di*phosphate (ADP), because it now has only two phosphate groups attached to it (di = 2; tri = 3). However, the cell needs only to re-attach another phosphate group (carried out as part of the cell's metabolic processes) and energy can be stored once more as ATP.
- *Ribosomes* – these float free in the cytoplasm and are the site for protein synthesis within the cell.

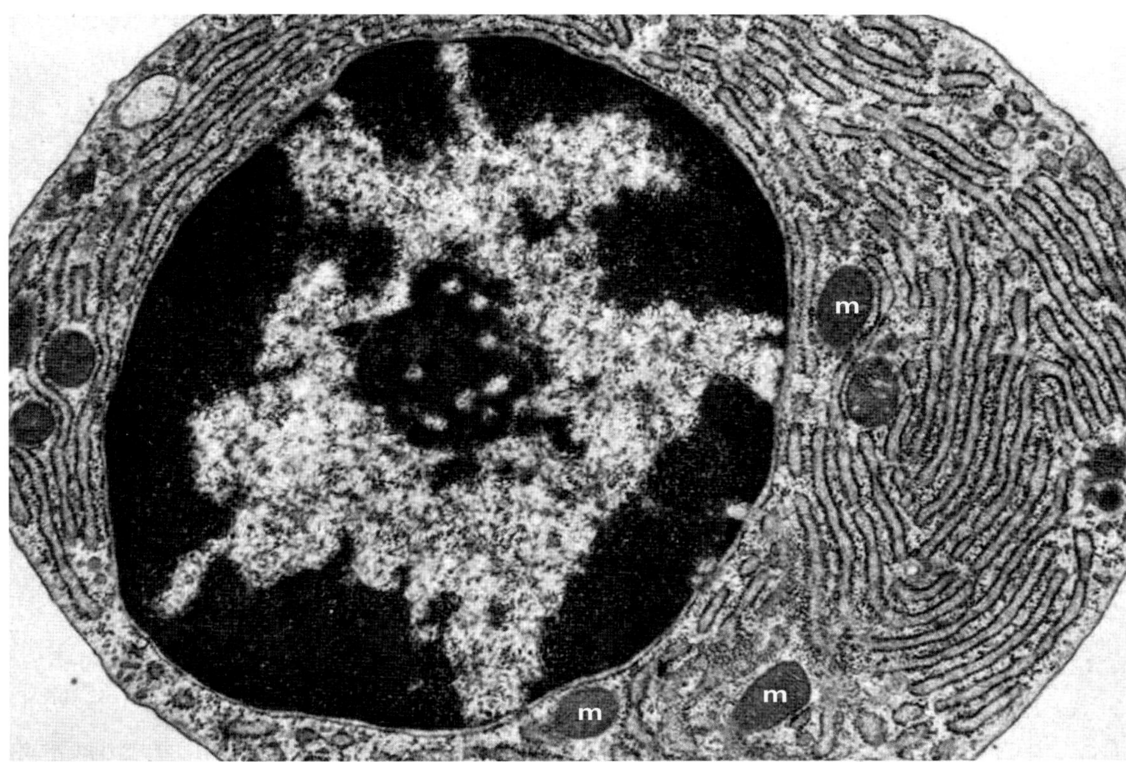

Fig. 1.3 Transmission electron micrograph of a plasma cell showing extensive rough ER and scattered mitochondria (m). (With permission from DA Samuelson, 2007. Textbook of veterinary histology. St Louis, MO: Saunders-Elsevier, p. 86.)

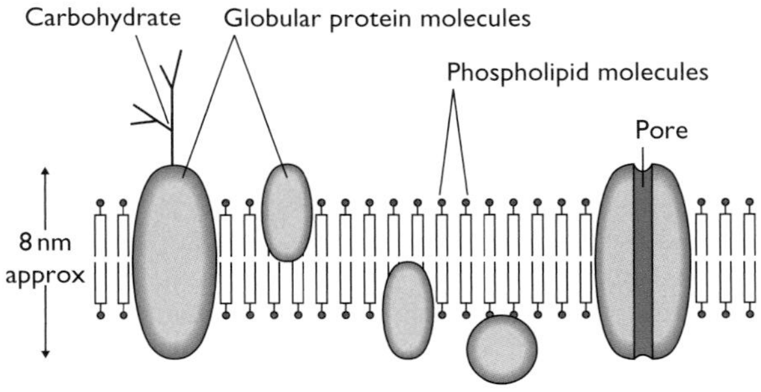

Fig. 1.4 Structure of the cell membrane showing the phospholipid bilayer. This structure is also known as the 'fluid mosaic model'.

- *Endoplasmic reticulum (ER)* – this is a network of membrane-lined interconnected tubes and cavities within the cytoplasm of the cell. There are two types of ER:
  - *Rough ER* (Fig. 1.3) is so called because it has numerous ribosomes attached to its surface and thus appears 'rough' when viewed under a microscope. The function of rough ER is to transport the proteins that have been synthesised by ribosomes. Some of these proteins are not required by the cell in which they are made but are 'exported' outside the cell (e.g., digestive enzymes and hormones).
  - *Smooth ER* is so called because it does not have ribosomes on its surface; its functions include the synthesis and transport of lipids and steroids.

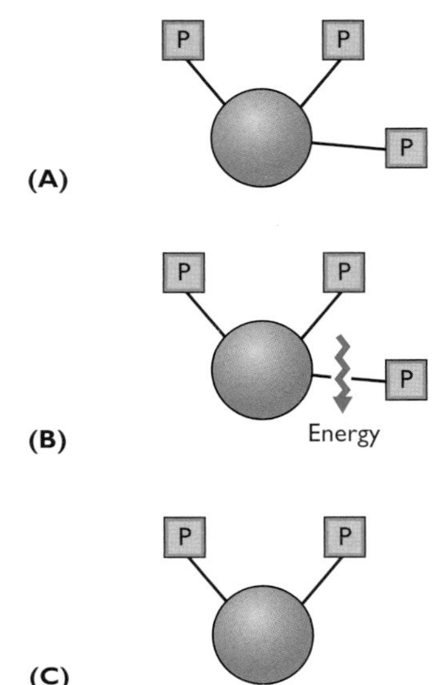

Fig. 1.5 The conversion of ATP to ADP to release energy. **(A)** The ATP molecule has three phosphate groups (P) attached by chemical bonds; energy is stored within the bonds. **(B)** One of the phosphate groups is 'snapped off', releasing energy. **(C)** The remaining molecule (ADP, with two phosphate groups) goes back into the metabolic cycle and has a phosphate group reattached, becoming ATP again.

- *The Golgi apparatus* or body – this is a stack of flattened sacs within the cytoplasm (Fig. 1.2). Its function includes the modification of some of the proteins produced by the cell (adding a carbohydrate component) and it plays a part in the formation of lysosomes.
- *Lysosomes* – these are membrane-bound sacs that contain lysozymes or digestive enzymes. Their function is to digest materials taken in by the cell during the process of phagocytosis or endocytosis (Fig. 1.6). Lysosomes also destroy worn-out organelles within the cell and, in some cases, the cell itself.

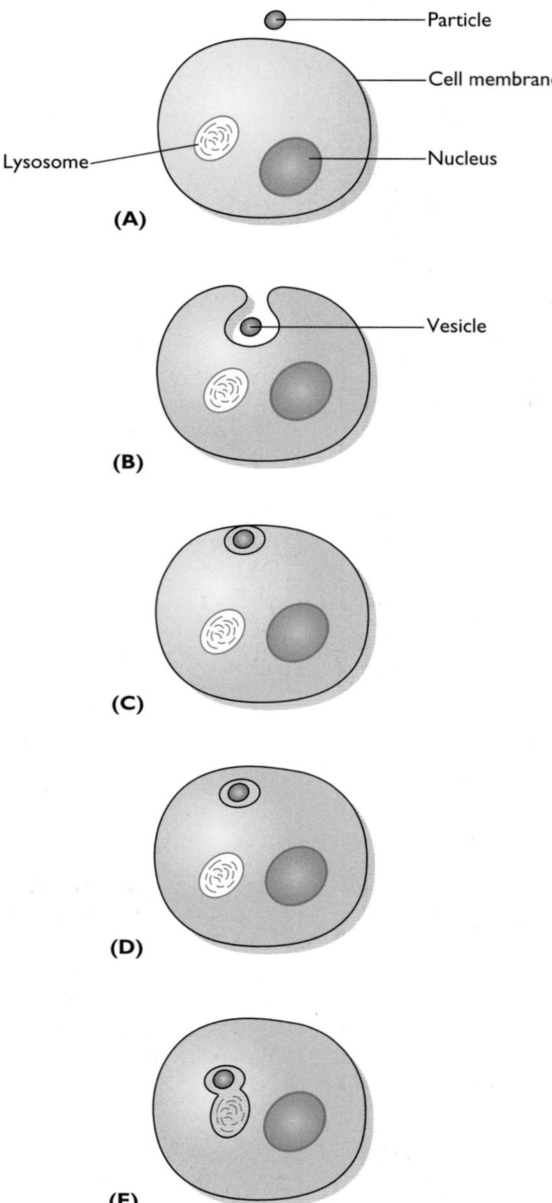

Fig. 1.6 Phagocytosis. **(A)** A small particle (e.g., bacterium) is present outside the cell. **(B)** The cell membrane invaginates and starts to enclose the particle. **(C)** The cell membrane completely surrounds the particle and seals it off in a vesicle. **(D)** The vesicle detaches from the membrane and enters the cell. **(E)** A lysosome, containing digestive enzymes, fuses with the phagocytic vesicle containing the particle and the particle is destroyed.

Lysosomal storage disease – this occurs if there is a dysfunction of the enzyme in the lysosomes resulting in the accumulation of waste substances. 'Lysosomal storage disease' is seen more commonly in cats. Storage diseases usually occur in young animals and present with clinical signs such as skeletal abnormalities, mental retardation and neurological and ocular disorders.

- *Centrosome and centrioles* – the centrosome contains a pair of rod-like structures called centrioles. These lie at right angles to each other and are involved in cell division (see mitosis).
- *Cilia and flagella* – these are extensions of the plasma membrane seen on some cells of the body. Cilia are found in large numbers on the outer surface of the cells and are responsible for creating a wave-like motion that moves fluid such as mucus and debris over the cell surface. Flagella are usually single and longer than cilia and move the cell along by undulating movements. The only example of a flagellum in mammals is the tail of a spermatozoon.

Materials can either be taken into the cell or exported out of it. These processes are called *endocytosis* and *exocytosis*, respectively. There are two types of endocytosis: phagocytosis or 'cell eating' and pinocytosis or 'cell drinking'. During both these processes the cell surface folds to make a small pocket that is lined by the cell membrane (Fig. 1.6). The pocket seals off, forming a vesicle that contains the material being brought into the cell. This separates from the cell surface, moves into the cell's interior and fuses with a lysosome, containing lysozymes, which digest the vesicle contents. The process of phagocytosis is also used by some white blood cells to remove foreign particles such as invading bacteria (see Chapter 7 on blood cells).

Cell division

The cells of the body are classified into two types:

- *Somatic cells* – these include all the cells of the body except those involved in reproduction. Somatic cells divide by *mitosis* and contain the *diploid number* of chromosomes.
- *Germ cells* – these are the ova (within the ovaries) and the spermatozoa (within the testes). Germ cells divide by *meiosis* and contain the *haploid number* of chromosomes.

Mitosis

The tissues of the body grow, particularly when the animal is young, and are able to repair themselves when damaged. This is achieved by the process of mitosis in which the somatic cells of the body make identical copies of themselves. The cells replicate by dividing into two – a process called *binary fission*. However, before they can do this they must first make a copy of all the hereditary or genetic information that the new cell will need in order to function normally. This information is carried in the DNA (deoxyribonucleic acid) of the chromosomes within the nucleus of the parent cell. The normal number of chromosomes is described as the diploid number and before cell division takes place the chromosomes are duplicated (Fig. 1.7).

Mitosis can be divided into four active stages, followed by a 'resting' stage (called *interphase*), during which the new daughter cells grow and prepare for the next division. Interphase is not

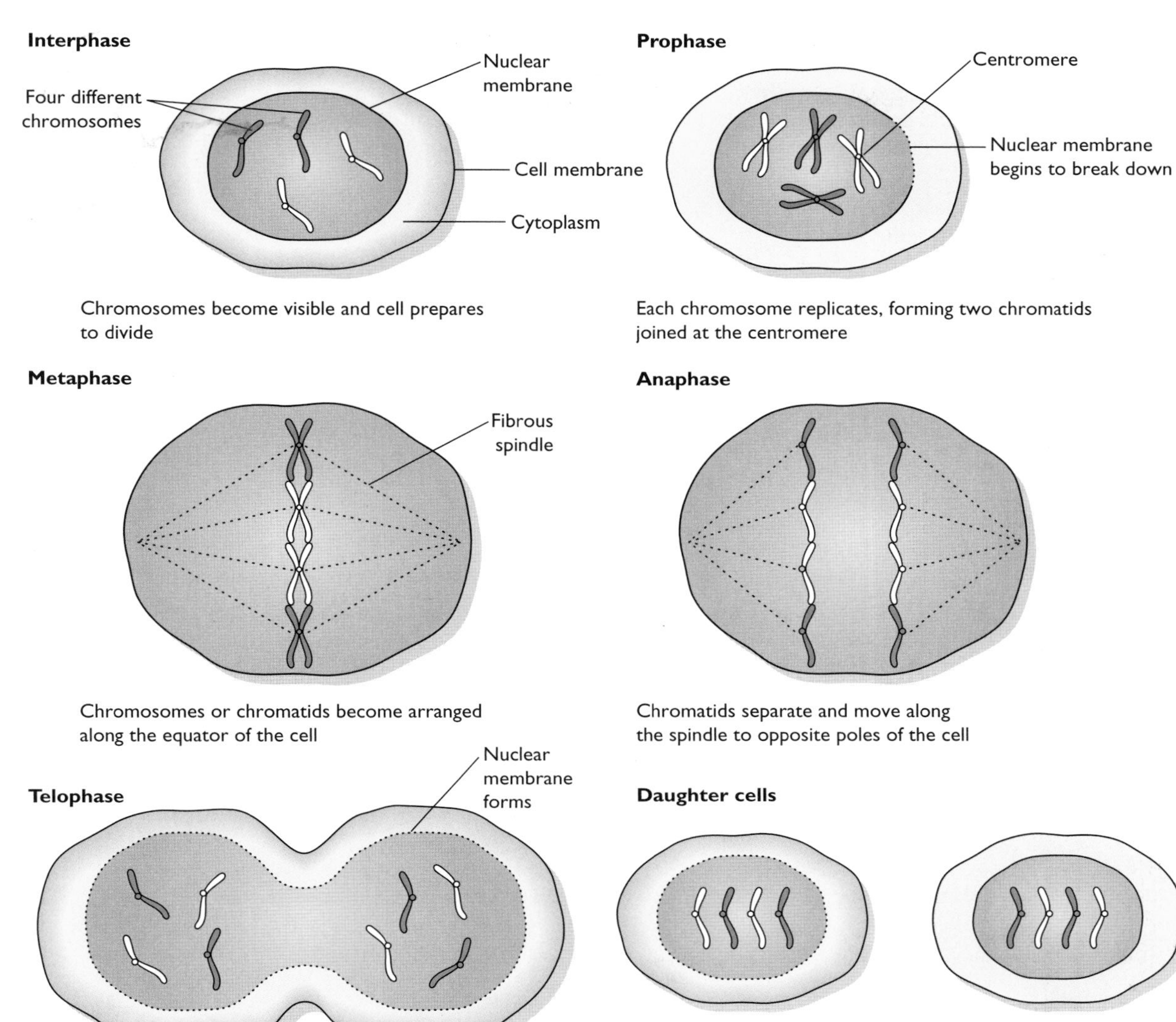

Fig. 1.7 Mitosis – the cell division seen in somatic cells.

actually a resting stage because it is during this stage that the DNA replicates in preparation for the next mitosis. The centrioles have also replicated by the start of the new mitotic division. The four active stages of mitosis are:

1. *Prophase* – the nuclear membrane breaks down and the chromosomes contract and become shorter, fatter and more distinct. The identical pairs of chromosomes have not yet separated and are referred to as the *chromatids*. The chromatids are held together at a region called the centromere. The centrioles are now found at the opposite poles or ends of the cell and spindle fibres start to form. These are 'threads' passing from the centriole at one pole to the centriole at the other pole.
2. *Metaphase* – the chromosomes line up in the middle of the cell (known as the equator) and the chromatids draw apart at the centromere.
3. *Anaphase* – the chromosomes attach to the spindle fibres and as these contract it moves the chromatids towards the opposite poles of the cell.
4. *Telophase* – the chromatids will be the chromosomes of the daughter cells. The spindle fibres break down and the nuclear membrane reforms. The cell starts to constrict across the middle and continues until it is divided into two. Each of the new daughter cells is genetically identical to the original parent cell, and both contain the full set of chromosomes, known as the diploid number. The chromosomes then unravel and the cell returns to interphase.

Mitosis results in the production of two identical daughter cells, each of which is identical to the parent cell and contains the diploid number of chromosomes.

Meiosis

This is the process by which the germ cells divide within the ovary of the female and the testis of the male. Meiosis results in the production of ova or sperm containing *half* the normal number of chromosomes (the haploid number). Meiosis must occur before fertilisation, when a sperm penetrates the ovum and the two nuclei fuse. If those two nuclei had the diploid number of chromosomes then the nucleus of the resulting gamete would have twice the normal number and abnormalities would develop.

The resting cell is in interphase before meiosis begins. The eight stages are as follows (see also Fig. 1.8):

1. *Prophase* – this takes longer than prophase in mitosis. The homologous (identical) chromosomes lie side by side and duplicate; each pair is joined at the centromere. These chromosomes may become entangled and pieces of one chromosome may become attached to another – this process is known as 'crossing over' and may influence the characteristics of the offspring.
2. *Metaphase I* – the homologous pairs of chromosomes come to lie along the line of the equator of the cell and the fibrous spindle starts to form.
3. *Anaphase I* – the pairs separate and the chromatids migrate along the spindle fibres towards the poles of the cell.

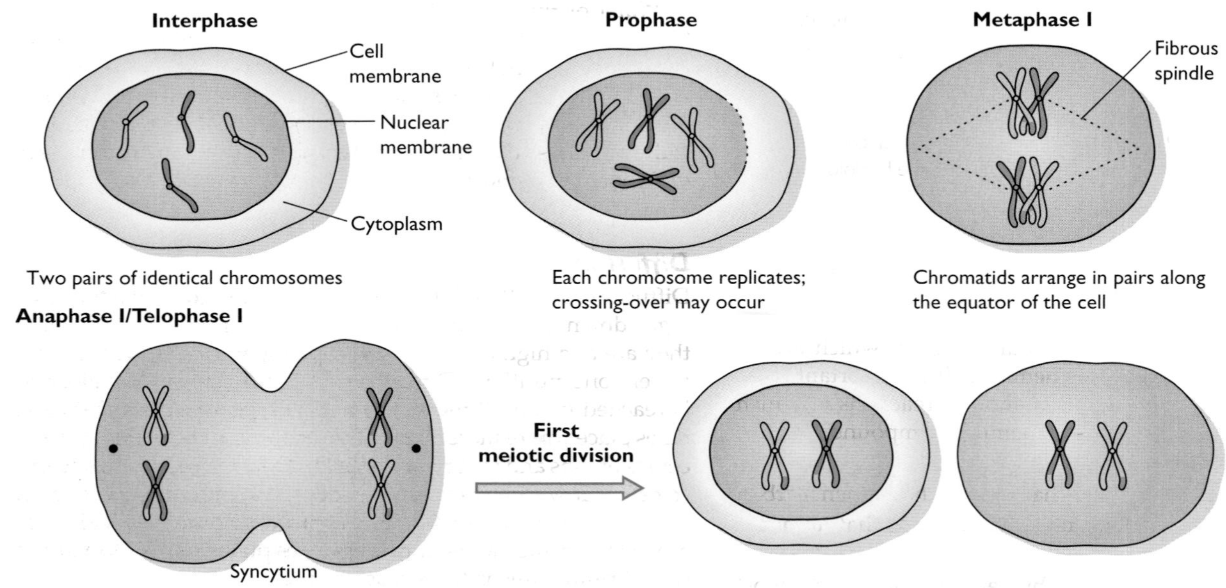

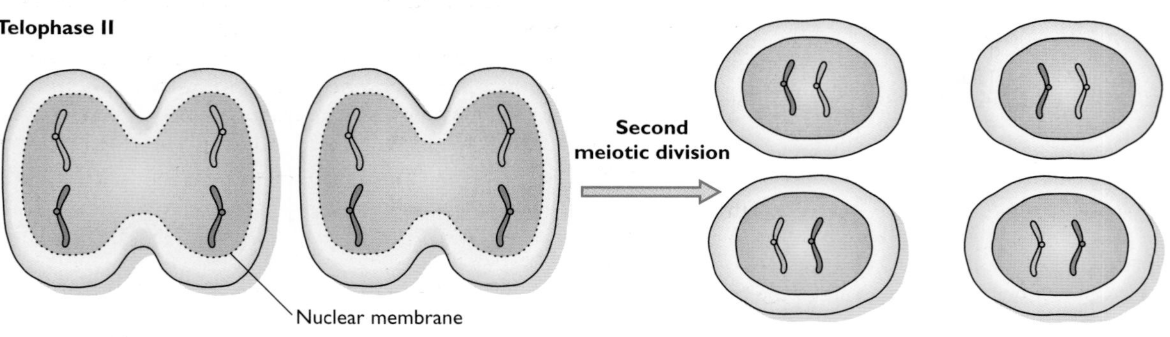

Fig. 1.8 Meiosis – the cell division seen in the germ cells.

4. *Telophase I* – the cytoplasm begins to divide but the nuclear membrane does not reform. In some cells, the cytoplasm does not divide completely and a dumb-bell shaped cell is seen – this is known as a *syncytium*. Telophase I is the *first meiotic division.*
5. *Prophase II* – this may be transitory as there is no need to replicate the chromosomes.
6. *Metaphase II* – the chromosomes arrange themselves along the equator and the spindle fibres appear.
7. *Anaphase II* – the chromatids pull apart and migrate towards the poles of the cells.
8. *Telophase II* – the cytoplasm begins to divide, the nuclear membrane reforms and four identical daughter cells are formed. Telophase II is the *second meiotic division*.

Meiosis results in the production of four identical daughter cells, each of which is non-identical to the parent cell and contains the haploid number of chromosomes.

The chemistry of the body

The cells, and therefore the tissues and organs, which are all made of cells, are composed of chemicals. It is important to be able to understand these chemicals and the reactions in which they take part within the body. Chemical compounds can be divided into two groups:

- *Organic* compounds are those that contain the element carbon
- *Inorganic* compounds are all those compounds that do not contain carbon.

Both groups are found in the body, but let us first look at the most biologically important inorganic compound of the body – water (H_2O).

Water content of the body

An individual mammalian cell contains ~80% water. In fact, 60–70% of the whole body's weight is water, which is divided into two main body compartments: *intracellular* (ICF) and *extracellular* (ECF) water.

ICF is that which is found inside the cells of the body and can be subdivided into the fluid within the blood cells and the fluid in all other cells. ICF takes up 40% of total body weight.

ECF is that which lies outside the cells (i.e., the surrounding environment of the cells). ECF takes up 20% of total body weight and includes the fluid in which the blood cells are suspended (the plasma), the fluid within the lymphatic system and the cerebrospinal fluid (the transcellular fluid) and the fluid that surrounds all the other cells of the body (the interstitial or tissue fluid).

Plasma takes up about 5% of body weight. It forms the medium in which the blood cells are transported within the blood–vascular system. It is rich in proteins, termed plasma proteins. *Transcellular fluid* is formed by active secretory mechanisms and its volume varies. It is considered to take up about 1% of body weight and it includes fluids such as cerebrospinal fluid, digestive juices and lymph. *Interstitial fluid* takes up 15% of body weight and lies outside the blood vascular system, surrounding the cells. It is formed from the blood by a process of ultrafiltration – small molecules and ions are separated from larger molecules and cells. The pressure in the blood vascular system forces the fluid through the walls of the capillaries. This acts like a sieve, holding back the large plasma protein molecules and the cellular components of the blood and allowing everything else to go through. Thus, interstitial fluid is similar to plasma but *without* the blood cells and protein molecules. Interstitial fluid is the medium in which the cells are bathed and from it the cells extract all that they need, such as oxygen and nutrients. They get rid of all their unwanted waste products into it.

Water or fluid provides the medium in which all the body's biochemical reactions take place and is thus essential to maintain the body's internal environment in a state of balance – this is a process known as *homeostasis*. Body water and the chemical substances within it constantly move around the body. The biological processes that are responsible for this movement are diffusion and osmosis.

Diffusion

Diffusion (Fig. 1.9A) is the movement of molecules of a liquid or a gas down a concentration gradient (i.e., from a region where they are at a high concentration to a region where they are at a lower concentration). Diffusion will occur until an equilibrium is reached (i.e. until the concentration equalises out). Diffusion takes place where there is no barrier to the free movement of molecules or ions and is very important in their movement in and out of cells. However, it can only occur if the particle size is small enough to pass through the cell membrane. If the molecules are too large, then another process takes place in order to achieve equilibrium – this is known as osmosis.

Osmosis

Osmosis (Fig. 1.9B) is the movement of water through a *semi-permeable membrane* from a fluid of low concentration to one of a higher concentration, which continues until the two concentrations are equal. The water can be considered to be diffusing along a concentration gradient. A semi-permeable membrane allows some substances through but not others. Osmosis is responsible for water movement from the interstitial fluid into the cells.

A solution consists of the molecules of one substance (the solute) dissolved in another substance (the solvent). In the body, the solvent is water so osmosis is a significant factor in the maintenance of the fluid volume within the body fluid compartments. A solution can be described as having an *osmotic pressure*. This is the pressure needed to prevent osmosis from occurring and is dependent on the number of particles, both dissolved and undissolved, in the solution; in other words, if the osmotic pressure of the plasma is high, water will flow into the blood to equalise the concentration; if the osmotic pressure of the plasma is low, water will flow out of the blood into the tissue spaces.

The osmotic pressure or tonicity of a rehydrating fluid is described relative to the osmotic pressure of blood plasma as follows:

- *Isotonic* – fluid has the same osmotic pressure as plasma
- *Hypotonic* – fluid has a lower osmotic pressure than plasma
- *Hypertonic* – fluid has a higher osmotic pressure than plasma.

This is important in selecting fluids for rehydration therapy – most fluids used are isotonic. The replacement fluid must be as close as possible in tonicity and electrolyte content to what has been lost from the body.

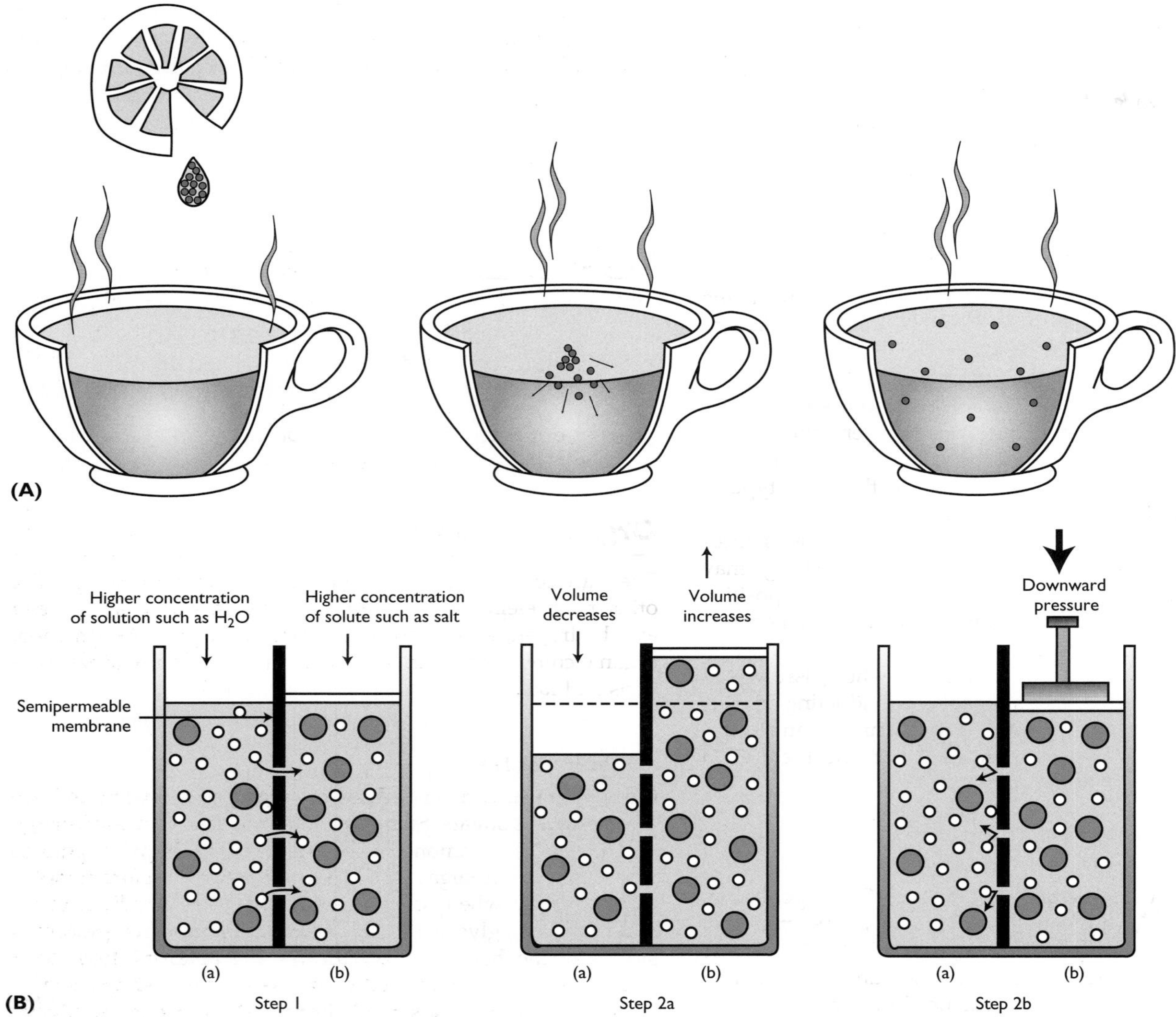

Fig. 1.9 (A) Diffusion. Molecules in solution are active and constantly collide into one another. With time, they become evenly distributed throughout the liquid, having moved down concentration gradients from areas of high concentration to those of low, until equilibrium is reached. Diffusion occurs when there is no barrier to free movement and it occurs more rapidly in hot liquids than in cold ones as molecules are more active at higher temperatures. (With permission from T Colville, JM Bassett, 2001. Clinical anatomy and physiology for veterinary technicians. St Louis, MO: Mosby, p. 24.) **(B)** Osmosis. Step 1: Smaller molecules of solution in side (a) can pass through the semi-permeable membrane into side (b), but the larger molecules of solute cannot. Step 2a: As solution moves from side (a) to side (b), the volume of side (b) increases until the concentration of solute is the same on both sides. Step 2b: Osmosis can be reversed by filtration, when hydraulic pressure is placed on side (b). This forces solution back through the semi-permeable membrane to side (a). (With permission from T Colville, JM Bassett, 2001. Clinical anatomy and physiology for veterinary technicians. St Louis, MO: Mosby, p. 25.)

Fluid balance

Water is constantly moving within the body – from the interstitial fluid into the cells, from the plasma to the tissue fluid, and so on – but it is also continually lost from the body and must be replaced to ensure that the total fluid balance in the body is maintained. Water is lost through the respiratory system (expired air contains water vapour), and in the urine and faeces. Dogs and cats do not sweat appreciably but do lose heat and water through panting. Water is also lost in the tears, which are produced constantly to moisten the eye, and in vaginal secretions. Water is taken into the body through drinking fluids and from the water content of food.

Fluid losses may be increased in sick or injured animals, through vomiting, diarrhoea, vaginal discharge (as seen with an open pyometra) or blood loss. This can lead to dehydration, which may have serious consequences, such as reduction of the circulating blood volume, known as hypovolaemic shock. In a normal adult animal, about 60% of the total bodyweight is water. This percentage will be slightly lower if the animal is old or very obese (fatty tissue contains little water) and slightly higher in young or thin animals.

Typical daily water loss is: 20 mL/kg bodyweight in the urine; 10–20 mL/kg bodyweight in the faeces; and 20 mL/kg bodyweight through the loss of water vapour in expired air and panting and in body secretions – a total of 50–60 mL of water per kg of bodyweight daily. Thus an adult healthy animal should take in 50–60 mL of water per kg bodyweight per day to balance the normal fluid loss (e.g., an animal weighing 20 kg will need 1000–1200 mL of water each day).

Inorganic compounds

A number of other inorganic compounds are also essential to the functions of the body: minerals, acids and bases. It is important to be familiar with some basic chemical definitions when considering these substances. Everything is composed of *atoms*, and an *element* is a substance that is composed of only one kind of atom (e.g., the element oxygen consists only of oxygen atoms). *Molecules* consist of two or more atoms linked by a chemical bond. A substance whose molecules contain more than one type of atom is called a *compound*.

When dissolved in water, the molecules of many substances break apart into charged particles, called *ions*. This charge may either be negative or positive: ions with one or more positive charges are called *cations* and ions with one or more negative charges are called *anions*.

An *electrolyte* is a chemical substance that, when dissolved in water, splits into ions and is thus capable of conducting an electric current. Sodium chloride (NaCl) is an example of an electrolyte in the body, its ions being sodium (Na^+) and chloride (Cl^-) in solution.

Minerals

The principal cations in the body are sodium (Na^+), potassium (K^+), calcium (Ca^{2+}) and magnesium (Mg^{2+}). The principal anions include chloride (Cl^-) and bicarbonate (HCO_3^-). These ions are essential to the functions of the body and it is vital that they are present in sufficient and balanced quantities. Sodium and chloride are mainly found in the ECF, while potassium is mainly found in the ICF (i.e., inside the cells). The concentration of these ions is important in the regulation of fluid balance between the intracellular and ECF. This balance is maintained by special 'pumps' in the cell membrane. An imbalance will lead to significant problems; for example, sodium affects the osmotic pressure of the blood and so influences blood volume and pressure; a high concentration of potassium in the ECF can disrupt heart function.

Calcium, phosphorus and magnesium are important minerals that are found in storage in bone tissue. Calcium is essential for many processes in the body, such as muscle contraction, nerve conduction and blood clotting. Iron and copper are also essential to normal body function, iron being an essential component of the haemoglobin in red blood cells.

Acids and bases

An *acid* is a compound that can release hydrogen ions when dissolved in solution. Compounds that can accept or take in hydrogen ions are called *bases* or *alkalis*. The acidity of a solution is expressed as its pH, which is the measure of the hydrogen ion concentration. The pH scale is from 0 to 14, with a pH of 7 being neutral. A solution with a pH less than 7 is acidic (the lower the number the higher the acidity, i.e., the greater the concentration of hydrogen ions). A solution with a pH above 7 is basic or alkaline (the higher the number the more alkaline the solution).

The pH of body fluids is 7.35 and it is important that the body maintains this level. Within the respiratory system and kidneys there are homeostatic processes to maintain the correct acid/base balance.

Acid/base balance – when the normal pH of the body is disrupted the animal may show an acidosis (i.e., a decreased blood pH), or an alkalosis (i.e., an increased blood pH). A respiratory acidosis may develop if the animal holds its breath, allowing carbon dioxide levels to rise and oxygen levels to fall; a respiratory alkalosis occurs during rapid panting, which lowers carbon dioxide levels. A metabolic acidosis may occur as a complication of diabetes mellitus and a metabolic alkalosis as a result of excessive vomiting and diarrhoea.

Organic compounds

These are compounds that are based on the element carbon. The other main elements found in organic compounds are oxygen and hydrogen, and in some instances nitrogen. The principal organic compounds found in the body are carbohydrates, proteins and fats.

Carbohydrates

Carbohydrates contain carbon, hydrogen and oxygen and are also known as sugars. Sugars are an important source of energy and the most common simple sugar in the body is glucose (Fig. 1.10). Simple sugars can join together to form more complex carbohydrates; when many sugars join together they form a *polysaccharide* (e.g., glycogen, which is the form in which glucose is stored in the body). Carbohydrates are obtained from food and are then broken down during digestion into simple sugars so that they can be absorbed through the mucous membrane of the digestive system into the blood and utilised by the body.

Lipids

Lipids include the fats, which are compounds of fatty acids and glycerol (Fig. 1.11) and are also made up of carbon, hydrogen and

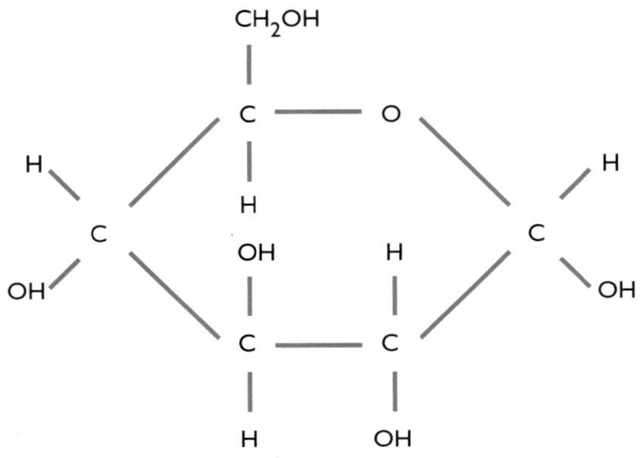

Fig. 1.10 Chemical structure of a simple carbohydrate – the sugar glucose.

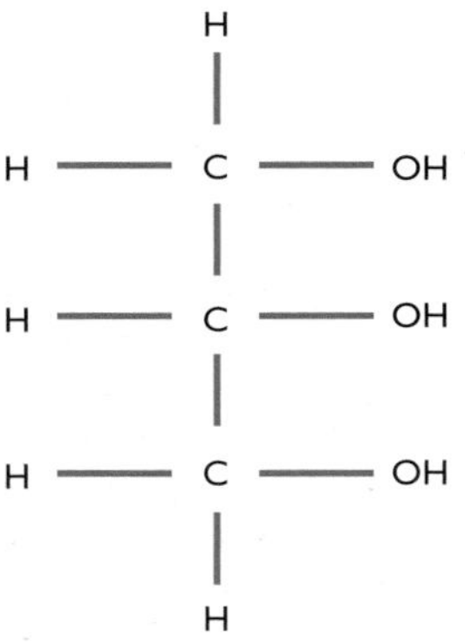

Fig. 1.11 Chemical structure of glycerol.

oxygen. Fatty acids are the main form in which fats are transported in the blood after the breakdown of lipids obtained from food. Although carbohydrates provide the most direct source of energy for the body, fats can also yield a large amount of energy. They are an important means of energy storage for the body, to be used when required. Other functions of lipids include insulation of the body itself and of nerves, and in the formation of cell membranes and synthesis of steroids.

Proteins

Proteins are built up from subunits called *amino acids* (Fig. 1.12). Proteins differ from carbohydrates and lipids in that they always contain nitrogen in addition to carbon, hydrogen and oxygen. They may also contain other elements such as sulphur, phosphorus and iodine. When two amino acids are joined together by a peptide link they form a dipeptide. The addition of more amino acids (a process called *polymerisation*) leads to the formation of a polypeptide. A protein consists of one or more polypeptide chains, which are then coiled and folded to give the specific structure of a particular protein (Fig. 1.13).

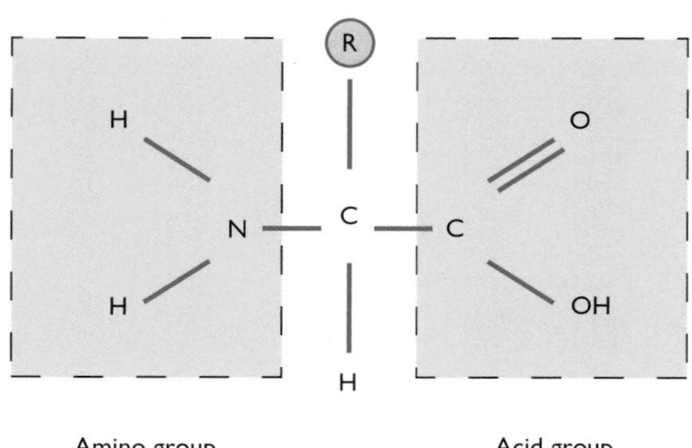

Fig. 1.12 General structure of an amino acid. The 'R' group varies from amino acid to amino acid. **Primary structure** – The linear sequence of amino acids in a peptide, **Secondary structure** – The repeating pattern in the structure of the peptide chain, e.g. an α-helix, **Tertiary structure** – The three-dimensional folding of the secondary structure, **Quaternary structure** – The three-dimensional arrangement of more than one tertiary polypeptide.

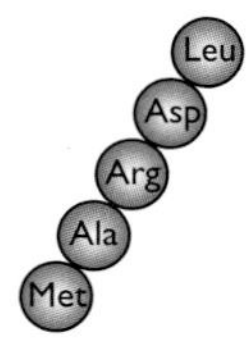

Primary structure –
the linear sequence of amino acids in a peptide

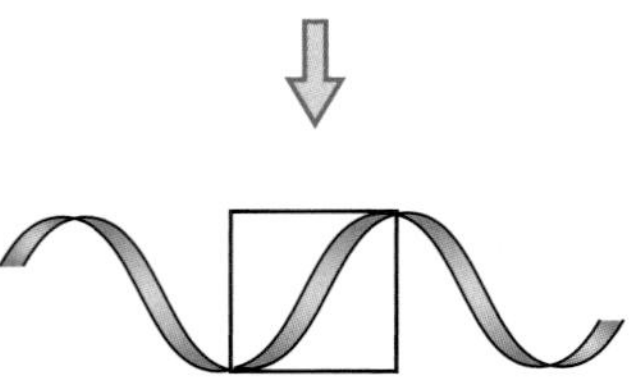

Secondary structure –
the repeating pattern in the structure of the peptide chain, e.g., an α-helix

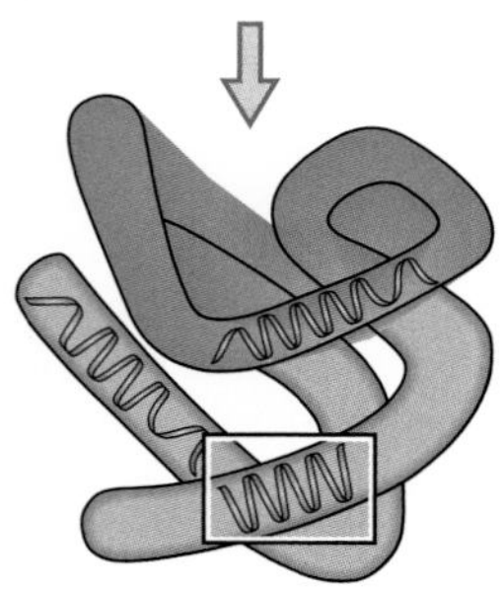

Tertiary structure –
the three-dimensional folding of the secondary structure

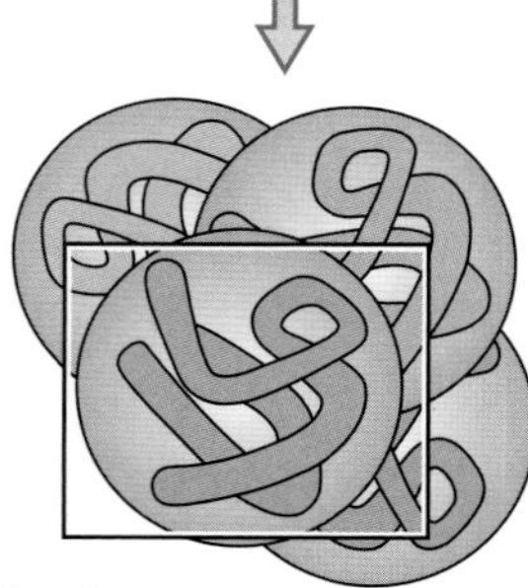

Quaternary structure –
the three-dimensional arrangement of more than one tertiary polypeptide

Fig. 1.13 The structure of a protein. It is not only the sequence of amino acids, but also the arrangement of the polypeptide chains, which determine the characteristics of a protein.

Proteins generally fall into one of two groups:

- *Globular* – the functional proteins. These are associated with cellular chemical reactions and include hormones and enzymes.
- *Fibrous* – the structural proteins. These are insoluble and are part of the composition of various structures in the body. They include keratin, collagen and elastin.

By means of digestive enzymes the body breaks down the proteins acquired from the diet into their constituent amino acids, which can then be absorbed through the mucous membrane of the digestive system into the blood.

Chemical reactions in the body

Most of the chemical reactions that take place in the body require the presence of a functional protein compound called an *enzyme*. Enzymes are organic catalysts that speed up and control chemical reactions in the body. Enzymes are involved in the breakdown of food in the digestive system but are also involved in the many metabolic processes that are carried out within cells.

A chemical reaction that requires an input of energy is called an *anabolic* reaction. A chemical reaction that releases energy is a *catabolic* reaction. The sum of the energy use (i.e., the gain and loss), is the *total metabolism*.

All animals require energy and this is provided by raw materials obtained from food. This is then converted by the body into a form that it can use – ATP. Energy cannot be created or destroyed, it is just moved around or else changes its form; for example, electrical energy can be converted to heat energy or it can be stored as potential energy that is released when the compound in which the energy is stored is broken down. In the body of an animal, energy comes from the oxidation of glucose (i.e., a reaction involving oxygen and glucose).

CHAPTER 2

Tissues and body cavities

KEY POINTS

- The cells of the body are arranged into four basic tissue types: epithelial, connective, muscle and nervous tissue.
- Epithelial tissue covers the outside of the body and lines all the body cavities and the structures within them. Its primary function is to protect but in some areas it may also be absorbent or secretory. Secretory epithelial tissue forms glands.
- Connective tissue is found in varying forms such as blood, fibrous connective tissue, cartilage and bone. Its main function is to connect and support the parts of the body, but it also carries nutrients to the tissues and conducts waste material away.
- Muscle tissue brings about the movement of the body. It is found as striated muscle attached to the skeleton, smooth muscle within the internal organs of the body and cardiac muscle found only in the myocardium of the heart wall. Control of striated muscle is voluntary, while that of smooth and cardiac muscle is involuntary and brought about by branches of the autonomic nervous system.
- Nervous tissue is found all over the body and its function is to conduct nerve impulses to and from parts of the body and the central nervous system.
- The body is divided into three body cavities, which contain the visceral systems. The thoracic and abdominal cavities are lined with a single layer of serous epithelial tissue, which is named according to its location within the cavity.

Within the body individual cells are grouped together to form tissues and organs. Thus:

- A *tissue* is a collection of cells and their products in which one type of cell predominates (e.g., epithelial tissue or muscle tissue).
- An *organ* is a collection of tissues forming a structure within an animal that is adapted to perform a specific purpose (e.g., liver, larynx, kidney).
- A *system* is a collection of organs and tissues that are related by function (e.g., the respiratory system).

Body tissues

Each tissue type consists of three main components:

- Cells: One type forms the majority of the cells and gives the tissue type its name (e.g., muscle tissue consists mainly of muscle cells).
- Intercellular products: These are produced by the cells and lie in the spaces between them.
- Fluid: Interstitial fluid flows through specialised channels running through the tissue.

There are four main types of tissue:

- *Epithelial:* protects the body; may also be secretory and absorbent
- *Connective:* binds the tissues together
- *Muscle:* brings about movement
- *Nervous:* conveys nerve impulses from one area to another and coordinates the response

Epithelial tissue

Epithelial tissue, or *epithelium,* covers the surface of the body and the organs, cavities and tubes within it – the internal and external surfaces of the body. Its main function is to protect delicate structures lying beneath it but in some areas the epithelium may be secretory (e.g., glands) or absorbent (e.g., in the small intestine). The epithelium lining structures such as the inside of the heart, blood vessels and lymph vessels is referred to as *endothelium.*

Epithelium may be described according to the number of layers of cells (i.e., its thickness):

- If an epithelium is one cell thick it is said to be *simple* (Fig. 2.1).
- If there is more than one layer it is said to be *stratified* or *compound* (Fig. 2.1).

The thickness of the epithelium reflects its ability to protect: the more layers of cells, the more protection is provided. The epithelium on the footpads consists of many layers of cells providing protection when walking on rough surfaces, while the epithelium over the abdominal wall is only a few cells thick and additional protection is provided by fur. Further protection may be provided by the presence of the protein keratin. The epithelium is described as being a *keratinised stratified* epithelium and this type can be seen in claws and nails.

Epithelium may also be described according to the shape of the cells within it (Fig. 2.1). There are three basic shapes of epithelial cell:

- *Squamous* cells: flattened in shape
- *Cuboidal* cells: square or cube-shaped
- *Columnar* cells: column-shaped (the height is greater than the width) (Fig. 2.2)

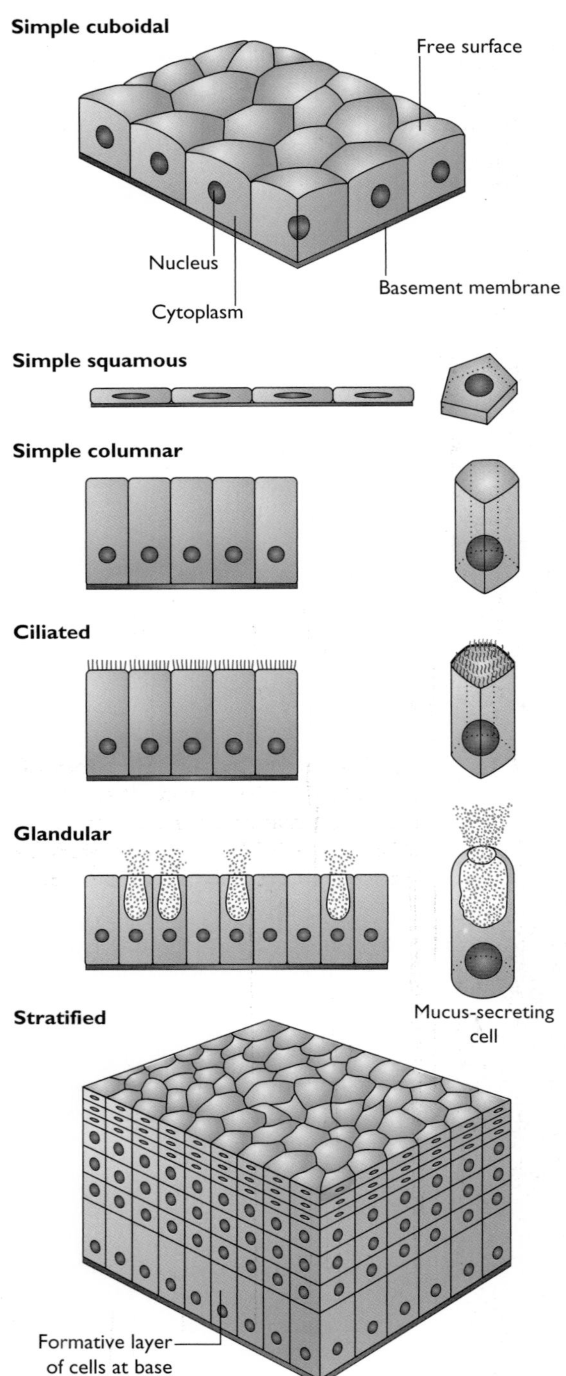

Fig. 2.1 The different types of epithelium found in the body.

> Some types of tumour originate from a specific type of tissue in the body and their names provide an indication of the cellular source. For example, a squamous cell carcinoma originates from squamous cells found in the skin, an adenoma develops in glandular tissue and a transitional cell carcinoma develops in the bladder wall.

The full classification of the type of epithelium is based upon the shape of the cell and the number of layers present. There are a number of different types of epithelial tissue in the body including:

- *Simple cuboidal epithelium* is the least specialised type of epithelium. It is one cell thick and the cells are cube-shaped. Cuboidal epithelium lines many of the glands and their ducts. This type of epithelium has an absorptive or secretory function depending on its location in the body (e.g., lining the renal tubules).
- *Simple squamous epithelium* has flattened cells and is one layer thick. Simple squamous epithelium is thin and delicate and is found in areas of the body where the covering surface needs to be easily permeable to molecules such as oxygen (e.g., lining the blood vessels and the alveoli of the lungs).
- *Simple columnar epithelium* has tall narrow cells and is one layer thick. Generally, simple columnar epithelium lines organs which have an absorptive function (e.g., the small and large intestines) or a secretory function (e.g., digestive glands) (Fig. 2.2).
- *Ciliated epithelium* is a more specialised epithelium consisting of a single layer of column-shaped cells (Figs. 2.1 and 2.3). The free surface of the cells has tiny hair-like projections called *cilia* whose function is to 'waft' foreign particles along the epithelial surface and out of the body. Ciliated epithelium lines the upper respiratory tract, where it helps to trap solid particles that have been inhaled, preventing them from entering the more distal parts of the respiratory system. The uterine tubes are also lined with ciliated epithelium, which helps to move the fertilised egg along the reproductive tract.
- *Stratified epithelium* is composed of a number of layers of cells and is thicker and tougher than the other types of epithelium. It is found in areas that are subjected to wear and to friction and shearing forces (e.g., the epidermis of the skin). Pseudostratified epithelium (Fig. 2.3) appears to be multilayered because of the irregular positioning of the nuclei but is actually a single layer of cells. This may be found in areas such as the trachea.
- *Transitional epithelium* is a type of specialised stratified epithelium found lining parts of the urinary system (i.e. structures and tubes that are capable of considerable distension and variations in internal pressure and capacity, such as the bladder and ureters). The cells are able to change their shape according to circumstances and thus their appearance varies with the degree of distension of the structure.

Glands

Glandular tissue is a modification of epithelial tissue. The epithelium, in addition to its protective function, may also be a secretory membrane. Glands are either unicellular or multicellular.

- *Unicellular glands* have individual secretory cells that are interspersed throughout the tissue. The most common type is the *goblet cell* (Fig. 2.4), which secretes clear sticky mucus directly on to the membrane surface. The epithelium is known as a *mucous membrane.* Mucus traps particles, providing extra protection, and also lubricates the epithelial surface. Mucous membranes are found covering the oral cavity, lining the vagina and the trachea and in many other parts of the body.
- *Multicellular glands* consist of many secretory cells folded to form more complex glands. They vary in shape and intricacy relating to their position and function in the body. Examples of some of the types of gland found in the body are shown in Fig. 2.5.

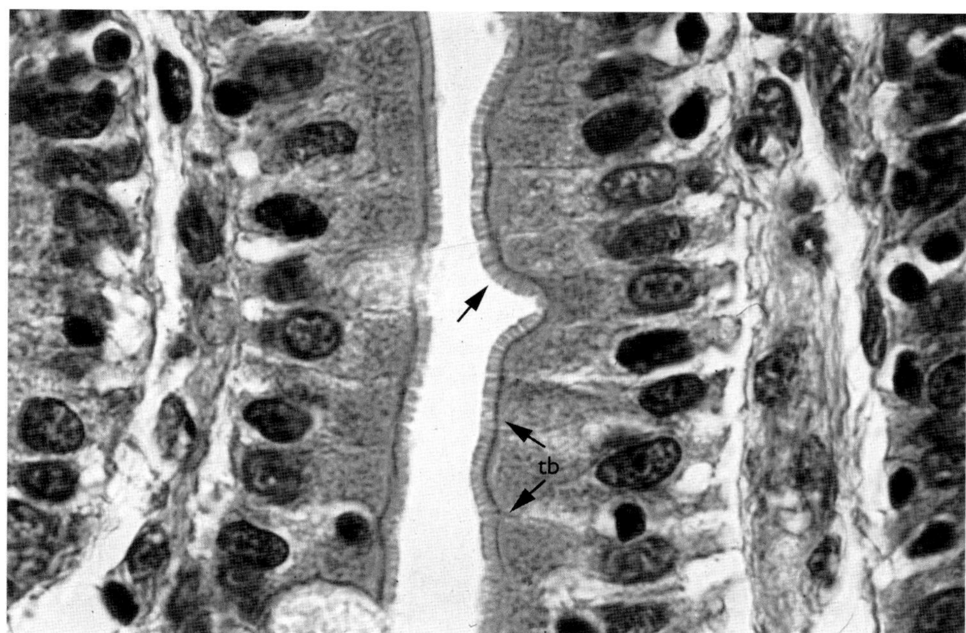

Fig. 2.2 Light micrograph of the mucosa of the small intestine showing a simple columnar epithelium with a border of microvilli that increase the surface area for absorption. (Taken from D Samuelson, 2007. Textbook of veterinary histology. St Louis, MO: Saunders, p. 42.)

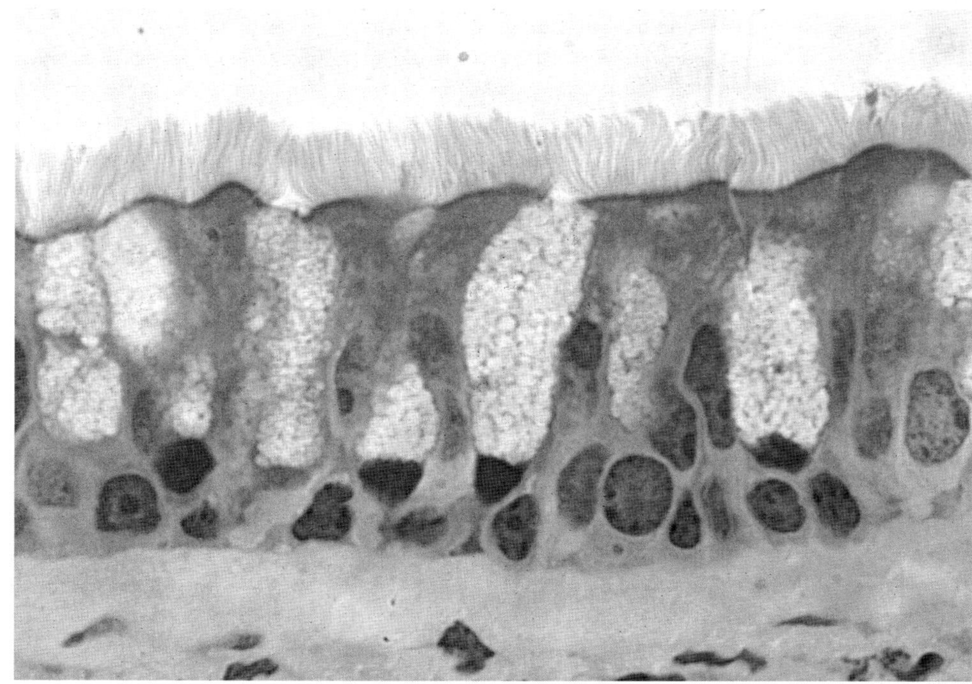

Fig. 2.3 Photomicrograph of the lining of the trachea showing a pseudostratified ciliated columnar epithelium. (Taken from D Samuelson, 2007. Textbook of veterinary histology. St Louis, MO: Saunders, p. 43.)

Glands may be categorised as either exocrine or endocrine.

- *Exocrine glands* have a system of ducts through which their secretory products are transported directly to the site where they will be used.
- *Endocrine glands* do not have a duct system (ductless glands) and their secretions, known as hormones, are carried by the blood to their target organ, which may be some distance away (see Chapter 6).

Connective tissue

Connective tissue is responsible for supporting and holding all the organs and tissues of the body in place. It also provides the transport system within the body, carrying nutrients to the tissues and waste products away. Connective tissue consists of cells embedded in an extracellular *matrix* or *ground substance*. The properties of this ground substance depend on the type of

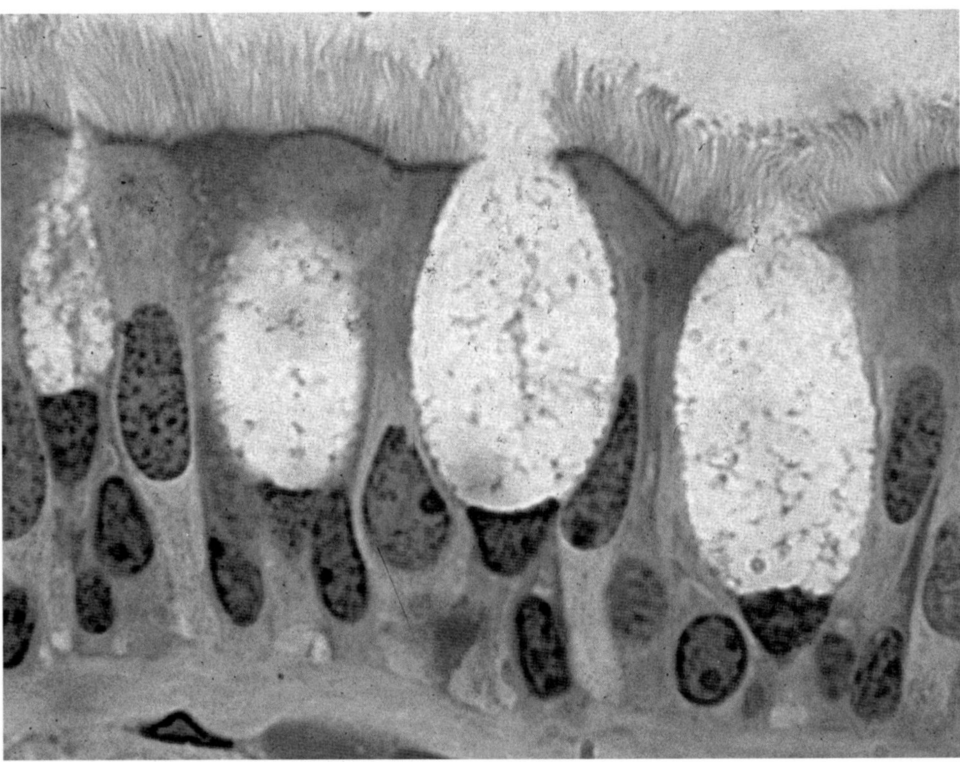

Fig. 2.4 Photomicrograph of goblet cells within a pseudostratified ciliated columnar epithelium. (Taken from D Samuelson, 2007. Textbook of veterinary histology. St Louis, MO: Saunders, p. 64.)

connective tissue. There are many types of connective tissue which, in order of increasing density are:

1. Blood
2. Haemopoietic tissue
3. Areolar tissue or loose connective tissue
4. Adipose or fatty tissue
5. Fibrous connective tissue or dense connective tissue
6. Cartilage
7. Bone

Blood

Blood is a specialised connective tissue that circulates through the blood vessels to carry nutrients and oxygen to the cells, and waste products to the organs of excretion. It consists of a number of different types of blood cells within a fluid ground substance – the plasma. (This is covered in more detail in Chapter 7.)

Haemopoietic tissue

This jelly-like connective tissue forms the bone marrow within the long bones and is responsible for the formation of the blood cells (see Chapter 7).

Areolar tissue

Areolar (meaning spaces) or loose connective tissue (Figs. 2.6 and 2.7) is the most widely distributed type of connective tissue and is found all over the body (e.g., beneath the skin, around blood vessels and nerves, between and connecting organs and between muscle bundles). The ground substance contains a loose weave work of two types of protein fibre: *collagen* fibres, with a high tensile strength secreted by the main cell type (the fibroblast), and *elastic* fibres, which enable the tissue to stretch and return to its former shape. Fat cells may be present in varying quantities depending on location and the degree of obesity of the animal. *Macrophages* – cells capable of phagocytosis – are also present.

Adipose tissue

Adipose tissue (Fig. 2.8) is similar to areolar tissue but its matrix contains mainly fat-filled cells, closely packed together, giving it the name fatty tissue. These fat cells act as an energy reserve and, in the dermis of the skin, the tissue insulates the body to reduce heat loss. In some areas, such as around the kidney, adipose tissue provides a protective layer.

A lipoma is a very common benign tumour that develops in adipose tissue. These are seen as the 'fatty lumps' frequently found on older dogs. They can become very large if not removed and depending on their position may cause some discomfort.

Dense connective tissue

Dense or fibrous connective tissue consists of densely packed collagen fibre bundles with relatively few fibroblasts and other cells in between them (Fig. 2.9). The fibres may be arranged in two ways:

- *Parallel arrangement* is known as regular fibrous connective tissue: tendons, which are strong bands of fibrous tissue

Shape of gland		Type of gland	Location of gland
Tubular (single, straight)	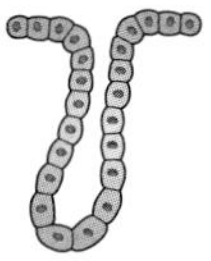	Simple tubular	Stomach, intestine
Tubular (coiled)	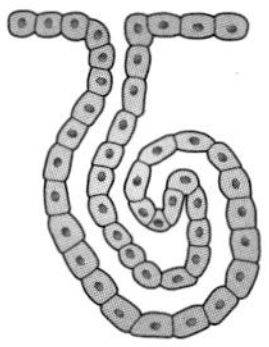	Simple coiled tubular	Sweat glands
Tubular (multiple)	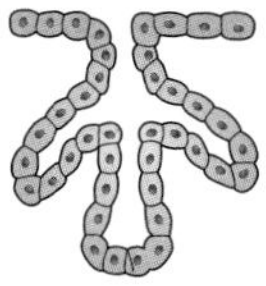	Simple branched tubular	Stomach, mouth, tongue, oesophagus
Alveolar (single)	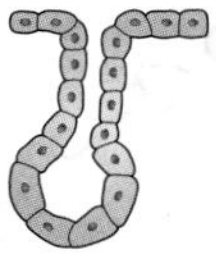	Simple alveolar	Sebaceous glands
Alveolar (multiple)	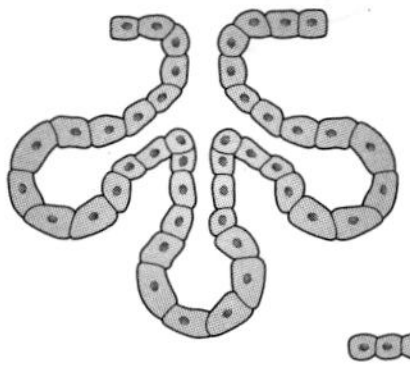	Branched alveolar (acinar)	Sebaceous glands
Tubular (multiple)	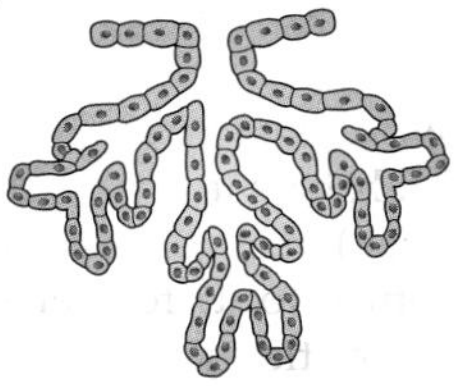	Compound tubular	Bulbourethral glands, mammary glands, kidney tubules, testes, mucous glands of the mouth
Alveolar (multiple)	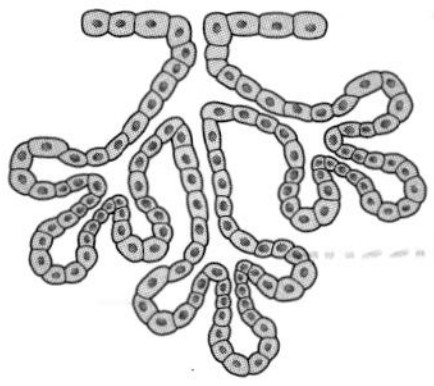	Compound alveolar (acinar)	Mammary glands
Some tubular; some alveolar	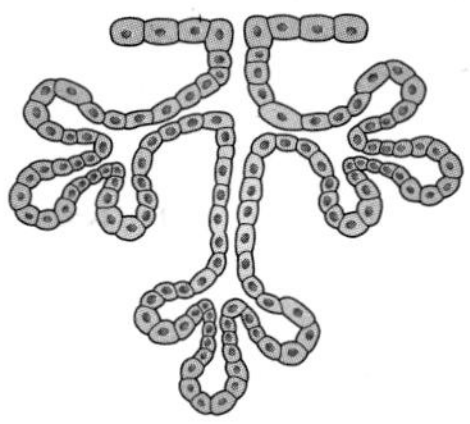	Compound tubuloalveolar	Salivary glands, pancreas, respiratory passages

Fig. 2.5 The different types of gland found in the body.

linking muscles to bone, and ligaments, which link bone to bone.

- *Irregularly interwoven fibres* are seen in the dermis of the skin and in the capsules of joints, as well as in organs such as the testes and lymph nodes. Irregular dense connective tissue is often found in sheets and forms the basis of most fascias and aponeuroses.

Cartilage

Cartilage is a specialised connective tissue which is rigid but flexible and resilient and is able to bear weight (Fig. 2.10). It is composed of cells (known as *chondrocytes*) and fibres within a gel-like ground substance. Cartilage has no blood supply and its nutrition is supplied by the fibrous sheath or perichondrium that surrounds it.

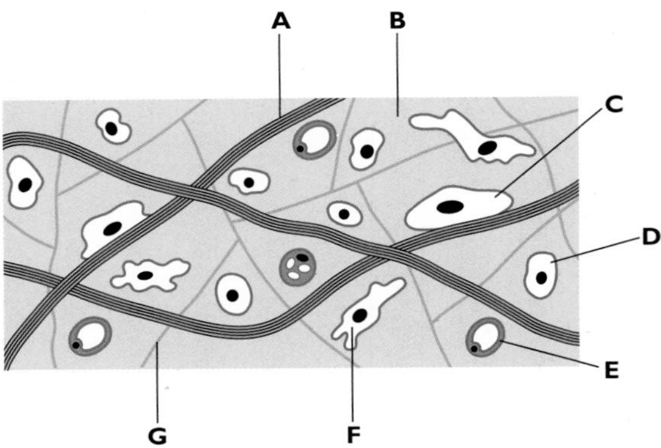

Fig. 2.6 Composition of areolar tissue. **(A)** Collagen fibres: flexible but very strong and resistant to stretching. **(B)** Ground substance: this contains the different fibres and cells of the tissue. **(C)** Fibroblast: long, flat cell that produces collagen and elastic fibres. **(D)** Mast cell: secretes an anticoagulant. **(E)** Fat cell: stores fat. **(F)** Macrophage: large cell capable of phagocytosis of foreign particles. **(G)** Elastic fibres: form a loose and stretchable network.

There are three types of cartilage:

- *Hyaline cartilage* has a translucent, bluish-white appearance. The randomly arranged collagen fibres are not easily visible under the microscope because they have the same refractive index as the gel matrix. Hyaline cartilage is the most common type of cartilage in the body, and it forms the articular surfaces of joints and provides support in the nose, larynx, trachea and bronchi. It also forms the skeleton of the embryo before it becomes ossified by the process known as *endochondral ossification*.
- *Elastic cartilage* has chondrocytes within a matrix and numerous elastic fibres. Elastic cartilage occurs in places where support with flexibility is required (e.g., the external ear and epiglottis).
- *Fibrocartilage* has a similar basic structure but has a higher proportion of collagen fibres, giving it great strength (e.g., in the intervertebral discs and in the menisci of the stifle joint). It also attaches the tendons and ligaments to bone.

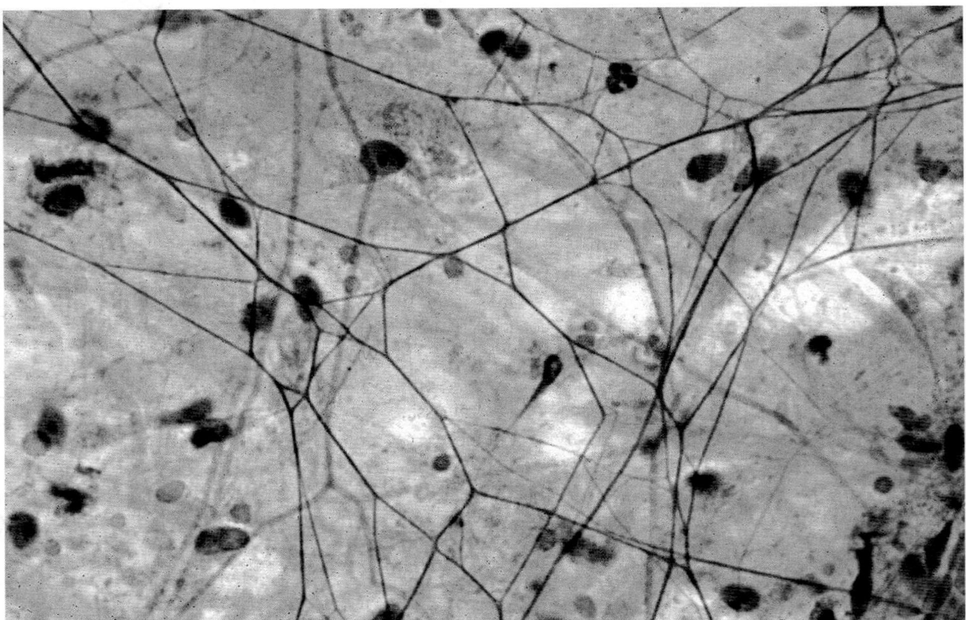

Fig. 2.7 Light micrograph of loose connective or areolar tissue showing a delicate network of collagen and elastic fibres in a piece of mesentery. (Taken from D Samuelson, 2007. Textbook of veterinary histology. St Louis, MO: Saunders, p. 92.)

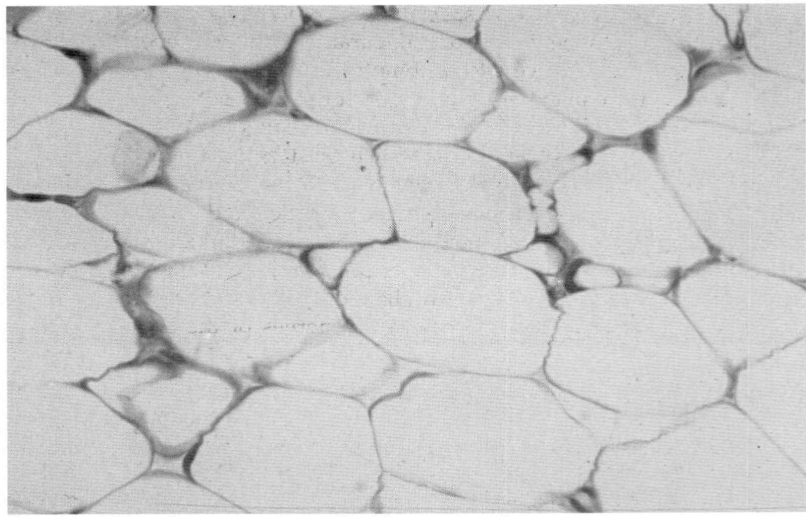

Fig. 2.8 Light micrograph of adipose tissue. (Taken from D Samuelson, 2007. Textbook of veterinary histology. St Louis, MO: Saunders, p. 98.)

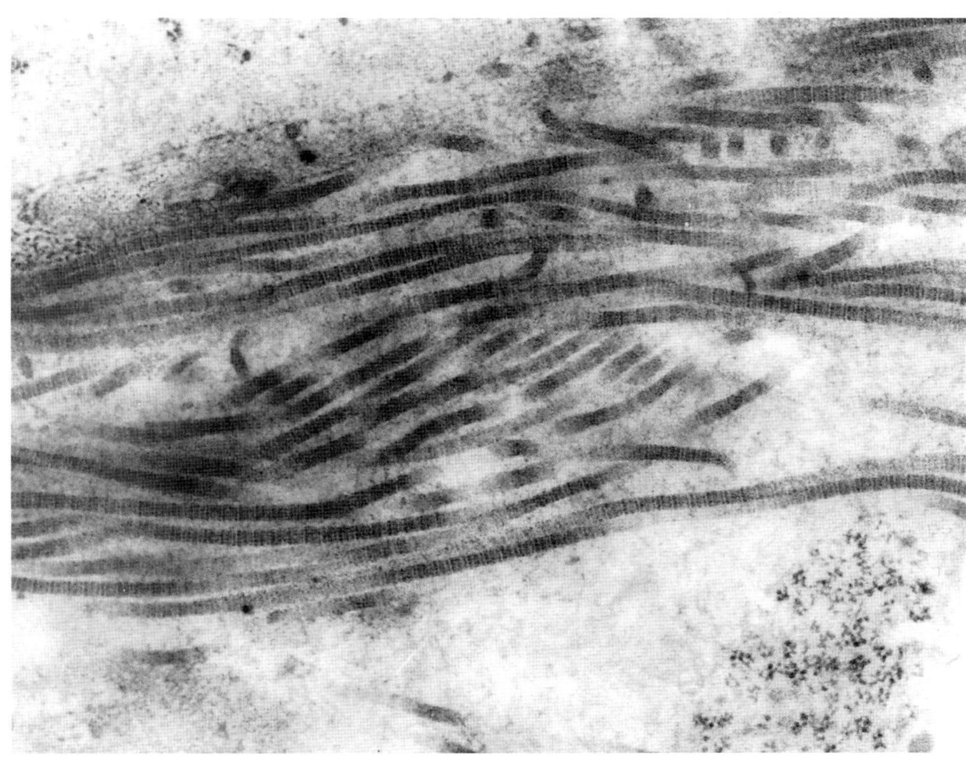

Fig. 2.9 Transmission electron micrograph (×25,000) of collagen fibres. (Taken from D Samuelson, 2007. Textbook of veterinary histology. St Louis, MO: Saunders, p. 87.)

Abnormalities in the formation and structure of cartilage and bone may lead to a variety of clinical conditions. One of the most common associated with degeneration of the articular cartilage is *osteoarthritis*. *Rickets*, seen in young animals on a diet in which there is an imbalance of calcium and vitamin D, causes signs resulting from problems with ossification of growing bones. *Osteochondritis dissecans (OCD)* is a general term describing disturbance in endochondral ossification and causes intermittent lameness in the shoulder and elbow joints of large breeds of dog such as the Great Dane. *Panosteitis* is a condition that occurs in young dogs and is an idiopathic inflammation of all bone tissues presenting as pain in the long bones.

Bone

Bone is a living tissue that is capable of remodelling and repairing itself when damaged. It is a specialised type of connective tissue, which provides the rigid supportive framework of the body and forms a system of levers for locomotion.

Bone consists of an extracellular matrix or ground substance that contains the protein osteonectin and collagen fibres. Together these form *osteoid*, within which crystals of insoluble calcium phosphate are deposited as the bone tissue becomes calcified. Calcification gives bone its characteristic rigidity and hardness. As the ground substance becomes calcified, the bone cells or *osteocytes* are trapped in spaces called *lacunae*. Running through the bone matrix are fine channels, called *Haversian canals*, which carry the blood vessels and nerves of the bone (Figs. 2.11 and 2.12). Each Haversian canal is surrounded by a series of concentric cylinders of matrix material called *lamellae* and the osteocytes within their lacunae. Each series of these cylinders, together with the canal, is called a *Haversian system* (Figs. 2.11 and 2.12). A fibrous membrane, the *periosteum*, covers the outer surface of all types of bone.

There are two types of bone tissue:

- *Compact bone* is solid and hard and is found in the outer layer or cortex of all types of bone. The Haversian systems of compact bone are densely packed together.
- *Cancellous or spongy bone* consists of an internal meshwork of bony 'struts' or *trabeculae* with interconnected spaces between filled with red bone marrow. Cancellous bone is found in the ends of long bones, and in the core of short, irregular and flat bones.

Muscle tissue

Muscle tissue is responsible for organised movement in the body.

Skeletal or striated muscle

This type of muscle is found attached to the skeleton and brings about movement (Fig. 2.13). It is under voluntary or conscious control, meaning that an animal uses its brain to move its limbs.

The muscle cells or fibres are long and cylindrical and lie parallel to each other. Each individual muscle fibre is composed of bundles of microfilaments known as *myofibrils* that are made of two contractile proteins called *actin* (thin filaments) and *myosin* (thick filaments). Their highly regular arrangement gives the muscle its striated or striped appearance when viewed under a microscope. Each fibre has several nuclei, which lie on the outer surface of the cell as the presence of the myofibrils pushes all the cell structures to the outer margins.

The muscle fibres are grouped together in bundles or *fascicles* by connective tissue. Groups of fascicles are then held together by connective tissue and form a large muscle. The whole muscle is surrounded by the *muscle sheath*, which is continuous with the tendons that connect the muscle to a bone.

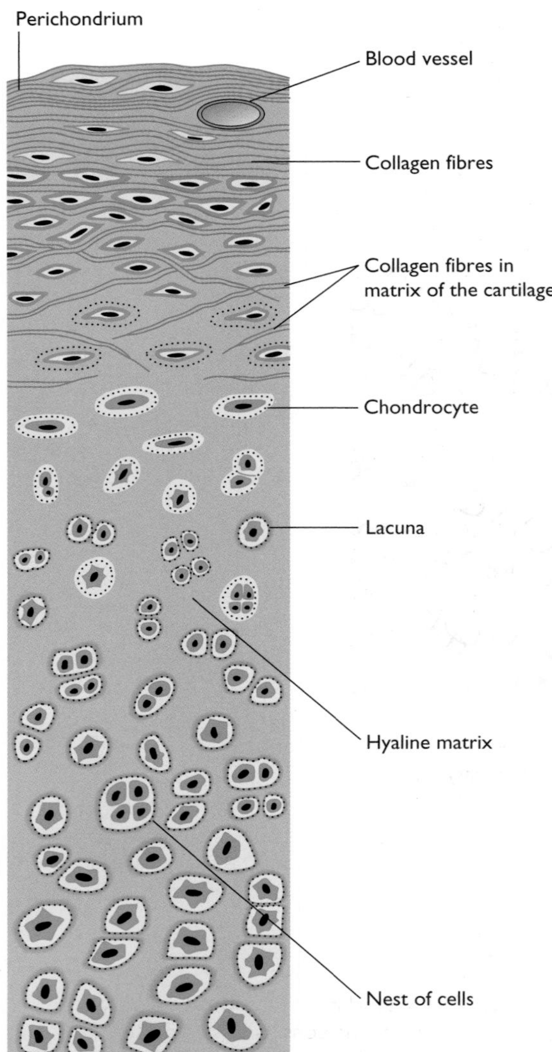

Fig. 2.10 The structure of hyaline cartilage.

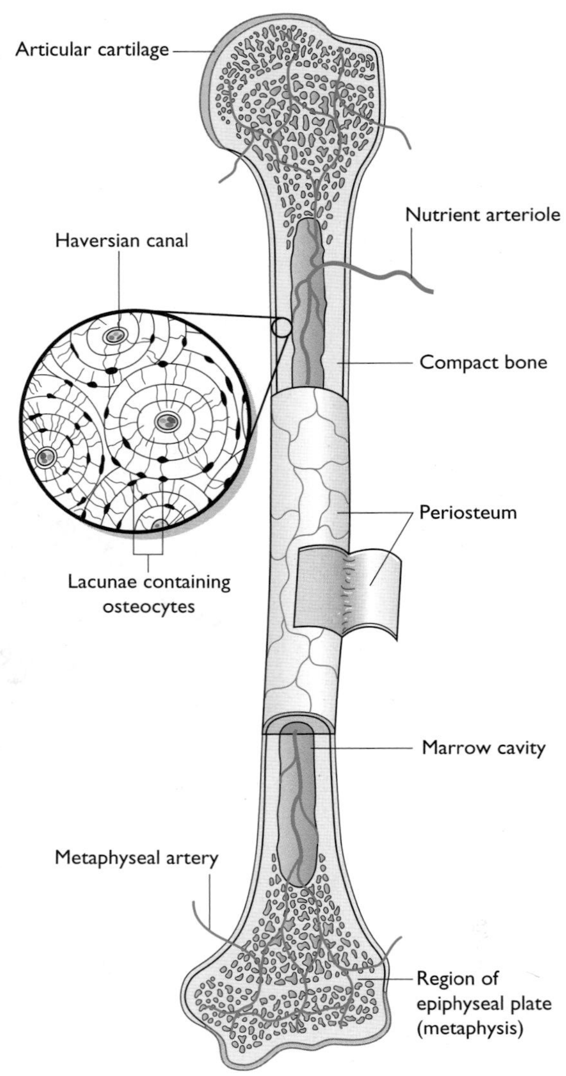

Fig. 2.11 The structure of compact bone.

Smooth muscle

Smooth muscle is also called unstriated, involuntary and visceral muscle. It is found in regions of the body that are under involuntary control (e.g., in the walls of the blood vessels, digestive tract, respiratory tract, bladder and uterus). It is therefore responsible for moving food through the digestive system, controlling the flow of blood through blood vessels and other unconscious processes. Smooth muscle is controlled by the autonomic nervous system.

The cells of smooth muscle are long and spindle-shaped (Fig. 2.14) and are surrounded by small amounts of connective tissue that bind the cells into sheets, or layers. The nucleus in each cell lies in its centre. Smooth muscle does not appear 'striped' when viewed under the microscope, hence its name.

Cardiac muscle

This type of muscle is found only in the heart and forms the *myocardium.* It is responsible for the rhythmic and automatic contraction of the heart that continues throughout an animal's life. This inherent contractibility is increased or slowed down by nerves supplying the heart according to the requirements of the body. Control of cardiac muscle is therefore involuntary or unconscious.

Cardiac muscle cells are striated and cylindrical in shape (Fig. 2.15). Unlike the cells of striated muscle, they branch to create a network of fibres, which are linked by *intercalated discs.* These enable nerve impulses to be conveyed across the myocardium extremely quickly, producing a rapid response to the changing needs of the body.

Muscle disease: Some disease conditions may affect muscle tissue. *Toxoplasmosis*, caused by the protozoan parasite *Toxoplasma gondii*, may result in inflammation of muscle tissue, or myositis. Metabolic disorders, such as *Cushing's disease*, may cause a generalised myopathy, resulting in muscular weakness and muscle wastage or atrophy. *Myasthenia gravis*, which presents as chronic fatigue, is a result of a lack of receptors for acetyl choline at the neuromuscular junctions.

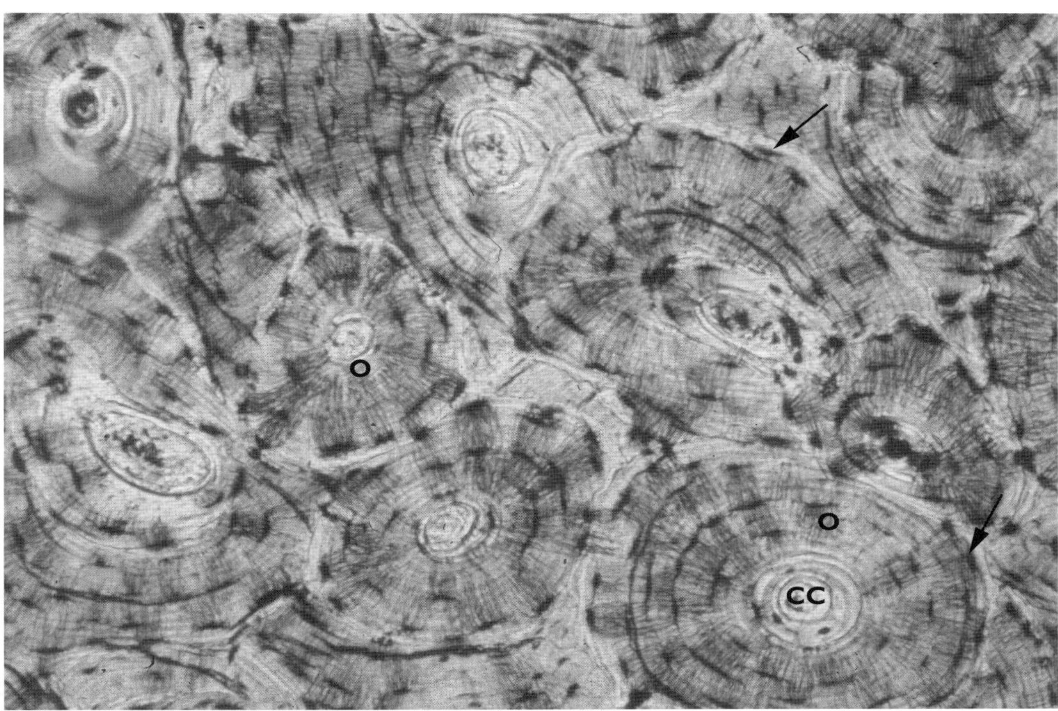

Fig. 2.12 Light micrograph (×100) of compact bone showing Haversian canals (CC) surrounded by lamellae of osteocytes (O) within their lacunae. (Taken from D Samuelson, 2007. Textbook of veterinary histology. St Louis, MO: Saunders, p. 122.)

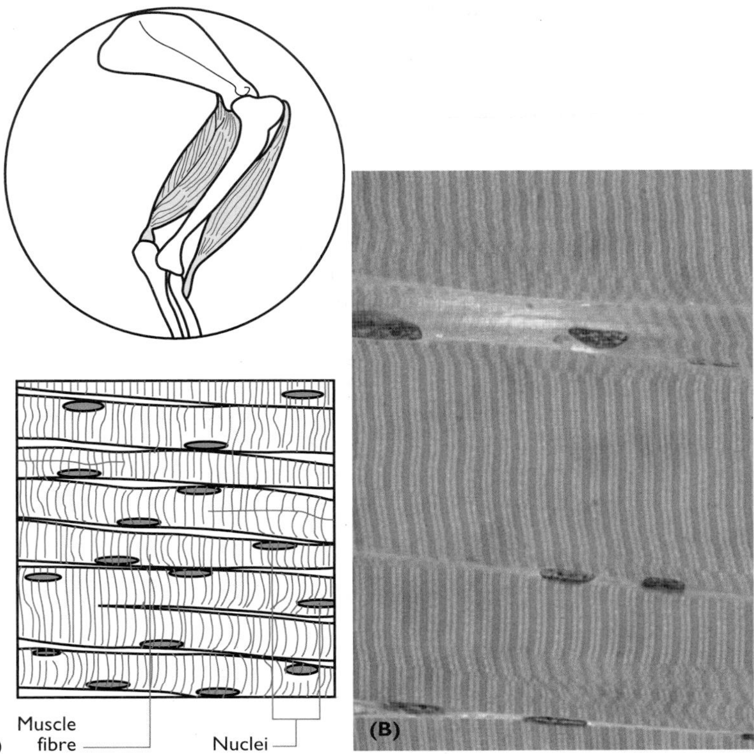

Fig. 2.13 **(A)** Skeletal muscle, as found attached to the bones. It is voluntary and consists of striped (striated) cells, which are long and cylindrical in shape. Each cell has several nuclei. **(B)** Light micrograph (×1000) of skeletal muscle showing characteristic bands and lines and nuclei located at the edges of the fibres. (Taken from D Samuelson, 2007. Textbook of veterinary histology. St Louis, MO: Saunders, p. 165.)

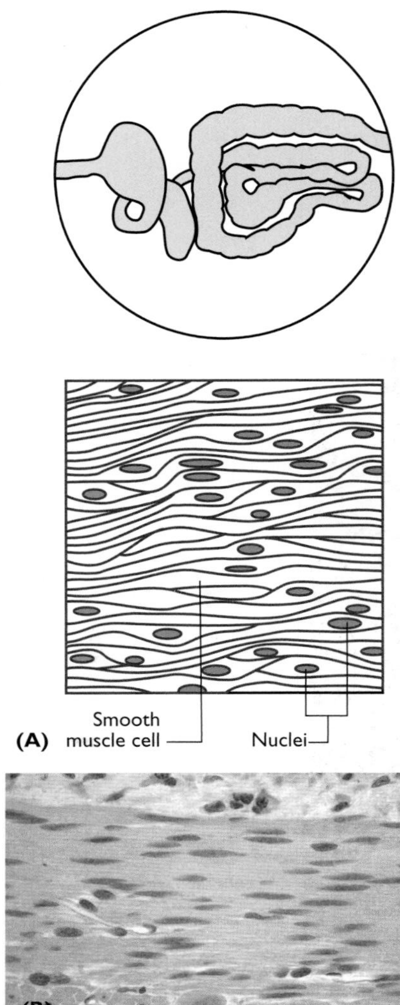

Fig. 2.14 **(A)** Smooth muscle, as found in the gastrointestinal tract and other viscera. It is involuntary and consists of small spindle-shaped cells without striations (hence 'smooth'). Each cell has one nucleus in the centre. **(B)** Light micrograph (× 1000) of smooth muscle cells showing the long spindle shaped cells with no striations. (Taken from D Samuelson, 2007. Textbook of veterinary histology. St Louis, MO: Saunders, p. 161.)

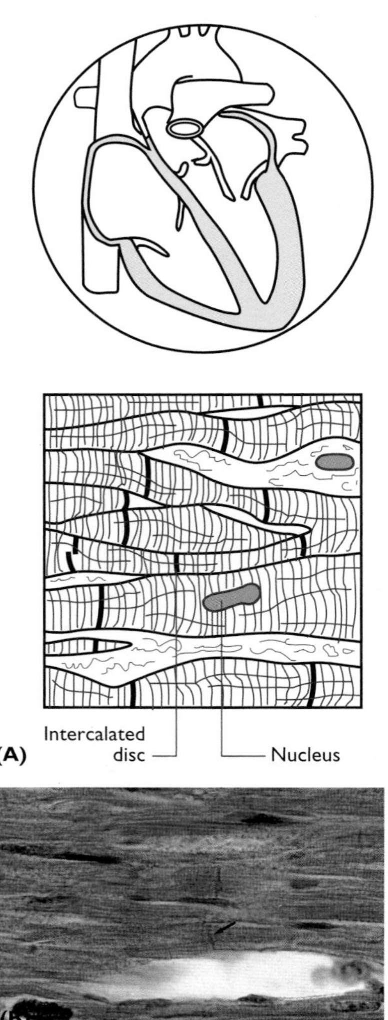

Fig. 2.15 **(A)** Cardiac muscle, found in the heart. It is involuntary and consists of striated, cylindrical cells. Cells are connected by intercalated discs. **(B)** Light micrograph (× 1000) of cardiac muscle cells. Arrow indicates intercalated discs. (Taken from D Samuelson, 2007. Textbook of veterinary histology. St Louis, MO: Saunders, p. 173.)

Nervous tissue

The main cell of nervous tissue is the *neuron* (Fig. 2.16), whose function is to transmit nerve impulses from one area to another. Each neuron consists of a *cell body*, containing the nucleus, several short processes known as *dendrons* and one long process known as an *axon*. Dendrons carry information towards the cell body, while the axon carries information away from it and towards its destination. Many axons within the body are covered in fatty material known as *myelin*. This is secreted by specialised cells wrapped around each axon – the *Schwann cells* – and it increases the speed of transmission of nerve impulses from one place to another. Myelin also provides protection and maintains the 'health' of the axon.

Dendrons and axons are referred to as nerve fibres and the whitish structures identified by the naked eye as 'nerves' within the body are collections of large numbers of nerve fibres.

Nerve impulses are transferred from one neuron to another by means of button-like structures known as *synapses*. All nerve pathways consist of neurons and synapses. (Nervous tissue is covered in more detail in Chapter 5.)

Some inflammatory diseases, which are often immune mediated, affect the myelin sheath. The loss of myelin surrounding the nerve, described as *demyelination*, slows down the rate of transmission of the nerve impulse, resulting in problems such as muscle weakness or *paresis*.

The body cavities

The body is divided into separate areas referred to as the body cavities (Fig. 2.17). They are described as 'potential' spaces because, although they are completely filled with the visceral organs and fluid, there is only a very small amount of free space.

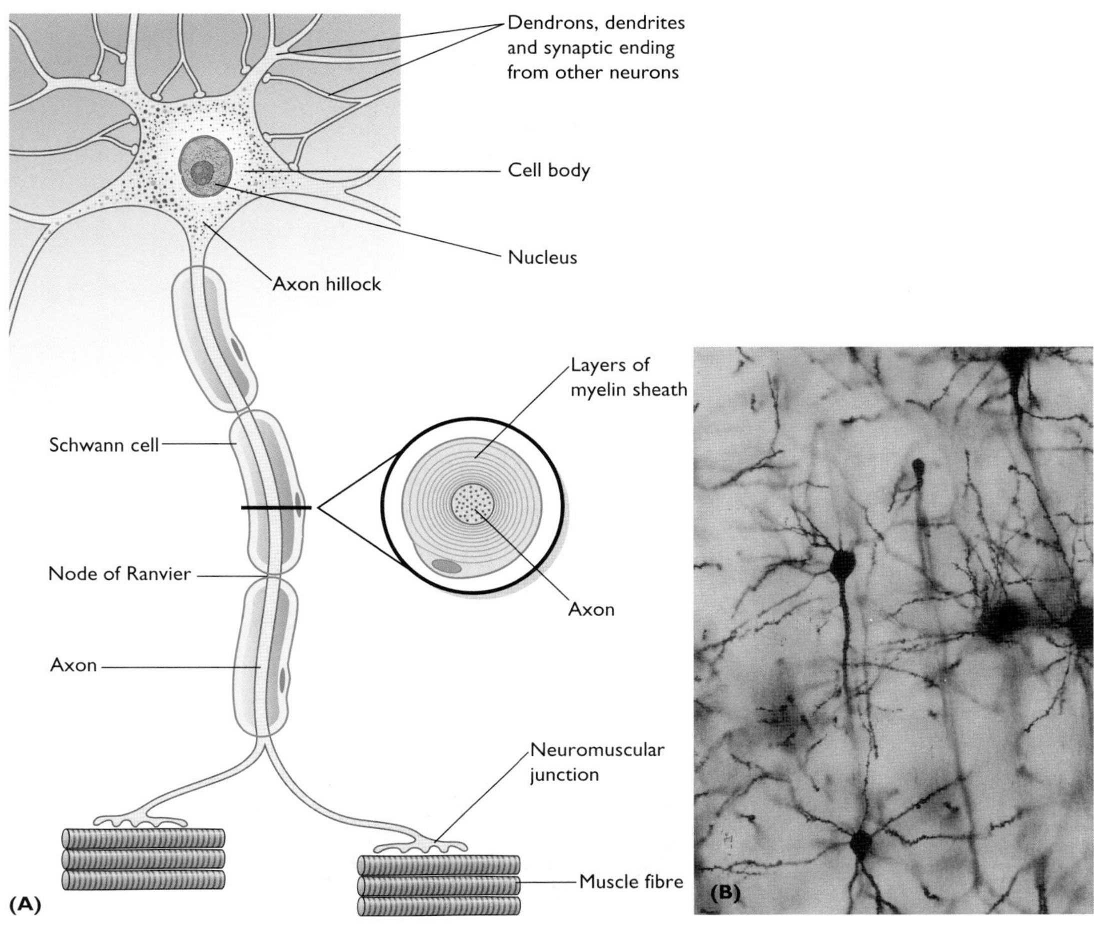

Fig. 2.16 **(A)** The structure of a neuron (nerve cell). **(B)** Light micrograph of nervous tissue. (Taken from D Samuelson, 2007. Textbook of veterinary histology. St Louis, MO: Saunders, p. 182.)

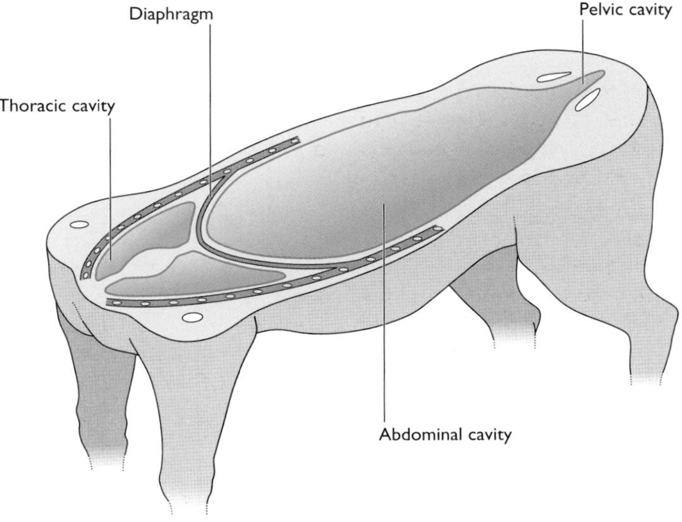

Fig. 2.17 Longitudinal section through the body showing the three body cavities.

All the body cavities are lined with a *serous membrane* or endothelium, which is a single continuous layer of epithelium that produces a watery or serous lubricating fluid. This is different from the thicker, more proteinaceous secretion *mucus*, which has a protective function. Serous fluid acts as a lubricant between the surfaces of the cavity and the organs and structures within it.

Each part of the serous membrane is a continuous layer, named according to its position within the cavity:

- *Parietal* describes the serous membrane that lines the boundaries or sides of the cavity.
- *Visceral* describes the serous membrane that covers all the organs within the cavity.

There are three body cavities:

- Thoracic
- Abdominal
- Pelvic

The thoracic cavity

The thoracic cavity (Table 2.1) contains the heart, lungs and other associated structures. Its skeletal walls are formed by the bony

Table 2.1 Summary of the boundaries of the body cavities

Anatomical boundary	Thoracic cavity	Abdominal cavity	Pelvic cavity
Cranial	Thoracic inlet	Diaphragm	Pelvic inlet (continuous with abdominal cavity)
Caudal	Diaphragm	Pelvic inlet (abdominal and pelvic cavities are not separated by a physical barrier)	Pelvic outlet
Dorsal	Thoracic vertebrae and hypaxial muscles	Lumbar vertebrae and hypaxial muscles	Sacrum
Ventral	Sternum	Muscles of ventral abdominal wall	Floor of pelvis
Lateral	Ribs and intercostal muscles	Muscles of lateral abdominal wall	Lateral wall of pelvis

thoracic cage consisting of the ribs, thoracic vertebrae and sternum. The 'entrance' into the cavity is known as the *cranial thoracic inlet* and is formed by the first thoracic vertebra, the first pair of ribs and the manubrium. The exit or caudal border is filled by the *diaphragm*.

The serous membrane lining the thoracic cavity and covering the organs within it is called the *pleura* (Fig. 2.18). The parietal pleura lines the inside of the thoracic cavity but is named according to which part of the walls it covers (i.e., the *diaphragmatic pleura* covers the diaphragm and the *costal pleura* covers the ribs). The thoracic cavity is divided into two *pleural cavities* by a continuation of the parietal pleura. Each cavity contains one of the lungs and serous pleural fluid. The lungs themselves are covered in visceral pleura, called the *pulmonary pleura*. Between the two pleural cavities, the thorax is divided into right and left sides by a vertical connective tissue septum called the *mediastinum*, which is covered in the *mediastinal pleura*. The mediastinum is the potential space formed by the double layer of parietal pleura that separates the two pleural cavities. It contains the pericardial cavity, containing the heart, aorta, trachea, oesophagus and the thymus gland in young animals.

The *pericardial cavity* lies within the mediastinum in the thoracic cavity and is the space in which the heart sits. The heart is contained within the *pericardium*, which is a double-layered membranous sheath that completely surrounds it. Between the two layers of membrane is serous fluid that acts as a lubricant, enabling the heart to beat freely.

Some disease processes affect the cavities, resulting in an accumulation of fluids. An example of this is *pleuritis*, which is an inflammation of the serous membrane that lines the thoracic cavity. Pleuritis may be caused by a number of conditions (e.g., bacterial infection) and results in pleural effusion, which leads to respiratory problems. *Peritonitis* may be caused by infection (e.g., by damage to the abdominal wall from an external wound), as the result of a perforation of the intestinal wall by an ingested foreign body.

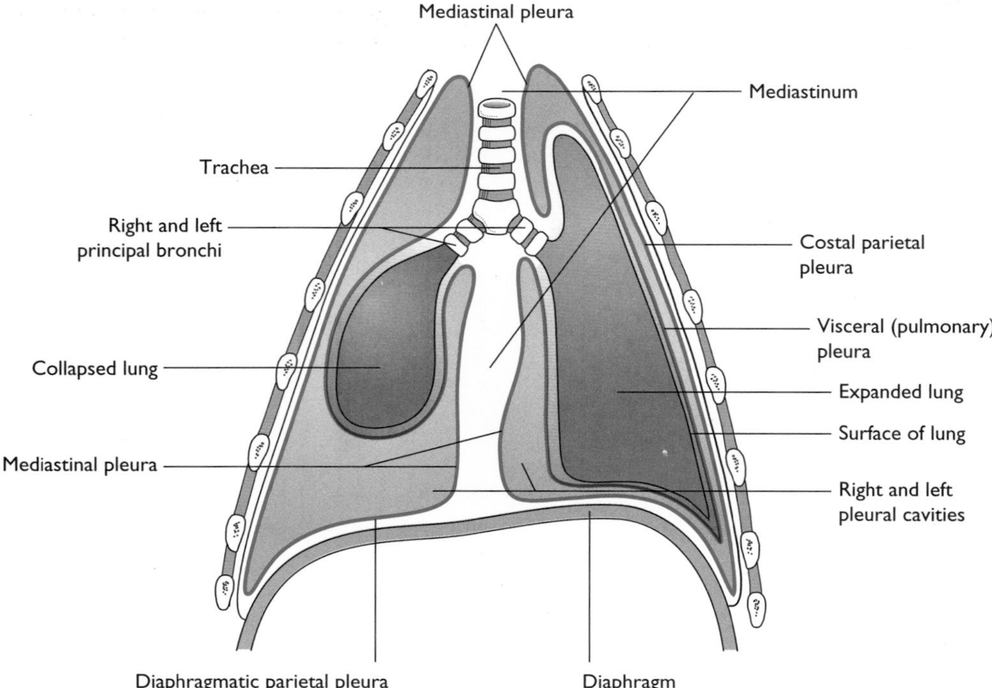

Fig. 2.18 The anatomy of the thoracic cavity showing the mediastinum and pleura.

The abdominal cavity

The abdominal cavity (Table 2.1) lies caudal to the thoracic cavity and contains the abdominal viscera (Fig. 2.17). These include the organs of the digestive system and related glands, the urogenital system and all the associated vessels and nerves that supply these systems. The abdominal cavity is bounded cranially by the diaphragm and caudally by the pelvic inlet (there is no actual physical division between the abdominal and pelvic cavities). Dorsally, the boundary is the lumbar vertebrae and the hypaxial muscles. The muscles of the abdominal walls form the dorsolateral, ventral and lateral limits.

The internal surface of the abdominal cavity is lined with a serous membrane called the *peritoneum* (Fig. 2.19). This is a continuous sheet that forms a closed cavity, the peritoneal cavity. The peritoneal cavity is the potential space between the parietal peritoneum that lines the abdominal walls and the visceral peritoneum that covers the organs. The peritoneal cavity contains only a small volume of lubricating serous fluid known as *peritoneal fluid*, which allows friction-free movement of the organs and prevents adhesions forming between the organs and the peritoneum.

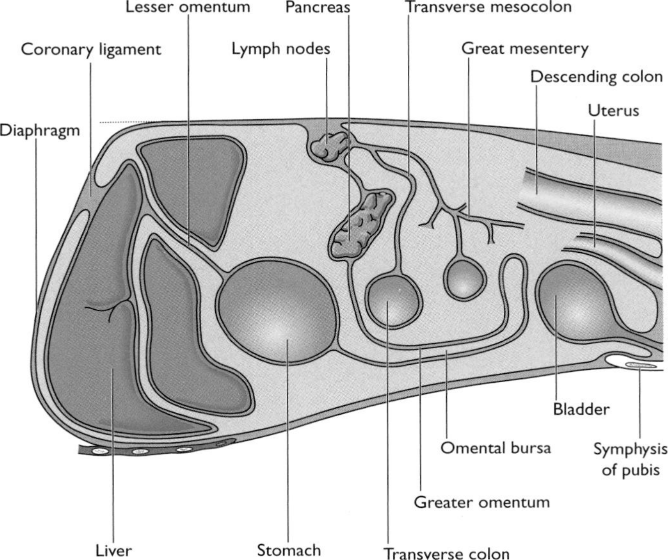

Fig. 2.19 Sagittal section through the abdominal cavity showing the reflections (folds) of the peritoneum.

The visceral peritoneum is folded on itself in a way that keeps the organs separate, suspending the organs within the abdominal cavity and carrying the various vessels and nerves that serve the viscera. This area of peritoneum is collectively known as the *mesentery*. The folds of mesentery have different names depending on their position (e.g., the mesentery suspending the duodenum is called the *mesoduodenum*, while the one suspending the ovary is the *mesovarium*). The *omentum* is a mobile fold of peritoneum that contains a 'lacy' network of fine vessels and fat and is divided into the *greater omentum*, arising from the greater curvature of the stomach, and the *lesser omentum*, arising from the lesser curvature of the stomach.

The pelvic cavity

The pelvic cavity (Table 2.1) lies caudal to the abdominal cavity (Fig. 2.17) and contains the urinary bladder, the rectum and the reproductive organs. There is no physical separation between the two as there is between the thoracic and abdominal cavities. The cavity is bounded cranially by the pelvic inlet and caudally by the caudal pelvic aperture. The sacrum and the first few coccygeal vertebrae form the dorsal boundary and the pubis and ischium form the floor of the cavity. The walls are formed by muscles and ligaments. A continuation of the peritoneum extends into the cranial parts of the cavity and covers the organs that lie in both cavities (e.g., bladder and reproductive tract).

CHAPTER 3

Skeletal system

KEY POINTS

- The skeletal system provides a supporting framework for the body, a firm base to which the muscles of locomotion are attached, and protects the softer tissues enclosed within the framework.
- The skeleton can be considered to be made up of three parts:
  - *Axial skeleton*, forming the central axis of the animal and comprising the skull, vertebral column and the rib cage
  - *Appendicular skeleton*, comprising the fore and hind limbs and the limb girdles, which attach them to the body
  - *Splanchnic skeleton*, which in the dog and cat consists only of the os penis found within the soft tissues of the penis
- Each part of the skeleton consists of many bones, each of which plays an important part in the function of the skeletal system.
- Bones are covered in 'lumps, bumps and holes'. Each has a specific descriptive name and a function, which contributes to movement (i.e., muscle attachment), or to maintaining the health of the tissue (i.e., blood or nerve supply).
- Bones are linked together by means of joints.
- Joints can be classified according to the type of tissue from which they are made (e.g., fibrous, cartilaginous or synovial joints), or according to the type of movement they allow (e.g., hinge or gliding joints).

The skeletal system is the 'framework' upon which the body is built – it provides support, protection and enables the animal to move (Fig. 3.1). The joints are considered to be an integral part of the skeleton. The skeletal system is made of the specialised connective tissues, bone and cartilage.

The functions of the skeletal system are:

1. *Support*: It acts as an internal 'scaffold' upon which the body is built.
2. *Locomotion*: It provides attachment for muscles, which operate a system of levers (i.e., the bones), to bring about movement.
3. *Protection*: It protects the underlying soft parts of the body (e.g., the brain is encased in the protective bony cranium of the skull).
4. *Storage*: It acts as a store for the essential minerals calcium and phosphate.
5. *Haemopoiesis*: Haemopoietic tissue forming the bone marrow manufactures the blood cells.

Bone structure and function

Bone shape

Bones can be categorised according to their shape:

- *Long bones* are typical of the limb bones (e.g., femur, humerus), and also include bones of the metacarpus/metatarsus and phalanges; long bones have a *shaft* containing a *medullary cavity* filled with bone marrow (Fig. 3.2).
- *Flat bones* have an outer layer of compact bone with a layer of cancellous or spongy bone inside; there is no medullary cavity (e.g., flat bones of the skull, scapula and ribs).
- *Short bones* have an outer layer of compact bone with a core of cancellous bone and no medullary cavity (e.g., carpal and tarsal bones).
- *Irregular bones* have a similar structure to short bones but a less uniform shape; they lie in the midline and are unpaired (e.g., vertebrae).

Some specialised types of bone are:

- *Sesamoid bones* are sesame-seed-shaped bones that develop within a tendon (and occasionally a ligament) that runs over an underlying bony prominence; they serve to change the angle at which the tendon passes over the bone and thus reduce 'wear and tear' (e.g., the patella associated with the stifle joint) (Fig. 3.1).
- *Pneumatic bones* contain air-filled spaces known as *sinuses* that have the effect of reducing the weight of the bone (e.g., maxillary and frontal bones).
- *Splanchnic bone* is bone that develops in a soft organ and is unattached to the rest of the skeleton (e.g., the os penis, the bone within the penis of the dog and cat).

Development of bone

The process by which bone is formed is called *ossification* and there are two types: *intramembranous* and *endochondral* ossification. The cells responsible for laying down new bone are called *osteoblasts*; the cells that destroy or remodel bone are called *osteoclasts*.

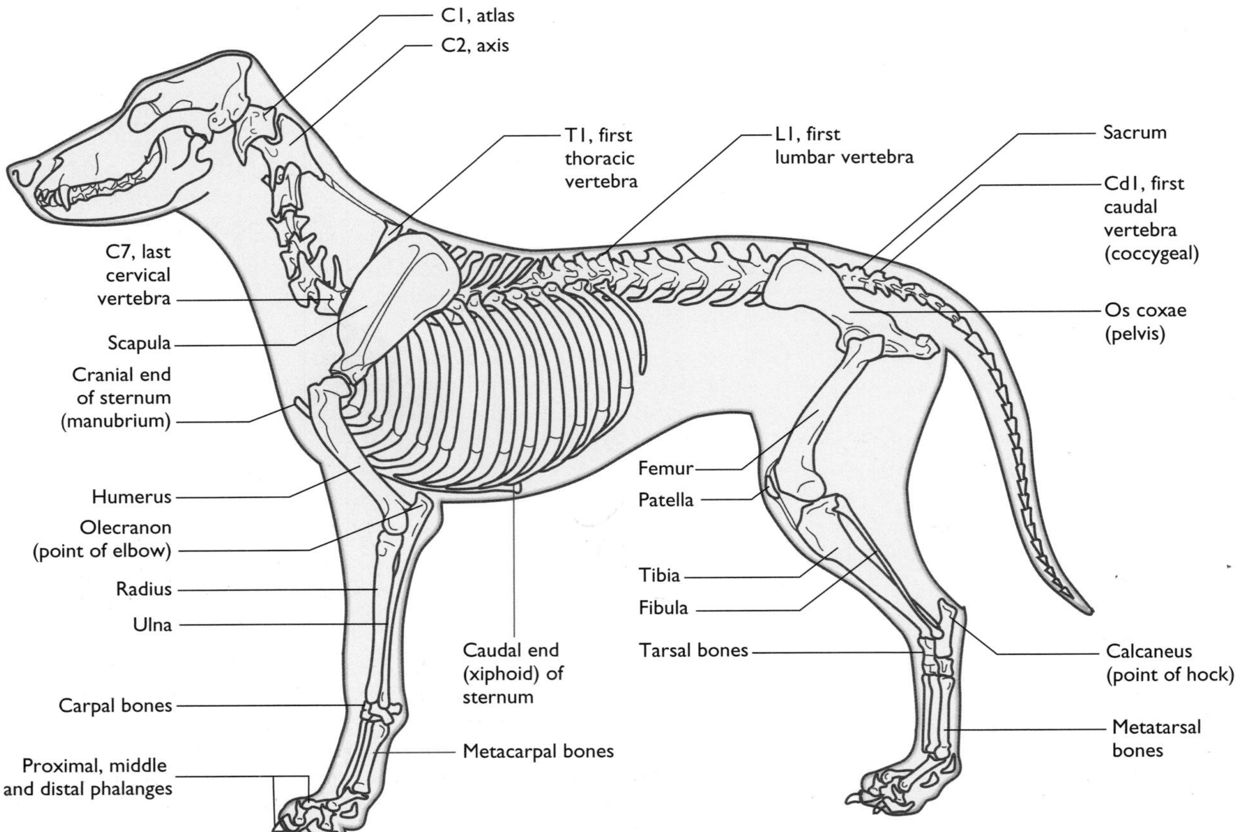

Fig. 3.1 The skeleton of the dog showing the major bones. (With permission from T Colville, JM Bassett, 2001. Clinical anatomy and physiology for veterinary technicians. St Louis, MO: Mosby, p. 102.)

- *Intramembranous ossification* is the process by which the flat bones of the skull are formed. The osteoblasts lay down bone between two layers of fibrous connective tissue. There is no cartilage template.
- *Endochondral ossification* involves the replacement of a hyaline cartilage model within the embryo by bone. The process starts in the developing embryo but is not completed fully until the animal has reached maturity and growth has ceased. The long bones of the limb develop by this method.

Endochondral ossification

The process of endochondral ossification (Fig. 3.3) is as follows:

1. A cartilage model develops within the embryo.
2. Primary centres of ossification appear in the *diaphysis* or shaft of the bone. The cartilage is replaced as the osteoblasts lay down bone, which gradually extends towards the ends of the bone.
3. Secondary centres of ossification appear in the *epiphyses* or ends of the bone, continuing the bone development.
4. Osteoclasts then start to remove bone from the centre of the diaphysis to form the marrow cavity, while the osteoblasts continue to lay down bone in the outer edges.
5. Between the diaphysis and epiphyses, a narrow band of cartilage persists. This is the *growth plate* or *epiphyseal plate,* which allows the bone to lengthen while the animal is growing. Eventually, when the animal has reached its final size, this will be replaced by bone and growth will no longer be possible. The epiphyseal plate is then said to have 'closed' and the time at which it happens is different for each type of bone.

Rickets is a disease of young growing animals caused by a nutritional deficiency of vitamin D or phosphorus. The bones fail to calcify and become bowed, and the joints appear swollen because of enlargement of the epiphyses. Any animal kept permanently inside is at risk of developing rickets because vitamin D is formed by the action of ultraviolet light on the skin.

The skeleton

The skeleton (Fig. 3.1) can be divided into three parts.

1. *Axial skeleton* runs from the skull to the tip of the tail and includes the skull, mandible, vertebrae and sternum.
2. *Appendicular skeleton* consists of the pectoral (front) and pelvic (hind) limbs and the shoulder and pelvic girdles that attach (or append) them to the body.
3. *Splanchnic skeleton* in the dog and cat is represented by the os penis within the tissue of the penis.

When studying the anatomy of the skeletal system it is helpful to understand the terms that are used to describe the various projections, passages and depressions that are found on and within bones.

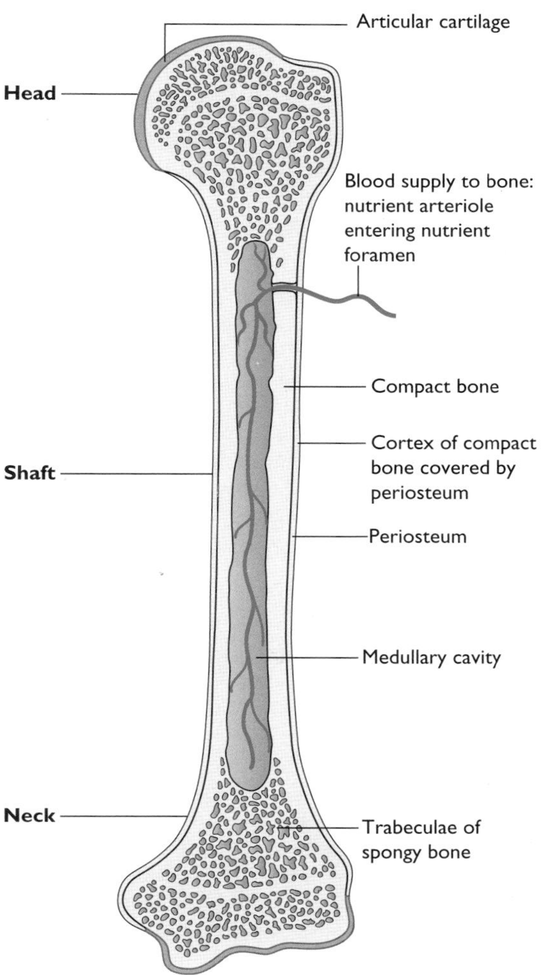

Fig. 3.2 Structure of a typical long bone.

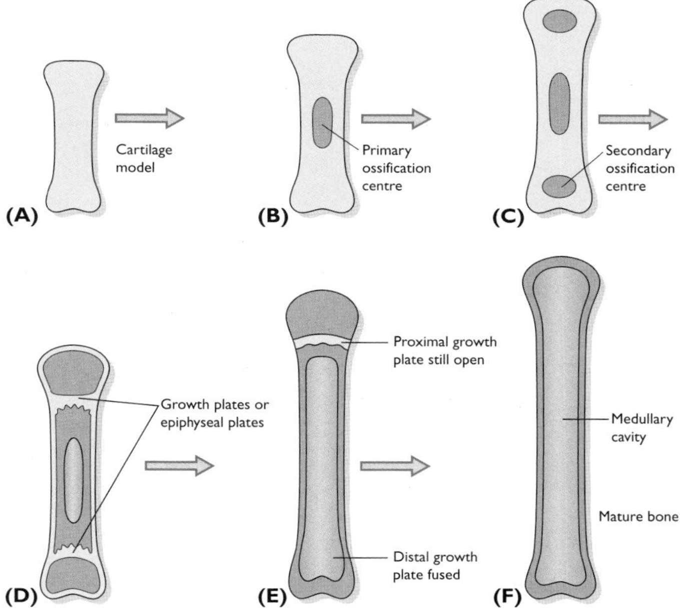

Fig. 3.3 Stages of endochondral ossification. **(A)** A cartilage model of the bone exists in the embryo. **(B)** Ossification begins from the primary ossification centre in the shaft (diaphysis). **(C)** Secondary ossification centres appear in the ends of the bone (epiphyses). **(D)** Ossification continues in primary and secondary centres; osteoclasts start to break down bone in the shaft, creating the marrow cavity. **(E)** The first growth plate fuses and growth is now only possible at the proximal growth plate; the medullary cavity extends into the epiphysis. **(F)** The proximal growth plate fuses and bone growth ceases.

- *Tuberosity/trochanter/tubercle*: protuberances on bones, which are usually for the attachment of muscles
- *Trochlea*: bony structures through or over which tendons pass; usually grooves in the bone and allow tendons to act as pulleys
- *Condyle*: a rounded projection on a bone, usually for articulation with another bone
- *Epicondyle*: a projection of bone on the lateral edge above its condyle
- *Foramen* (pl. *foramina*): an opening or passage into or through a bone (e.g., to allow the passage of blood vessels and nerves)
- *Fossa*: a hollow or depressed area on a bone
- *Head, neck* and *shaft*: used to describe parts of a long bone (Fig. 3.2)
- *Tendon*: connects muscle to bone
- *Ligament*: connects one bone to another bone

The axial skeleton

The skull

The bones of the head include the skull, nasal chambers, mandible or lower jaw and hyoid apparatus. The functions of the skull are:

1. To house and protect the brain
2. To house the special sense organs – eye, ear, nose and tongue
3. To house and provide attachment for parts of the digestive system (teeth, tongue, etc.)
4. To provide attachment for the hyoid apparatus and the numerous muscles of mastication and facial expression
5. To provide a bony cavity through which air can enter the body
6. To communicate (the muscles of facial expression are found on the head and are an important means of communication)

Cranium

The caudal part of the skull that provides the bony 'case' in which the brain sits is called the cranium (Figs. 3.4 and 3.5). The bones of the cranium include:

- *Parietal*: forms much of the dorsal and lateral walls of the cranium.
- *Temporal*: lies below the parietal bone on the caudolateral surface of the skull. The most ventral part of the temporal bone forms a rounded prominence called the *tympanic bulla*, which houses the structures of the middle ear. There is an opening into the tympanic bulla, called the *external acoustic meatus*, which in life is closed by the tympanic membrane or eardrum. The cartilages of the external ear canal are attached to this region.

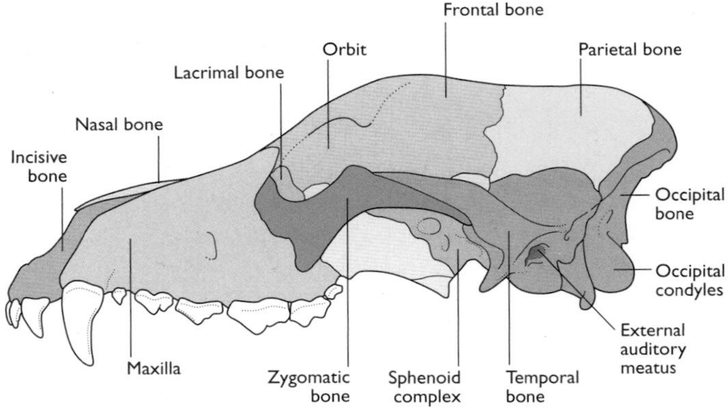

Fig. 3.4 Lateral view of the dog skull showing main bony features.

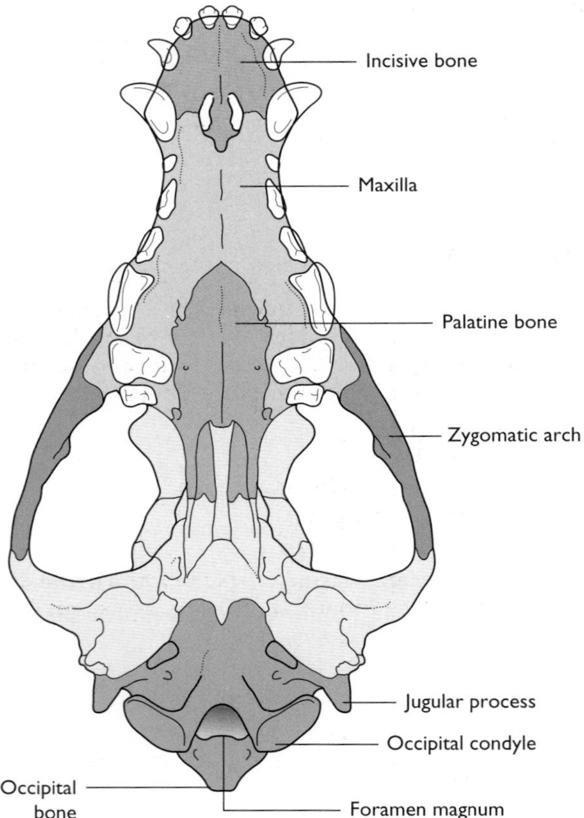

Fig. 3.5 Ventral view of the dog skull showing main bony features.

- *Frontal* forms the front aspect of the cranium or 'forehead' and contains an air-filled chamber called the *frontal sinus*, which connects to the nasal chamber.
- *Occipital* lies at the base of the skull on the caudal aspect. In this region there is a large hole called the *foramen magnum*, through which the spinal cord passes. On either side is a pair of bony prominences, the *occipital condyles*. These articulate with the first cervical vertebra or atlas (Fig. 3.1). At the side of the occipital condyles are the *jugular processes*, which are sites for muscle attachment.
- *Sphenoid* lies on the ventral aspect of the skull, forming the floor of the cranial cavity. It is penetrated by many small foramina through which nerves and blood vessels pass.
- *Sagittal crest* is a ridge of bone on the dorsal midline surface of the skull, which can be prominent in muscular dogs.
- *Zygomatic arch* is an arch of bone that projects laterally from the skull, forming the 'cheekbone'.
- *Lacrimal* lies at the base of the orbit, which houses the eye, and is the region through which the tears drain from the eye into the nose.

In some breeds, such as the Cavalier King Charles Spaniel, poor development of the skull can result in a small cranium, which is insufficient in size to accommodate the brain. The result of this is the herniation of the cerebellum through the foramen magnum (see Chapter 5), causing a number of problems including hydrocephalus (fluid on the brain), and syringomyelia (fluid filled cavities of the spine). Affected dogs may show an extremely painful reaction to touch and may have an uncoordinated gait (ataxia).

Nasal chambers

The most rostral part of the skull carries the *nasal chamber*, the sides of which are formed by the *maxilla* and the roof by the *nasal bone*. The nasal chamber is divided lengthways into two by a cartilaginous plate called the *nasal septum*. Each of the chambers is filled with delicate scrolls of bone called the *nasal turbinates* or *conchae*. These are covered in ciliated mucous epithelium (see Chapter 8). At the back of the nasal chamber, forming a boundary between the nasal and cranial cavities, is the *ethmoid bone*. In the centre of this bone is the *cribriform plate*, a sieve-like area perforated by numerous foramina through which the olfactory nerves pass from the nasal mucosa to the olfactory bulbs of the brain (see Chapter 5).

The roof of the mouth is called the *hard palate* and is formed from three bones on the ventral aspect of the skull: the *incisive bone* or premaxilla, part of the *maxilla* and the *palatine*. The incisive bone is the most rostral and carries the incisor teeth (Fig. 3.5).

Many of the bones of the skull are joined together by fibrous joints called *sutures*. Sutures are firm and immovable joints but allow for expansion of the skull in a growing animal.

Mandible

The mandible or lower jaw comprises two halves or *dentaries*, joined together at the chin by a cartilaginous joint called the *mandibular symphysis*. Each half is divided into a horizontal part, the *body*, and a vertical part, the *ramus* (Fig. 3.6). The body carries the sockets or *alveoli* for the teeth of the lower jaw. The ramus articulates with the rest of the skull at the *temporomandibular joint* via a projection called the *condylar process*. A rounded *coronoid process*, which projects from the ramus into the temporal fossa, is the point to which the temporalis muscle attaches (Fig. 3.6). There is a depression on the lateral surface of the ramus, the *masseteric fossa*, in which the masseter muscle lies.

The mandibular symphysis is a common fracture site in cats when they are involved in a collision with a car. It can be relatively easily repaired by wiring the two sides together and patients usually make a good recovery.

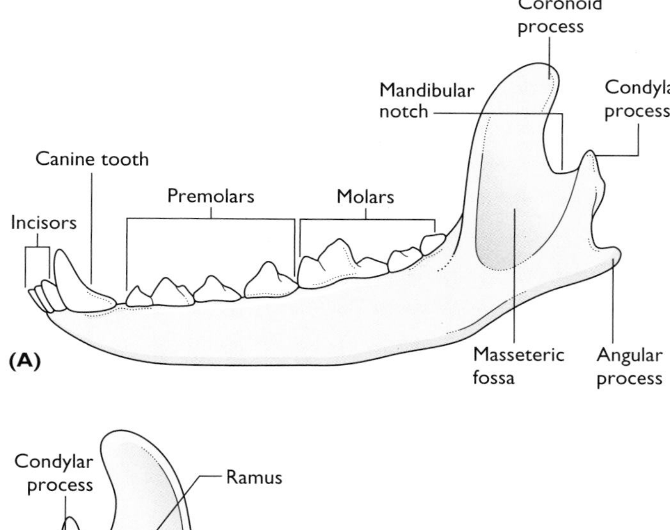

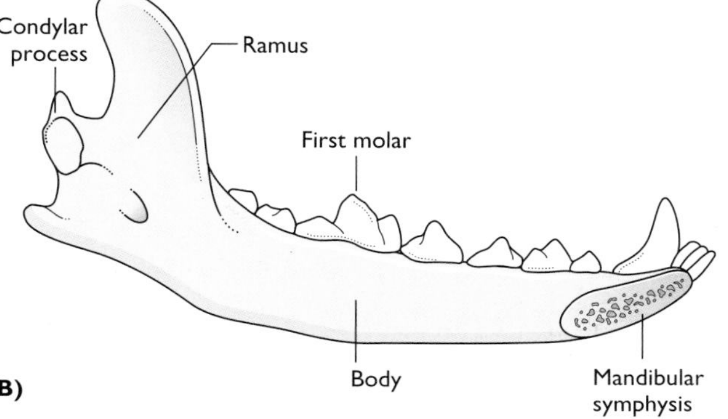

Fig. 3.6 Lateral **(A)** and medial **(B)** views of the dog mandible.

Hyoid apparatus

The hyoid apparatus lies in the intermandibular space and consists of a number of fine bones and cartilages joined together in an arrangement that resembles a trapeze (Fig. 3.7). The hyoid apparatus is the means by which the larynx and tongue are suspended from the skull. The apparatus articulates with the temporal region of the skull in a cartilaginous joint.

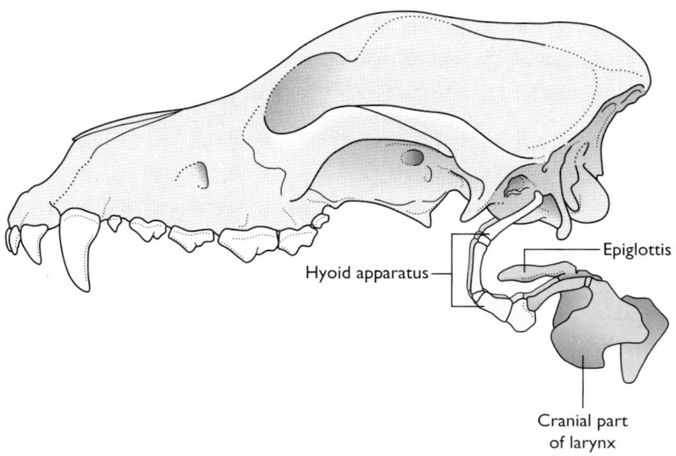

Fig. 3.7 The trapeze-like hyoid apparatus suspended from the skull (dog).

Skull shapes

The shape of the skull varies among species. In the domestic cat the skull is much more rounded or 'apple-shaped' than it is in the dog, and there is little difference between the various cat breeds. In the dog, although the basic anatomy remains the same, the overall appearance differs greatly among the different breeds (Fig. 3.8).

Three morphological forms of dog skull are recognised:

- *Dolichocephalic*: The head, particularly the nose, is long and narrow (e.g., Greyhound, Borzoi, Afghan hound).
- *Mesaticephalic*: This is the 'normal' or average shape of the dog skull (mes meaning 'middle'; e.g., Beagle, Labrador; Pointer).
- *Brachycephalic*: The cranium is often more rounded and the nose is short and may be pushed in, because of shortening of the nasal chambers, hard palate and mandible (e.g., Bulldog, Pekinese, Boxer, Pug).

> The shape of the skull, particularly in brachycephalic breeds such as the Bulldog or the Boxer, can lead to a variety of clinical conditions (e.g., snoring respiration, difficulty in breathing). The relative size of the head can also cause difficulties with whelping. Breeds with a mesaticephalic shape of skull (e.g., Labradors) are much less likely to exhibit these conditions.

The vertebrae

The vertebral column consists of a number of bones arranged in a series along the midline of the body and extending from the base of the skull to the tip of the tail. The vertebrae are divided into regions depending upon their position in the body:

- *Cervical* (C): neck region
- *Thoracic* (T): thoracic region
- *Lumbar* (L): lower back or abdominal region
- *Sacral* (S): croup or pelvic region
- *Caudal* (Cd) or *coccygeal*: in the tail

Each species has a characteristic number of vertebrae within each region, which is written as a formula. In the dog and cat this formula is C7, T13, L7, S3, Cd20-23 (Fig. 3.1).

The functions of the vertebral column are:

1. To stiffen the body axis and help maintain posture
2. To enclose and protect the spinal cord
3. To shield and protect the softer underlying structures of the neck, thorax, abdomen and pelvis

Basic plan of a vertebra

The vertebrae within all regions of the vertebral column are basically similar in structure, although each region shows slight differences related to function. A typical vertebra (Fig. 3.9) consists of a roughly cylindrical ventral *body* with a convex cranial end and a concave caudal end. This arrangement enables the bodies to fit together, creating a flexible rod. The body is topped by an arch, called the *vertebral* or *neural arch*, which forms a tunnel-like *vertebral foramen* through which the spinal cord passes. When linked together, the vertebral foramina constitute the *spinal canal*.

The neural arch has a dorsal projection called the *spinous process* or *neural spine*, which varies in height and size from one region of the vertebral column to another. On either side of the

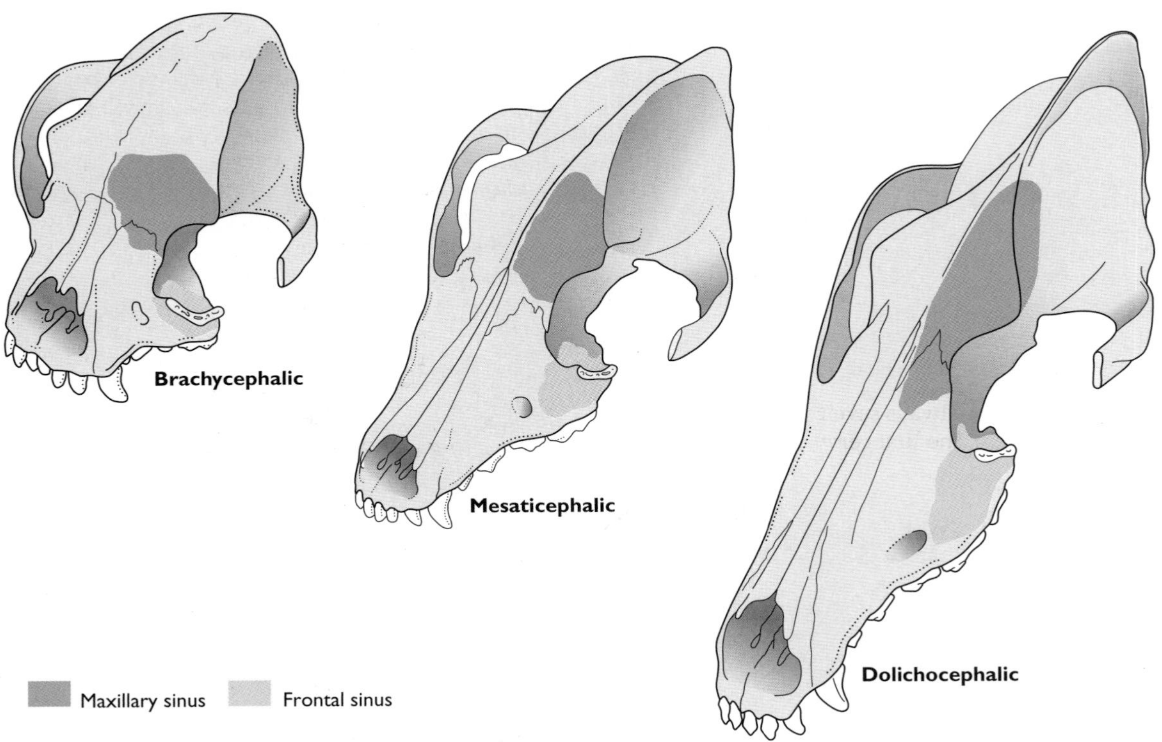

Fig. 3.8 The three basic shapes of the dog skull seen in common breeds. Also shows the positions of the maxillary and frontal sinuses.

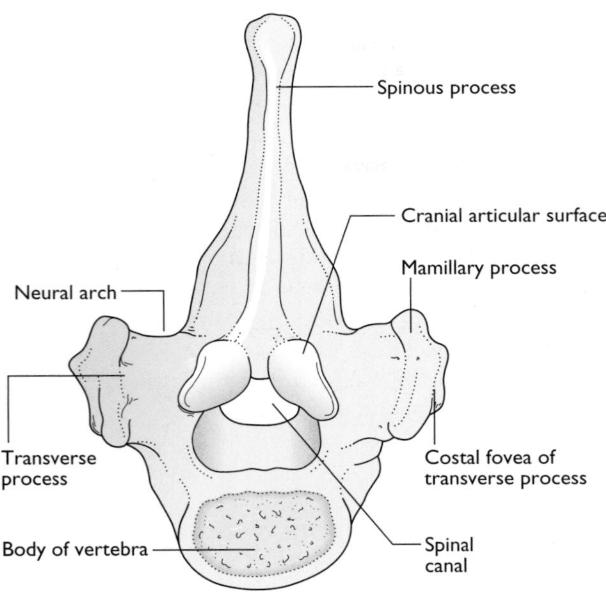

Fig. 3.9 Basic structure of a typical vertebra.

vertebra there are laterally projecting processes, the *transverse processes*, which also vary in shape and size between regions. The transverse processes divide the muscles of the vertebral column into dorsal or *epaxial* and ventral or *hypaxial* divisions (see Chapter 4 – Muscles of the trunk).

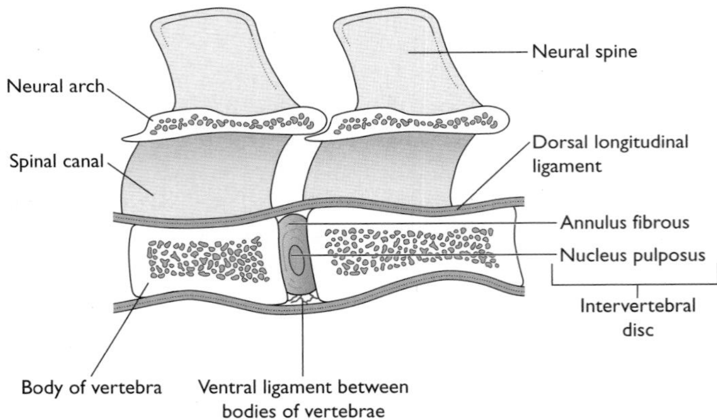

Fig. 3.10 The intervertebral disc, positioned between vertebrae and acting as a 'cushion'.

On the cranial and caudal edges of the arch of each vertebra there are *cranial* and *caudal articular processes*. These form a synovial joint with those of the adjacent vertebrae, creating a flexible rod running in the midline of the body. There are also a number of other processes, which are sites for muscle attachment. Lying between the bodies of each pair of vertebrae is a fibrocartilaginous *intervertebral disc*, which acts as a 'shock absorber', preventing damage to the spinal cord (Fig. 3.10). The intervertebral disc is composed of a tough fibrous connective tissue outer area, called the *annulus fibrosus*, and a core of gelatinous material called the *nucleus pulposus*.

The vertebrae are linked by ligaments that run between them and they articulate with one another by two types of joint:

- *Cartilaginous*: between the bodies of each vertebra
- *Synovial*: between the cranial and caudal articular processes

Prolapsed or 'slipped' disc. In this condition, the annulus fibrosus ruptures and the pulpy centre of the disc protrudes outward. This puts pressure either on the spinal cord or on the associated nerves leaving the cord, causing the animal to show symptoms ranging from pain to paralysis due to the loss of motor function.

Regional variations

- *Cervical vertebrae* (Fig. 3.11A). There are always seven cervical vertebrae in the neck of all mammals. The first cervical vertebra, or *atlas*, has a unique and distinctive shape. The atlas does not have a body or a spinous process, but consists of two large wing-like lateral masses joined by a ventral and dorsal arch. The second cervical vertebra, or *axis*, is also unusual and has an elongated, blade-like spinous process, which serves as a point of attachment for neck muscles. A strong ligament, called the *nuchal ligament*, also attaches to the spinous process and extends from the axis to the first thoracic vertebra. On the cranial aspect of the axis, a projection of bone called the *dens* or *odontoid process* fits into the vertebral foramen of the atlas and serves as a pivot around which the atlas can be rotated. The remaining cervical vertebrae (C3–C7) follow the basic vertebral plan, and get progressively smaller as they advance towards the junction with the thoracic vertebrae.
- *Thoracic vertebrae* (Fig. 3.11B). There are usually 13 thoracic vertebrae. Their distinguishing feature is their tall spinous

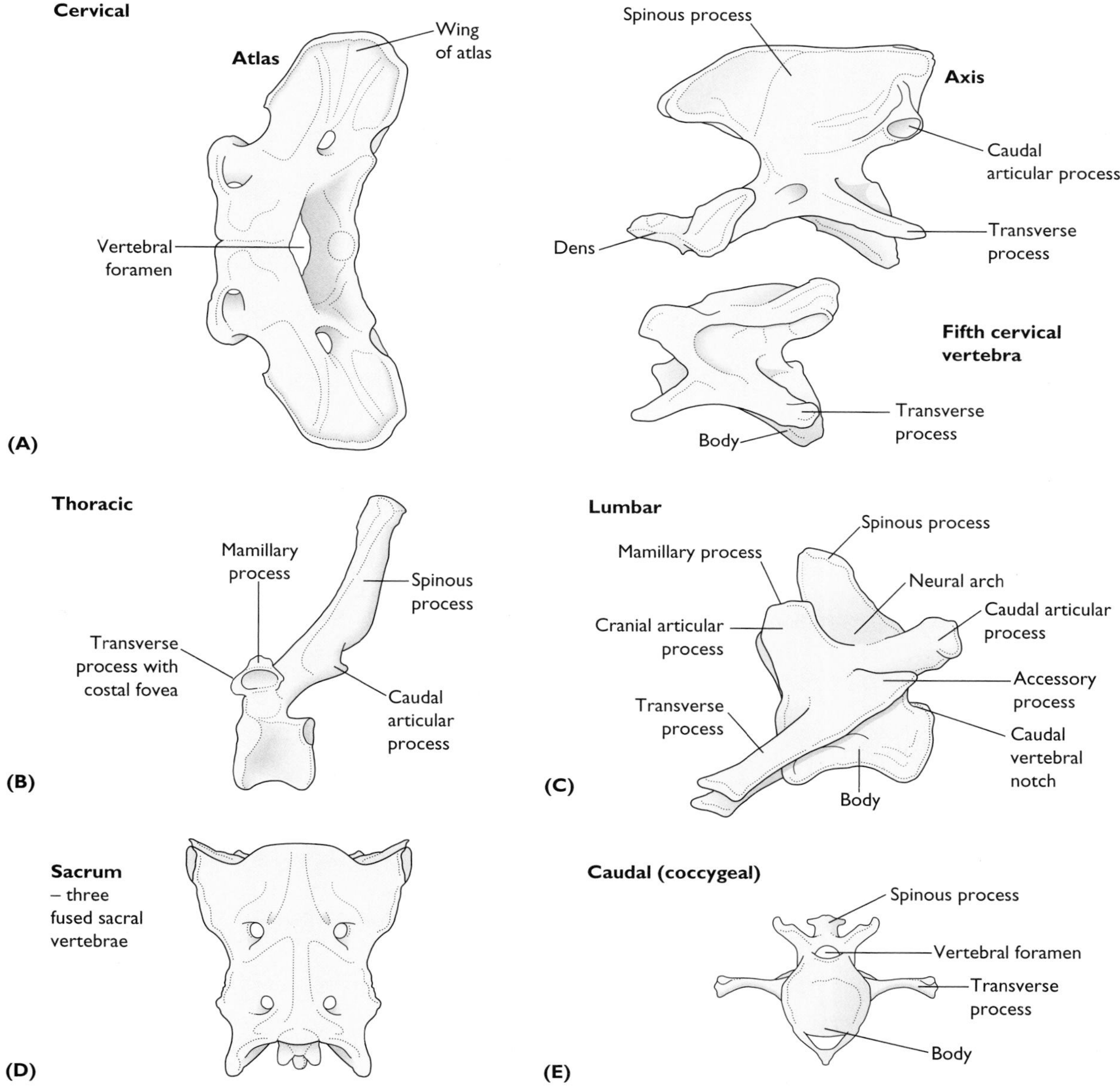

Fig. 3.11 Variations in the shape of vertebrae. **(A)** Cervical. **(B)** Thoracic. **(C)** Lumbar and **(D)** Sacral (the three sacral vertebrae are fused into one bone). **(E)** Caudal/coccygeal.

processes and short bodies. They articulate with the ribs at two sites: the *costal fovea*, which forms a synovial joint with the *head* of the rib, and the *transverse fovea*, which forms a synovial joint with the *tubercle* of the rib. The height of the spinous processes decreases as the series progresses towards the lumbar region.
- *Lumbar vertebrae* (Fig. 3.11C). There are usually seven lumbar vertebrae. These vertebrae have large bodies and long transverse processes angled cranioventrally, to which the lumbar muscles attach.

The synovial joint between the atlas (C1) and the occipital condyles of the skull allows nodding movements of the head, and the synovial joint between the atlas and axis (C1–C2) allows a pivotal movement so that the head can turn in all directions.

- *Sacral vertebrae* (Fig. 3.11D). These three vertebrae are fused together to form the *sacrum* in the adult dog and cat. The sacrum forms a fibrosynovial joint with the wing of the ilium of the pelvic girdle: the *sacroiliac joint*.
- *Caudal or coccygeal vertebrae* (Fig. 3.11E). These vary in number and shape according to the length of the tail. The first few resemble the lumbar vertebrae, but they get progressively smaller and simpler throughout the series. The last few caudal vertebrae are reduced to little rods of bone.

During parturition, under the influence of the hormone relaxin, the sacroiliac ligament relaxes and softens so that the pelvis can stretch, enabling the fetuses to pass out through the birth canal. In some species, particularly larger ones such as cattle, relaxation of the ligaments causes the tail to droop.

The ribs and sternum

The ribs form the walls of the bony thoracic cage that protects the organs of the chest. There are 13 pairs of ribs in the dog and cat, which articulate with the thoracic vertebrae (Fig. 3.12). A rib is a flat bone consisting of compact bone on the outside packed with cancellous bone on the inside. Each rib has a bony dorsal part and a cartilaginous ventral part, the *costal cartilage*. The most dorsal part of the bony rib has two projections: the *head*, which articulates with the *costal fovea* of the vertebra, and the *tubercle* or *neck*, which articulates with the *transverse fovea* of the appropriate thoracic vertebra.

The costal cartilage articulates with the sternum, either directly or indirectly. The first eight pairs of ribs attach directly to the sternum and are called the *sternal ribs*. The ribs from pairs 9 to 12 are called *asternal* or *'false' ribs*, and they attach via their costal cartilages to the adjacent rib, forming the *costal arch*. The last ribs (pair 13) have no attachment at their cartilaginous ends, which lie free in the abdominal muscle – this pair are called the *'floating' ribs*. The space between each successive pair of ribs is called the *intercostal space* and is filled by the *intercostal muscles* of the trunk (Fig. 3.13).

The sternum forms the floor of the thoracic cage (Fig. 3.13) and is composed of eight bones, the *sternebrae*, and the intersternebral cartilages. The most cranial sternebra is the *manubrium*, which projects in front of the first pair of ribs and forms part of the cranial thoracic inlet. Sternebrae 2–7 are short cylindrical bones. The last sternebra is longer and dorsoventrally flattened and is

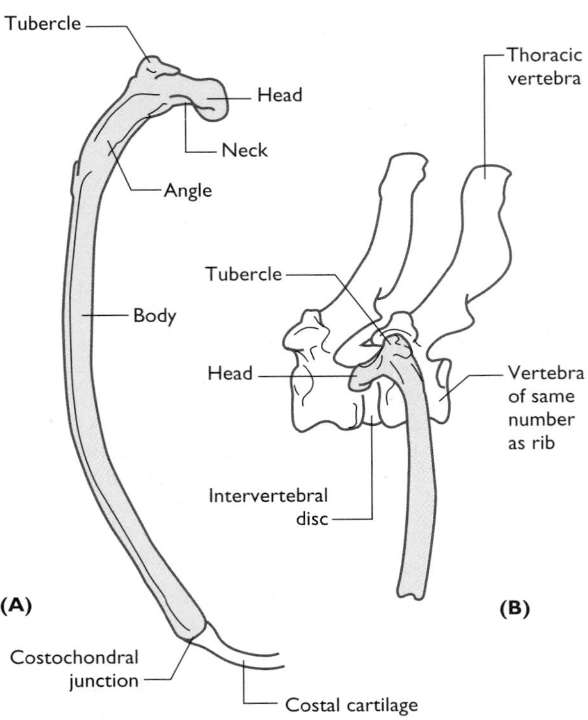

Fig. 3.12 Structure of the canine rib. **(A)** Caudal view. **(B)** Lateral view showing articulation with a thoracic vertebra. (With permission from T Colville, JM Bassett, 2001. Clinical anatomy and physiology for veterinary technicians. St Louis, MO: Mosby, p. 112.)

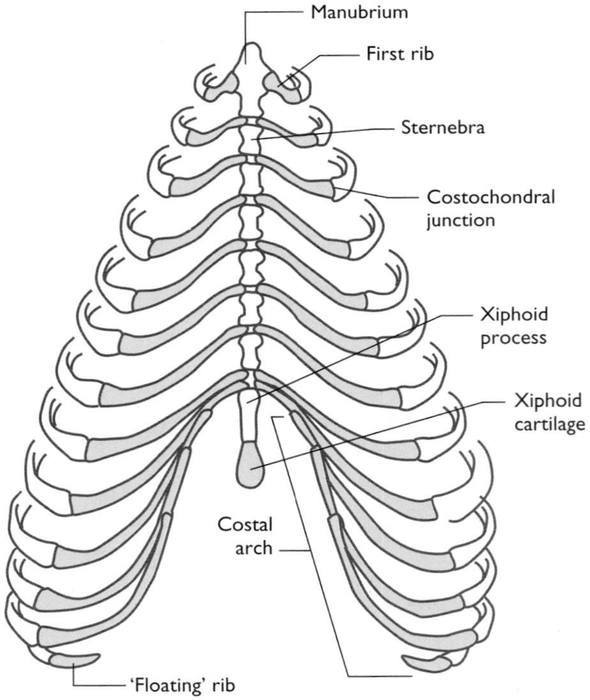

Fig. 3.13 The rib cage of the dog, showing sternal, asternal and 'floating' ribs. (With permission from T Colville, JM Bassett, 2001. Clinical anatomy and physiology for veterinary technicians. St Louis, MO: Mosby, p. 112.)

called the *xiphoid process*. Attached to the xiphoid process and projecting caudally is a flap of cartilage called the *xiphoid cartilage*. The linea alba attaches to this. Between each pair of sternebrae are cartilaginous discs called the *intersternebral cartilages*.

The appendicular skeleton

The appendicular skeleton is composed of the pectoral (or fore) limb and the pelvic (or hind) limb and the shoulder and pelvic girdles that attach these to the body. The forelimb has no bony connection to the trunk, only being attached by muscles. This absorbs the 'shock' at the point when the limb takes the animal's weight in four-legged animals or running quadrupeds. This differs from primates, which generally walk on their hind legs and so have evolved a pectoral girdle with a clavicle. However, the hind limb does have a bony articulation in the pelvic girdle, which forms the platform for the muscles that provide the propulsive force as the animal is running.

Bones of the forelimb

The bones of the forelimb (Fig. 3.1) are:

- *Clavicle*: This is frequently absent in the dog. When present, it is just a remnant of bone that lies in the muscles cranial to the shoulder joint; it is described as being *vestigial*. The clavicle is normally present in the cat but does not articulate with other bones.
- *Scapula*: This is also called the shoulder blade (Fig. 3.14). It is a large, flat bone found on the lateral surface of the trunk at the junction of the neck and ribs. It has a prominent ridge or *spine* running down the middle of its lateral surface. This divides the lateral surface into two regions: the *supraspinous fossa* and *infraspinous fossa*. On the distal end of the spine there is a bony projection called the *acromion*. At the distal end of the scapula the bone narrows at the *neck* and there is a shallow articular socket, called the *glenoid cavity*, which forms the shoulder joint with the head of the humerus. The medial surface of the scapula is flat and comparatively smooth.
- *Humerus*: This is a long bone forming the upper forelimb (Fig. 3.15). It articulates proximally with the scapula at the *shoulder joint*, and distally with the radius and ulna at the *elbow joint*. The proximal end of the humerus consists of a large rounded projection, the *head*. Cranial and lateral to the head there is a large prominence, called the *greater tubercle*. Another prominence, the *lesser tubercle*, lies medial to the head. Both of these are sites for attachment of the muscles that support the shoulder joint. Distal to the head is the *neck*, attached to the slightly twisted *shaft* of the bone. On the distal end of the humerus are the *medial* and *lateral epicondyles*, between which is the *condyle*. Just proximal to this is a deep hollow called the *olecranon fossa*. This receives the anconeal process of the ulna. There is also a hole in the centre of the condyle called the *supratrochlear foramen*. Note that there is no supratrochlear foramen in the cat.
- *Radius and ulna*: These are both long bones that lie side by side in the forearm (Fig. 3.16). At the proximal end of the ulna is a projection known as the *olecranon*, which forms the point of the elbow (Fig. 3.17). In front of this is a crescent-shaped

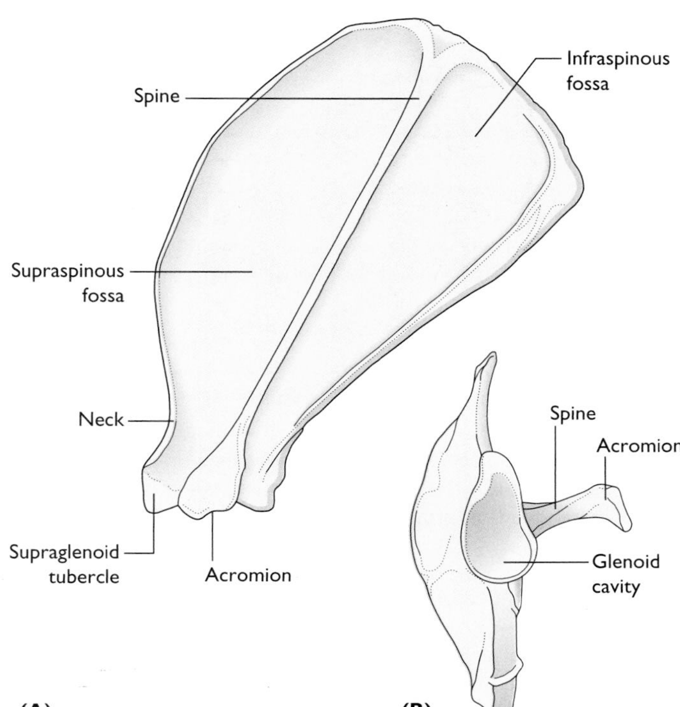

Fig. 3.14 The dog scapula. **(A)** Lateral view. **(B)** Ventral view.

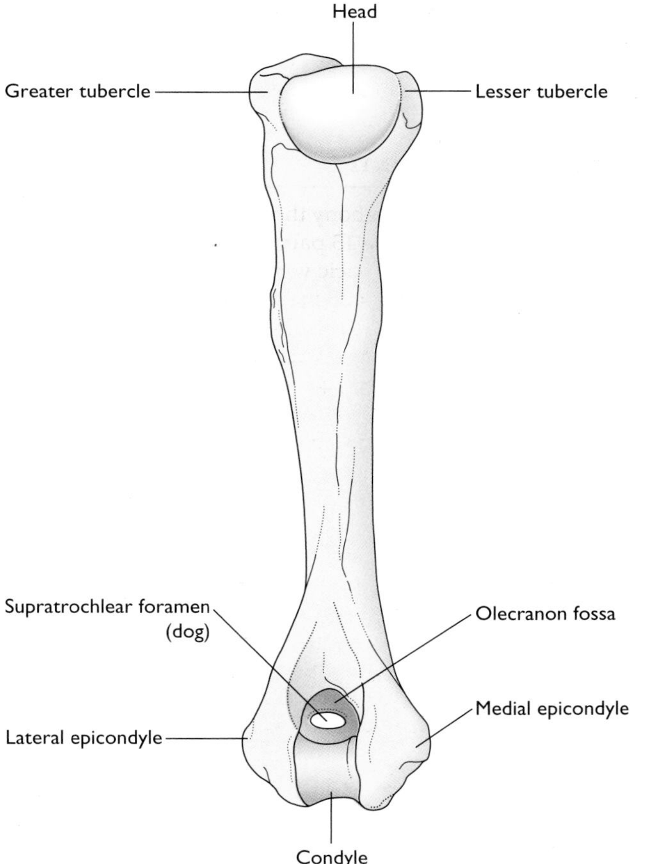

Fig. 3.15 The dog humerus. (Cats do not have a supratrochlear foramen.)

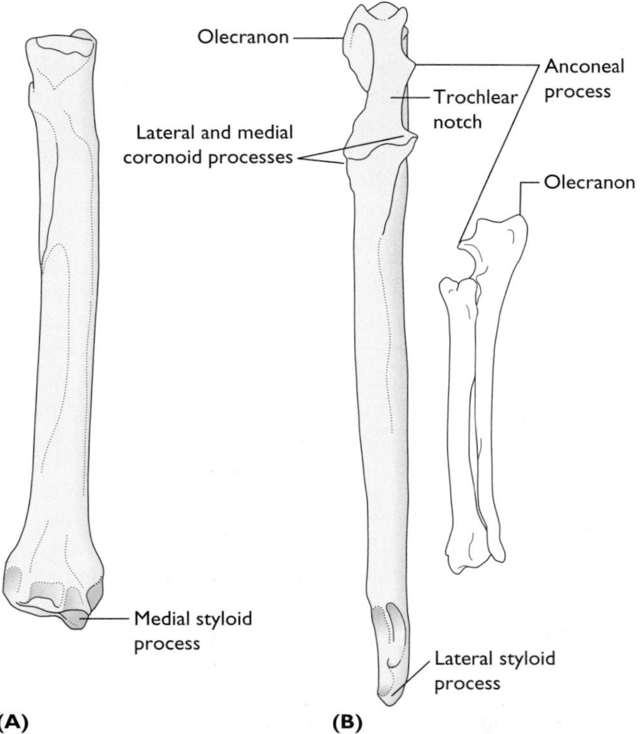

Fig. 3.16 **(A)** The dog radius. **(B)** The dog ulna (cranial and lateral views).

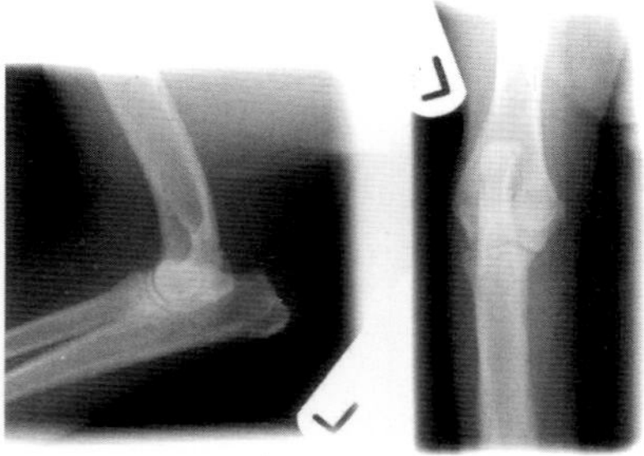

Fig. 3.17 Lateral and craniocaudal views of the canine elbow. (Courtesy of Panagiotis Mantis.)

concavity called the *trochlear notch*, which articulates with the distal humerus. At the top of the trochlear notch is a beak-like projection called the *anconeal process*, which sits within the olecranon fossa of the humerus when the elbow is extended. Distally, the ulna narrows to a point called the *lateral styloid process*. The *radius* is a rod-like bone, shorter than the ulna (Fig. 3.16). At the proximal end is a depression, the *fovea capitis*, which articulates with the humerus. At the distal end of the radius there is a pointed projection called the *medial styloid process*.

The shaft of the humerus has a slight twist on it and is known as the musculo-spiral groove. If the humerus is broken, the resulting fracture is often in the form of a spiral and may affect the radial nerve that runs within the spiral, causing temporary or permanent radial nerve paralysis. This is indicated by the animal 'knuckling' over on its lower forelimb (see Chapter 5).

Elbow dysplasia is a common condition of the heavier breeds of dog (e.g., Newfoundland, St Bernard, Rottweiler, Basset hound). It encompasses a number of developmental conditions, such as an ununited anconeal process and detached olecranon process, which result in instability of the elbow joint, leading to osteoarthritis. The disease can be inherited and there is a BVA/KC scheme to identify affected individuals and to help breeders select the most suitable dogs for breeding.

- *Carpus*: This is composed of seven short bones, the carpal bones, arranged in two rows (Fig. 3.18). The proximal row has three bones, the most medial being the *radial carpal bone*, which articulates proximally with the radius. The *ulnar carpal bone* articulates proximally with the ulna. The *accessory carpal bone* lies on the lateral edge and projects caudally. Distally, the first row of carpal bones articulates with the second row of four carpal bones. The carpal bones also articulate with each other within the row.
- *Metacarpus*: This is composed of five small long bones (Fig. 3.18). In the dog and cat the first metacarpal bone (I) – the most medial – is much smaller than the other metacarpal bones (II–V), and is non-weight bearing. This forms part of the *dew claw*. The metacarpals articulate proximally with the distal row of carpal bones and distally with the phalanges.
- *Digits*: These are composed of the *phalanges*, which are long bones (Fig. 3.18). Each digit has three phalanges, except digit I – the dew claw – which has only two. The proximal phalanx articulates with a metacarpal bone. The middle phalanx articulates with the phalanx above and below it. The distal phalanx ends in the *ungual process*, which forms part of the *claw*.
- There are pairs of small *sesamoid bones* behind the metacarpophalangeal joints and the distal joints between the phalangeal bones.

A common injury of racing greyhounds is stress fracture of the metacarpal and metatarsal bones, due to the strenuous forces of running at speed around a circular track. Fractures most frequently occur to the right central tarsal bone from running round an anticlockwise track. Sadly, owners are often reluctant to pay for treatment, and in addition the dog is unable to race while the bone is healing, so individuals are often put down.

Bones of the hind limb

The bones of the hind limb (Fig. 3.1) are:

- *Pelvis*: This is the means by which the hind limb connects to the body (Fig. 3.19). It consists of two hip bones or *ossa coxarum*, which join together at the *pubic symphysis*. They form a firm articulation with the sacrum at the *sacroiliac joint*. Each hip bone is formed from three bones – the *ischium, ilium* and *pubis* – grouped around one very small bone called the *acetabular bone*. The largest of these bones is the ilium, which has a broad cranial expansion called the *wing*. The ischium has a prominent caudal projection called the *ischial tuberosity*. The ilium, ischium and pubis meet each other at the *acetabulum*, which is the articular socket in which the head of the femur sits, forming the hip joint. The hip joint is a ball-and-socket joint.

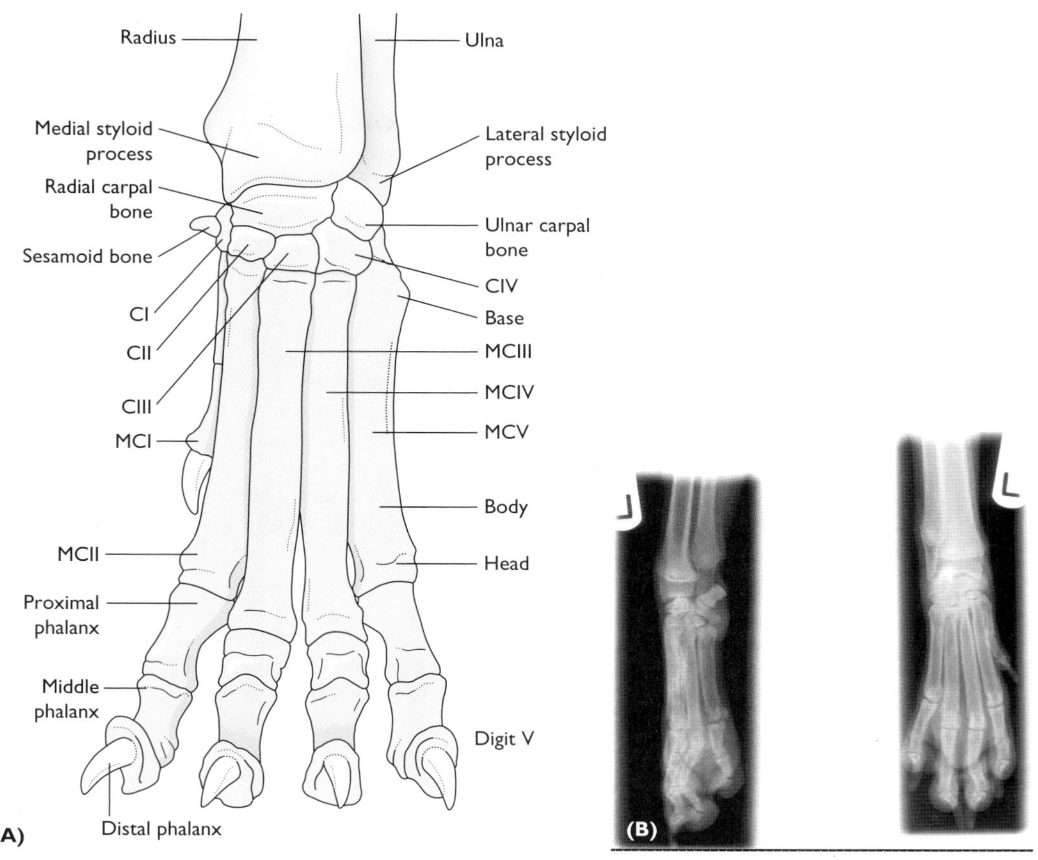

Fig. 3.18 (A) Bones of the distal forelimb in the dog. CI, CII, etc. = carpal bones 1, 2, etc. MC, metacarpal bones. Metacarpal bone 1 is the dew claw. **(B)** Lateral and dorsopalmar views of the canine carpus and distal forelimb. (Courtesy of Panagiotis Mantis.)

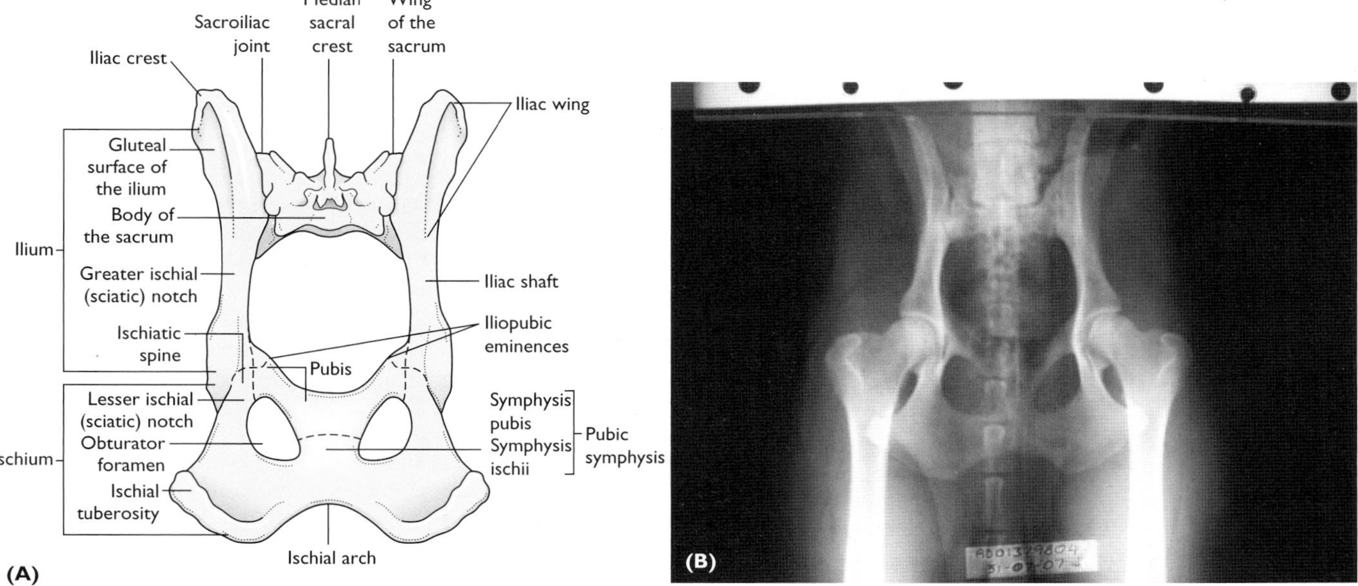

Fig. 3.19 (A) Bones and bony features of the dog pelvis. **(B)** Ventrodorsal view of the canine pelvis. (Courtesy of Richard Aspinall.)

Hip dysplasia is an inherited condition that affects a range of larger breeds of dog (e.g., Labradors, Retrievers, German Shepherds). It is caused by malformation of the femoral head and/or a shallow or malformed acetabulum, resulting in subluxation of the hip joint leading to osteoarthritis. There is a BVA/KC scheme to help identify affected dogs and to advise breeders on the choice of breeding stock.

- The head of the femur is held in place by a ligament known as the *teres* or *round ligament*, which attaches to a non-articular area within the joint cavity called the *acetabular fossa*. On either side of the pubic symphysis is a large hole called the *obturator foramen* that serves to reduce the weight of the pelvic girdle and to provide extra surface area for the attachment of muscles and ligaments.
- *Femur*: This is a long bone that forms the thigh (Fig. 3.20). On the proximal femur the articular head faces medially to articulate with the acetabulum of the pelvis. The head is joined to the shaft by a *neck*. Lateral to the head is a projection called the *greater trochanter* and on the medial side is another smaller projection called the *lesser trochanter*. Both of these are sites for muscle attachment. The femur has a strong shaft and on its distal extremity it has two caudally projecting *condyles*: the *medial condyle* and the *lateral condyle*, which articulate with the tibia at the *stifle joint* (Fig. 3.21). The *patella* runs between these condyles in the *trochlea groove*.

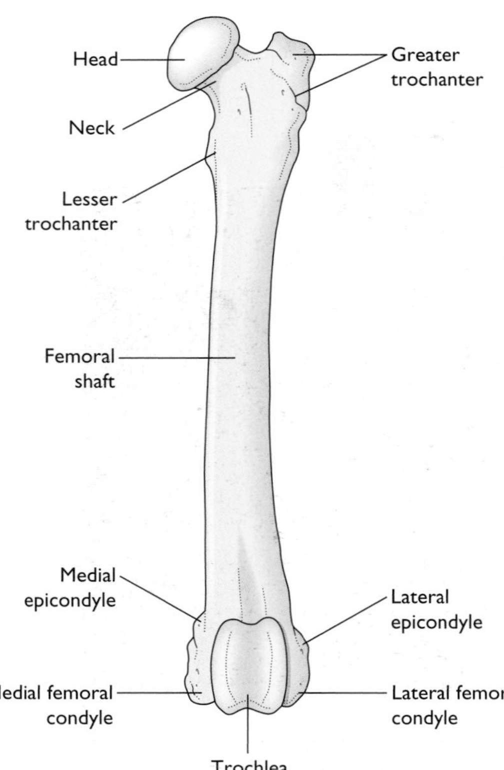

Fig. 3.20 The dog femur.

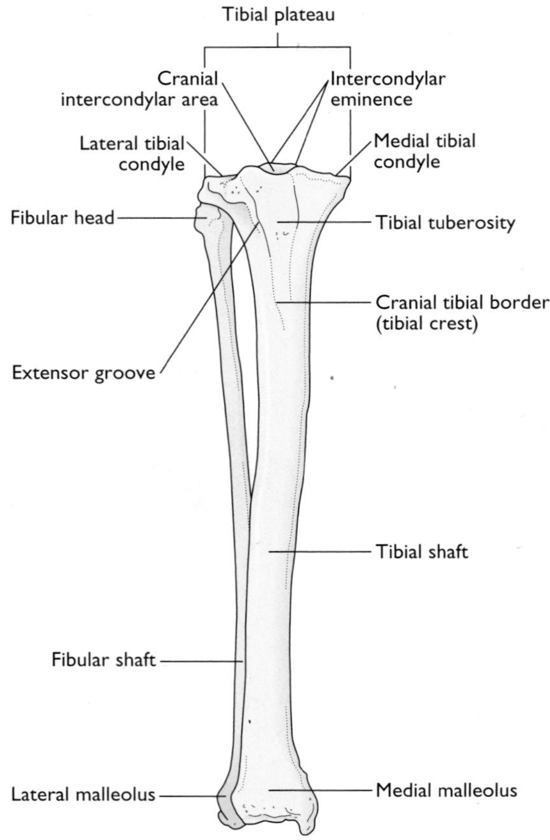

Fig. 3.21 Lateral view of the canine stifle joint.

Legg-Calve-Perthes Disease is a disease seen in small dogs, such as West Highland Terriers, Yorkshire Terriers and Jack Russells, that presents as a lameness of the hip joint. It is not fully understood what causes this condition but it affects young dogs and begins with the interruption of the blood supply to the head of the femur, which results in the disintegration of the femoral head.

- *Patella*: This sesamoid bone is found within the tendon of insertion of the *quadriceps femoris* muscle, which is the main extensor of the stifle (see Chapter 4 and Fig. 3.21). Two more sesamoid bones, called the *fabellae*, are found behind the stifle in the origin of the *gastrocnemius* muscle. They articulate with the condyles of the femur.
- *Tibia and fibula*: These long bones form the lower leg (Fig. 3.22). The tibia and fibula lie parallel to each other; the more medial bone, the tibia, is the much larger of the two. The tibia is expanded proximally where it articulates with the femur. On the dorsal surface there is a prominence called the *tibial crest* for attachment of the quadriceps femoris muscle. Distally, the tibia has a prominent protrusion, the *medial malleolus*, which can be palpated on the medial aspect of the hock. The fibula is a thin long bone lying laterally to the tibia. It ends in a bony point called the *lateral malleolus*.

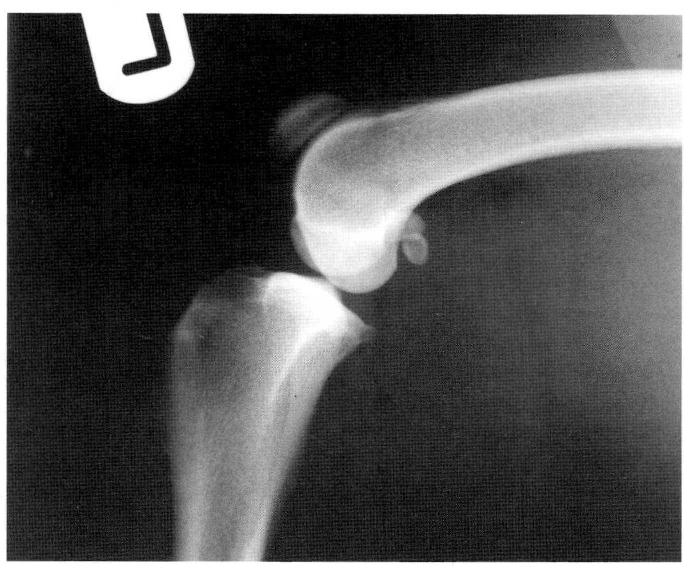

Fig. 3.22 The dog tibia and fibula. (Courtesy of Richard Aspinall.)

- *Tarsus*: This is formed from seven short bones, the *tarsal bones*, arranged in three rows (Fig. 3.23). The two bones forming the proximal row, the *talus* and *calcaneus*, articulate with the distal end of the tibia and fibula at the hock joint (Fig. 3.23; see also Fig. 3.25). The talus, or tibial tarsal bone, is the most medial and has a proximal trochlea, which is shaped to fit the end of the tibia. The calcaneus, or fibular tarsal bone, is positioned laterally and has a large caudal projection known as the *tuber calcis*, which forms the 'point' of the hock.

In some small breeds of dog (e.g., Yorkshire Terrier), the patella may slip out of place, causing extreme pain and difficulty in extending the stifle joint. This is an inherited condition and is due to malpositioning of the tibial crest or too shallow a trochlear groove on the distal end of the femur.

- *Metatarsus and digits*: These closely resemble the pattern of the metacarpus and digits in the forepaw. The metatarsus is composed of four metatarsal bones, although some breeds possess five, having a small metatarsal I or hind dew claw (Fig. 3.23).

Splanchnic skeleton

This is composed of the splanchnic bones. A splanchnic bone is a bone that develops in soft tissue and is unattached to the rest of the skeleton. The only example of a splanchnic bone in the dog and cat is the bone of the penis, the *os penis*. The urethra lies in the *urethral groove*, on the ventral surface of the os penis in the dog. In the cat the urethral groove is on the dorsal surface of the os penis, because of the different orientation of the penis (see Chapter 11).

The cow has a splanchnic bone in its heart, called the *os cordis*, while birds have splanchnic bones forming a rim around the eye to provide strength to the large eyeball (see Chapters 13 and 17).

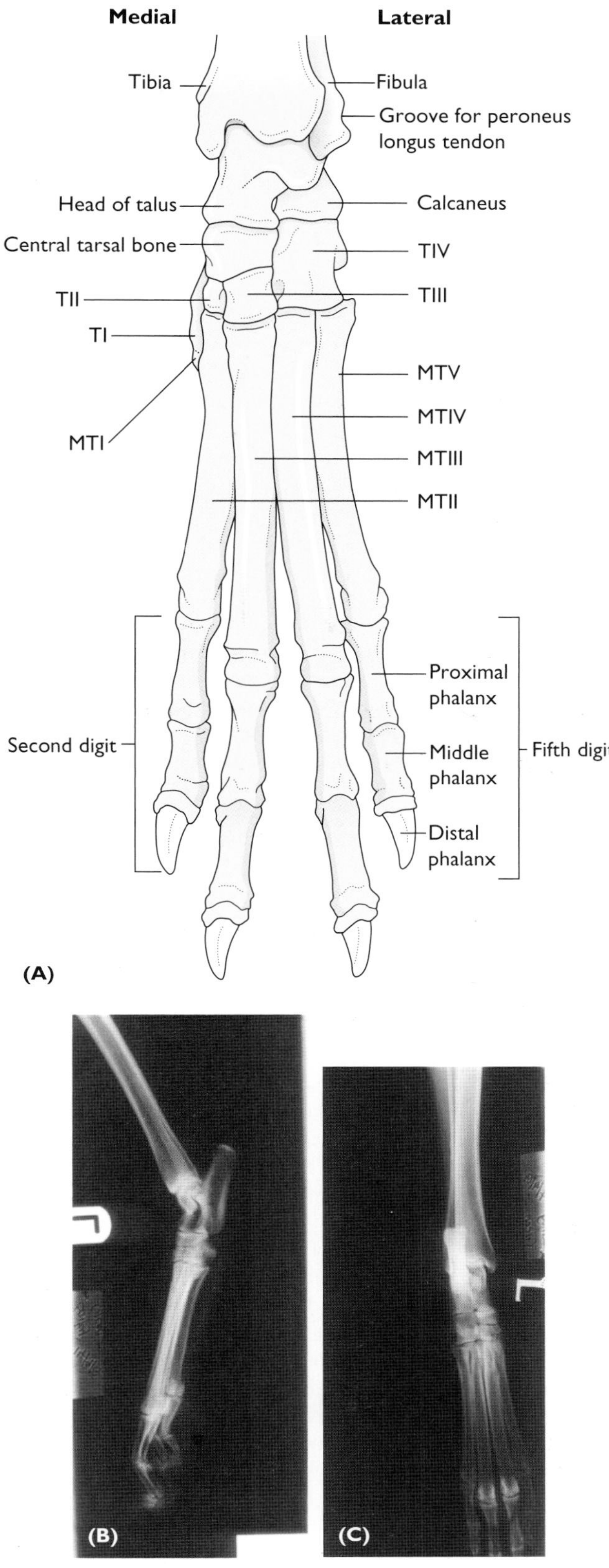

Fig. 3.23 **(A)** The dog tarsus or hindpaw. TI, TII, etc. = tarsal bones 1, 2, etc. MT, metatarsal bones. **(B)** Lateral and **(C)** dorsoplantar views of the canine tarsus and distal hind limb. (Courtesy of Panagiotis Mantis.)

Joints

When one bone connects to another they form an articulation, also known as an arthrosis or *joint*. Joints allow variable degrees of movement and can be categorised into one of three groups:

- Fibrous joints
- Cartilaginous joints
- Synovial joints

Fibrous joints

Fibrous joints are immovable joints and the bones forming them are united by dense fibrous connective tissue, e.g., in the skull fibrous joints unite the majority of the component bones and are called *sutures*. The teeth are attached to the bony sockets in the jaw bone by fibrous joints.

Fibrous joints are also classed as *synarthroses*, meaning a type of joint that permits little or no movement. Some cartilaginous joints also fall into this category.

Cartilaginous joints

Cartilaginous joints allow limited movement or no movement at all and are united by cartilage, such as the *pubic symphysis* connecting the two hip bones and the *mandibular symphysis* joining the two halves of the mandible. Both these joints are also classed as *synarthroses*.

Some cartilaginous joint may also be classed as *amphiarthroses*, which allow some degree of movement between the bones, such as between the bodies of the vertebrae, allowing for limited flexibility of the spinal column.

Synovial joints

Synovial joints, or *diarthroses*, allow a wide range of movement. In synovial joints, the bones are separated by a space filled with synovial fluid known as the *joint cavity* (Fig. 3.24). A joint capsule surrounds the whole joint; the outer layer consists of fibrous tissue, which serves as protection, and the joint cavity is lined by the *synovial membrane*, which secretes *synovial fluid*. This lubricates the joint and provides nutrition for the hyaline articular cartilage covering the ends of the bone. Synovial fluid is a straw-coloured viscous fluid that may be present in quite large quantities in large joints, especially in animals that have a lot of exercise.

Some synovial joints may have additional stabilisation from thickened *ligaments* within the fibres of the joint capsule. These are most commonly found on either side of the joint, where they are called *collateral ligaments*. However, other synovial joints have stabilising ligaments attached to the articulating bones within the joint. These are known as *intracapsular ligaments* and examples include the cruciate ligaments within the stifle joint (Fig. 3.25).

A few synovial joints possess one or more intra-articular fibrocartilaginous *discs* or *menisci* within the joint cavity. These are found in the stifle joint, which has two crescent-shaped menisci, and in the temporomandibular joint between the mandible and the skull. These structures help to increase the range of movement of the joint and act as 'shock absorbers', reducing wear and tear.

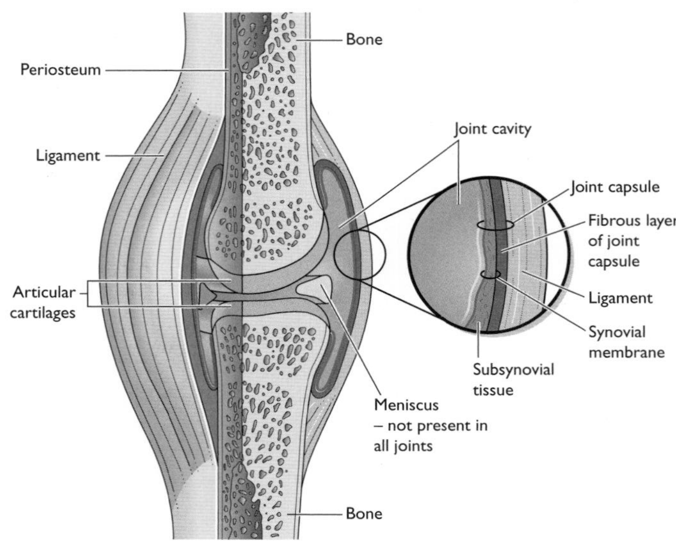

Fig. 3.24 Structure of a typical synovial joint.

Ruptured cruciate ligament. The two cruciate ligaments provide stability to the stifle joint. In large- and medium-breed dogs this ligament may rupture as a result of severe joint torsion during exercise, causing joint instability and lameness. The cranial cruciate ligament is the most commonly affected, and surgical intervention to stabilise the stifle joint is often required to resolve the problem. If the ligament is not repaired, the resulting joint laxity may lead to osteoarthritis.

Synovial joints allow considerable freedom of movement between the articulating bones, the extent of which depends upon the type of synovial joint. The movement allowed by a synovial joint may be in a single plane only, or in multiple planes.

The range of movements that are possible in synovial joints is:

- *Flexion/extension*: These are antagonistic movements of a joint.
  - Flexion *reduces* the angle between two bones (i.e., bends the limb).
  - Extension *increases* the angle between two bones (i.e., straightens the limb).
- *Abduction/adduction*: These movements affect the whole limb.
  - Abduction (meaning to 'take away') moves a body part *away* from the median plane or axis (e.g., moving the leg out sideways).
  - Adduction moves a body part back *towards* the central line or axis of the body (e.g., moving the leg back to standing position).
- *Rotation*: The moving body part 'twists' on its own axis, meaning that it rotates either inwardly or outwardly
- *Circumduction*: The movement of an extremity (i.e., one end of a bone) in a circular pattern
- *Gliding/sliding*: The articular surfaces of the joint slide over one another.
- *Protraction*: The animal moves its limb cranially, meaning advances the limb forward, as when walking.
- *Retraction*: The animal moves the limb back towards the body.

Synovial joints can be further classified into subcategories based upon the types of movement that they allow (Table 3.1).

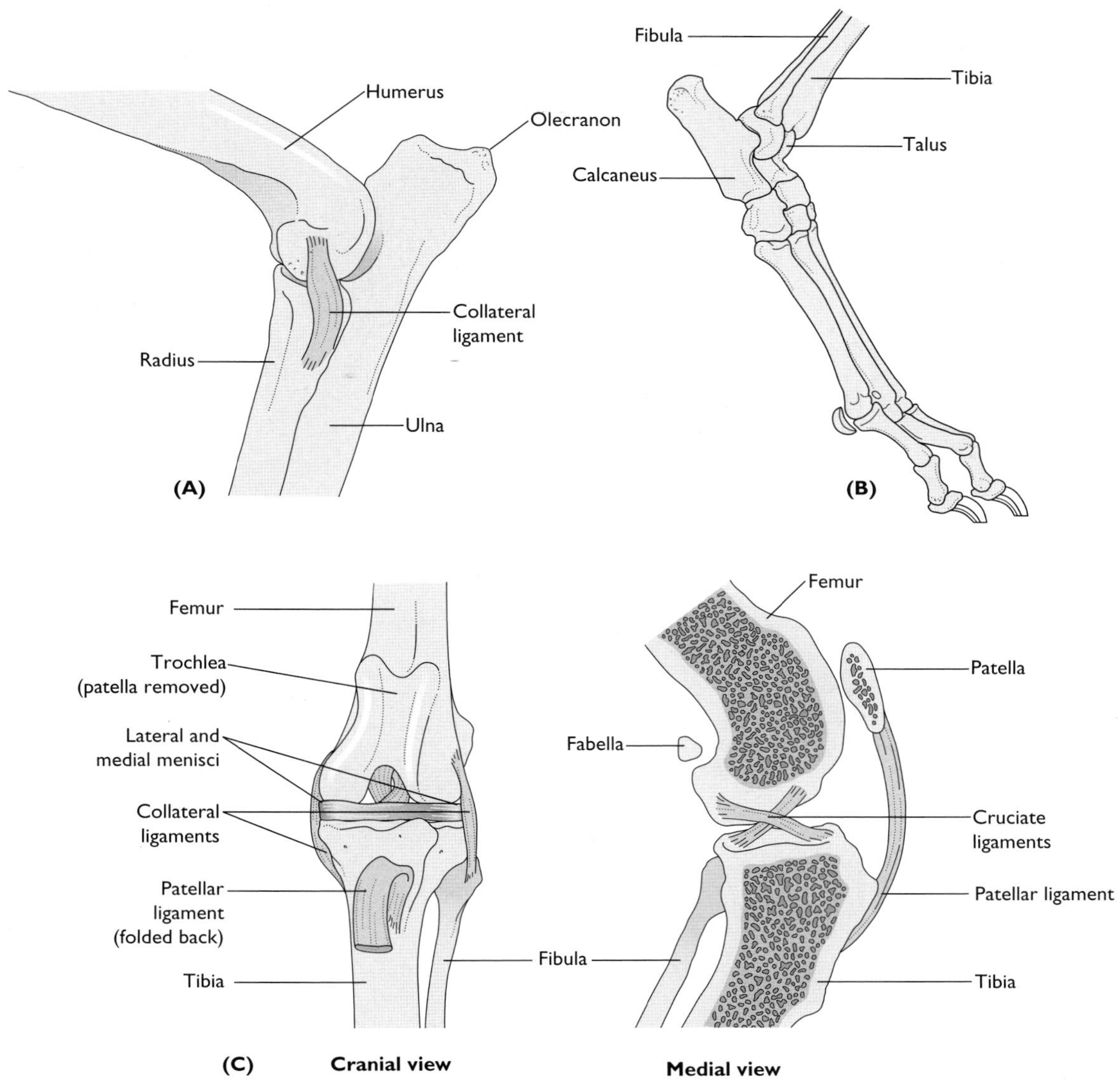

Fig. 3.25 **(A)** The elbow joint, lateral view. **(B)** The tarsus or hock joint, lateral view. **(C)** The stifle joint, cranial and medial views.

Table 3.1 Properties of different synovial joint types

Type of synovial joint	Description	Example of joint
Plane/gliding	Allows sliding of one bony surface over the other	Joints between the rows of carpal and tarsal bones
Hinge	Allows movement in one plane only (i.e., flexion and extension)	Elbow; stifle
Pivot	Consists of a peg sitting within a ring; allows rotation	Atlantoaxial joint (between C1 and C2)
Condylar	Consists of a convex surface (condyles) that sits in a corresponding concave surface; allows movement in two planes (flexion, extension and overextension)	Hock or (tarsus)
Ball and socket	Consists of a rounded end or ball, sitting within a socket or cup; allows a great range of movement	Hip; shoulder

CHAPTER 4

Muscular system

KEY POINTS

- The muscular system comprises striated or skeletal muscle, which is muscle attached to the skeleton that brings about movement of a region.
- Each striated muscle fibre is filled with myofibrils made of two contractile proteins, actin and myosin. At the cellular level, muscle contraction results from the formation of cross-bridges between the actin and myosin molecules.
- Muscle fibres are stimulated to contract by nerve impulses carried by nerve fibres. The number of muscle fibres supplied by a single nerve fibre is called a motor unit. In muscles that perform accurate and delicate movements, a nerve fibre will supply a few muscle fibres, but in muscles that perform less accurate movements a nerve fibre will supply many muscle fibres.
- Muscle tissue is always under a degree of tension, known as muscle tone. The tone increases when an animal is alert or frightened and decreases when it is relaxed or asleep.
- All muscles consist of a central belly and, at the point of attachment to a bone, an origin (often called the head), and an insertion.
- Skeletal muscles may be either:
- Extrinsic muscles are attached from one major structure, such as the trunk, to another structure, such as a limb. These muscles bring about movement of the *whole* limb in relation to other body parts.
- Intrinsic muscles are attached at both ends within the one structure, such as a limb. These muscles bring about movement *within* the individual limb (e.g., bending an elbow).
- Each area has a range of specialised muscles designed to bring about the specific types of movement necessary for the animal's normal function.

The muscular system includes all the skeletal or striated muscles within the body. Striated muscle is that tissue attached to the skeleton that is under voluntary or conscious control (for microscopic structure see Chapter 2).

Muscle structure and function

Contraction

Muscle is stimulated to contract when it receives a nerve impulse from the central nervous system. Each striated muscle fibre is composed of myofibrils made of thin *actin* filaments and thick *myosin* filaments. These fibres overlap in such a way that under the microscope muscle has the appearance of alternating light and dark bands or striations. These bands are separated into units called *sarcomeres*, which are the units of contraction.

During contraction, the actin and myosin filaments slide over one another and cross-bridges form between the heads of the myosin filaments and the heads of the actin filaments. The cross-bridges swing through an arc, pulling the thin filaments past the thick ones, and the sarcomere shortens. Once this movement is completed the cross-bridge detaches itself from the thin filament and reattaches itself further away – in other words, the cross-bridges between the myosin and actin filaments act as a ratchet mechanism, thus shortening the muscle (Fig. 4.1). This process requires energy input, which is provided by adenosine triphosphate molecules; calcium ions are also essential to the process of muscle contraction.

The nerve that stimulates the muscle to contract enters the muscle and then splits up into many fibres to innervate the bundles of muscle fibres. The number of muscle fibres supplied by one nerve fibre will vary depending on the type of movement for which the muscle is responsible. If it is a delicate movement then a nerve fibre may only innervate a small number of muscle fibres. However, in larger movements, such as those made by the muscles of the limbs, one nerve fibre may supply 200 or more muscle fibres. A single nerve together with the muscle fibres that it supplies is called a *motor unit.* The junction between the nerve fibre and the muscle is called the neuromuscular junction and a chemical called acetyl choline transmits the impulse across this gap.

Myasthenia gravis is an immune mediated disease that affects the acetyl choline receptors of the neuromuscular junction. This causes severe muscle weakness, which leads to symptoms that include exercise intolerance, regurgitation and drooling.

Muscle tone

Many of the skeletal muscles in the body are always in a slight state of tension, known as *muscle tone.* Even when an animal is at rest, muscles, such as those responsible for maintaining posture, will not be truly relaxed. Muscle tone is achieved by a proportion of the motor units within the muscle being activated so that some of the muscle fibres are contracting while others are relaxed. The nervous system can adjust this, and the number of motor units stimulated will increase when the animal is in an anxious state; in other words, the muscles become 'twitchy' or 'jumpy'. Thus, muscles undergo two types of contraction:

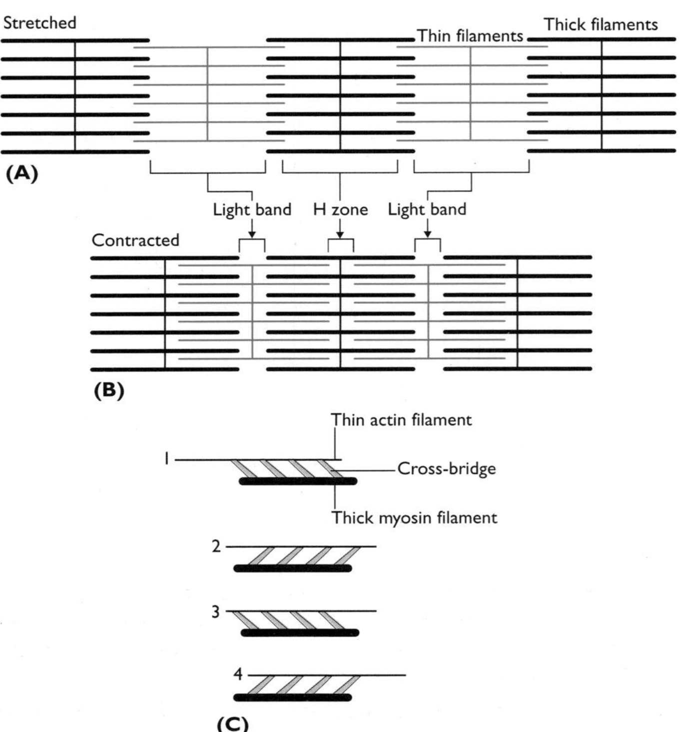

Fig. 4.1 The 'ratchet mechanism' involving actin and myosin within striated muscle fibres. **(A)** Muscle before contraction (shortening). **(B)** When the muscle shortens, the thick and thin filaments slide in between one another. The dark bands remain the same width in the shortened (contracted) muscle but the light bands and 'H zones' get narrower. **(C)** Close-up view of the 'ratchet mechanism', showing cross-bridges between the thin actin and thick myosin filaments.

- *Isometric* contraction happens when tension is generated in the muscle – muscle tone is increased, but the muscle does not shorten
- In *isotonic* contraction, the muscle actually moves or shortens.

The more a muscle is used or exercised, the larger it will become – it is said to be *hypertrophied.* However, if a muscle is not used for some reason (e.g., due to injury or illness when the animal may be recumbent, or if a limb is in a cast), it will wither or shrink in size; it is said to be *atrophied.*

Muscle atrophy or wasting may be the result of many factors, such as lack of use as a result of lameness, fracture, denervation (injury to the nerve that supplies it) or a generalised disease condition, such as neoplasia. Muscle enlargement or hypertrophy may result from overexercise or overuse. This may be seen where a patient has fractured a limb and the muscles in the other limb must work harder to support it.

Anatomy of a muscle

A 'classically' shaped muscle (Fig. 4.2) has a thick, fleshy central part called the *belly* and tapers at each end – the *head.* Here, the connective tissue muscle sheath is continuous with the dense fibrous connective tissue of the tendon that attaches the muscle to a bone. A muscle is attached to a bone at two points: its starting point is called its *origin;* this moves least during contraction.

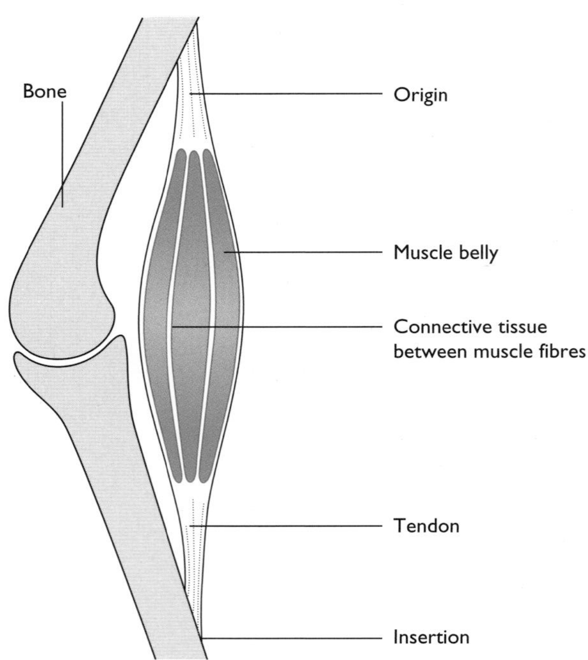

Fig. 4.2 Basic structure of a muscle. The connective tissue between the muscle fibres is continuous with that of the tendon.

The opposite end, where the muscle inserts on the bone, is called the *insertion.* However, a muscle can have more than one belly, all inserting at one point, in which case the muscle is said to have a number of heads (e.g., the biceps muscle has two heads). The length of the tendon attaching the muscle to a bone will vary, and in some cases tendons are far longer than the muscle itself (e.g., flexor and extensor tendons running over the digits).

Not all muscles take the 'classical' shape described above. Sometimes they are present in flat sheets, in which case the tendon is also drawn out into a flat sheet of connective tissue – this type of arrangement is called an *aponeurosis* (e.g., the muscles of the abdominal wall). Some muscles form a circular ring and serve to control the entrance or exit to a structure (e.g., the stomach and the bladder). These are called *sphincter muscles.*

A *bursa* is a connective tissue sac lined with synovial membrane and filled with synovial fluid. These typically develop between a bony prominence and a tendon, ligament or muscle and their function is to reduce friction between the associated structure and the bone. Sometimes a bursa completely wraps around a tendon forming a *synovial* or *tendon sheath* (Fig. 4.3).

The skeletal muscles of the body can be classed as either intrinsic or extrinsic:

- *Intrinsic muscles* lie completely within one region of the body where they have their origin and insertion. They act on the joints in that part only; for example, when a dog bends its elbow it is using the intrinsic muscles of the forelimb.
- *Extrinsic muscles* run from one region of the body to another and alter the position of the whole part (e.g., a limb) in relation to the other. The muscles that attach the foreleg of the dog to the trunk are extrinsic muscles; they move the whole foreleg in relation to the trunk.

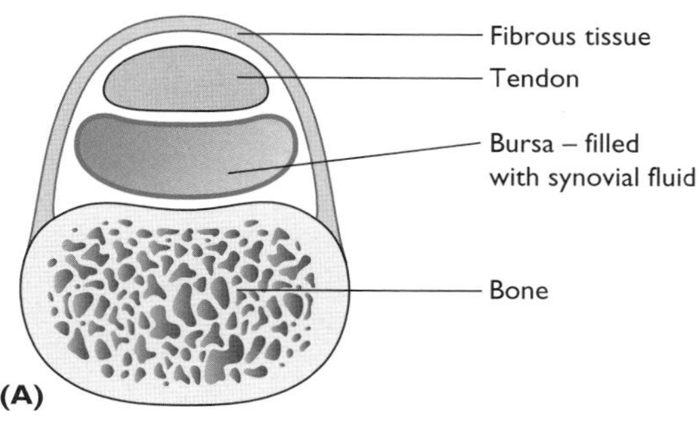

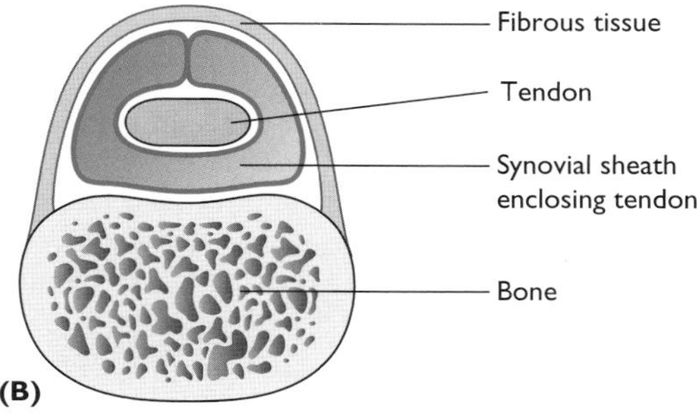

Fig. 4.3 **(A)** Structure of a bursa. **(B)** Structure of a synovial sheath.

The skeletal muscles

To simplify the study of these muscles we can look at one area of the body at a time.

Muscles of the head

Muscles of facial expression

The muscles of facial expression are intrinsic muscles that move the lips, cheeks, nostrils, eyelids and external ears. A number of muscles are responsible for these movements, all of which are **innervated by the *facial nerve* (cranial nerve VII).**

Paralysis of the facial nerve will cause a drooping of the ear, lip and eyelid, inability to blink (palpebral reflex) and drooling. This is most commonly seen on one side of the face only, which gives an asymmetric appearance to the face. The nerve could be damaged by the edge of a door slamming on the dog's face or even by the dog hanging its head out of the car window when it is driving along.

Muscles of mastication

The main muscles responsible for the masticatory or 'chewing' action of the jaw (Fig. 4.4) are:

- *Digastricus:* This muscle opens the jaw, aided by gravity, and is located on the caudoventral surface of the mandible. Its origin is the jugular process of the occipital bone and it inserts on the angle and ventral surface of the mandible
- *Masseter:* This muscle closes the jaw and lies lateral to the mandible. It originates from the zygomatic arch and inserts on the masseteric fossa on the lateral surface of the mandible
- *Temporalis:* This muscle also closes the jaw and is the largest and strongest muscle of the head. It covers much of the dorsal and lateral surfaces of the skull. It fills the temporal fossa of the skull and inserts on the coronoid process of the mandible

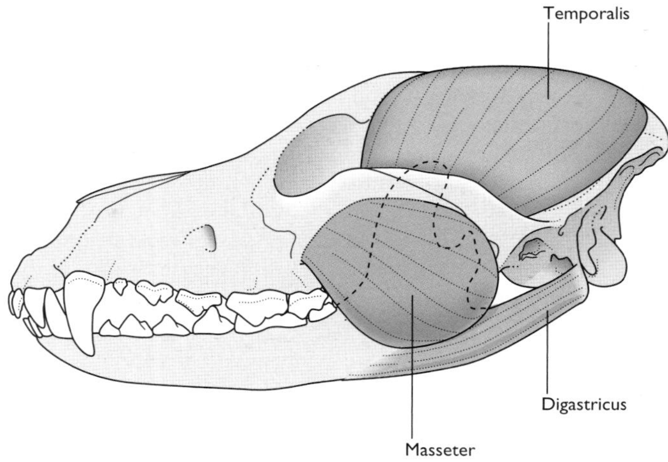

Fig. 4.4 The muscles of mastication.

- *Medial and lateral pterygoids:* These are deep muscles that lie medial to the mandible. They aid the temporalis and masseter muscles in closing the jaw, but they are also responsible for the side to side movements of the mouth.

The tone in the muscles of the jaw responsible for closure – the temporalis and the masseter – is what keeps the mouth closed when it is not in use.

Muscles of the eye

The extrinsic muscles of the eye (Fig. 4.5), also called the *extra-ocular* muscles, are responsible for moving the eye within its bony socket. These muscles are:

- Four *RECTUS* muscles: *dorsal rectus, ventral rectus, medial rectus, lateral rectus.* These four muscles all insert on the *sclera* of the eyeball near the 'equator', at the surface that corresponds to

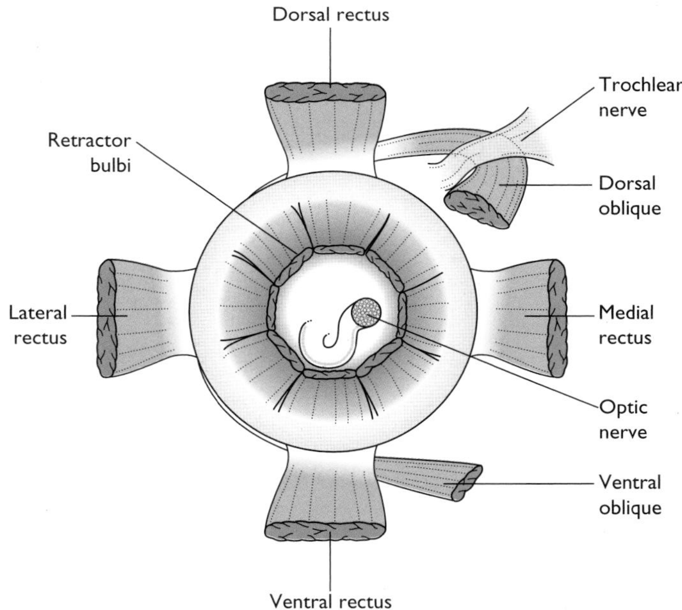

Fig. 4.5 The positions of the extraocular muscles, viewed from behind the eyeball.

their name (i.e., the dorsal rectus muscle inserts on the upper part of the sclera). Their name also reflects their action: the dorsal rectus muscle turns the eye upward; the ventral rectus turns the eye downward; the medial rectus turns the eye inward; the lateral muscle turns the eye outward
- Two *OBLIQUE* muscles: *dorsal oblique* and *ventral oblique*. These two muscles are positioned as their name describes and they act to rotate the eye about its visual axis
- *Retractor bulbi:* This muscle forms a muscular cone around the optic nerve at the back of the eye and its action is to pull the eye deeper into the socket.

Other muscles of the head include:

- Intrinsic and extrinsic muscles in the tongue enable the tongue to carry out a wide range of delicate movements.
- Many muscles are found in the pharynx, larynx and soft palate, which enable these structures to carry out their specific functions (e.g., swallowing and sound production).
- Extrinsic muscles attach the head to the neck and move it in relation to the neck.

Muscles of the trunk

Muscles of the vertebral column

Groups of muscles lie above and below the vertebral column (Fig. 4.6). These are:

- *Epaxial muscles* lie dorsal to the transverse processes of the vertebrae (above the vertebral column). The epaxial muscles are numerous and are arranged in three longitudinal groups, which together span the length of the vertebral column. Their functions are to support the spine, extend the vertebral column and allow lateral flexion
- *Hypaxial muscles* lie ventral to the transverse processes of the vertebrae (below the vertebral column). One region is associated with the neck, another with the back. The hypaxial muscles flex the neck and tail, and contribute to flexion of the vertebral column.

Intramuscular injections. The epaxial muscles are a common site for giving intramuscular injections, because they are easily accessible and not associated with any vital nerves. Other muscles include the quadriceps femoris, the biceps femoris and the gluteals.

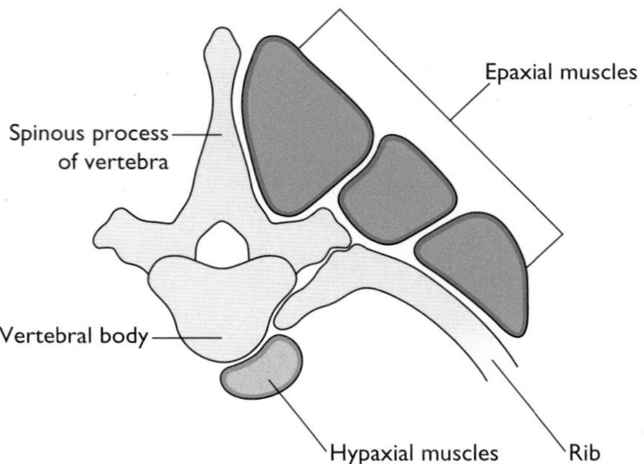

Fig. 4.6 The positions of the muscles around the vertebral column.

Muscles of the thorax

The muscles of the thoracic wall are mostly involved in respiration. The main muscles are:

- *External intercostals* are the most superficial, originating from the caudal border of one rib and insert on the cranial border of the rib behind it. Thus, each muscle is confined to one intercostal space. These muscles assist in inspiration.
- *Internal intercostals* lie below the external intercostals within the intercostal spaces and originate from the cranial surface of one rib and insert on the caudal border of the rib in front of it. These muscles assist in expiration, which is a largely passive movement.

The diaphragm

The diaphragm is the sheet of muscle that separates the thoracic and abdominal cavities (Fig. 4.7). It consists of a *central tendon* and a *muscular periphery* that arises from the lumbar vertebrae, caudal ribs and sternum. The lumbar portion of the muscle consists of thickened muscular bundles called the right and left *crura* (singular: crus).

The diaphragm is the main muscle of *inspiration.* When it contracts, the lungs expand and draw in air (see Chapter 8). In the centre of the diaphragm there are three openings that allow through structures that pass from the thoracic region into the abdomen. These openings are:

- *Aortic hiatus* transmits the aorta, azygous vein and thoracic duct.
- *Oesophageal hiatus* transmits the oesophagus and vagal nerve trunks.
- *Caval foramen* lies within the central tendon and transmits the caudal vena cava.

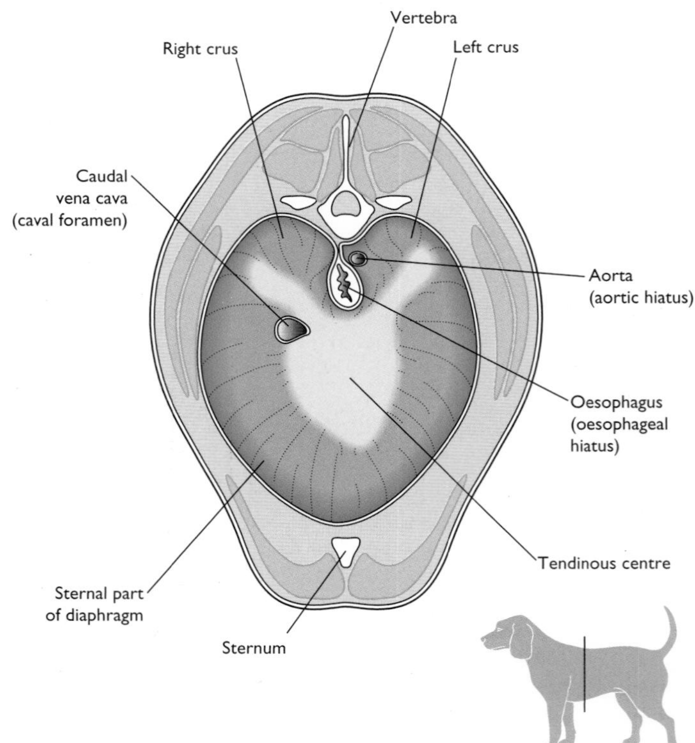

Fig. 4.7 Structure of the diaphragm, viewed from abdominal side.

Ruptured diaphragm or diaphragmatic hernia. A sudden change in pressure in the abdominal cavity (e.g., due to trauma from a road accident) could cause rupture of the diaphragm and migration of the abdominal organs into the thoracic cavity. This presents as sudden dyspnoea or difficulty in breathing, which can be life threatening if untreated.

Abdominal muscles

The abdominal wall on each side of the body is composed of four muscles, which form broad, flat sheets (Fig. 4.8). Their fibres run in all directions, which gives the abdominal wall great strength. Their function is to protect the organs and structures of the abdomen. The muscles of the abdominal wall are:

- *External abdominal oblique* is the most superficial of the lateral abdominal muscles. It originates from the lateral surfaces of the ribs and lumbar fascia and terminates in a wide aponeurosis in the midline known as the *linea alba.*
- *Internal abdominal oblique* is the intermediate muscle of the lateral abdominal wall, which also terminates in an aponeurosis on the linea alba.
- *Transversus abdominis* is the deepest of the lateral abdominal muscles, which also terminates in an aponeurosis on the linea alba.
- *Rectus abdominis* is a broad band of muscle on each side of the linea alba that forms the floor of the abdomen. The rectus abdominis originates on the first rib and sternum and inserts on the pubis by means of the *prepubic tendon.*

The linea alba, or white line, is the combined aponeuroses of the three lateral abdominal muscles. It extends along the ventral midline from the xiphoid process of the sternum to the pubic symphysis.

The linea alba can easily be seen when a vet makes a midline incision in the abdomen (e.g., during a bitch spay or any type of laparotomy). Because it is tough, it provides a good tissue in which to place sutures without the risk of them pulling out.

The *inguinal ring* is a slit-like opening in the aponeurosis of the external abdominal oblique muscle, in the region of the groin. This allows the passage of blood vessels from the abdomen to the external genitalia and mammary glands, and transmits the structures of the spermatic cord to the scrotum.

Inguinal hernia. This results from the passage of structures such as a loop of intestine or a pad of fat through the inguinal ring into the scrotum. There is always a risk that these structures can twist and the hernia then becomes *strangulated.* There is also an inguinal ring in female animals and there have been cases in which a loop of uterus has passed through.

Muscles of the forelimb

The muscles of the forelimb can be divided into extrinsic and intrinsic muscles.

Extrinsic group

The extrinsic muscles of the forelimb (Fig. 4.9) attach the forelimb to the trunk forming a *synsarcosis* (the attachment of a structure to the skeleton by muscles instead of the more conventional joint).

- *Trapezius* is a triangular sheet of muscle that originates from the dorsal midline from C2 to C7 and inserts on the spine of the scapula.

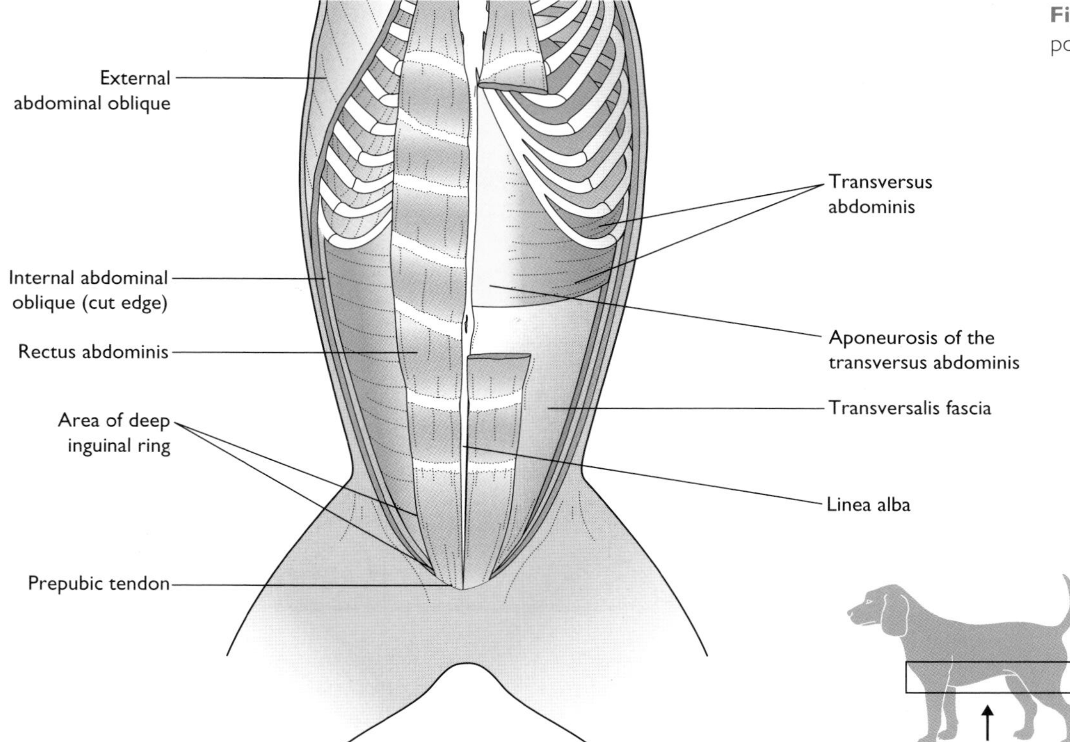

Fig. 4.8 The abdominal muscles and position of the linea alba.

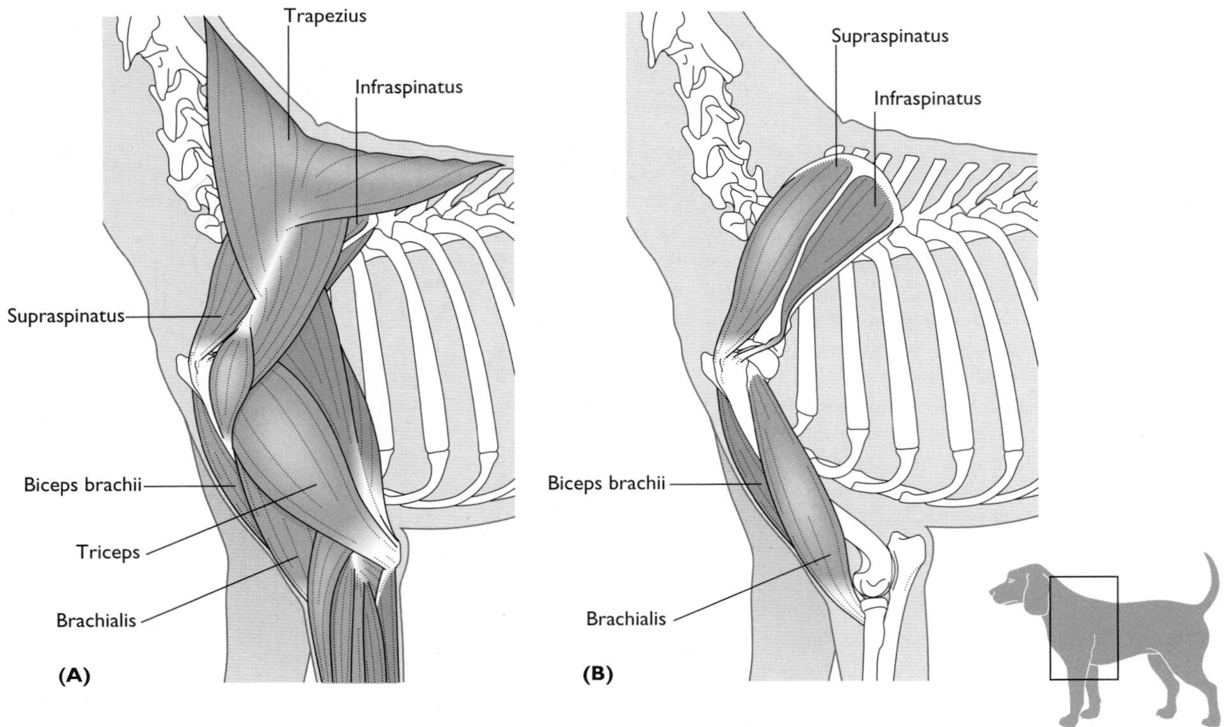

Fig. 4.9 Muscles of the upper forelimb. **(A)** Superficial muscles. **(B)** Deep muscles.

Action: draws the leg forward and protracts the limb

- *Pectoral* muscles run from the ribs and sternum and insert on the humerus.
  Action: adduct the limb and hold the forelimb against the body wall
- *Latissimus dorsi* is a large, fan-shaped muscle, which has a very broad origin on the thoracic spine and inserts on the humerus.
  Action: retracts the forelimb
- *Brachiocephalicus* muscle runs from the base of the skull to an insertion on the cranial aspect of the humerus.
  Action: when the limb is on the ground, it flexes the neck and bends the neck laterally; when the limb is not taking weight, it draws the foreleg forwards or protracts the limb.

Intrinsic group

The intrinsic muscles of the forelimb all originate and insert on the forelimb. They include:

- *Supraspinatus* arises from and fills the supraspinous fossa of the scapula and inserts on the greater tubercle of the humerus.
  Action: extends the shoulder and stabilises the shoulder joint
- *Infraspinatus* arises from and fills the infraspinous fossa of the scapula and inserts on the greater tubercle of the humerus.
  Action: helps to stabilise the shoulder joint and flexes the shoulder joint

Elbow region (*Fig. 4.10*)

- *Triceps brachii* muscle has four heads with separate origins. Three of the heads originate from the proximal humerus and the fourth head originates from the scapula. However, they all share a common insertion on the olecranon of the ulna. A bursa lies between the bone and the tendon to prevent friction.
  Action: extends the elbow joint
- *Biceps brachii* originates from the supraglenoid tubercle of the scapula and inserts on the radius and ulna.
  Action flexes the elbow joint
- *Brachialis* muscle originates from the humerus and inserts on the radius and ulna.
  Action: flexes the elbow joint

Carpus and digits

There are many muscles responsible for flexing and extending the carpus and the digits. The muscle bellies are grouped around the radius and ulna and communicate with the digits by means of long tendons.

The main flexors and extensors are:

- *Two carpal extensors* originate from the humerus and insert on the carpals; they run in front of the lower limb and foot.
- *Two digital extensors* originate from the humerus and insert on the third phalanx; they run in front of the lower limb and foot.
- *Two carpal flexors* run behind the carpus and foot.
- *Two digital flexors:* The *superficial digital flexor* inserts on the second phalanx and the *deep digital flexor* inserts on the third phalanx.

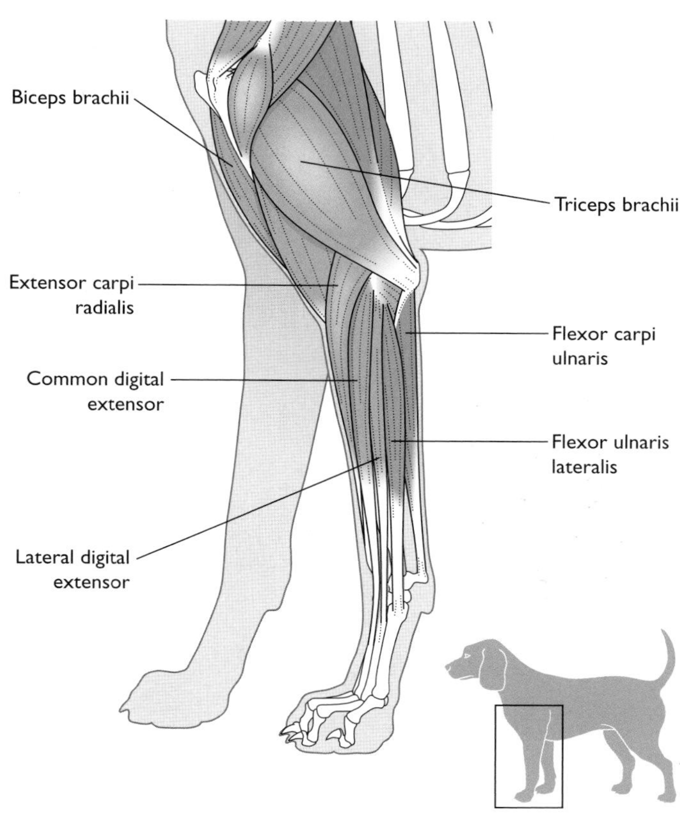

Fig. 4.10 Some of the muscles of the lower forelimb.

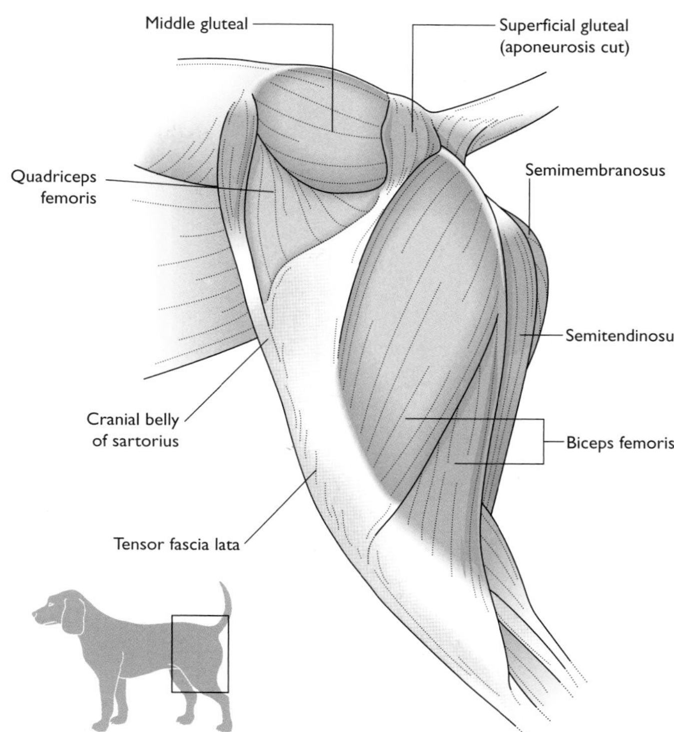

Fig. 4.11 Superficial muscles of the left lateral thigh area.

Muscles of the hind limb

The hind limb is attached to the pelvic girdle by a mobile ball and socket joint, the hip joint. The *sublumbar hypaxial muscles* of the vertebral column are extrinsic muscles attached to the vertebral column and to the pelvic girdle.

The intrinsic muscles of the hind limb all insert on the hind limb itself or on the pelvic girdle and are described below.

Muscles of the thigh

These originate on the pelvic girdle and insert on the femur.

- *Gluteals:* Three muscles, the *superficial, middle* and *deep gluteals*, and the *tensor fascia latae* form the curve of the rump and are powerful extensors of the hip joint.
  Action: extend the hip joint and abduct the thigh
  - *Hamstring group* forms the caudal aspect of the thigh and act together to propel and extend the whole limb backwards (Fig. 4.11), providing the main propulsive force of the animal. The group consists of three muscles:
  - *Biceps femoris* is the most lateral muscle in this group (Fig. 4.11). It originates from the pelvis and runs over the femur to the tibia and inserts on the calcaneus of the hock.
    Action: extends the hip, flexes the stifle and extends the hock
  - *Semitendinosus* runs from the pelvis and inserts on the tibia and calcaneus.
    Action: extends the hip, flexes the stifle and extends the hock
  - *Semimembranosus* is the most medial muscle of the hamstring group. It runs from the pelvis to the femur and tibia.
    Action: extends the hip and flexes the stifle
- *Quadriceps femoris* is a large muscle that runs down the cranial aspect of the thigh. It consists of four parts, all of which insert at the same point on the tibial tuberosity or crest. The tendon of this muscle contains the *patella*, which articulates with the femur at the stifle joint.
  Action: extends the stifle joint
- Adductor muscles lie on the medial aspect of the thigh and hold the limb close into the body (Fig. 4.12). The group consists of three muscles:
  - *Pectineus* muscle runs from the pubis to the distal femur.
    Action: adducts the limb
  - *Sartorius* inserts on the cranial border of the tibia with the gracilis muscle.
    Action: adducts the limb
  - *Gracilis* forms the caudal half of the medial surface of the thigh.
    Action: adducts the limb

The tendon of the pectineus muscle is sometimes transected to relieve pressure on the hip joint of dogs with hip dysplasia. Pectineotomy does not cure the problem but may provide a degree of pain relief, particularly in young dogs.

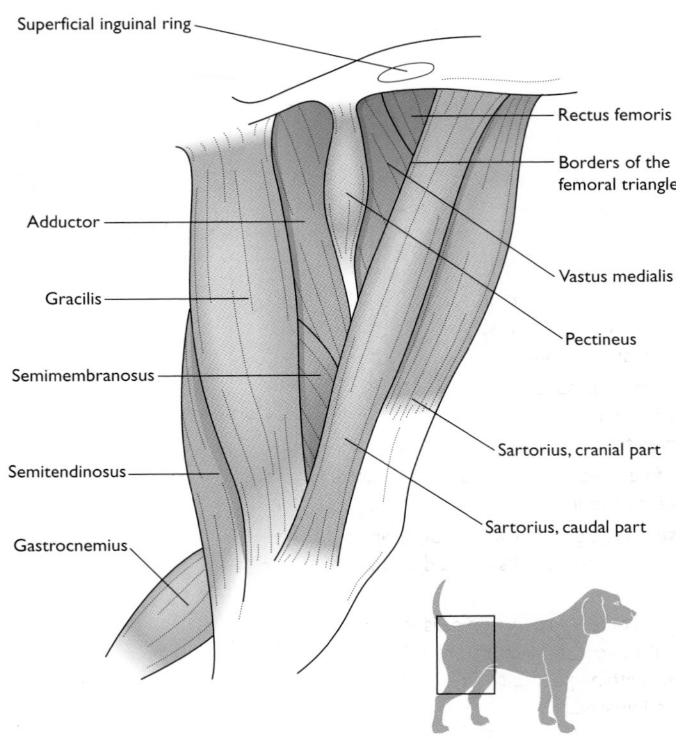

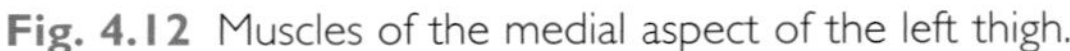

Fig. 4.12 Muscles of the medial aspect of the left thigh.

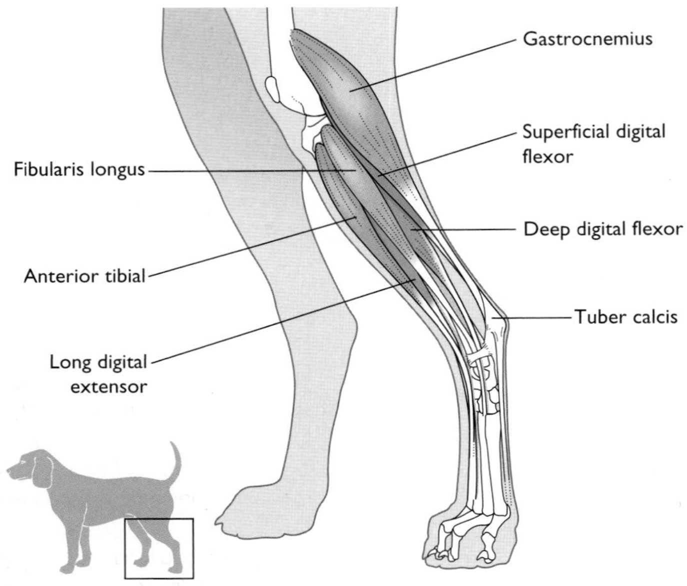

Fig. 4.13 Muscles of the lower left hind limb.

Muscles of the lower hind limb

These muscles act mainly on the hock joint (Fig. 4.13). They include:

- *Gastrocnemius* muscle originates from the caudal aspect of the femur and inserts on the calcaneus of the hock. The tendons of this muscle contain two small sesamoid bones or fabellae that articulate with the caudal aspect of the stifle joint.
  Action – extends the hock and flexes stifle
- *Achilles tendon* is the large, strong tendon that runs down the back of the leg to the point of the hock. It includes the tendons of insertion of the gastrocnemius, biceps femoris and semitendinosus, all of which insert on the calcaneus, and also of the superficial digital flexor muscle, which continues over the point of the hock and down to its insertion on the digits. There is a bursa at the point of insertion on the calcaneus.

The popliteal lymph node lies within the fibres of the gastrocnemius muscle and can be palpated just caudal to the stifle joint. Normally it is about 2 cm long but if it is enlarged it may indicate some form of infection or tumour in the distal extremity.

Muscles of the hock and digits

As is seen in the forelimb, a number of muscles are responsible for flexing and extending the hock and the digits:

- *Anterior tibialis* runs from the proximal end of the tibia to the tarsus.
  Action: flexes the hock and rotates the paw medially
- *Three digital extensors* run in front of the hock and foot.
- *Two digital flexors* run behind the foot. The *superficial digital flexor* runs from the femur to the phalanges and is one of the components of the Achilles tendon.

CHAPTER 5

Nervous system and special senses

KEY POINTS

- The functional unit of the nervous system is the neuron. Neurons connect with each other by synapses to create a complex network that conveys electrical impulses all around the body. The function of this system is to take in information from the external and internal environments, analyse it and then initiate an appropriate response.
- The brain and spinal cord form the control centre of this network and consist of dense accumulations of nervous tissue.
- The brain can be seen to be divided into fore, mid- and hindbrains. Each part of the brain performs a different function and is vital for the survival of the animal.
- To ensure that the brain functions normally it is protected externally by a bony cranium and three layers of meninges, and internally by the ventricular system consisting of canals filled with cerebrospinal fluid (CSF). In addition, every blood vessel entering the brain is wrapped in a layer of protective cells forming the blood–brain barrier, which prevents potentially harmful substances from reaching the brain tissue.
- The whole body is supplied by the peripheral nerves. These are given off as cranial nerves from the brain and spinal nerves from the spinal cord.
- There are five special senses, each of which is vital for the survival of the individual.
- External stimuli (e.g., sight and sound) are perceived by specialised receptor cells located within the special sense organs.
- Information from the receptor cells is transmitted by nerve impulses to the brain by cranial nerves. It is interpreted within specific centres in the brain and a response is initiated.

The presence of a nervous system allows an animal to respond, in a coordinated manner, to both the demands of the external environment and the internal changes within its body. The functions of the nervous system are:

- To receive stimuli from the external and internal environment
- To analyse and integrate these stimuli
- To bring about the necessary response

Although the nervous system works as a well-integrated composite unit within the body, for descriptive purposes, it can be divided into:

- Central nervous system (CNS): the brain and spinal cord
- Peripheral nervous system: all the nerves given off from the CNS:
  - Cranial nerves: leaving the brain
  - Spinal nerves: leaving the spinal cord
  - Autonomic nervous system: nerves that supply the viscera; can be further divided into:
    - sympathetic nervous system
    - parasympathetic nervous system

Nervous tissue

Neuron structure

The main cell of the nervous system is the *neuron* (see Chapter 2, Fig. 2.16). Neurons are responsible for the transmission of nerve impulses throughout the nervous tissue. Nerve impulses pass from one neuron to another by means of structures known as *synapses*. All nerve pathways are made up of neurons and synapses. Complex nervous tissue, such as that of the brain and spinal cord, is made of neurons supported by connective tissue and *neuroglial cells*, whose function is to supply nutrients to and carry waste materials away from the neurons.

Each neuron consists of the following parts:

- A *cell body* containing a nucleus.
- Several short processes called *dendrons*, which are formed from many finer *dendrites*. These carry nerve impulses *towards* the cell body. A single cell body may receive as many as 6000 dendrons from other neurons.
- One long process called an *axon*. These carry nerve impulses *away* from the cell body. The axon leaves the cell at a point known as the *axon hillock*.

Nerve impulses from the dendrons are directed across the cell body towards the axon hillock and continue down the axon, reaching their final destination very rapidly. The speed of transmission along the axon is increased by the presence of a *myelin sheath*. Myelin is a lipoprotein material made by *Schwann cells* surrounding the axon. Its whitish appearance contributes to the colour of the more visible nerves in the body and to the white matter of the CNS. The myelin sheath is interrupted at intervals of about 1 mm by spaces known as the *nodes of Ranvier* and it is through these that the axon tissue receives its nutrient and oxygen supply. Nonmyelinated fibres are embedded within the Schwann cells (Fig. 5.1) and despite their name are actually covered in a single layer of myelin. Totally uncovered fibres are rare and may be found in areas such as the cornea of the eye.

Neurons vary in size; the diameter of the axons and dendrons may be a few micrometres and the length depends on the destination

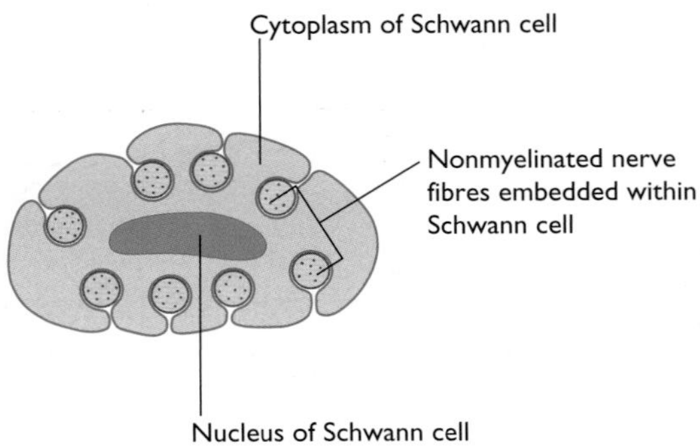

Fig. 5.1 Cross-section through a Schwann cell showing nonmyelinated nerve fibres embedded within the cytoplasm.

of the nerve fibre. This may be anything from a few millimetres to more than a metre long. Neurons also vary in shape (Fig. 5.2).

Synapses

Each axon terminates in a structure called a *synapse* (Fig. 5.3). Where an axon terminates on an individual muscle fibre, the synapse is referred to as a *neuromuscular junction* and the nerve impulse stimulates contraction of the muscle fibre. Within the button-like presynaptic ending are vesicles containing chemical transmitter substances. The most common chemical is *acetylcholine* but others found in the body include adrenaline (epinephrine), serotonin and dopamine.

As the nerve impulse travels down the axon, the vesicles drift towards the *presynaptic membrane* (Fig. 5.3) and release the transmitter into the *synaptic cleft*. It diffuses rapidly across this gap and combines with the *postsynaptic membrane*, making the membrane more 'excitable' and allowing the transmission of the nerve impulse to continue on down the nerve fibre. The effect is stopped by the release of cholinesterases – enzymes that destroy any acetylcholine remaining in the synaptic cleft – and the synapse returns to its resting state ready for the next nerve impulse. Effective transmission of a nerve impulse across the synapse will only occur in the presence of *calcium ions*.

The nervous symptoms of eclampsia in the bitch, which include shaking, disorientation and eventual collapse and milk fever in the cow, are caused by low levels of calcium in the blood, affecting the transmission of nerve impulses.

Generation of a nerve impulse

Nerve impulses transmitted along axons and dendrites can be considered to be electrical phenomena. An impulse changes the electrical charge of the neuron by altering the relationship

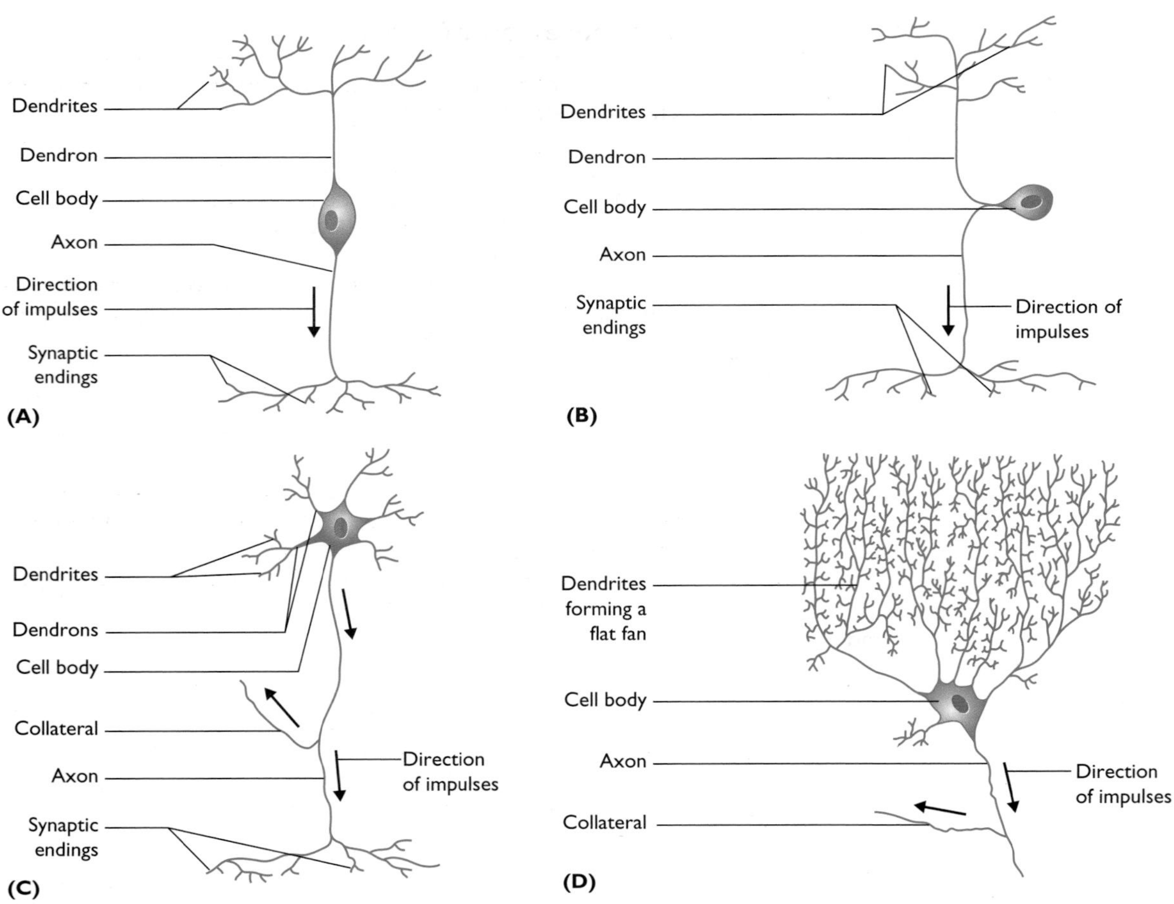

Fig. 5.2 The variation in shape of neurons. **(A)** Bipolar neuron. **(B)** Pseudo-unipolar neuron (e.g., a sensory neuron). **(C)** Multipolar neuron (e.g., a motor neuron). **(D)** Multipolar neuron (e.g., Purkinje cell from the cerebellum of the brain).

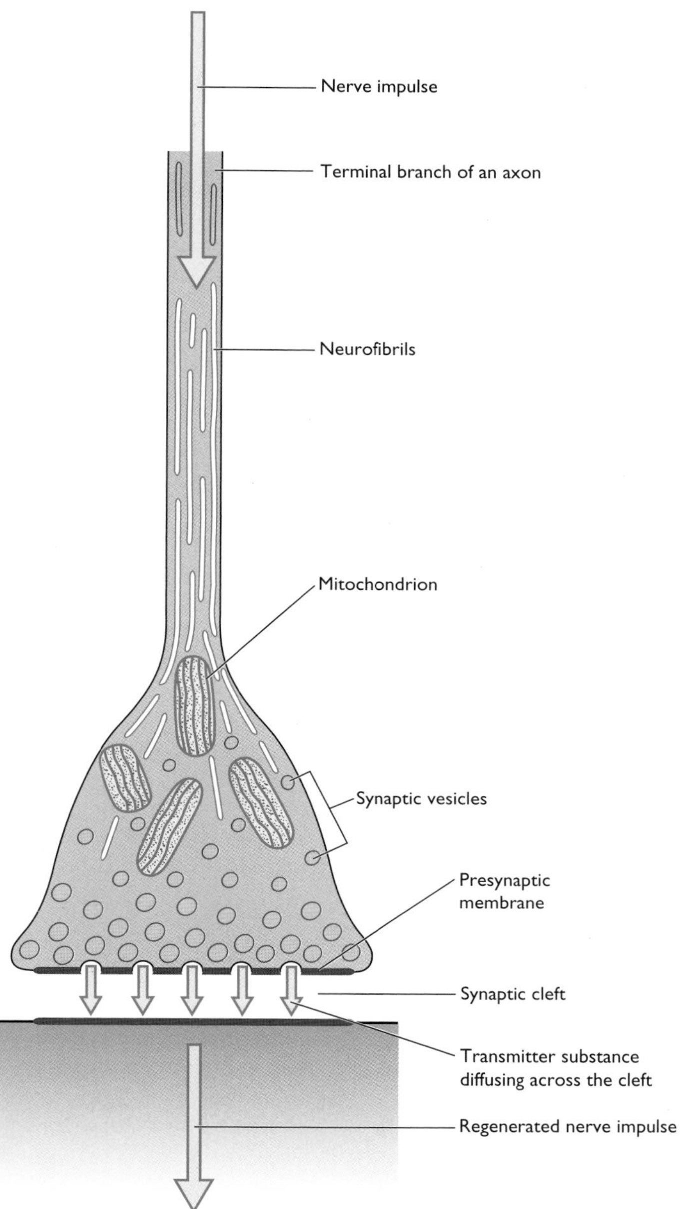

Fig. 5.3 The structure of a synapse.

between the negative charge of the cell contents and the positive charge of the cell membrane. This results from a change in the permeability of the cell membrane to sodium and potassium ions, causing an exchange of ions between the inside and the outside of the neuron (Fig. 5.4).

For a short time after the impulse has passed, the nerve fibre becomes refractive, meaning that it cannot be reactivated by another impulse until the permeability of the cell membrane returns to normal. This ensures that the flow of impulses travels only in one direction.

A nerve impulse is an *all-or-nothing phenomenon:* the nerve is either stimulated or it is not; there is no gradation of impulse. A particular neuron will always transmit with the same power or the same speed. The different effects of the nervous system depend on:

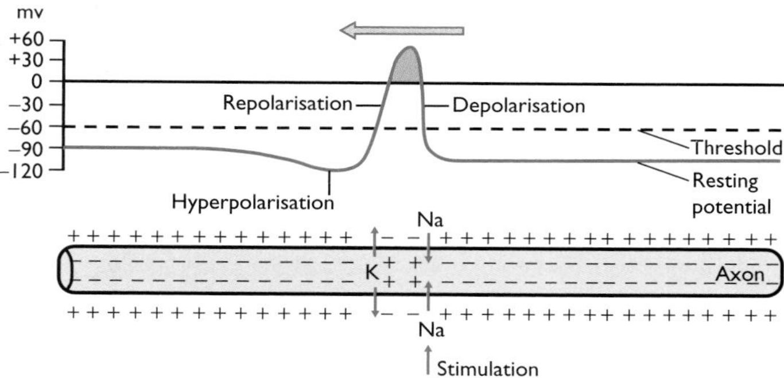

Fig. 5.4 The alterations in electrical charge that occur in an axon as a nerve impulse travels along it from right to left. The charge differences are brought about by movement of sodium and potassium ions across the axon membrane.

- The *number of nerve impulses* transmitted per second: a weak stimulus produces few impulses at long intervals, while a strong stimulus produces rapid impulses at shorter intervals.
- The *number of neurons* activated by a single stimulus: a strong stimulus produces activity in a large number of neurons and a weak stimulus produces activity in a small number.
- The *type of neuron* stimulated: some have an excitatory effect while others have an inhibitory effect.

Classification of nerves

Peripheral nerves can be classified according to their function and to the structures they supply.

- *Sensory nerves* carry impulses towards the CNS.
- *Motor nerves* carry impulses away from the CNS.
- *Mixed nerves* carry both sensory and motor fibres.

An *intercalated neuron* is one that lies between a sensory neuron and a motor neuron. Such neurons may not always be present within a nerve pathway.

- *Afferent nerves* carry impulses towards a structure, usually in the CNS.
- *Efferent nerves* carry impulses away from a structure, usually in the CNS.

Afferent and efferent are also terms used within other systems (e.g., the blood vascular system) to describe blood and lymphatic capillaries going to and leaving organs.

Nerve fibres may be further classified according to the organ with which they are associated.

- *Visceral* sensory and motor nerves are associated with the visceral body systems – the heart, digestive, respiratory, urinary and reproductive systems. Stimuli are carried by visceral sensory nerves from blood vessels, mucous membranes and the visceral organs to the CNS. Impulses are transmitted from the CNS by visceral motor nerves to smooth muscle and glandular tissue, where they initiate a response.
- *Somatic* sensory and motor nerves are associated with the somatic structures in the body – receptors in the skin, muscles, joints and tendons and in specialised somatic organs such as the ear and eye. Stimuli are carried by somatic sensory nerves towards the CNS and nerve impulses are carried by somatic motor nerves to skeletal muscles, where they initiate a response.

The central nervous system

During embryonic development of the CNS, a hollow neural tube forms from the ectodermal layer of the inner cell mass of the embryo. This neural tube runs along the dorsal surface of the embryo and, as it develops, nerve fibres grow out laterally extending to all parts of the body and eventually forming the peripheral nervous system. The anterior end of the tube becomes the *brain* and the remaining tube becomes the *spinal cord*. The brain and spinal cord are hollow and are filled with CSF.

The brain

The function of the brain is to control and coordinate all the activities of the normal body. The brain is a hollow, swollen structure lying within the cranial cavity of the skull, which protects it from mechanical damage. In many species, three distinct areas can be identified: the forebrain, midbrain and hindbrain. In mammals, this arrangement may be difficult to recognise because the right and left cerebral hemispheres of the forebrain are enlarged and overlie the midbrain (Fig. 5.5).

Forebrain

This consists of the cerebrum, thalamus and hypothalamus.

The *cerebrum* – or right and left *cerebral hemispheres* – takes up the greater part of the forebrain and contains up to 90% of all the neurons in the entire nervous system (Fig. 5.5). The right and left sides are linked by the *corpus callosum,* a tract of white matter whose nerve fibres run across the brain between the right and left hemispheres. It is found in the roof of the *third ventricle*, which is part of the hollow ventricular system inside the brain and contains CSF.

The surface of the hemispheres is deeply folded, which enables a large surface area to be enclosed within the small cranial cavity and allows nutrients in the CSF to reach the cell bodies of neurons lying deep inside the brain tissue. The folds are known as *gyri* (upfolds), *sulci* (shallow depressions) and *fissures* (deep crevices). The two hemispheres are divided by the *longitudinal fissure.* Each cerebral hemisphere consists of four lobes, each of which contains specific *centres* or *nuclei* with specific functions related to conscious thought and action.

The tissue of the cerebral hemispheres consists of:

- An outer layer of *grey matter* known as the *cerebral cortex*, containing millions of cell bodies of neurons. Deeper in the brain are groups of cell bodies forming *centres* or *nuclei*, which act as relay stations collecting information and sending out impulses to a variety of areas.
- An inner layer of *white matter* made of tracts of myelinated nerve fibres linking one area to another. Histologically the tissue appears white because of the high proportion of the white lipoprotein myelin.

The *thalamus* is found deep in the tissue of the posterior part of the forebrain. Its function is to process information from the sense organs and relay it to the cerebral cortex.

The *hypothalamus* lies ventral to the thalamus and has several functions:

1. It acts as a link between the endocrine and nervous systems by secreting a series of releasing hormones that are then stored in the pituitary gland.
2. It helps to control the autonomic nervous system by influencing a range of involuntary actions such as sweating, shivering, vasodilation and vasoconstriction.
3. It exerts the major influence over homeostasis in the body by influencing osmotic balance of body fluids, the regulation of body temperature, and control of thirst and hunger centres in the brain.

On the ventral surface of the forebrain (Fig. 5.6) the following structures can be seen:

- *Optic chiasma:* Nerve impulses, carried by the optic nerve (cranial nerve II) from the right eye, pass to the right side of the brain and to the left side via the optic chiasma (and similarly for the left eye). This ensures that information from each eye reaches both sides of the brain.
- *Pituitary gland:* is an endocrine gland attached below the hypothalamus by a short stalk (see Chapter 6).

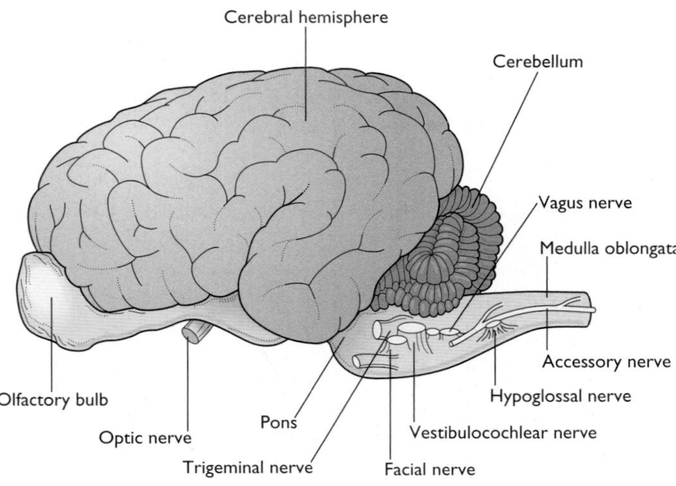

Fig. 5.5 Left lateral view of the canine brain.

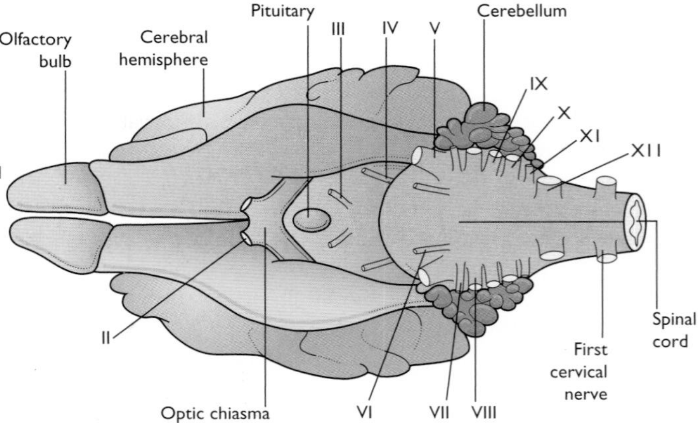

Fig. 5.6 View of the ventral surface of the canine brain.

- *Olfactory bulbs:* are a pair of bulbs that form the most rostral part of the brain. They are responsible for the sense of smell or olfaction. Their size is determined by the sense of smell in a particular species. Fish have very large olfactory bulbs and hence an excellent sense of smell, while humans have very small olfactory bulbs. The cat has larger olfactory bulbs than the dog, and, in fact, cats have a much better sense of smell.

Midbrain

This is a short length of brain lying between the forebrain and the hindbrain. It is overhung by the cerebral hemispheres and is not easy to see in the gross specimen. It acts as a pathway for fibres running from the hindbrain to the forebrain carrying the senses of hearing and sight.

Hindbrain

This consists of the cerebellum, pons and medulla oblongata.

The *cerebellum* lies on the dorsal surface of the hindbrain (Fig. 5.5). Its name means 'little brain' as it was originally thought to be a smaller version of the cerebrum. It has a globular appearance and is covered in deep fissures. In cross-section, the tissue is very obviously divided into an outer cortex of grey matter and an inner layer of white matter. The grey matter consists of numerous Purkinje cells (Fig. 5.2), each of which forms thousands of synapses with other neurons.

The cerebellum controls balance and coordination. It receives information from the semicircular canals of the inner ear and muscle spindles within skeletal muscles. Voluntary movements are initiated by the cerebrum and fine adjustments are made and coordinated by the cerebellum.

The *pons* lies ventral to the cerebellum and forms a bridge of nerve fibres between the cerebellar hemispheres. It contains centres that control respiration.

The *medulla oblongata* extends from the pons and merges into the spinal cord (Fig. 5.5). It contains centres responsible for the control of respiration and blood pressure.

Injury or malformation of the cerebellum results in incoordination and spasticity. Kittens whose dam was infected with the feline enteritis virus during pregnancy may be born with **cerebellar hypoplasia** (underdevelopment) and will never be able to walk in a normal coordinated fashion.

The medulla oblongata and the pons form part of the brain stem that is responsible for the vital control of respiration and blood pressure. If the brain stem is damaged, such as by brain stem herniation through the foramen magnum, which may occur if the brain swells as a result of inflammation or traumatic damage, then respiration and blood pressure will be affected and the animal will die; this is often described as being 'brain stem dead'.

Epilepsy is a disorder of the CNS. It results from an irritable focus in the brain, which causes disorganized electrical activity resulting in convulsions or 'fits'. The convulsions may be described as being *clonic*, in which muscular contractions are interspersed with periods of relaxation, or *tonic*, where the contractions are sustained.

Protection of the brain

Normal brain function is essential for the maintenance of an animal's life. If it is damaged mechanically or chemically, function will be impaired and the animal may die. Several structures have evolved within the brain to protect it from harm.

Cranium

This bony structure forms a tough outer shell to protect the soft brain tissue from physical damage.

Ventricular system

The ventricular system (Fig. 5.7) is derived from the hollow neural tube of the embryo. The lumen of this tube develops into a series of interconnecting canals and cavities or ventricles found inside the brain and spinal cord. The ventricles and the central canal are filled with CSF. This also surrounds the outside of the brain, lying in the subarachnoid space (Fig. 5.8). CSF is secreted by networks of blood capillaries known as *choroid plexuses* lying in the roofs of the ventricles. It is a clear fluid, resembling plasma, but has no protein in it – it is an example of a transcellular fluid. The function of CSF is to protect the CNS from damage by sudden movement or knocks and to provide nutrients to the nervous tissue of the brain and spinal cord.

Samples of CSF can be collected from the cisterna magna, lying between the cerebellum and the medulla oblongata. The patient is anaesthetised and restrained in sternal or lateral recumbency, with its chin touching its chest. A spinal needle is slowly advanced into the space until CSF begins to drip from the hub.

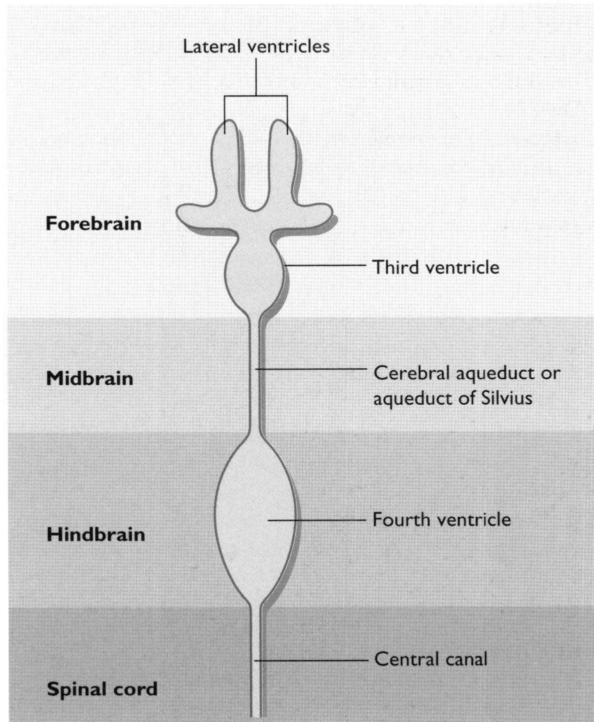

Fig. 5.7 Dorsal view of the ventricular system of the brain and its relationship to the areas of the brain (not to scale).

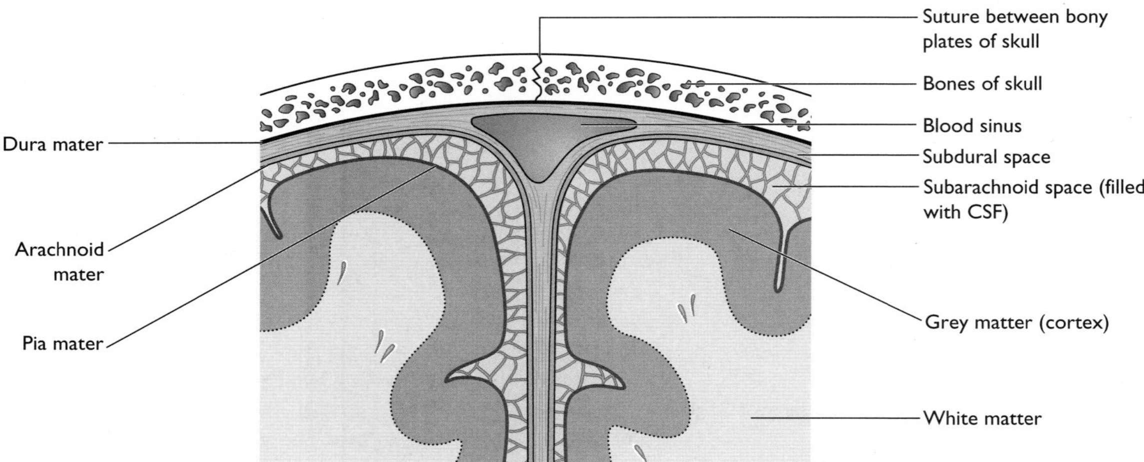

Fig. 5.8 Cross-section through the cerebral hemispheres to show the meninges of the brain.

Meninges

The meninges (Fig. 5.8) consist of three protective layers around the brain and spinal cord. From the outermost layer inwards, they are:

1. *Dura mater* is a tough fibrous layer of connective tissue continuous with the periosteum of the bones of the cranium. Below the dura mater is the *subdural space,* which is filled with fat, connective tissue and blood capillaries.
2. *Arachnoid mater* is a network of collagen fibres and larger blood vessels that supply the adjacent area of nervous tissue with nutrients. Below the arachnoid mater is the *subarachnoid space,* in which the CSF flows.
3. *Pia mater* is a delicate membrane that closely adheres to the brain and spinal cord and follows all the gyri and sulci.

Blood–brain barrier

This is a modification of the neuroglial tissue that connects and supports all the neurons within the nervous tissue. Different types of neuroglial cells surround the blood capillaries, creating an almost impermeable layer, to protect the brain from substances that are harmful to or not needed by the brain. These include urea, certain proteins and antibiotics. Other materials such as oxygen, sodium and potassium ions and glucose can pass rapidly through the barrier to be used for brain metabolism.

> The action of general anaesthetic agents relies on their ability to pass through the blood–brain barrier and affect the neurons in the brain. Drugs that affect the brain must be in a lipophilic form (soluble in lipids), so that they are able to pass through the phospholipid cell membranes of the neuroglial cells.

The spinal cord

The spinal cord is a glistening white tube running from the medulla oblongata of the brain to the level of the sixth or seventh lumbar vertebra, where it breaks up into several terminal spinal nerves forming a structure known as the *cauda equina* (Fig. 5.9). It leaves the skull through the largest foramen in the body, the *foramen magnum,* and runs through the vertebral canal formed by the interlinking vertebrae that protect it. The cord decreases in size from its cranial to caudal end, but in the caudal cervical and midlumbar regions it may be thicker because these correspond to areas where collections or plexuses of nerves leave the spinal cord to supply the fore and hind limbs.

The spinal cord develops segmentally in the embryo and, although this is difficult to see in the adult, each segment corresponds to a different vertebra and gives off a pair of *spinal nerves* – one to the right and one to the left. The spinal nerves leave the vertebral canal through the appropriate *intervertebral foramen.*

In cross-section (Fig. 5.10) the spinal cord consists of:

- *Central canal* leads away from the ventricular system of the brain and contains CSF.
- *Grey matter* forms a 'butterfly'-shaped core of tissue surrounding the central canal. It consists of the cell bodies of neurons and nonmyelinated nerve fibres. Most of the synaptic contact in the cord occurs in the grey matter.
- *White matter* surrounds the grey matter and is coloured white by the myelin around the nerve fibres. It is organised into tracts of fibres carrying information towards the brain *(ascending tracts)* or away from the brain *(descending tracts).* Each tract has an origin and a destination, which ensures that transmission of nerve impulses is efficient and very rapid.

The spinal cord is protected by three meninges arranged in a similar pattern to those surrounding the brain. There is a space between the periosteum of the vertebrae and the dura mater. This is the *epidural space* and is the site into which local anaesthetic is introduced to achieve regional anaesthesia of the spinal cord. Small amounts of CSF runs in the *subarachnoid space* which protects the cord from mechanical damage and supplies the nervous tissue with nutrients.

The peripheral nervous system

The peripheral nervous system consists of all the nerves given off from the CNS. These are:

- *Cranial nerves:* leaving the brain
- *Spinal nerves:* leaving the spinal cord

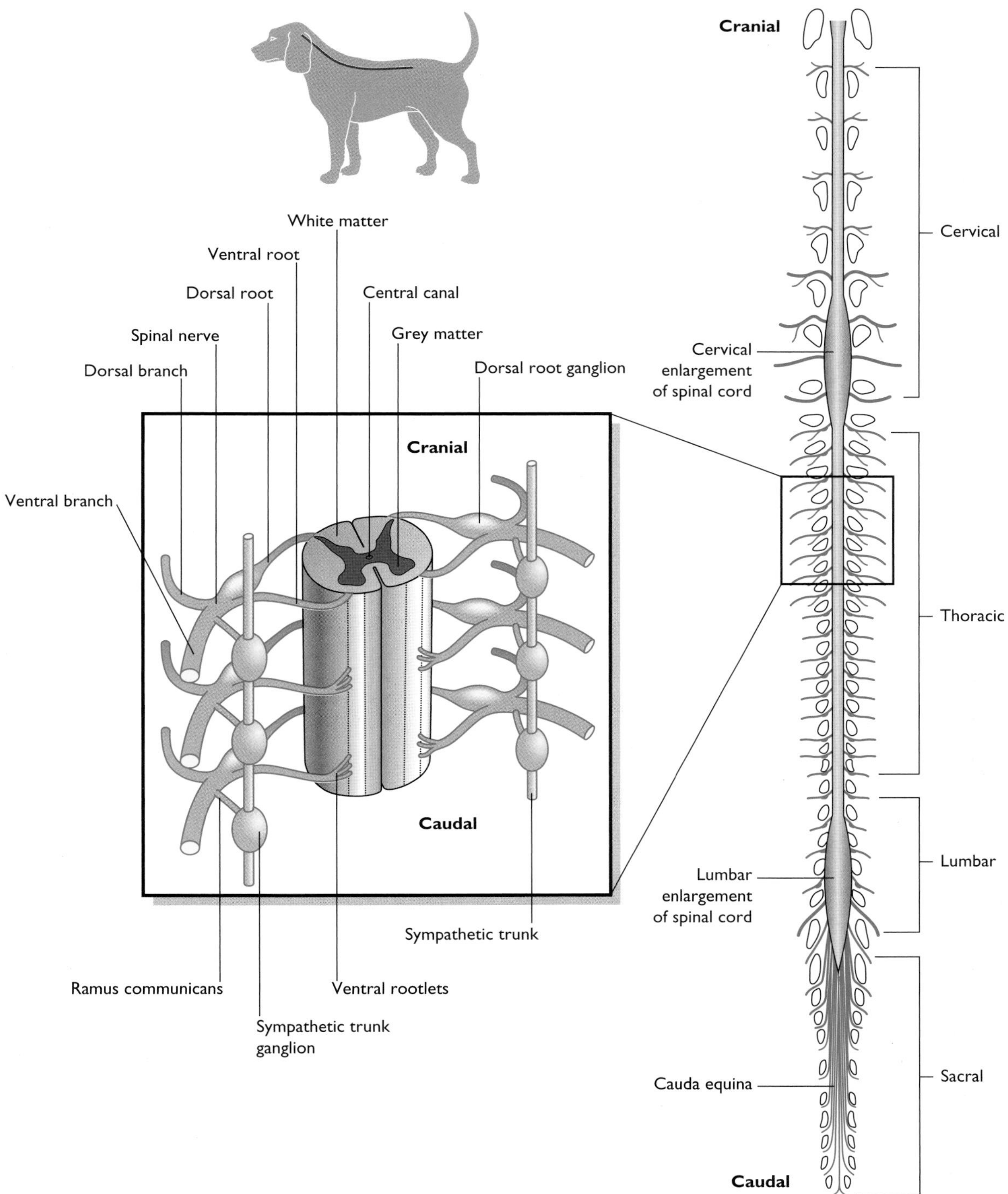

Fig. 5.9 View of the spinal cord of the dog with vertebrae removed.

- *Autonomic nervous system:* contains some nerve fibres from the brain, but most nerves arise from the spinal cord.

Cranial nerves

The 12 pairs of cranial nerves arise from the brain (Fig. 5.6) and leave the cranial cavity by various foramina. The majority of these nerves supply structures around the head and are relatively short, but some supply structures at some distance from the point at which they leave the brain, such as the vagus nerve (cranial nerve X), which is the longest nerve in the body.

Cranial nerves are referred to by their name and by a Roman numeral (Table 5.1). They may carry:

- Only *sensory* fibres, from the organs to the brain
- Only *motor* fibres, from the brain to the organs
- Both sensory and motor fibres, which are *mixed* nerves

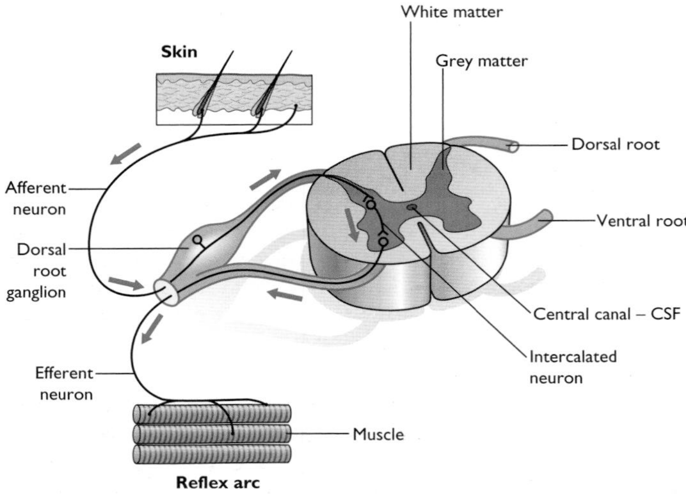

Fig. 5.10 Transverse section through the spinal cord showing reflex arc.

Spinal nerves

As the spinal cord passes down the vertebral canal each segment, corresponding to a vertebra, gives off a pair of spinal nerves, one to the right side and one to the left (Fig. 5.9). These nerves are numbered according to the number of the spinal vertebra in front. However, there are eight cervical nerves but only *seven* cervical vertebrae; the first cervical nerve (Ce1) leaves the spinal cord in front of C1; Ce7 leaves in front of C7 and Ce8 leaves behind it. From then on, each nerve leaves from behind the appropriate vertebra.

Each spinal nerve consists of two components (Fig. 5.10):

- A *dorsal root* carries *sensory* fibres *towards* the spinal cord. Several millimetres from the cord is a small swelling containing the cell bodies of the sensory neurons, the *dorsal root ganglion*. The efferent fibres from the cell bodies run into the spinal cord and synapse in the grey matter.
- A *ventral root* carries *motor* fibres *away* from the spinal cord. There are no ganglia outside the cord, the ganglia of the ventral root are in the grey matter of the cord.

In some nerve pathways, there may be one or more *intercalated neurons* lying in the grey matter between the sensory and motor neurons. The sensory and motor nerve fibres of each spinal nerve come together in the same myelin sheath and leave the vertebral column via the relevant intervertebral foramen as a *mixed* nerve (Fig. 5.9).

Examples of major peripheral nerve pathways within the limbs

Pectoral limb

Most structures within the pectoral limb are supplied by the brachial plexus, which lies above the area of the axilla and just below the spinal cord. It is formed by the spinal nerves from C6, C7, C8, T1 and T2, which combine to form various named nerves within the limb.

Table 5.1 Cranial nerves

Cranial nerve	Type of nerve fibre	Function
I. Olfactory	Sensory	Carries the sense of smell or olfaction from the olfactory bulbs to the brain
II. Optic	Sensory	Carries information about sight from the eyes to the brain; some nerve fibres from each eye cross over, via the optic chiasma, to the opposite side of the brain; in this way each side of the brain receives information from both eyes
III. Oculomotor	Motor	Supplies the extrinsic muscles of the eye, enabling the eye to make minute, delicate movements; accurate movement of the eye is essential for survival
IV. Trochlear	Motor	Supplies the extrinsic muscles of the eye
V. Trigeminal	Mixed	Sensory fibres are carried from the skin around the eye and the face; motor fibres supplied to the muscles of mastication, mainly the temporal and masseter
VI. Abducens	Motor	Supplies the extrinsic muscles of the eye
VII. Facial	Motor	Supplies the muscles of facial expression including those associated with the movement of the lips, ears and skin around the eyes
VIII. Vestibulocochlear (auditory)	Sensory	Vestibular branch carries the sensation of balance from the semicircular canals of the inner ear; cochlear branch carries the sensation of hearing from the cochlea of the inner ear
IX. Glossopharyngeal	Mixed	Carries the sensation of taste from the taste buds on the tongue and pharynx; supplies motor fibres to the muscles of the pharynx
X. Vagus	Mixed	Carries sensory fibres from the pharynx and larynx; supplies motor fibres to the muscles of the larynx; parasympathetic visceral motor fibres to the heart and various thoracic and abdominal organs including the gastrointestinal tract down to the descending colon
XI. Accessory (spinal accessory)	Motor	Supplies the muscles of the neck and shoulder
XII. Hypoglossal	Motor	Supplies the muscles of the tongue

- The *radial nerve* is the largest nerve of the brachial plexus. It runs laterally from the brachial plexus and follows the musculospiral groove of the humerus. At the level of the lateral head of the triceps it divides into deep and superficial branches. Before it divides it supplies the *extensors* of the elbow and after it divides it supplies the *extensors* of the carpus and digits. The superficial branch carries sensation from the dorsal surface of the forepaw and lower forelimb.

Radial nerve paralysis. If an animal damages the radial nerve in its forelimb it will knuckle over on its forepaw, leading to excessive wear of the skin on the dorsal surface of the paw; the ventral surface is protected from normal wear by the pads. This occurs because the animal is unable to use the extensor muscles that bring the limb into its normal position. The damaged nerve may recover but if it has been severed the only treatment may be to amputate the forelimb.

- The *median nerve* runs caudal to the brachial artery and vein on the medial side of the forelimb. It supplies the *flexors* of the carpus and digits and carries sensation from the joint capsule of the elbow.
- The *ulnar nerve* shares some fibres with the median nerve and for much of its length it follows its route. It also supplies the *flexors* of the carpus and digits but carries sensation from the caudolateral parts of the lower forelimb and the paw.

Pelvic limb

Structures within the hind limb are supplied by nerves from the lumbosacral plexus formed by the spinal nerves from L3, L4, L5, L6, L7, S1 and S2. These combine to form the variously named nerves of the hind limb.

- The *femoral nerve* is the main nerve of the hind limb and is the equivalent of the radial nerve in the fore limb. After leaving the plexus it runs deep within the tissue of the quadriceps femoris muscle, which makes it less prone to traumatic damage. It supplies the *extensors* of the stifle joint.
- The *saphenous nerve* is given off by the femoral nerve and is more superficial. It supplies the sartorius muscle (adductor) and carries sensation from the dorsomedial aspect of the thigh, stifle and lower limb.
- The *sciatic nerve* is the largest nerve of the lumbosacral plexus. It leaves the plexus running over the ischium and along the lateral surface of the thigh deep within the biceps femoris. It supplies the muscles of the hamstring group (i.e., *extensors* of the hip and *flexors* of the stifle), and it carries sensation from the caudolateral regions of the thigh.
- The *tibial nerve* is given off by the sciatic nerve and supplies the *flexor* muscles on the caudal surface of the lower limb and the plantar surface of the hind foot.

The term 'sciatica' implies pain sensation in the areas supplied by the sciatic nerve (i.e., the caudolateral regions of the thigh).

Reflex arcs

A reflex arc is a fixed involuntary response to certain stimuli. The response is always the same. It is rapid and automatic and involves only nerve pathways in the spinal cord, using the appropriate spinal nerve. Reflex arcs are a means of protection and produce a prompt response to potentially damaging phenomena such as heat or sharp objects.

Common reflexes observed in the dog and cat are:

- Withdrawal or pedal reflex
- Anal reflex
- Patellar reflex
- Panniculus reflex
- Palpebral reflex

Using the patellar reflex as an example, we can follow the pathway taken by the nerve impulse (Fig. 5.10). The tendon of the quadriceps femoris muscle passes over the patella as the straight patellar ligament and inserts on the tibial tuberosity of the proximal tibia. Within the muscle fibres are stretch receptors known as muscle spindles, whose function is to monitor muscle tone. The nerve pathway is as follows:

1. When the tendon is lightly tapped, the muscle fibres stretch.
2. This initiates a response in the muscle spindles and a nerve impulse passes along the sensory nerve to the spinal cord.
3. Within the grey matter of the spinal cord, the sensory nerve synapses with the motor nerve and an impulse passes along it to the muscle fibres of the quadriceps femoris, causing contraction.
4. This extends or kicks out the leg, completing the reflex arc.

This is an example of a *monosynaptic reflex* because there is only one set of synapses. A *polysynaptic reflex* (e.g., the withdrawal reflex) involves one or more intercalated neurons and several synapses within the grey matter.

A reflex is unconscious and will still occur even if the spinal cord has been severed. However, if the web of the dog's foot is pinched and it withdraws its foot and then yelps or bites you, this indicates that it has felt pain. There is *conscious perception*, involving the transmission of impulses up the tracts of white matter of the spinal cord to the brain and back to the muscles of the jaw, as well as along the pathway of the reflex arc. A conscious response indicates that the spinal cord is intact.

Reflexes may be described as being:

- *Unconditional* reflexes: unconscious and automatic (the type already described). They cannot be overcome.
- *Conditional* reflexes: overcome by conscious thought; keeping your hand on a hot iron, for example, requires a determined effort to prevent your muscles contracting and pulling the hand away. The phenomenon known as Pavlov's dogs is an example of a conditioned reflex. In this experiment the Russian physiologist Ivan Pavlov (1849–1936) observed that his dogs salivated at the sight and smell of food. He started to ring a bell every time he fed the dogs and over a period of weeks he found that if he rang the bell the dogs would salivate even if no food was offered. He had modified the salivation reflex by altering the stimulus.

Conditioned reflexes are the basis of toilet training and of obedience training using 'clickers'.

Autonomic nervous system

This can be considered to consist almost entirely of *visceral motor nerves* supplying cardiac muscle, smooth muscle and glandular tissue (including the liver and pancreas) of all the internal organs and of blood vessels. Control of the system is unconscious; an animal does not have to push food along its intestine or constrict its blood vessels by conscious thought (Fig. 5.11).

The autonomic nervous system can be divided into two parts: the *sympathetic nervous system* and the *parasympathetic nervous system*. The division is based on the anatomical derivation of the

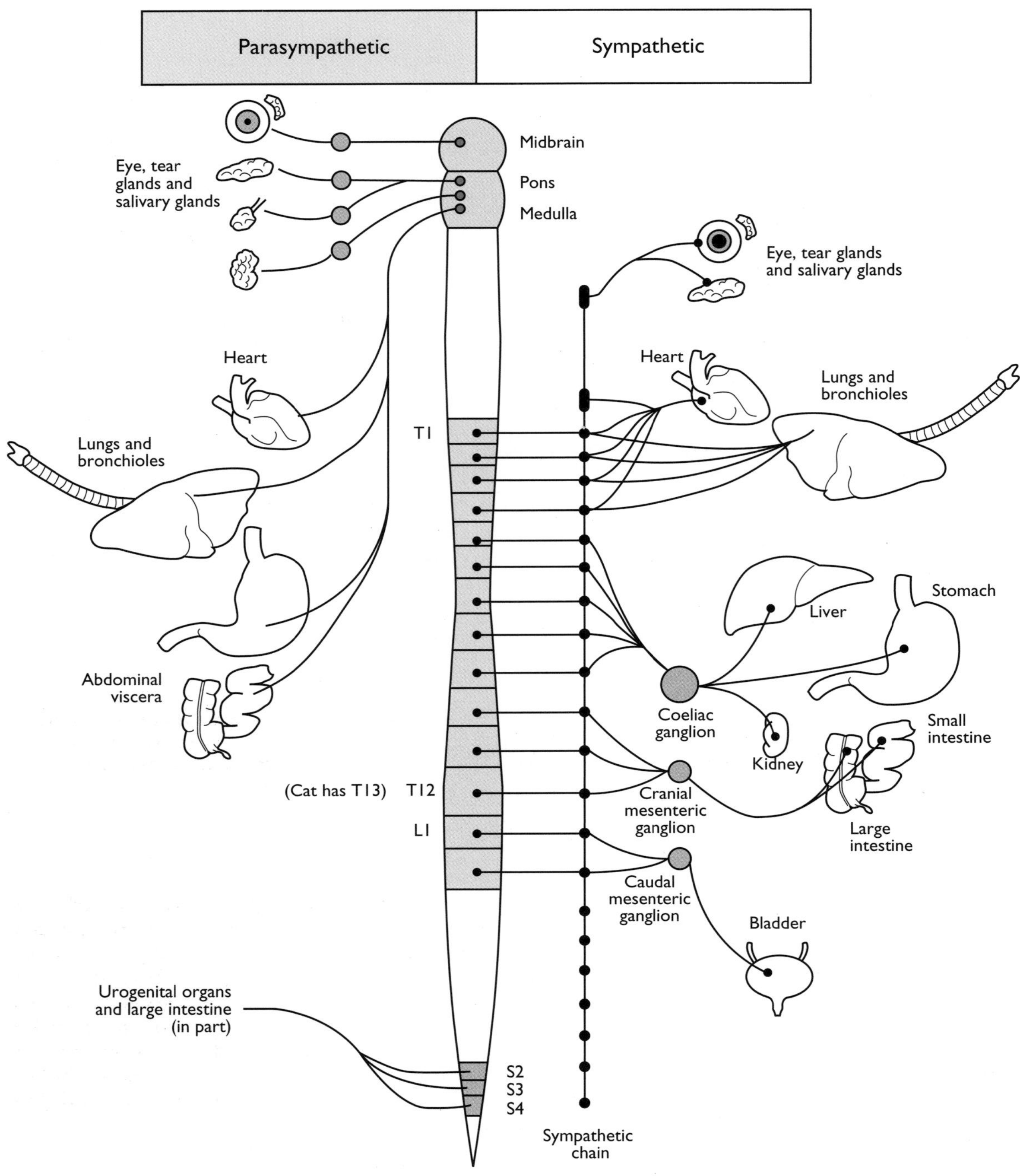

Fig. 5.11 Outline of the autonomic nervous system. (With permission from T Colville, JM Bassett, 2001. Clinical anatomy and physiology for veterinary technicians. St Louis, MO: Mosby, p. 156.)

spinal nerves and on their differing effects. Most organs are supplied by both types and control involves a balance between the two (Table 5.2).

Special senses

The special senses are:

- Taste
- Smell
- Sight
- Hearing
- Balance

Specialised receptor cells are adapted to respond to a particular stimulus and convey the information to the CNS. Information is processed within the CNS and an appropriate response is initiated. Mammals have evolved specialised organs in which to house the receptor cells; these are the *special sense organs*.

Table 5.2 The autonomic nervous system

	Sympathetic system	**Parasympathetic system**
Origin of nerve fibres	Vertebrae TI to L4 or L5	Cranial nerves III, VII, IX, X; vertebrae SI, S2
Preganglionic nerve fibres	Short; each nerve leads to a ganglion containing cell bodies and lying close under the vertebral column; there is a chain of ganglia – the sympathetic chain – one on each side of the vertebral column	Long; ganglia lie close to the organ they supply; there is no chain of ganglia
Postganglionic nerve fibres	Long; lead away from the sympathetic chain and travel towards the organ it supplies; usually follow the path of blood vessels	Short; fibres run a short distance from the ganglion to the organ
Areas supplied	Viscera in thorax, abdomen and pelvis; also supply sweat glands, blood vessels and piloerector muscles associated with hair follicles. Most ganglia are paired, but three are unpaired: 1. Coeliac: supplies stomach, small intestine, pancreas, large intestine and adrenal medulla 2. Cranial (superior) mesenteric: supplies large intestine 3. Caudal (inferior) mesenteric: supplies bladder and genitals	Structures in the head including the eye and salivary glands; vagus (X) supplies the heart, lungs, stomach, small intestine, pancreas and large intestine
Transmitter substances		
A. Within the system (i.e., between cell body and dendron)	Acetylcholine	Acetylcholine
B. At the terminal synapses (i.e., between the axon and the effector organ)	Noradrenaline (norepinephrine)	Acetylcholine
General effect	Prepares the body for 'fear, flight, fight'; heart and respiratory rates are increased, blood vessels to skeletal muscle are dilated, blood glucose levels rise, piloerector muscles to the hairs contract so hackles are raised, gastrointestinal tract activity decreases	Animal is more relaxed; heart rate is slowed, respiratory bronchioles constrict, gastrointestinal tract activity increases – digestive juices and salivary secretion increases, peristalsis increases

Taste buds: taste

The sensation of taste is known as *gustation* and the organs used to detect it are the taste buds (Fig. 5.12) found on the dorsal surface of the tongue, the epiglottis and the soft palate and covered in moist mucous membrane. Taste buds are *chemoreceptors* stimulated by the chemicals responsible for smell dissolved in the mucus around the oral cavity.

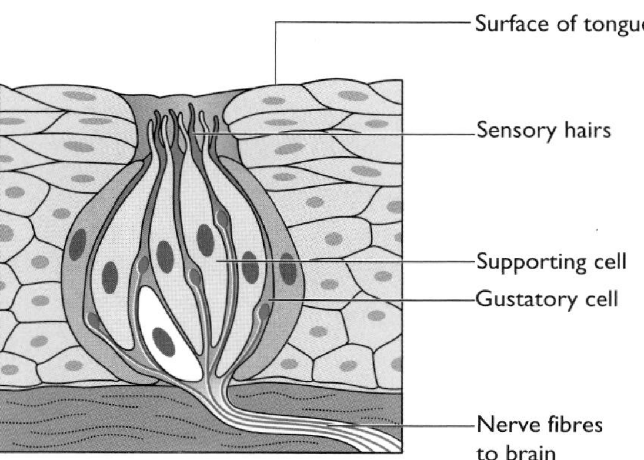

Fig. 5.12 Cross-section through a taste bud.

Each taste bud consists of receptor or *gustatory cells* surrounded by *sustentacular* or supporting cells. Projecting from the upper surface of each taste bud are hair-like processes. Fine nerve fibres, which are branches of the facial (VII), glossopharyngeal (IX) and vagus (X) nerves, conduct impulses away from the gustatory cells towards the brain, where they are interpreted as taste. The sensation of taste in animals is difficult to quantify. It is thought to be directed more towards selecting tastes that are harmless or harmful to them rather than to enjoyment or dislike, as in humans.

Nasal mucosa: smell

The sensation of smell is known as *olfaction*. The receptor cells are also chemoreceptors and the sensation is closely allied to gustation; the two sensations often work together. The receptor cells are rod-shaped bipolar neurons, which are distributed throughout the mucosa covering the caudal part of the nasal cavities and the turbinate bones. The axon leaving each receptor cell combines with other axons to form the *olfactory nerve fibres* (I). Chemicals responsible for smell dissolve in the mucus of the nasal cavity and stimulate the production of nerve impulses. These are transmitted along the olfactory nerve fibres, through the *cribriform plate* of the *ethmoid bone* (dividing the nasal and cranial cavities) and into the *olfactory bulbs* of the forebrain, where they are interpreted as smell.

The eye and sight

The eye is the organ of sight. *Photoreceptor cells* adapted to respond to the stimulus of light are found in the innermost layer of the eye, the *retina.* All mammals have a pair of eyes, each of which lies within a deep bony cavity of the skull known as the *orbit.* Each eye lies rostral to the cranial cavity, lateral to the nasal cavities and dorsal to the mouth. The dog and the cat are predatory species and their eyes point forwards (Fig. 5.13). This provides a wide area of binocular or 3D vision, enabling them to pinpoint the position of their prey accurately. Prey species such as the rabbit or the mouse have prominent eyes set on the sides of the head. These provide a wide area of monocular or 2D vision, which enables the animal to see the predator but not to fix its position; this does not matter, the important factor is that the predator is nearby and that the prey animal runs away.

Each eye consists of three main parts: the eyeball, the extrinsic muscles and the eyelids.

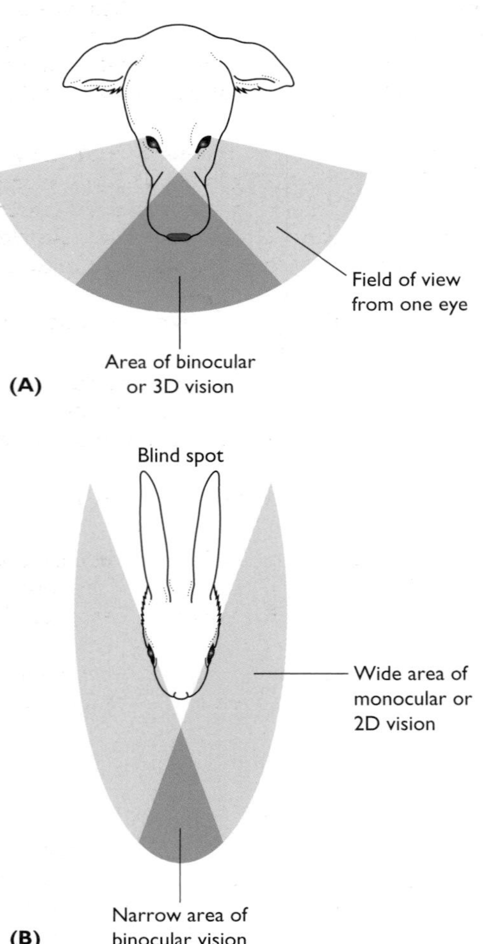

Fig. 5.13 Fields of vision. **(A)** Predator animal (e.g., dog). **(B)** Prey animal (e.g., rabbit).

The eyeball

The eyeball (Fig. 5.14) is a globe-shaped structure made of three layers:

1. The *sclera*
2. The *uvea*
3. The *retina*

Sclera

The *sclera* forms the fibrous outer covering of the eye, in conjunction with the *cornea.*

- *Cornea* forms the transparent anterior part of the eye and bulges slightly outwards from the orbit. It has a poor blood supply but is well supplied with sensory nerve fibres. The outer surface is covered in a layer of squamous epithelium, the *conjunctiva.* The cornea is the first part of the eye to be hit by rays of light and is involved in focusing these on to the retina.
- *Sclera* is dull white in colour and consists of dense fibrous connective tissue and elastic fibres into which the extrinsic muscles insert. Its function is to protect the delicate internal structures of the eye and to maintain the eye shape.

The junction between the cornea and sclera is known as the *limbus.* This is the drainage point for the aqueous humour of the anterior chamber of the eye.

Uvea

The *uvea*, a vascular pigmented layer, is firmly attached to the sclera at the exit of the optic nerve but is less well attached in other areas (Fig. 5.14). It is made up of the following parts:

- *Choroid* is the darkly pigmented vascular lining of the eye which takes up approximately two-thirds of the uvea. It contains the blood vessels supplying all the internal structures of the eyeball. The pigmented cells prevent light rays escaping through the eyeball.

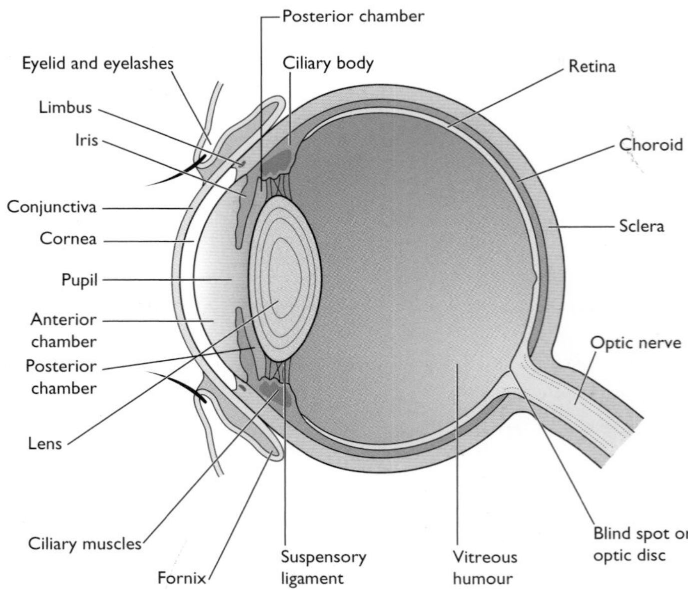

Fig. 5.14 Structure of the canine and feline eye.

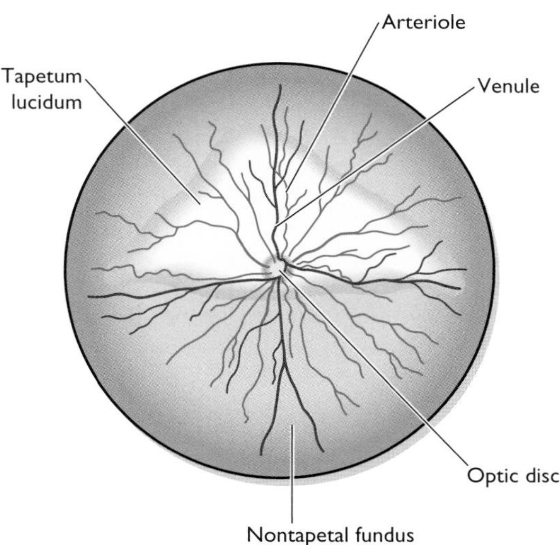

Fig. 5.15 The retina of the canine eye, showing the area of the tapetum lucidum.

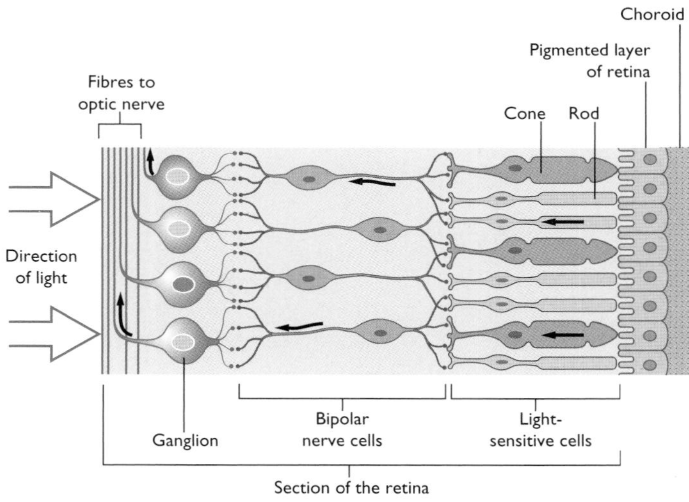

Fig. 5.16 Structure of the retina (cross-section).

- *Tapetum lucidum* is a triangular area of yellow-green iridescent light-reflecting cells lying dorsal to the point at which the optic nerve leaves the eye (Fig. 5.15). Its function is to reflect light back to the photoreceptor cells of the retina, making use of low light levels and improving night vision. The tapetum lucidum is well developed in carnivores but is present in most mammals except humans and pigs.
- *Ciliary body* is a thickened structure projecting towards the centre of the eye. It contains smooth muscle fibres – the *ciliary muscle* – that control the thickness and shape of the lens.
- *Suspensory ligament* is a continuation of the ciliary body forming a circular support around the perimeter of the lens.
- *Iris* is an anterior continuation of the ciliary body containing both radial and circular smooth muscle fibres (Fig. 5.14). Its free edge forms the hole in the centre, the *pupil.* The dog has a circular pupil while the cat has a vertical slit. Pigmented cells in the iris give it a characteristic range of colours. The nerve supply to the iris is from the oculomotor nerve (III) and it also receives sympathetic and parasympathetic nerve fibres. The function of the iris is to regulate the amount of light entering the eye.

Retina

The retina is the innermost layer of the eye. Light is focused onto the photoreceptor or light-sensitive cells of the retina by the lens and information is transmitted to the brain via the optic nerve (II). The retina is made of several layers (Fig. 5.16). Light travels through the outer layers before it stimulates the deeper photoreceptor cells.

From the layer closest to the choroid the retina layers are as follows:

- *Pigmented layer* prevents light leaking out of the eyeball. This augments the effect of the pigments cells within the choroid.
- *Photoreceptor cells* are named according to their shape:
  - *Rods* are sensitive to low light levels but not to colour; they provide black and white and night vision.
  - *Cones* are sensitive to bright light; they provide colour vision.

The photoreceptor cells of dogs and cats are made up of 95% rods and 5% cones. This means that they see different degrees of light and shade, but colour vision is poorly developed.

- *Bipolar neurons* gather information from the rods and cones and transmit it to the next layer.
- *Ganglion cells* may be as many as 1×10^6 cells. Their axons travel across the surface of the retina towards the *optic disc,* where they form the optic nerve (II). At this point there are no rods and cones and for this reason it is also known as the *blind spot* (Fig. 5.14).

Within the centre of the eye is the *lens,* a transparent biconvex disc surrounded by the suspensory ligament and the ciliary body (Fig. 5.14). The tissue of the lens is crystalline and elastic, and its shape is altered by the contraction of the ciliary muscles around it. This enables the lens to focus rays of light onto the retina.

The iris divides the anterior part of the eye into two chambers:

- *Anterior chamber* lies between the iris and the cornea. It contains a clear watery fluid known as *aqueous humour,* which is secreted by the ciliary body and drains out of the eye via the limbus.
- *Posterior chamber* lies between the iris and lens and also contains *aqueous humour.*

The posterior part of the eye lying between the lens and the retina is known as the *vitreous chamber.* This occupies 80% of the volume of the eye and contains a clear, jelly-like substance known as *vitreous humour.*

The function of both the aqueous and vitreous humours is to provide nutrients for the structures within the eye and to maintain the shape of the eye.

The extrinsic muscles

The eyeball is well supplied with extrinsic muscles (see Chapter 4, Fig. 4.5). These originate on the connective tissue of the sclera and insert on the periosteum of the bones forming the orbit of the skull. They are essential for the fine movements of the eyeballs, which must be coordinated so that the eyes work together to achieve accurate binocular or 3D vision. The nerve supply to the extrinsic muscles is via the oculomotor (III), trochlear (IV) and abducens (VI) nerves.

In some medical conditions, such as diabetes mellitus, or as a result of old age or genetic factors, the lens may develop a **cataract**. The lens becomes opaque, which interferes with the passage of light rays to the retina, and the animal becomes blind. In some cases, the condition may be able to be treated by removal of the lens but the animal will then only have distance vision.

Glaucoma, or an increase in intraocular pressure, results if there is overproduction of aqueous humour or blockage of the fluid drainage point at the limbus of the eye. It may also be a symptom of hypertension, as seen in cats with chronic renal failure. Intraocular pressure is measured using a tonometer.

The eyelids

The bony orbit of the skull protects the majority of the eyeball but the anterior third is soft, relatively protuberant and at risk from mechanical damage. It is protected by a set of eyelids and associated glands. Each eye has an upper and lower eyelid joined at the *medial canthus* adjacent to the nose and at the *lateral canthus* (Fig. 5.17). The upper eyelid is more mobile than the lower one. Each eyelid is covered by hairy skin on the outer surface and lined by a layer of mucous membrane on the inner surface. This layer is continuous with the conjunctiva covering the cornea. The point where it reflects back is known as the *fornix* (Fig. 5.14). The inner surface of the eyelids is protected and lubricated by the *Meibomian glands.* Growing from the outer edge of the upper eyelids are well-defined *cilia*, resembling human eyelashes. These may be present but less obvious on the lower lids. Associated with these are sebaceous and rudimentary sweat glands.

In the dog, the following conditions associated with the eyelashes may be inherited characteristics:

- **Entropion**: The edges of the eyelids turn inwards, causing the eyelashes to scratch the cornea; seen in the Labrador, Cocker Spaniel and Sharpei.
- **Ectropion**: The edge of the eyelid droops down, revealing an area of mucous membrane, which becomes dry and inflamed; seen in soft-eyed breeds such as the St Bernard and Bloodhound.
- **Distichiasis**: Extra or ectopic eyelashes grow along the margin of the eyelids and scratch the cornea.

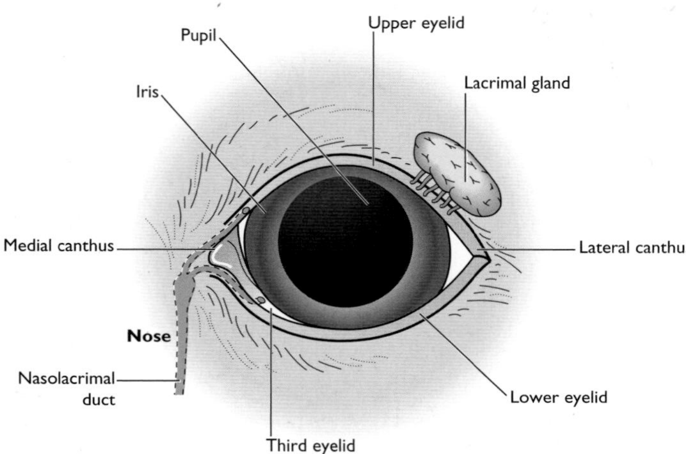

Fig. 5.17 External anatomy of the left eye.

Within the tissue of the eyelids are the *palpebral muscles* responsible for eyelid movement. The palpebral or blink reflex protects the eye from damage and is a useful means of assessing the depth of anaesthesia; it disappears as the level of anaesthesia deepens. Deep to the upper and lower eyelids, and lying in the medial canthus of each eye, is the *third eyelid* or *nictitating membrane.* In the dog, it is a T-shaped piece of hyaline cartilage and smooth muscle; in the cat it is made of elastic cartilage and smooth muscle. The third eyelid is covered on both sides by mucous membrane, which is continuous with the lining of the eyelids and the cornea. It is supplied with glandular and lymphoid tissue to protect the eye and keep it moist. Nerve supply to the third eye is via the sympathetic system.

The surface of the cornea is kept moist and protected from damage by the *lacrimal gland,* a modified cutaneous gland lying on the dorsolateral surface of eyeball beneath the upper eyelid (Fig. 5.17). This produces secretions known as tears, which flow over the anterior surface of the eye and drain into two small openings in the area of the medial canthus. These openings lead into the *nasolacrimal duct,* which leaves the bony orbit and runs through the nasal cavity to open into the nostril.

The **Harderian glands** lie underneath the third eyelid and contribute to the lubricating and protective function of tears. In some dogs, particularly in brachycephalic breeds such as the bulldog, the Harderian glands may become enlarged and protrude from under the third eyelid. This is a condition often referred to as 'cherry eye' because the inflamed gland resembles a cherry. The treatment may be to attempt to push the gland back behind the eyelid or to remove it completely.

Formation of an image

The function of the eye is to conduct rays of light from an object and form an image on the retina (Fig. 5.18). This occurs in the following stages:

1. The light rays pass through the cornea, which plays some part in directing them onto the retina.
2. The light rays pass through the pupil. The size of the pupil is controlled by the iris in response to the intensity of the light; this is the *pupillary reflex.* Constriction and dilation of the pupil are controlled by the autonomic nervous system.
3. The light rays strike the lens. The curvature of the lens is altered by the ciliary muscles and the rays converge to a sharp point on the retina; they are said to be *focused.*
4. The light rays strike the retina and pass through the layers of cells until they hit the *photoreceptor cells.* These are stimulated and send nerve impulses along the nerve fibres that form the optic nerve (II). Information is carried to the visual cortex of the cerebral hemispheres and is interpreted as an image. The image formed on the retina is inverted but the brain processes the information making use of other sensations and interprets it as the correct way up.
5. Some of the light is reflected back to the photoreceptor cells by the *tapetum lucidum.* This makes optimum use of lower light levels.

The ability to *accommodate*, or change the shape of the lens to focus on near and far objects, develops soon after birth. As the lens ages and becomes less flexible, the time taken for accommodation increases. In humans this can be corrected by the use of

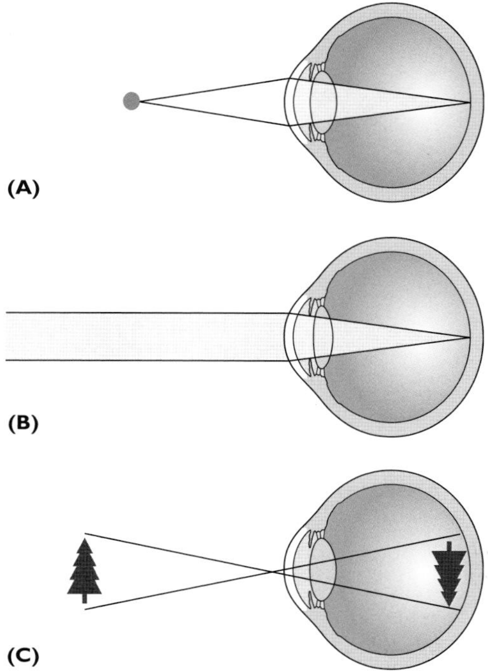

Fig. 5.18 Formation of the visual image. **(A)** Light rays from close objects are diverging (spreading out) as they reach the eye. The light is focussed by contraction of the ciliary muscles, which causes the lens to shorten and flatten, bending the light onto the retina. **(B)** Light rays from distant objects are effectively parallel as they reach the eye. These rays are focussed by relaxation of the ciliary muscles, which causes the lens to elongate and thin. **(C)** The image on the retina is upside down when it forms; the brain inverts this, allowing normal perception of the image the correct way up.

glasses, but animals must learn to adapt their behaviour to cope with this 'old age' change.

The ear: hearing and balance

The ear is the organ of hearing and balance. Receptor cells adapted to respond to sound waves and to the movement of the body are located within the inner ear. All mammals have a pair of ears located on the dorsal part of the head. Each ear can be divided into three parts:

- External ear
- Middle ear
- Inner ear

The external ear

This consists of the following structures:

- The *pinna* is a funnel-shaped plate of cartilage whose functions are:
  - To guide sound waves picked up from the external environment down the external auditory meatus to the tympanic membrane (ear drum)
  - To act as a means of facial expression and communication between animals of the same species. Pinnae are used in conjunction with other parts of the body (e.g., the eyes and tail) to communicate dominance, fear, acceptance, and so on.

The pinna varies in size and shape between breeds and has been altered by generations of selective breeding, leading to the development of characteristics many of which predispose to ear disease. The original wolf-like dog, from which all breeds are thought to be derived, has upright V-shaped ears; this is still seen in German Shepherds, Chows and Huskies. All cats have upright pointed ears that, until the recent introduction of the Scottish Fold with its twisted, flattened ear pinnae, have been left untouched by selection.

Each pinna is formed from a sheet of elastic cartilage known as the *auricular cartilage*. This continues as an incomplete tube known as the *external auditory meatus* linked at the base to the *annular cartilage*. This in turn articulates with the external acoustic process of the *tympanic bulla*, forming a series of interlinking cartilages that enable the pinna to move freely to pick up sound waves.

Both sides of the auricular cartilage are covered in hairy skin; in most breeds the outer side is more hairy than the inner side. The covering of skin continues into the external auditory meatus where there are fewer hair follicles; the Poodle is particularly noted for its hairy ear canals. The skin is well supplied with *ceruminous glands*, modified sebaceous glands that secrete wax and protect the ear canal from damage and infection.

- The *external auditory meatus* may also be called the external ear canal. The opening of the canal faces dorsolaterally; it runs vertically down the side of the skull – the *vertical canal* – and then turns inwards to run horizontally – the *horizontal canal*. The canal ends at a delicate sheet of tissue known as the *tympanic membrane* or *ear drum*.

Otitis externa, or infection of the ear canal, is a common condition in dogs and cats. It may be caused by a variety of microorganisms, such as ear mites (*Otodectes cynotis*), bacteria and fungi, such as *Malassezia pachydermatis*. The shape of the pinna and the presence of hair may predispose to infection by creating a hot, airless environment within the ear canal. Infection results in pain, aural discharge, self-trauma and, in some cases, aural haematoma.

The ear canal is lined in normal skin. If an animal is suffering from a skin condition, the ear canal may also be affected. This is particularly true of hormonal skin conditions, such as that seen in Cushing's disease, when the patient may also have otitis externa.

The middle ear

The middle ear (Fig. 5.19) consists of:

- The *tympanic cavity*, which lies within the *tympanic bulla* of the petrous temporal bone of the skull. It is lined with ciliated columnar mucous membrane and is filled with air. In the dorsal part of the cavity are the *auditory ossicles*. Opening into the cavity is the *Eustachian* or *auditory tube*. This is a short canal that connects the nasopharynx to the middle ear and whose function is to equalise air pressure on either side of the tympanic membrane.
- The *tympanic membrane* or ear drum forms the boundary between the external and middle ears at the end of the external auditory meatus. It is a thin, semi-transparent, oval membrane whose function is to convey the vibrations caused by sound waves from the external auditory meatus to the auditory ossicles.

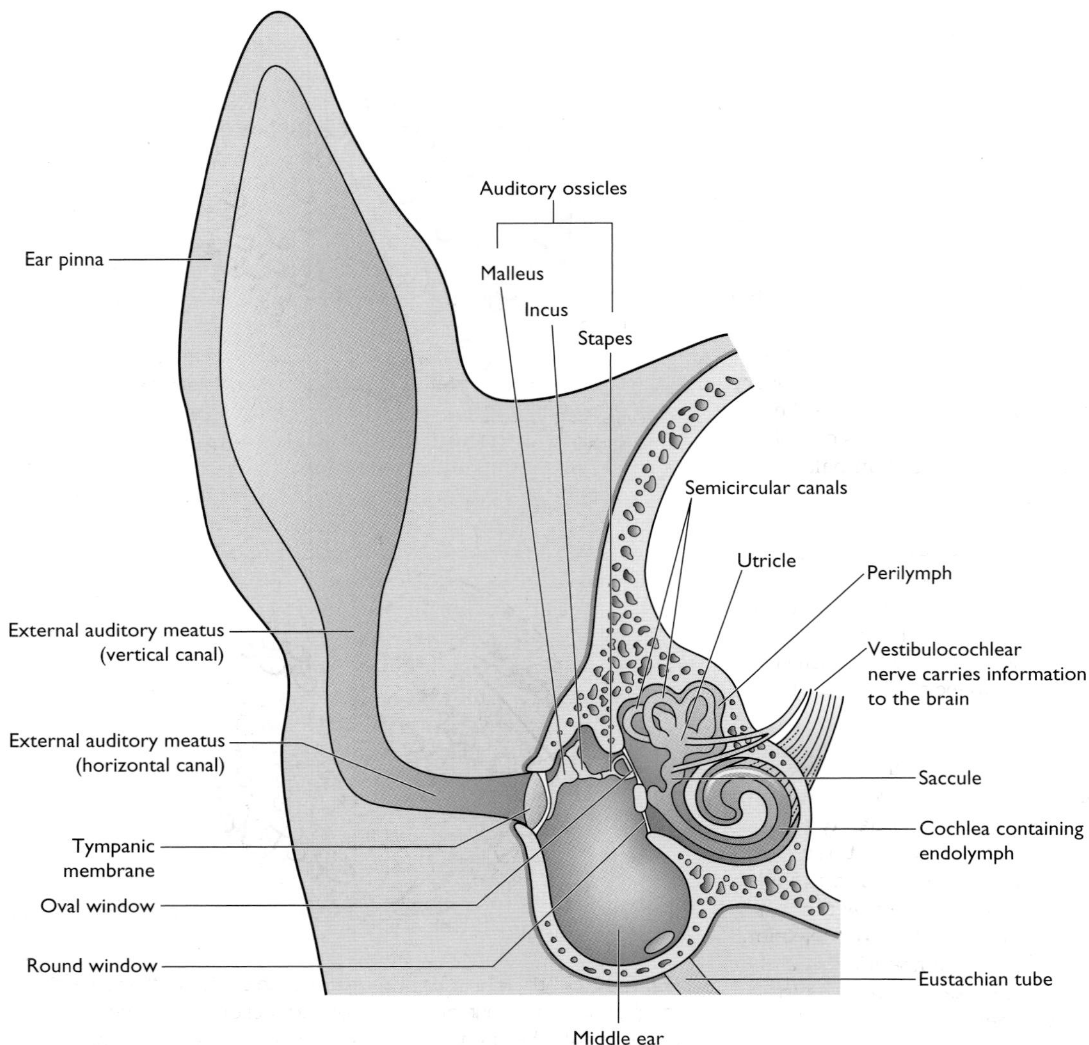

Fig. 5.19 Section through the canine or feline ear.

- The *auditory ossicles* are three small bones forming a flexible chain that connect the tympanic membrane to the oval window of the inner ear. The bones are linked by synovial joints and are known as:
  - *Malleus*, or hammer, in contact with the tympanic membrane
  - *Incus*, or anvil
  - *Stapes*, or stirrup, in contact with the oval window

The function of the ossicles is to transmit the vibrations caused by sound waves across the middle ear to the inner ear.

The inner ear

The inner ear (Fig. 5.19) consists of:

- The *bony labyrinth*, which lies within the petrous temporal bone. It is divided into three areas – the bony cochlea, bony vestibule and bony semicircular canals – each of which contains a corresponding part of the membranous labyrinth. It contains *perilymph*, which flows around the outside of the membranous labyrinth. The bony labyrinth is linked to the middle ear by two membranes:
  - *Round window*, also called the cochlear window, lies between the bony cochlea and the centre of the tympanic cavity.
  - *Oval window*, also known as the vestibular window, lies between the bony vestibule and the dorsal part of the tympanic cavity; the stapes is in contact with this membrane.
- The *membranous labyrinth* is a system of interconnecting tubes filled with a fluid known as *endolymph*. Inside the structure are sensory receptor cells adapted to respond to sound and movement. The shape of the membranous labyrinth corresponds to the bony labyrinth but does not completely fill it. There are three parts:
  - *Membranous cochlea* has a similar shape to a snail's shell. It forms a blind-ending ventral spiral and is filled with endolymph. Within the cochlea are a group of sensory receptor cells forming the spiral *organ of Corti*, whose function is to detect sound. Projecting from each receptor cell is a sensory hair and at the base is a nerve fibre that is part of the cochlear branch of the vestibulocochlear nerve (VIII).

Perception of sound. Sound waves, picked up by the pinna and transmitted across the ear by the tympanic membrane and auditory ossicles to the oval window, set up vibrations or ripples first in the perilymph and then the endolymph. These ripples move the sensory hairs of the receptor cells in the organ of Corti, and this sends nerve impulses along their associated nerve fibres. The impulses are carried by the cochlear branch of the vestibulocochlear nerve (VIII) to the auditory cortex of the cerebral hemispheres, where they are interpreted as sound.

- *Membranous vestibule* is made of two sac-like structures, the utricle (Fig. 5.20) and saccule, which connect with the cochlea and the semicircular canals and are filled with endolymph. Both these structures contain areas of sensory hair cells known as maculae, surrounded by jelly-like material containing calcium carbonate particles or *otoliths*. The function of these structures is to maintain balance when the animal is standing still.

Static balance. When an animal is *standing still*, the head still makes minute movements. The pull of gravity moves the jelly-like material within the maculae of the utricle and saccule. This moves the sensory hairs, which transmit nerve impulses to the brain via the vestibular branch of the vestibulocochlear nerve (VIII). The brain interprets this information in terms of the position of the body in relation to the space around it.

- *Membranous semicircular canals* are three canals filled with endolymph, each of which describes two-thirds of a circle. The plane of each circle is approximately at right angles to the other two; in this way, the three dimensions of movement are monitored. Each canal is connected to the utricle by a swollen area known as an *ampulla*. Inside each ampulla is a cone-shaped projection or *crista* containing sensory hair cells embedded in a jelly-like *cupula*. The function of these structures is to maintain balance during movement.

Dynamic balance. As the animal *moves*, the endolymph in the semicircular canals moves and stimulates the cristae within the ampullae. Nerve impulses are transmitted by the hair cells to the brain via the vestibular branch of the vestibulocochlear nerve (VIII). Within the brain, they are passed to the cerebellum, where the information is coordinated.

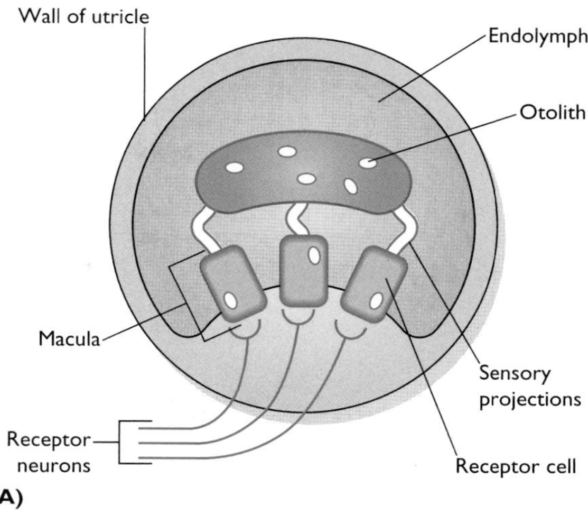

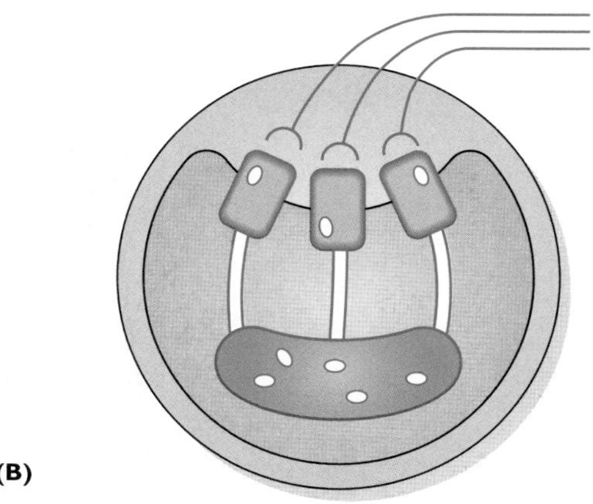

Fig. 5.20 Simplified section through an utricle. **(A)** With the head upright, there is no pull on the sensory projections of the utricle. **(B)** When the head is tilted or upside down, the otoliths fall away from the macula. The sensory projections become stretched and this causes impulses to be set up in the receptor cells. These are transmitted to the brain in the receptor neurons, giving information about the orientation of the head.

Endocrine system

KEY POINTS

- The endocrine system is part of the regulatory system of the body and works in conjunction with the nervous system. The nervous system produces an immediate response while the endocrine system produces a slower but longer-lasting effect.
- Endocrine glands secrete hormones, which are carried by the blood to specific target organs.
- Each target organ responds only to a particular hormone or to a group of hormones and is unaffected by other hormones.
- Hormonal secretion is controlled by different mechanisms (e.g., levels of a chemical in the blood), or by a feedback loop.
- Each hormone has a specific effect and many interrelate with other hormones to create a complex network that acts to maintain homeostasis.

Basic functions and hormones

The endocrine system forms part of the regulatory system of the body and works in conjunction with the other regulatory mechanism, the nervous system. A series of *endocrine glands* secrete chemical messengers known as *hormones*, which are carried by the blood to their *target organs*. These may be some distance away from the gland. In contrast, exocrine glands produce secretions that are released via ducts and lie close to their effector organs (e.g., sweat glands, gastric glands).

Chemically, hormones may be steroids, proteins or amines (derived from amino acids). They regulate the activity of the target organ, which responds to that particular hormone. All other organs are unaffected. The response produced by hormones is slower and lasts longer, and complements the rapid and relatively short-lived responses produced by the nervous system.

The endocrine glands are distributed throughout the body and may secrete more than one hormone (Fig. 6.1).

The glands are:

- Pituitary gland
- Thyroid gland
- Parathyroid glands
- Pancreas
- Ovaries
- Testes
- Adrenal glands

Secretion of a hormone occurs in response to a specific stimulus (Table 6.1). Stimuli may be:

- Nerve impulses: Adrenaline (epinephrine), for example, is released from the adrenal medulla in response to nerve impulses from the sympathetic nervous system.
- A stimulating or releasing hormone, e.g., TSH, thyrotrophic/thyroid-stimulating hormone, from the anterior pituitary gland activates the thyroid gland.
- Levels of certain chemicals in the blood, e.g., raised blood glucose levels, stimulate the release of insulin from the pancreas.
- Feedback loops prevent oversecretion or reduce secretion once the effect has been achieved; for example, oestrogen from the ovarian follicles prevents further secretion of follicle-stimulating hormone from the anterior pituitary gland, so preventing further follicular development (see Fig. 6.4).

Not all hormones are secreted by endocrine glands; some are produced from tissue within another organ, including:

- *Gastrin* is produced by the wall of the stomach. As food enters the stomach via the cardiac sphincter, gastrin stimulates the release of gastric juices from the gastric glands and digestion begins.
- *Secretin*, is produced by the wall of the small intestine. As food enters the duodenum from the stomach, secretin stimulates the secretion of intestinal and pancreatic juices, which continue the process of digestion.
- *Chorionic gonadotrophin* is produced during pregnancy by the ectodermal layer of the chorion surrounding the conceptus. It helps to maintain the corpus luteum in the ovary throughout gestation.
- *Erythropoietin* or *erythropoietic-stimulating factor* is produced by the kidney in response to low levels of blood oxygen. It stimulates the bone marrow to produce erythrocytes or red blood cells.

Endocrine glands

Pituitary gland

This is a small gland lying ventral to the hypothalamus in the forebrain (Fig. 6.1). It is also known as the hypophysis and is divided into two lobes, each of which acts as a separate gland. The pituitary gland is often referred to as the 'master gland' because its hormones control the secretions of many of the other endocrine glands.

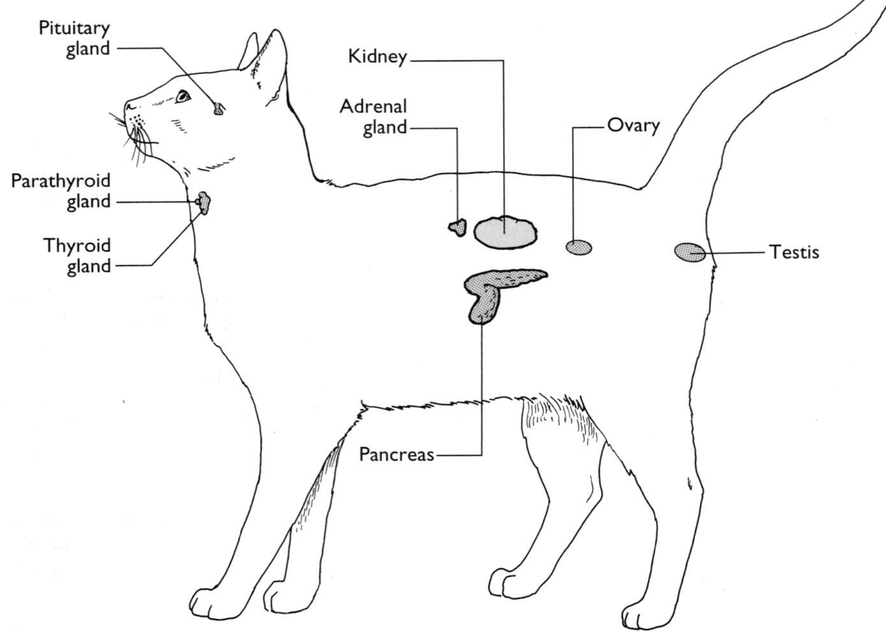

Fig. 6.1 Locations of important endocrine glands in the cat. (With permission from T Colville, JM Bassett, 2001. Clinical anatomy and physiology for veterinary technicians. St Louis, MO: Mosby, p 290.)

Anterior pituitary gland

Also known as the *adenohypophysis*, this produces:

- *Thyrotrophic/thyroid stimulating hormone* (TSH) stimulates the thyroid gland.
- *Growth hormone* or *somatotrophin* controls the rate of growth in young animals by:
  - Controlling the rate of growth at the epiphyses of the bones
  - Being involved in protein production from amino acids
  - Regulating the use of energy during periods of poor food supply. Glucose is conserved for use by the nervous system and fat is broken down to be used as a source of energy by the rest of the body.
- *Adrenocorticotrophic hormone* (ACTH) stimulates the adrenal cortex. Oversecretion may cause the symptoms of Cushing's disease.
- *Prolactin* stimulates the development of the mammary glands and the secretion of milk during the latter half of pregnancy. The milk cannot be released unless oxytocin is secreted at the end of the gestation period.
- *Follicle stimulating hormone* (FSH): At the start of the oestrous cycle, or at puberty, external factors, such as day length (photoperiod), temperature or pheromones secreted by the male or other females, affect the hypothalamus. This secretes *gonadotrophin-releasing hormone*, which stimulates the anterior pituitary gland to secrete FSH. FSH stimulates germ cells in the ovary to develop into follicles, each containing an ovum (Fig. 6.4; also see Chapter 11).
- *Luteinising hormone* (LH): Secretion is stimulated by the presence of oestrogen in the blood. LH stimulates the ripe follicles in the ovary to rupture and release their ova (ovulation). The remaining tissue becomes 'luteinised' to form the corpus luteum (Fig. 6.4.; also see Chapter 11).
- *Interstitial cell stimulating hormone* (ICSH) stimulates the interstitial cells or cells of Leydig in the testis to secrete testosterone. This is the male equivalent of LH.

Posterior pituitary gland

The posterior pituitary gland is also known as the *neurohypophysis*. The hormones associated with this part of the pituitary gland are secreted by the hypothalamus and only stored here. They are:

- *Antidiuretic hormone* (ADH), also called vasopressin, alters the permeability of the collecting ducts of the kidney to water. It is secreted in response to the changing volume of extracellular fluid (ECF) and helps maintain homeostasis (see Chapter 10).
- *Oxytocin* has two effects:
  - It acts on the mammary glands during late pregnancy and causes the milk to be released or 'let down' in response to suckling by the neonate.
  - At the end of gestation, oxytocin causes the contraction of the smooth muscle of the uterus, resulting in parturition and delivery of the fetuses.

Diabetes insipidus: This presents as polydipsia, polyphagia and production of urine with a specific gravity of around 1.00 (normal SG in the dog is 1.018–1.045). The condition may be a result of undersecretion of ADH from the posterior pituitary gland or failure of the renal tissue to respond to the hormone that controls the concentration of urine in the renal collecting ducts. Diagnosis is confirmed by the water deprivation test and treatment relies on the daily administration of ADH drops, which may not always be obtainable.

Thyroid glands

These lie in the midline on the ventral aspect of the first few rings of the trachea (Fig. 6.1). They are controlled by TSH from the anterior pituitary gland and secrete three hormones:

- *Thyroxin* (or T_4) and *tri-iodothyronine* (or T_3) have a similar effect. Tri-iodothyronine contains a high proportion of the trace element iodine; a lack of iodine in the diet can have a dramatic effect. Both hormones affect the uptake of oxygen by all the cells in the body and are essential for normal growth.

Table 6.1 Endocrine glands and their associated hormones

Endocrine gland	Hormone(s)	Stimulus for secretion	Main actions
Pituitary – anterior	1. TSH	Hypothalamus	Stimulates release of thyroid hormone
	2. Growth hormone (somatotrophin)	Hypothalamus	Controls epiphyseal growth and protein production; regulates the use of energy
	3. Adrenocorticotrophic hormone (ACTH)	Hypothalamus	Controls release of adrenocortical hormones
	4. Prolactin		
	5. Follicle-stimulating hormone (FSH)	Photoperiod, environmental temperature and pheromones all affect the hypothalamus	Stimulates development of mammary glands and secretion of milk Stimulates development of follicles in the ovary
	6. Luteinising hormone (LH)	Oestrogen secreted by the ovarian follicles	Causes rupture of the follicles (ovulation) and development of the corpus luteum
	7. Interstitial-cell-stimulating hormone (ICSH). Male equivalent of LH		Stimulates secretion of testosterone from interstitial cells of the testis
Pituitary – posterior	1. Antidiuretic hormone (ADH)	Status of extracellular fluid and plasma	Acts on collecting ducts of the kidney – alters permeability to water
	2. Oxytocin		Stimulates uterine contractions during parturition; milk 'let down'
Thyroid	1. Thyroxin	TSH	Controls metabolic rate and is essential for normal growth
	2. Calcitonin	Raised blood calcium levels	Decreases resorption of calcium from the bones
Parathyroid	Parathormone	Lowered blood calcium levels	Stimulates calcium resorption from bones; promotes calcium uptake from intestine
Pancreas	1. Insulin	Raised blood glucose levels – particularly after feeding	Increases uptake of glucose into the cells; stores excess glucose as glycogen in the liver
	2. Glucagon	Lowered blood glucose levels	Release of stored glycogen from the liver to be converted into glucose
	3. Somatostatin		Mild inhibition of insulin and glucagon; prevents wild swings in blood glucose levels
Ovary			
A. Follicle	Oestrogen	FSH	Signs of oestrus; preparation of the reproductive tract and external genitalia for coitus
B. Corpus luteum	1. Progesterone	LH	Preparation of reproductive tract for pregnancy; development of mammary glands; maintains the pregnancy.
	2. Relaxin		Released during late pregnancy; causes relaxation of pelvic ligaments prior to birth
Testis	Testosterone	ICSH	Male characteristics and behaviour; sperm development
Adrenal			
A. Cortex	Glucocorticoids	ACTH	Raises blood glucose levels; reduces the inflammatory response
	Mineralocorticoids – aldosterone	Status of ECF and plasma	Acts on distal convoluted tubules of the kidney – regulates uptake of sodium and hydrogen ions
	Sex hormones		Small quantities
B. Medulla	Adrenaline (epinephrine) and noradrenaline (norepinephrine)	Sympathetic nervous system	Fear, fright, flight syndrome

Undersecretion of thyroid hormones – *hypothyroidism* – is more common in dogs. In young animals, hypothyroidism causes dwarfism (stunted growth). In older animals, the condition is known as myxoedema: the dog becomes fat and sluggish, alopecic, the skin feels cold and clammy and the heart rate slows, all due to a reduced metabolic rate.

Oversecretion – *hyperthyroidism* – is more common in old cats. The affected animal is thin, active, often aggressive, has a good appetite and a fast heart rate, all due to a raised metabolic rate.

- *Calcitonin* lowers the levels of blood calcium by decreasing the rate of bone resorption. When levels of blood calcium are high (e.g., if a calcium-rich diet is eaten), calcium is deposited in the bone and acts as a reservoir for later use (Fig. 6.2). Calcitonin has an opposite effect to parathormone but is of less importance.

Parathyroid glands

These glands lie on either side of the thyroid gland and secrete the hormone *parathormone* (Fig. 6.1). Secretion is dependent on

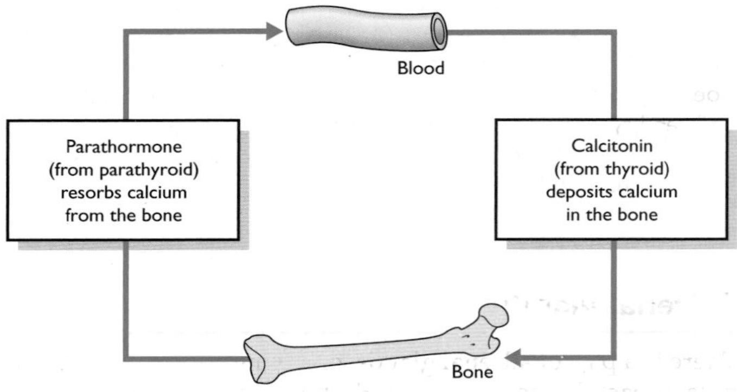

Fig. 6.2 Control of blood calcium levels by calcitonin and parathormone.

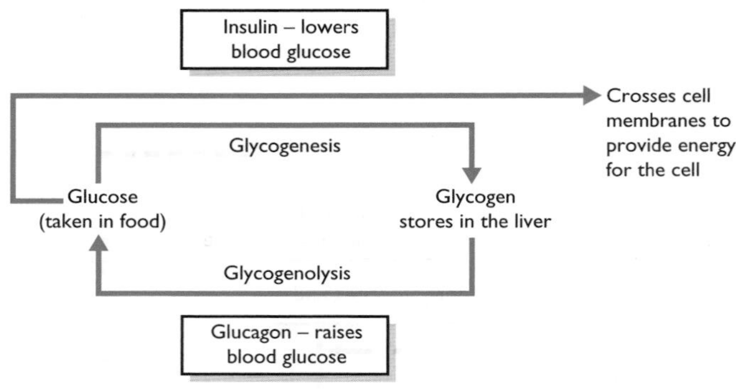

Fig. 6.3 Control of blood glucose levels.

the levels of calcium in the blood. If levels are low, calcium is resorbed from the bones and absorption of calcium from the intestine is increased (Fig. 6.2).

Oversecretion (*hyperparathyroidism*) occurs in:

- *Primary hyperparathyroidism*, due to neoplasia of the parathyroid glands. This causes bone resorption, bone weakness and pathological fractures.
- *Secondary hyperparathyroidism*, as seen in chronic renal failure. The calcium:phosphate ratio in the blood is altered by impaired kidney function. This leads to increased output of parathormone and consequently increased resorption of bone in an effort to maintain blood calcium levels. There is preferential resorption from the mandible and maxilla, producing a condition known as 'rubber jaw' – the jaw becomes pliable and fragile and the teeth may fall out.
- *Nutritional hyperparathyroidism* results from low-calcium diets (e.g., an all-meat diet). Parathormone is produced in an attempt to raise the blood calcium levels by bone resorption.

Pancreas

The pancreas is a pinkish lobular gland lying in the loop of the duodenum in the abdominal cavity (Fig. 6.1). It has an exocrine part and an endocrine part and is described as being a *mixed gland*. The exocrine secretions, which are digestive juices, enter the duodenum via the pancreatic duct (see Chapter 9). The endocrine secretions are produced by discrete areas of tissue within the exocrine tissue, known as the *islets of Langerhans*.

The islets of Langerhans secrete three hormones, each from a different type of cell:

- *Insulin* (from the beta cells) is secreted in response to high blood glucose levels. Insulin lowers blood glucose levels by:
  - Increasing the uptake of glucose into the cells, where it is metabolised to provide energy
  - Storing excess glucose as glycogen in the liver. Conversion of glucose to glycogen occurs by a process known as *glycogenesis* (Fig. 6.3).

Diabetes mellitus: This results from a lack of insulin and is a condition in which the animal suffers from hyperglycaemia and glucosuria (the presence of glucose in the urine). If left untreated, the condition may progress to a stage where the body uses its protein and fat stores as a source of energy. Daily insulin injections and dietary control are necessary to control the condition.

- *Glucagon* (from the alpha cells) is secreted in response to low blood glucose levels. Glucagon raises blood glucose levels by breaking down the glycogen stores in the liver. Conversion of glycogen to glucose occurs (Fig. 6.3).
- *Somatostatin* (from the delta cells) is mildly inhibitory to the secretions of insulin and glucagon and prevents wild fluctuations in blood glucose levels, which may damage the tissues. It also decreases gut motility and the secretion of digestive juices, which serve to reduce the efficiency of the digestive and absorptive processes.

The ovary

Female mammals have two ovaries, which lie one on each side of the dorsal abdominal cavity caudal to the kidneys. At the onset of sexual maturity, the two ovaries become capable of secreting two hormones:

- *Oestrogen* is produced by the walls of the developing *ovarian follicles*. Development of germ cells in the ovary into ripe follicles is the result of the secretion of FSH from the anterior pituitary gland. Oestrogen causes the behaviour associated with the oestrous cycle and prepares the reproductive tract and external genitalia for mating (see Chapter 11). Oestrogen also exerts negative feedback on the anterior pituitary gland, preventing further secretion of FSH and further follicular development (Fig. 6.4).
- *Progesterone* is secreted by the *corpus luteum*, which develops from the remaining follicular tissue after the follicle has ovulated. The corpus luteum develops as a result of the production of LH from the anterior pituitary gland. Progesterone prepares the reproductive tract for pregnancy and maintains the pregnancy (see Chapter 11). During pregnancy, progesterone exerts negative feedback on the hypothalamus and prevents secretion of *gonadotrophin-releasing hormone* and so prevents further oestrous cycles until parturition occurs. It also causes development of the mammary glands during pregnancy (Fig. 6.4).

In the later stages of pregnancy, the corpus luteum also secretes a hormone known as *relaxin*. This causes the sacroiliac and other ligaments around the birth canal to soften and relax in preparation for parturition.

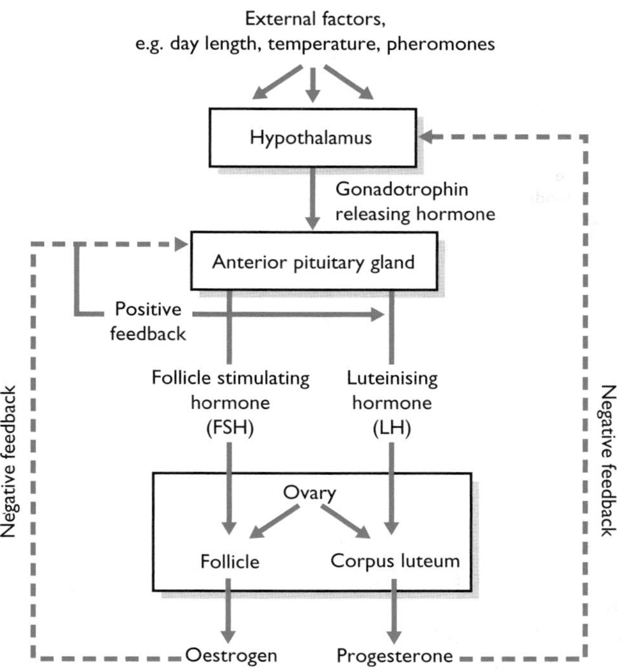

Fig. 6.4 Inter-relationships between the female reproductive hormones.

False or pseudopregnancy and pyometra are two conditions of the entire bitch that may result from the prolonged high levels of progesterone secreted by the corpus luteum of the bitch. The corpus luteum normally remains for about 42 days, which is much longer than in any other mammal. High levels of the hormone may cause a pregnancy-like state in some bitches, or in older individuals reduces the speed of the inflammatory response, resulting in failure to eliminate bacteria that may invade the uterine tissue, leading to the accumulation of pus and the absorption of bacterial toxins.

The testis

Male mammals possess a pair of testes, which are carried external to the abdominal cavity within the scrotum. At the start of sexual maturity, the testes begin to secrete two hormones:

- *Testosterone* is produced by the *interstitial cells* or *cells of Leydig* in response to the secretion of ICSH from the anterior pituitary gland. Testosterone is responsible for:
  - The development of male characteristics such as penis development, development of the barbs on the feline penis, muscle development, jowls on the face of a tomcat, size
  - Male behaviour patterns, such as sexual drive, aggression, territorial behaviour, courtship displays and mating behaviour
  - Development of spermatozoa
- *Oestrogen* is produced in small quantities by the *Sertoli cells* in the seminiferous tubules of the testes.

Sertoli cell tumour is a condition affecting older dogs or dogs with retained testes. The Sertoli cells proliferate and secrete high levels of oestrogen, resulting in feminisation syndrome. The clinical signs are bilateral symmetrical alopecia, gynaecomastia (enlarged mammary glands) and attractiveness to male dogs. The treatment is to castrate the patient.

Adrenal glands

There is a pair of adrenal glands, one lying close to the cranial pole of each kidney (Fig. 6.1). Each gland has an outer *cortex* and an inner *medulla*. There is no connection between the two parts and they can be considered as two separate glands.

Adrenal cortex

The hormones produced are known as *steroids* and have a similar structure based on lipid. There are three groups, each one being secreted by a different layer:

- *Glucocorticoids:* Secretion is regulated by ACTH from the anterior pituitary gland. The hormones are known as *corticosteroids*; the most important are *cortisol* and *corticosterone*. In the normal animal they are present in low levels but increase in response to stress. They have two main actions:
  - They increase blood glucose levels by reducing glucose uptake by the cells, increasing the conversion of amino acids to glucose in the liver (a process known as *gluconeogenesis*) and mobilising fatty acids from the adipose tissue ready for conversion to glucose.
  - When present in large quantities, they depress the inflammatory reaction, which delays healing and repair. This property is used therapeutically to reduce swelling and inflammation.

Cushing's disease is caused by oversecretion of glucocorticoids, or hyperadrenocorticalism. The clinical signs include polydipsia, polyuria, polyphagia, bilateral symmetrical alopecia, muscle wasting and a potbelly. The condition may result from oversecretion of ACTH from the anterior pituitary gland or from a tumour of the adrenal cortex. Treatment involves the removal of the neoplastic adrenal gland or suppression of the secretion of adrenocortical hormones by drugs such as trilostane.

- *Mineralocorticoids:* The most important is *aldosterone*. This acts on the distal convoluted tubule of the kidney where it regulates acid–base balance of the plasma and ECF by excretion of H^+ ions and also controls the excretion of Na^+ and K^+ ions (see Chapter 10).
- *Adrenal sex hormones:* Both male and female animals produce all types of sex hormones. They are secreted in insignificant quantities but may be the reason why some animals show a certain level of sexual behaviour despite being neutered.

Adrenal medulla

This produces two hormones with similar actions: *adrenaline* (epinephrine) and *noradrenaline* (norepinephrine). These hormones prepare the body for emergency action, known as the 'fear, flight, fight' syndrome, and are controlled by the sympathetic nervous system. Their actions are to:

- Raise blood glucose levels by the breakdown of glycogen stored in the liver – *glycogenolysis*. This increases the body's energy levels.
- Increase the heart rate and the rate and depth of respiration; this increases the amount of oxygen reaching the tissues.
- Dilate the blood vessels of the skeletal muscles; this enables the supply of glucose and oxygen to reach the areas where it is needed.
- Decrease the activity of the gastrointestinal tract and the bladder. In an emergency their functions are less important.

CHAPTER 7

Blood vascular system

KEY POINTS

- The blood vascular system consists of the blood, heart, circulatory system and lymphatic system.
- Blood is the liquid connective tissue that carries oxygen and nutrients to the tissues and returns waste products produced by the tissues during metabolism to the lungs, kidneys and liver.
- Blood is made up of a liquid part, plasma, containing all the dissolved substances carried around the body, and a cellular part. There are several types of blood cell, each of which differs in appearance and function.
- The blood is pumped around the body by a four-chambered muscular structure, the heart.
- The right side of the heart sends blood into the pulmonary circulation (i.e., the lungs), and the left side of the heart sends blood into the systemic circulation (i.e., the rest of the body).
- The right and left atria of the heart receive blood from the lungs or the rest of the body, while the right and left ventricles pump blood out to the lungs or the rest of the body.
- The circulatory system consists of a network of arteries, capillaries and veins that supply every tissue and organ of the body.
- Arteries have thick walls and carry oxygenated blood under pressure away from the heart. The exception is the pulmonary artery, which carries deoxygenated blood from the heart to the lungs.
- Veins have thinner walls and carry deoxygenated blood towards the heart. The exception is the pulmonary vein, which carries oxygenated blood from the lungs to the heart.
- All mammals have a double circulation – the systemic and the pulmonary circulations. Blood passes through the heart twice during one complete circuit of the body.
- The lymphatic system collects excess tissue fluid or lymph in a network of lymphatic vessels and returns it to the circulatory system close to the heart.
- As the lymph is carried along the vessels it passes through a series of lymph nodes, which filter out any foreign particles or pathogens. These are 'monitored' by lymphocytes within the lymphoid tissue and the immune system produces a specific response to combat any potential threat to the health of the animal.

The blood vascular system is made up of four parts:

1. *Blood* is a fluid connective tissue that transports oxygen and nutrients around the body and collects waste products produced by the tissues.
2. The *heart* is a hollow, muscular, four-chambered organ responsible for pumping blood around the body.
3. The *circulatory system* is a network of arteries, veins and capillaries in which the blood flows around the body.
4. The *lymphatic system* is a network of lymphatic vessels that transports lymph or excess tissue fluid around the body and is responsible for returning it to the circulation.

Blood

Blood is a highly specialised fluid connective tissue (see Chapter 2), consisting of several types of cell suspended in a liquid medium called *plasma*. Blood makes up about 7% of the total body weight and has a pH of about 7.4 (7.35–7.45).

Functions

Blood has many functions within the body but they can be broadly divided into two groups: transport and regulation.

Transport

- *Gases in solution*: Blood carries oxygenated blood from the lungs and delivers the oxygen to the tissues where it is used. It then collects deoxygenated blood containing carbon dioxide produced by the tissues during their metabolic processes, and carries it back to the lungs, where the carbon dioxide is exchanged for oxygen in the inspired air.
- *Nutrients*: Blood transports nutrients (e.g., amino acids, fatty acids and glucose), which result from the process of digestion, from the digestive system to the liver and to the tissues where they are needed.
- *Waste products*: Blood collects the waste products (e.g., urea and creatinine) resulting from metabolism in the tissues and transports them to the kidney and liver, where they are excreted from the body.
- *Hormones and enzymes*: Blood transports enzymes and hormones from the endocrine glands to their target tissues.

Regulation

Blood plays a vital role in homeostasis by regulating:

- *Volume and constituents of the body fluids*: Blood carries water in the form of plasma to the tissues and is responsible for maintaining the osmotic balance of the fluids and the cells.

The presence of plasma proteins, particularly albumin in the blood, controls the flow of fluid between the fluid compartments and is responsible for maintaining blood volume and blood pressure.

- *Body temperature*: Blood conducts heat around the body to the body surface where, if necessary, it is lost by peripheral vasodilation.
- *Acid–base balance*: Blood maintains a constant internal pH in the body by the presence of buffers, such as bicarbonate, which are able to absorb H^+ ions when the blood is acid (low pH) and give out H^+ ions when the blood is alkaline (high pH). In this way, all the processes of the body are able to function effectively.
- *Defence against infection*: Blood helps to prevent infection through the action of the white blood cells, which are part of the body's immune system. It also carries antibodies and antitoxins produced by the immune system around the body.
- *Blood clotting*: The clotting mechanism prevents excessive blood loss from wounds and other injuries and prevents the entry of infection.

Oedema is an abnormal accumulation of fluid in the cavities and intercellular spaces of the body. When oedematous fluid accumulates in the peritoneal cavity it is described as *ascites*. Oedema occurs when there is an imbalance between osmotic pressure and hydrostatic pressure. It can be caused by a number of factors – anything that increases osmotic pressure outside the blood vessels, such as inflammation, or reduces osmotic pressure in the blood, such as hypoproteinaemia. Increased hydrostatic pressure inside blood vessels resulting from heart failure may also cause oedema.

Composition of blood

Blood is a red fluid that is carried by the blood vessels of the circulatory system. It is composed of a fluid part, the *plasma*, and a solid part, the *blood cells* (Fig. 7.1). Plasma forms part of extracellular fluid (ECF) (see Chapter 1). Each constituent of the blood plays a specific part in the overall function of blood.

Plasma

Plasma is the liquid part of the blood that separates out when a blood sample is spun in a centrifuge. The main constituent is water (about 90%) in which are a number of dissolved substances being transported from one part of the body to another. These include carbon dioxide in solution, nutrients such as amino acids, glucose and fatty acids, waste materials such as urea, hormones, enzymes, antibodies and antigens.

In addition to these, plasma contains:

- *Mineral salts*: The main mineral salts found in ECF are sodium and chloride, but potassium, calcium, magnesium and bicarbonate are also present. The functions of these mineral salts include maintaining osmotic balance and maintaining pH by acting as buffers. Calcium has a number of essential roles in the body, including blood clotting, muscle contraction and nerve function.
- *Plasma proteins* help to maintain the osmotic pressure of the blood because they are too large to pass out of the circulation. This has the effect of retaining fluid in the blood by osmosis; in other words, it prevents too much water from 'leaking' out into the extracellular spaces. If this did occur then the volume

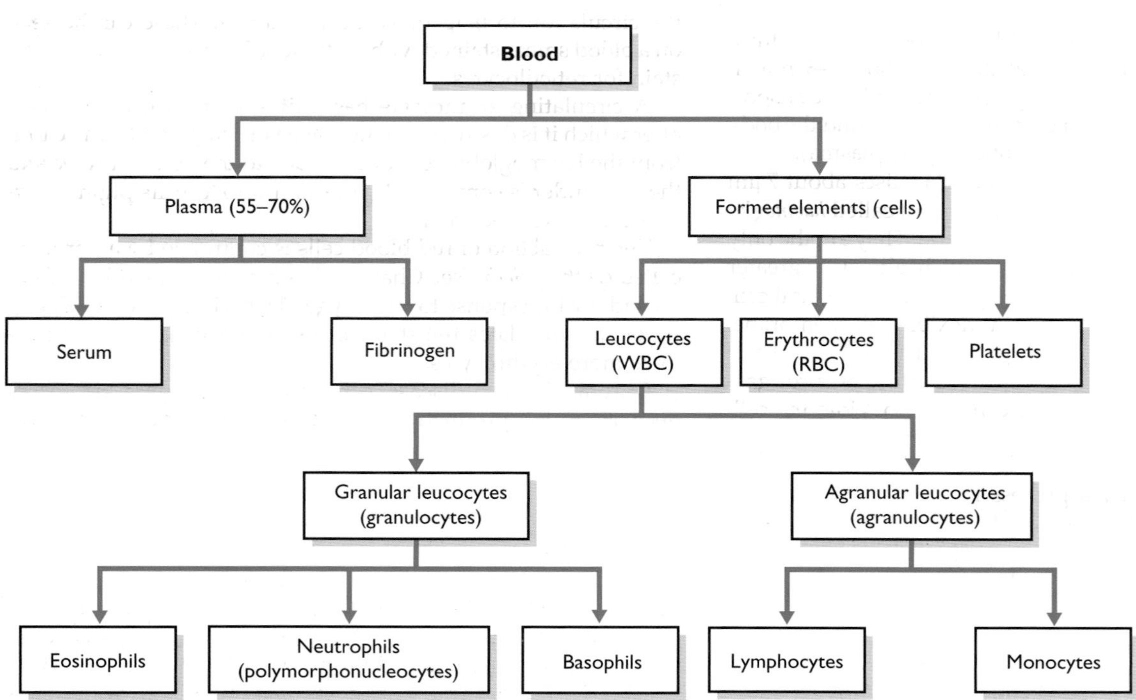

Fig. 7.1 The composition of blood.

of the blood would decrease and the blood pressure would fall, with serious consequences. The most important proteins are:

- *Albumin* helps to maintain the osmotic concentration of the blood (i.e., holds the water in the blood).
- *Fibrinogen* and *prothrombin* are involved in the clotting mechanism of the blood.
- *Immunoglobulins* are the antibodies produced by the immune system of the body.

Albumin, fibrinogen and prothrombin are produced by the liver, but the immunoglobulins are produced by the cells of the immune system.

Blood cells

The blood cells (Fig. 7.1) make up the solid component of blood and can be divided into three types:

- *Erythrocytes*: the red blood cells
- *Leucocytes*: the white blood cells
- *Thrombocytes*: the platelets, which are cell fragments

Before studying the different types of blood cell it is useful to understand a number of terms.

- *Haemopoiesis*: the formation of all types of blood cell
- *Erythropoiesis*: the formation of red blood cells or erythrocytes
- *Lymphoid tissue*: found in the lymph nodes and spleen and produces agranular leucocytes (i.e., lymphocytes and monocytes)
- *Myeloid tissue*: found in the red bone marrow and responsible for the formation of erythrocytes and granular leucocytes (i.e., neutrophils, eosinophils and basophils)
- *Serum*: plasma minus the clotting factors fibrinogen and prothrombin; can be obtained by allowing a blood sample to clot naturally

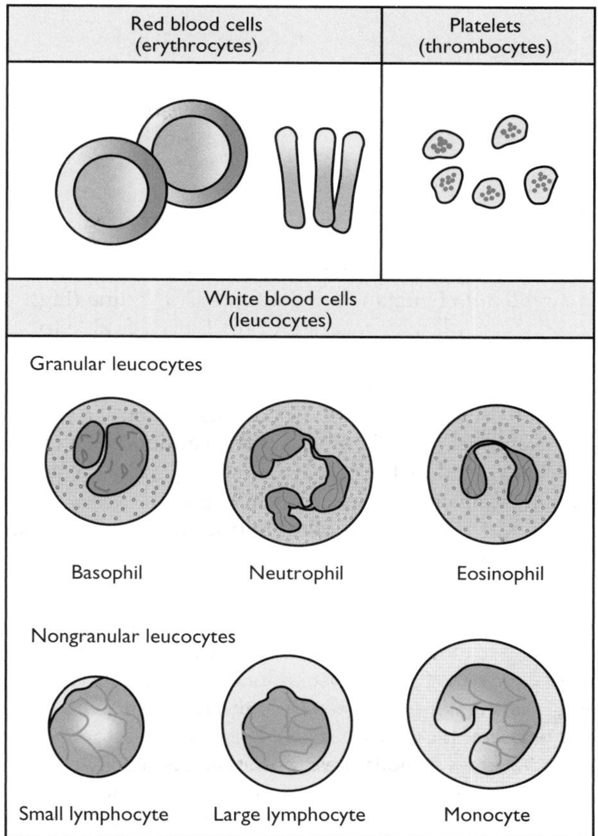

Fig. 7.2 The cellular components of blood. (With permission from T Colville, JM Bassett, 2001. Clinical anatomy and physiology for veterinary technicians. St Louis, MO: Mosby, p. 197.)

Erythrocytes

Also known as red blood cells or red blood corpuscles, erythrocytes are the most numerous blood cell; there are about 6–8 million per cubic millilitre of blood (Fig. 7.2). Their function is to transport oxygen and a small proportion of carbon dioxide around the body (most carbon dioxide is carried in solution in the plasma).

Mature erythrocytes are biconcave circular discs about 7 μm in diameter. Erythrocytes contain a red pigment called *haemoglobin*, which is a complex protein containing iron. They are the only cells in the body without a nucleus, which allows a greater amount of haemoglobin to be packed into a relatively small cell. Erythrocytes are surrounded by a thin, flexible cell membrane, which enables them to squeeze through capillaries. Their shape and thin cell membrane gives them a large surface area for gaseous exchange and allows oxygen to diffuse across into the cell, where it combines with the haemoglobin to form *oxyhaemoglobin*.

Erythrocytes are formed from undifferentiated *stem cells* within the bone marrow by a process known as *erythropoiesis*. The stem cells change into *erythroblasts*, which have a nucleus. The cell begins to acquire haemoglobin and its nucleus shrinks; it is now known as a *normoblast*. As the cell develops further it becomes a *reticulocyte*, at which point the nucleus consists only of fine threads in the cytoplasm known as *Howell–Jolly bodies*. Eventually, the nucleus disappears and the mature erythrocyte is released into the circulation. This process takes 4–7 days.

If there is a shortage of erythrocytes (e.g., acute haemorrhage or iron-deficiency anaemia), reticulocytes are also released into the circulation to help make up the deficit. These can be seen on a blood smear stained with methylene blue, which is a specific stain for reticulocytes.

A circulating erythrocyte has a lifespan of about 120 days, after which it is destroyed in the spleen or lymph nodes. The iron from the haemoglobin is recycled back to the bone marrow and the remainder is converted by the liver into the bile pigment *bilirubin* and excreted in bile.

The production of red blood cells is controlled by a hormone called *erythropoietin* (see Chapter 6), which is released by cells in the kidney in response to low oxygen levels in the tissues. Erythropoietin stimulates the stem cells in the bone marrow to produce more erythrocytes.

Chronic kidney disease can result in anaemia due to a decrease in the production of erythropoietin, and this form of anaemia is classed as non-regenerative.

Leucocytes

Also known as white blood cells, leucocytes are much less numerous than red blood cells and the cells contain nuclei. Leucocytes can be classified as either *granulocytes* or *agranulocytes* depending upon whether they have visible granules in their cytoplasm when stained and viewed under a microscope (Fig. 7.2). The function of leucocytes is to defend the body against infection.

Granulocytes

This type of leucocyte is produced within the bone marrow and makes up approximately 70% of all leucocytes. They have granules within their cytoplasm and have a segmented or lobed nucleus that can vary in shape. They are referred to as polymorphonucleocytes or PMNs (meaning many-shaped nuclei). They can be further classified according to the type of stain they take up: neutral, basic or acidic. There are three types of granulocyte:

- *Neutrophils* take up neutral dyes and the granules stain purple (Fig. 7.2). Immature neutrophils have a nucleus that looks like a curved band and are known as *band cells*. Neutrophils are the most abundant of the leucocytes, forming about 90% of all granulocytes. They are able to move through the endothelial lining of the blood vessels into the surrounding tissues and engulf invading bacteria and cell debris by phagocytosis, thus helping to fight disease. A *neutrophilia* or raised numbers of neutrophils indicates the presence of an infective process, while a *neutropenia* or lack of white cells may be characteristic of certain viral infections.
- *Eosinophils* take up acidic dye and the granules in their cytoplasm stain red (Fig. 7.2). They are involved in the regulation of the allergic and inflammatory processes and secrete enzymes that inactivate histamine. Eosinophils play a major role in controlling parasitic infestation. An *eosinophilia* or raised numbers of eosinophils occurs in response to parasitic infestation.
- *Basophils* take up basic or alkaline dyes and the granules in the cytoplasm stain blue (Fig. 7.2). Basophils secrete *histamine*, which increases inflammation, and *heparin*, which is a natural anticoagulant preventing the formation of unnecessary blood clots. Basophils are present in very small numbers in normal blood.

Agranulocytes

Agranulocytes have a clear cytoplasm. There are two types:

- *Lymphocytes* are the second most common type of white blood cell, forming 80% of all agranulocytes (Fig. 7.2). Lymphocytes are the main cell type of the immune system and are formed in lymphoid tissue, although they originate from stem cells in the bone marrow. Lymphocytes are responsible for the specific immune response, and there are two different types: the *B lymphocytes*, which produce antibodies and are involved in humoral immunity, and the *T lymphocytes*, which are involved in the cellular immune response.
- *Monocytes* have a horseshoe-shaped nucleus and are the largest of the leucocytes, although they are only present in small numbers (Fig. 7.2). They are *phagocytic* cells and when they migrate to the tissues they mature and become known as *macrophages*.

Lymphoma is a type of cancer that occurs when the B or T lymphocytes begin growing and multiplying uncontrollably. The abnormal lymphocytes collect in one or more of the lymph nodes or in lymphatic tissue (e.g., the spleen) and form a tumour.

Thrombocytes

Thrombocytes, or *platelets*, are cell fragments formed in the bone marrow from large cells called *megakaryocytes*. They are small discs with no nuclei and are present in the blood in large quantities. Platelets are involved in blood clotting.

Thrombocytopenia is the term used for a reduction in the number of platelets. Decreased production may be linked to a bone marrow dysfunction, which may be as a result of a viral infection, or if the animal is undergoing chemotherapy.

Blood clotting

The ability to form a blood clot is one of the most important defence mechanisms in the body. It means that injured blood vessels can be sealed and excessive blood loss can be prevented. Blood clotting is essential for wound healing and also prevents the entry of pathogenic microorganisms into the wound. The formation of a blood clot is complicated and involves a number of different chemical factors in the blood. It is described as a *cascade mechanism* because one step leads on to another in a similar way to a cascade of water.

To simplify the process we will only consider the main steps. When a blood vessel or a tissue is damaged the following happens:

1. Platelets stick to the damaged blood vessel and to one another to form a seal. The platelets release an enzyme called *thromboplastin*.
2. In the presence of thromboplastin and calcium ions, the plasma protein *prothrombin* is converted to the active enzyme *thrombin*. (Vitamin K is essential to the blood clotting mechanism and is required for the manufacture of prothrombin in the liver.)
3. Thrombin then converts the soluble plasma protein *fibrinogen* into a meshwork of insoluble fibres called *fibrin*. The presence of calcium is an essential factor.
4. The fibrin fibres form a network across the damaged area that traps blood cells and forms a *clot*. This seals the vessel in what is often called a 'scab' and further blood loss from the wound is prevented.

The normal *clotting time* in a healthy animal is 3–5 min but it may be affected by a number of factors. It may be reduced by:

- Surface contact with materials that will act as foundation for the clot (e.g., gauze swabs).
- Raising the environmental temperature: keeping the animal in a warm kennel.

Clotting time may be increased by:

- Lack of vitamin K, which is needed by the liver to form prothrombin in the blood (seen in warfarin poisoning, which interferes with levels of vitamin K).
- Liver disease: the liver manufactures the plasma proteins involved in clotting.
- Genetic factors (e.g., haemophilia), which affect the availability of some clotting factors.
- Systemic diseases such as anthrax, canine infectious hepatitis and viral haemorrhagic disease all cause subcutaneous haemorrhages due to interference with blood clotting.
- Thrombocytopenia: Lack of platelets may be seen in some forms of leukaemia.
- Lack of blood calcium: This feature is used in the lab to prevent blood samples clotting. Chemicals such as EDTA (ethylene diamine tetra-acetic acid), citrate and oxalate all

combine with calcium in the blood and prevent it being involved in the clotting process.
- Parasitic disease: Infestation with *Angiostrongylus vasorum* (lungworm) can cause clotting dysfunction and subsequent haemorrhage (e.g., in the eye, which is described as hyphaema).

The body has its own natural anticoagulant called *heparin*. This is secreted by the basophils and prevents unwanted clots forming in the blood vessels and organs. If part of a clot, referred to as an *embolus*, detaches, it may be carried around the body and block any of the vital blood vessels, killing the animal.

Heparin is added to a saline solution to make *heparinised saline*. This is used to flush intravenous catheters on their placement and to ensure their ongoing patency.

The heart

The heart is a muscular organ that contracts rhythmically, pumping the blood through the blood vessels and around the body (Fig. 7.3). The heart is enclosed within a double-layered serous sac, the *pericardium*. This lies in the *mediastinum*, the space that separates the two pleural cavities of the thorax (see Chapter 2).

The heart is conical in shape and lies slightly to the left of the midline. It lies obliquely in the thorax, with its attached portion or *base* positioned above and more cranially to its free portion or *apex*, which lies close to the sternum at the level of the caudal surface of the sixth rib. The heart has four chambers and is separated into right and left halves by the *septum*. The right side of the heart pumps blood into the pulmonary circulation; the left side of the heart pumps blood into the systemic circulation.

- The two upper chambers are the right and left atria (singular: atrium). These receive blood from the veins of the systemic and pulmonary circulations.
- The two lower chambers are the right and left ventricles. These pump out blood from the heart into the arteries of the pulmonary and systemic circulations.

The walls of the ventricles have a thicker muscle layer or *myocardium* than the atria, to assist them in pumping the blood into the arteries. The myocardium is thickest in the left ventricle, as this chamber must pump the blood into the aorta and all around the body in the systemic circulation. The wall of the heart consists of three layers:

1. The inner layer (*endocardium*) is continuous with the endothelial lining of the blood vessels.
2. The middle layer (*myocardium*) is made of cardiac muscle (see Chapter 2).
3. The outer layer (*epicardium*) forms the serous inner layer of the pericardium.

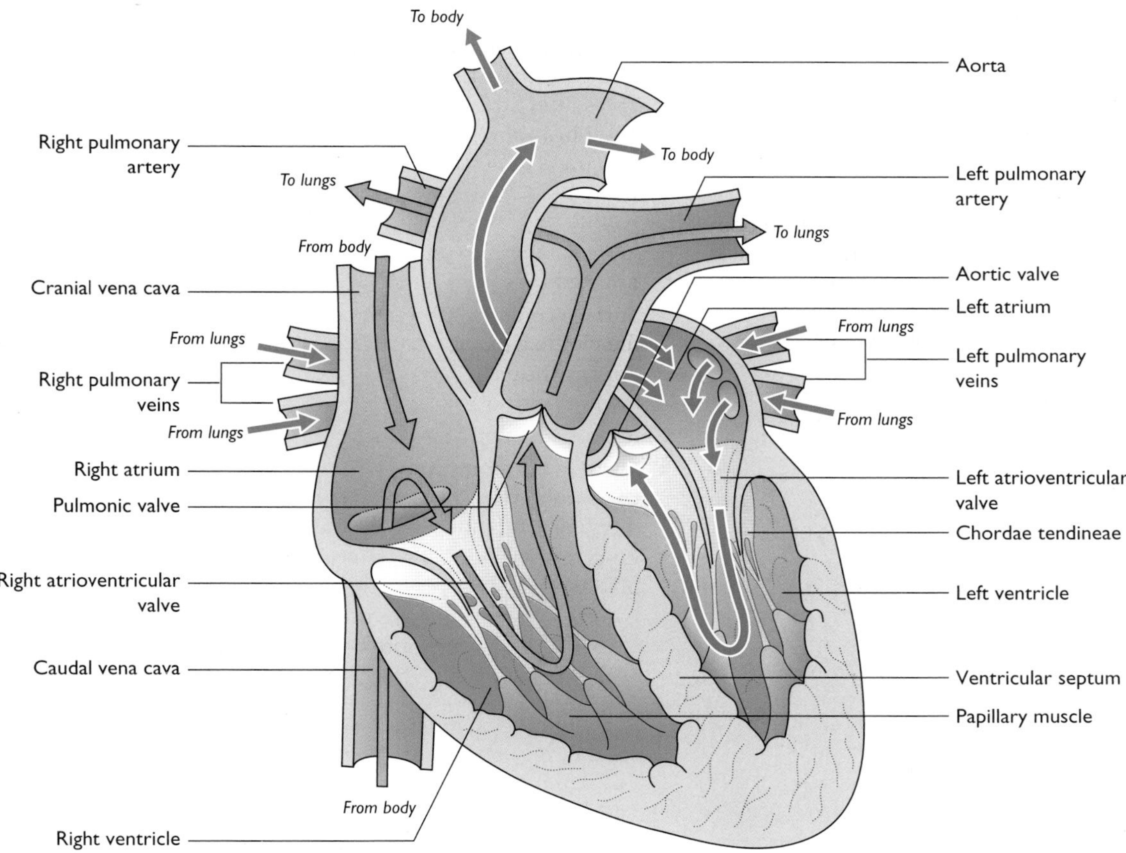

Fig. 7.3 The structure of the heart and direction of blood flow.

Bacterial infection may cause an inflammation of the endocardium, which is known as endocarditis. This can result in severe damage to parts of the heart such as the valves, distorting them and leading to leaky valves and cardiac insufficiency, which can be fatal.

Heart valves

Within the chambers of the heart there are two sets of valves that create a one-way flow of blood, preventing backflow from the atria to the ventricles as the blood circulates through the heart:

- The *right atrioventricular (AV)* or *tricuspid* valve lies between the right atrium and right ventricle and is composed of three fibrous flaps or *cusps* that attach to a fibrous ring encircling the opening to the right ventricle.
- The *left atrioventricular (AV)* or *bicuspid* or *mitral* valve lies between the left atrium and left ventricle and is composed of two cusps.

The free edges of the AV valves are attached to the *papillary muscles* of the walls of the ventricles by fibrous threads called the *chordae tendineae* (Fig. 7.3). The AV valves open to allow the blood to fill the ventricles from the atria; when the ventricles are full they close to prevent backflow of blood into the atria. The chordae tendineae prevent the valves everting as blood is pressed against them when the ventricles begin to contract. It is the closing of the AV valves that causes the first heart sound – 'lub'.

At the base of the major vessels leaving the ventricles are two more sets of valves, the *semilunar* valves, which prevent the flow of blood from the vessel back into the ventricle. They are composed of three half-moon-shaped cusps and when they shut it causes the second heart sound – 'dub'. The semilunar valves are as follows:

- The *pulmonary* valve lies at the base of the pulmonary artery as it leaves the right ventricle.
- The *aortic* valve lies at the base of the aorta as it leaves the left ventricle.

Mitral valve insufficiency is one of the most common causes of congestive heart failure in the dog. A damaged or poorly developed mitral valve results in alteration to the normal blood flow through the heart. This causes backing up of the blood in the left atrium and increased pressure in the pulmonary vein that drains into it. Oedematous fluid accumulates in the lung tissue, causing a 'heart cough'.

Circulation of blood through the heart

Deoxygenated blood returning from around the body is carried to the right side of the heart by the major veins: the *cranial vena cava* and *caudal vena cava* (Fig. 7.3). The blood enters the right atrium, which, when full, contracts and forces the blood into the right ventricle via the right AV valve. When the right ventricle is full it contracts and pumps the blood out of the heart into the pulmonary artery, via the pulmonary valve. The blood is now within the pulmonary circulation and is carried to the lungs, where it picks up oxygen from the inspired air – it becomes oxygenated.

From the lungs, the oxygenated blood is carried in the pulmonary veins back to the left side of the heart. The blood enters the left atrium, which contracts when full, forcing the blood through the left AV valve into the left ventricle. When the left ventricle is full it contracts and pumps the blood into the main artery of the body, the aorta, via the aortic valve. The blood is now in the systemic circulation and travels around the body in the arteries. Oxygen is given up to the tissues and carbon dioxide is collected from the tissues – the blood is said to be deoxygenated. Deoxygenated blood returns to the heart in the veins.

It is important to note that both atria contract at the same time, followed by the ventricles: the cardiac cycle consists of the contraction and relaxation of the two atria followed by the contraction and relaxation of the two ventricles. Within the cardiac cycle, the period of contraction is called *systole* and the period of relaxation is called *diastole*.

Any form of structural or functional defect in the heart valves will interfere with normal blood flow through the heart. This will create a turbulent flow, which may be audible and detectable by auscultation with a stethoscope. This condition is described as a *heart murmur.*

The conduction system of the heart

The myocardium of the heart is composed of a highly specialised type of muscle tissue – *cardiac muscle* (see Chapter 2). It is able to contract rhythmically and automatically without nervous input, meaning that it has an inherent contractibility. In order to satisfy the changing requirements of the body (e.g., when running or sleeping), the heart rate (the number of beats per minute) must be able to alter rapidly and this is brought about by nerve impulses from the autonomic nervous system which override the inherent rate. The mechanism that is responsible for initiating and coordinating the heartbeat is called the *conduction system* (Fig. 7.4).

The *heart rate* or *pulse* is the number of heartbeats per minute. It is measured by palpation of an artery and can be felt most easily in areas where a superficial artery runs over a bone, such as the femoral, brachial or coccygeal artery.

The sequence of this mechanism and the specialised structures involved are as follows:

1. The heartbeat begins in the *sinoatrial node*, which is referred to as the *pacemaker* of the heart. The sinoatrial node is an area of modified cardiac muscle cells in the wall of the right atrium, near its junction with the cranial vena cava. It is here that the autonomic nerves have their effect and the impulse to contract arises. The wave of contraction then spreads across both atria – *atrial systole.*
2. The myocardium in the walls of the ventricles is not in electrical continuity with that of the atria so the nerve impulse must now pass through another specialised group of cardiac muscle cells called the *AV node* at the top of the interventricular septum. When this node is excited it sends impulses along a specialised bundle of fibres, called the *bundle of His*, which runs down the interventricular septum.
3. At the bottom of the interventricular septum, the bundle of His divides into right and left branches, which spread into the two ventricles. These branches connect with a network of specialised neurons, the *Purkinje fibres,* which spread out through the ventricular muscle.
4. The wave of contraction starts in the myocardium at the apex of the heart (i.e., the bottom of the ventricles), and spreads upwards through the muscle of the ventricles, pushing the blood up towards the pulmonary artery and the aorta and out of the heart – *ventricular systole.*

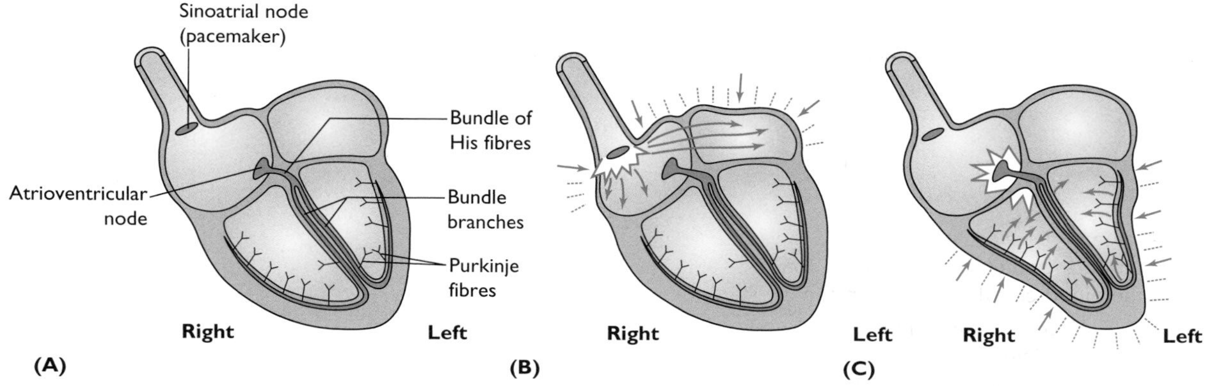

Fig. 7.4 The conduction mechanism of the heart. **(A)** The heart at rest. **(B)** The sinoatrial node fires and impulses spread across the atria, which contract. **(C)** The AV node fires, sending impulses along conducting fibres into the ventricles, causing them to contract.

- **Hypertrophic cardiomyopathy** is a disease that causes abnormal thickening of the heart muscle or myocardium. This results in a reduction in size of the ventricles and affects the blood flow into the chamber. It is a common chronic progressive disease of cats and causes lethargy, rapid and/or laboured breathing.
- **Dilated cardiomyopathy** is more commonly seen in dogs. The heart muscle becomes thin and weakened resulting in poor contraction. This is the second most common heart disease in dogs, after mitral valve disease and the clinical signs are similar to those of hypertrophic cardiomyopathy.

Electrocardiography, or ECG, is the technique in which the electrical conductivity of the heart is measured. Figure 7.5 illustrates a normal ECG wave, which may be recorded on a paper trace or on a monitor. The procedure is carried out in a conscious animal and is used as an aid to the diagnosis of abnormalities in heart rate and rhythm.

Blood pressure is a measurement of the force that pushes blood through the arterial circulation. It is governed by the heartbeat, the blood volume and the elasticity of the blood vessel walls. Blood pressure is at its highest during systole and lowest during diastole and the measurement is an average of the two values.

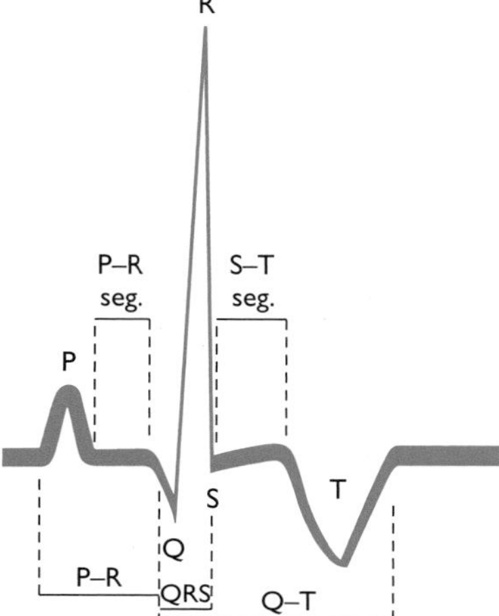

Fig. 7.5 Example of a lead II ECG trace with the major reflections (waves) and intervals marked.

Circulatory system

The circulatory system consists of a network of blood vessels whose function is to transport blood around the body. All mammals have a *double circulation*, which consists of:

- *Systemic circulation* carries blood from the heart around the majority of the body and back to the heart.
- *Pulmonary circulation* carries blood from the heart to the lungs and back to the heart.

The division of the circulation into two separate circuits allows the rapid distribution of oxygenated blood under high pressure, which is essential in an active endothermic animal. Blood passes through the heart twice during one complete circuit of the body.

Blood vessels

There are three types of blood vessel forming a continuous network throughout the body: the arteries, capillaries and veins (Fig. 7.6).

Arteries

Arteries carry blood *away* from the heart under pressure. The majority of the arteries transport oxygenated blood to the

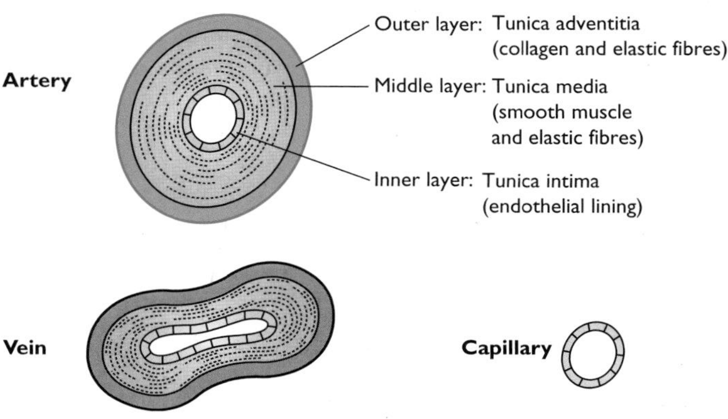

Fig. 7.6 The structure of blood vessels. Note that, in veins, the tunica media is thinner and contains fewer smooth muscle and elastic fibres than arteries. Capillaries only consist of a tunica intima.

capillary beds within the tissues. The exception is the *pulmonary artery*, which carries deoxygenated blood to the lungs. Arteries have relatively thick walls, which are composed of three layers:

1. *Tunica intima* consists of an endothelial lining, which is continuous throughout the entire circulatory system and is also continuous with the endothelial covering of the heart valves.
2. *Tunica media* consists of smooth muscle and elastic tissue.
3. *Tunica adventitia* is the fibrous outer coat of the vessel.

The elastic nature of the walls allows them to dilate or constrict and enables arteries to withstand blood under high pressure as it leaves the heart.

As the arteries enter the tissues they give off side or *collateral vessels*, which link up with one another to form a network or *anastomosis*. If any of the branches should become obstructed, the blood has an alternative route through the tissue and the cells will still receive oxygen and nutrients. Some tissues or organs, such as the brain, kidney and heart, do not have this system of collateral vessels but have *end arteries* as their sole blood supply. These form a pattern similar to the branches of a tree – they branch but never join up with each other. This mechanism prevents damage by a sudden drop in blood pressure, but if an end artery is occluded (e.g., by a blood clot), there is no alternative supply and the result may be fatal.

As the distributing arteries branch off in the tissues, they become smaller and narrower and are called *arterioles*. Their function is to regulate the blood flow to the capillary beds.

Capillaries

Capillaries are small, thin-walled, permeable vessels consisting of a single layer of endothelial cells. It is here that the exchange of gases, the uptake of nutrients and the removal of metabolic waste products take place. As the capillaries have a small diameter, blood flows slowly through them, allowing substances to diffuse between the blood and the tissues. The *capillary beds* are the networks of capillaries that extend between the arterioles and the *venules* (small veins) within the tissues.

Veins

Veins carry blood *towards* the heart. They have relatively thin walls and carry deoxygenated blood under low pressure. The exception is the *pulmonary vein*, which carries oxygenated blood from the lungs to the heart. Veins have a similar general structure to arteries but they have fewer smooth muscle and elastic fibres. Some veins carrying blood against the pull of gravity (e.g., those in the legs), possess semilunar *valves* to prevent the backflow of blood. As the walls of the veins are compressible, the action of the skeletal muscles around them helps to 'squeeze' the blood along.

> Selection of a suitable site for venepuncture (puncture of a vein for intravenous injection or collection of a blood sample) depends on the vein being relatively superficial and easily accessible. The most common veins used in the dog and the cat are the *cephalic vein* on the dorsal surface of the lower forelimb, the *lateral saphenous vein* running on the lateral side of the hock and the *jugular* vein running down either side of the neck in the jugular furrow.

The smallest veins are called *venules*, and these collect the deoxygenated blood from the capillary beds in the tissues and return it to the heart in the veins.

The systemic circulation

Arterial circulation *(Fig. 7.7)*

Oxygenated blood leaves the left ventricle in the *aortic arch*, which is the origin of the main artery of the body, the *aorta*. This gives off branches as follows:

- Two *coronary arteries* supply the tissues of the heart with oxygenated blood.
- The *brachiocephalic trunk* supplies blood to the head through the *common carotid arteries* and also gives off the *right subclavian artery*, which supplies the right forelimb and continues as the *right axillary artery* and then the *right brachial artery* within the limb.
- The *left subclavian artery*, which winds around the first rib to enter the left forelimb through the axilla; becomes the *left axillary artery* and then the *left brachial artery* to supply blood to the left forelimb.
- The aorta continues through the thorax, giving off paired *spinal arteries* to supply the various structures and muscles of the vertebral column and thorax.
- The aorta passes into the abdomen and gives off a number of paired arteries. These include:
  - The *renal arteries*, supplying the kidneys
  - The *ovarian* or *testicular arteries*, supplying the female or male gonads
  - Three large unpaired branches of the abdominal aorta, which supply the abdominal viscera: the *coeliac artery*, supplying the stomach, spleen and liver; the *cranial mesenteric artery*, supplying the small intestine; and the *caudal mesenteric artery*, supplying the large intestine
- The principal artery of the hind limb is the *external iliac artery*, which arises close to the termination of the aorta and branches into the *femoral artery*, supplying each of the hind limbs.
- The *internal iliac artery* is the branch of the aorta that supplies the pelvic viscera.

Venous circulation (Fig. 7.7)

The major veins that drain blood into the right atrium of the heart are:

- *Cranial vena cava* returns deoxygenated blood from the head, neck and forelimbs. The cranial vena cava receives blood from:
  - The *jugular veins*, which run down either side of the ventral surface of the neck in the jugular furrow and drain the head
  - The *subclavian veins*, which collect blood from the veins of the forelimb – the main ones being the *brachial vein* from the deeper tissues and the *cephalic vein* from the superficial tissues
- *Caudal vena cava* returns deoxygenated blood from the pelvic region, hind limbs and abdominal viscera. Many of the veins that join the caudal vena cava have the same name as the artery that supplies that region (e.g., *renal vein*, *hepatic vein*, *external iliac vein*).
- *Azygous vein* arises in the abdomen and runs towards the heart, passing through the diaphragm; in the thorax it runs

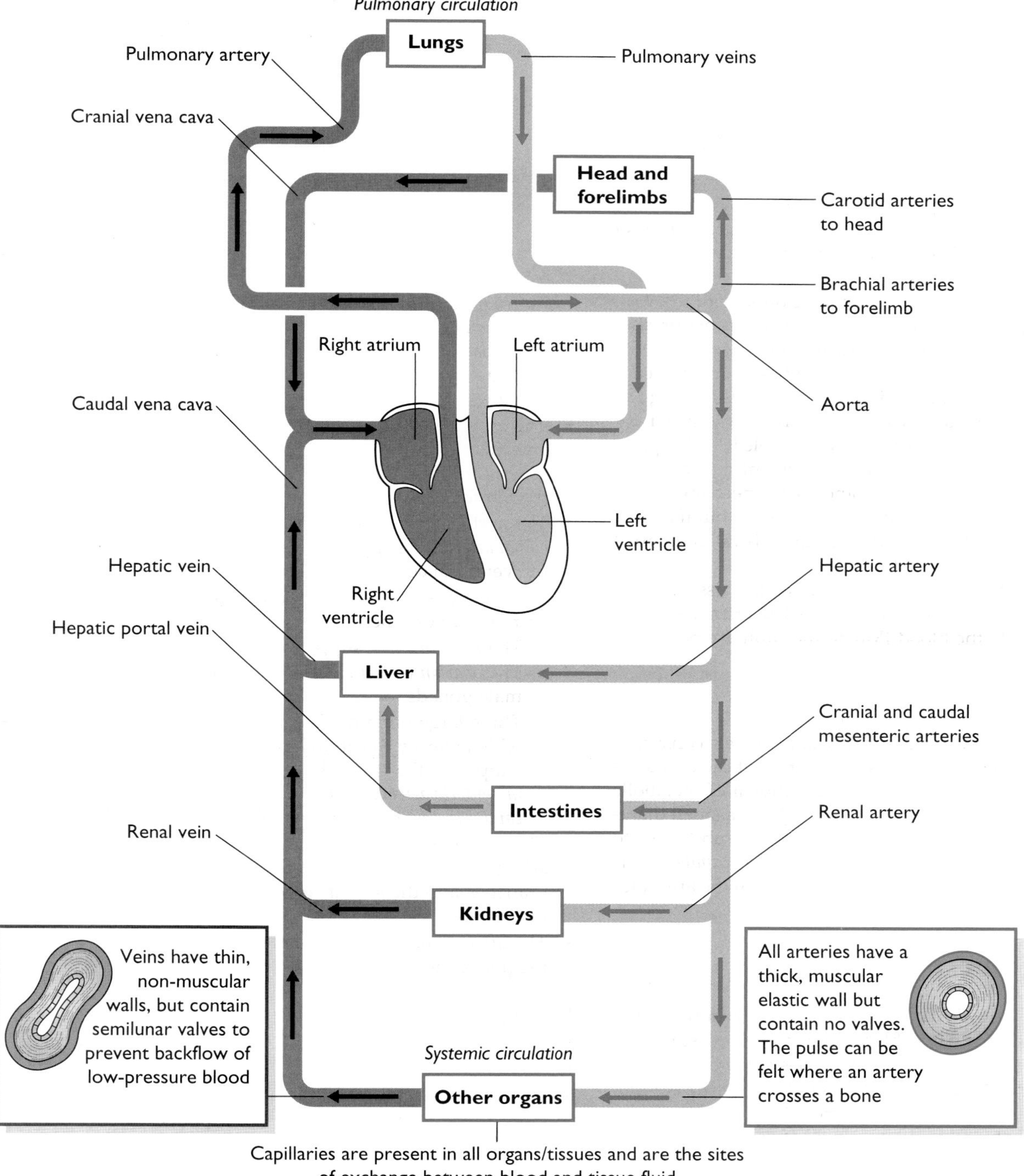

Fig. 7.7 Circulation of blood around the body.

dorsally and either joins the cranial vena cava or drains directly into the right atrium. The azygous vein drains venous blood from the thoracic body wall.

- The venous return from the heart itself is by the *coronary veins;* these join to form the *coronary sinus,* which then empties into the right atrium.

Occlusion of a vein or an artery by a blood clot is called a *thrombus*. This may be catastrophic, depending on the site and/or the size of the clot, particularly if it occurs in the brain or in the lungs. If part of the thrombus breaks off and becomes lodged in another capillary bed, it is described as being an *embolism*.

The hepatic portal system

Within the systemic circulation is a modified circulation system called the *hepatic portal system*. This takes blood straight from the digestive tract to the liver so that the products of digestion can be processed immediately (Fig. 7.7). The liver therefore has two blood supplies: one from the *hepatic artery* (oxygenated blood) and one from the *hepatic portal vein*. The veins that drain the digestive tract (e.g., stomach, intestine, pancreas), drain into the hepatic portal vein. The route to the heart taken by blood within the hepatic portal system is slightly different from that of the other parts of the systemic circulation. It passes through two capillary beds before returning to the heart – one in the structures of the digestive system and another in the liver. The venous blood from the liver then drains into the *hepatic veins*, which join the caudal vena cava.

A **portosystemic shunt** is a congenital malformation in the blood supply to the liver in which the venous blood coming from the digestive system bypasses the liver and does not enter the hepatic portal system. This results in raised levels of ammonia in the blood causing a number of clinical signs, such as stunted growth and neurological dysfunction (hepatic encephalopathy).

Fetal circulation

The fetal circulation differs from that of the neonate/adult mammal. During gestation, the *placenta* carries out the roles that are later performed by the lungs, kidneys and digestive tract. Blood circulating through the placenta provides oxygen and nutrients and removes waste products.

Blood is conducted to and from the placenta in the umbilical arteries and the umbilical vein. The *umbilical vein* carries oxygenated and nutrient-laden blood from the placenta to the fetus, passing to the fetal liver. The paired *umbilical arteries* carry deoxygenated blood, containing waste products, from the fetus back to the placenta and so to the circulation of the dam.

As gaseous exchange and nutrient transfer take place in the placenta, blood flow through the lungs and liver of the fetus is not as important and there are a number of *shunts* or bypasses:

In rare cases, the foramen ovale may remain open after birth. This is known as an **interventricular septal defect or a 'hole' in the heart**. Because of the greater pressure in the left ventricle, oxygenated blood passes through the defect from the left to the right side of the heart and pressure builds up on the right side (venous) of the systemic circulation. The animal shows symptoms of right-sided congestive heart failure such as ascites, enlarged liver and failure to thrive.

- *Foramen ovale* is an opening in the septum between the right and left atria and ventricles. Blood passes from the right ventricle to the left ventricle and into the systemic circulation, bypassing the lungs. The foramen ovale closes shortly after birth and the circulation becomes 'adult'.
- *Ductus arteriosus* is a vessel that forms a connection between the pulmonary artery and the aorta. Blood flows from the pulmonary artery to the aorta, bypassing the lungs. This closes shortly after birth as the lungs expand but remains as the *ligamentum arteriosus*.
- *Ductus venosus* is a venous shunt within the liver that connects the umbilical vein to the caudal vena cava. The nutrient- and oxygen-laden blood in the umbilical vein passes directly to the caudal vena cava and so to the fetal tissues instead of going through the fetal liver (the maternal liver has already metabolised the nutrients). This closes over at birth but remains as the *falciform ligament*.

The pulmonary circulation

Deoxygenated blood is pumped from the right ventricle of the heart in the pulmonary artery. Within the tissue of the lungs carbon dioxide diffuses from the blood in the thin-walled capillaries into the alveoli of the lungs. It then leaves the body in the expired air. Oxygen diffuses from the inspired air in the alveoli into the blood in the lung capillaries. These eventually combine to form the pulmonary veins, which carry oxygenated blood to the left atrium of the heart (Fig. 7.7).

Patent ductus arteriosus or PDA. In rare cases, the ductus arteriosus does not close at the moment of birth. As pressure in the aorta is greater than in the pulmonary artery, blood is diverted back into the lungs, avoiding the systemic circulation. The lungs become overperfused with blood and the animal shows symptoms of left-sided congestive heart failure such as a cough and exercise intolerance and it may have a 'machinery' heart murmur.

The lymphatic system

The lymphatic system is part of the circulatory system of the body and is responsible for returning the excess tissue fluid that has leaked out of the capillaries to the circulating blood. The fluid within the system is called *lymph* and is similar to plasma but without the larger plasma proteins. However, lymph contains more lymphocytes than are present in the blood. The lymphatic system is composed of both lymphatic vessels and lymphoid tissue, which are found in all regions of the body with a few exceptions such as the central nervous system and bone marrow.

The functions of the lymphatic system are:

- To return excess tissue fluid that has leaked out of the capillaries to the circulating blood
- To remove bacteria and other foreign particles from the lymph in specialised filtering stations known as lymph nodes
- To produce lymphocytes, which produce antibodies; the lymphatic system may also be considered as part of the immune system
- To transport the products of fat digestion and the fat-soluble vitamins from the lacteals of the intestinal villi to the circulation

The lymphatic system consists of the following parts:

- Lymphatic capillaries
- Lymphatic vessels
- Lymphatic ducts
- Lymph nodes
- Lymphatic tissues

Lymphatic capillaries

Excess tissue fluid is collected up by the smallest of the lymphatic vessels, the *lymphatic capillaries*. These are thin-walled, delicate tubes, which form networks within the tissues. In the villi of the small intestine the lymph capillaries are called *lacteals* and are responsible for collecting up the products of fat digestion (see Chapter 9).

Lymphatic vessels

The lymphatic capillaries merge to form the larger *lymphatic vessels*, which have a similar structure to veins and possess numerous closely spaced valves. Lymph flow is mainly passive and relies on the contraction of the surrounding muscles to move the lymph along. The valves prevent backflow and pooling of lymph in the vessels.

Lymphatic ducts

The lymphatic vessels enter the larger *lymphatic ducts* (Fig. 7.8), which drain lymph into blood vessels leading to the heart and so return it to the circulation. The major lymphatic ducts are:

- The *right lymphatic duct* is the smaller of the two major ducts and drains lymph from the right side of the head, neck and thorax, and right forelimb. It empties into the right side of the heart via either the right jugular vein or cranial vena cava.
- The *thoracic duct* is the main lymphatic duct and collects blood from the rest of the body. It arises in the abdomen, where it is called the *cisterna chyli*, and receives lymph from the abdomen, pelvis and hind limbs. As it passes through the aortic hiatus of the diaphragm and enters the thorax, it becomes known as the *thoracic duct* and receives lymph from the left side of the upper body and left forelimb. The thoracic duct empties into either the jugular vein or cranial vena cava, near the heart.
- There is also a pair of *tracheal ducts* that drain the head and neck and empty either into the thoracic duct or one of the large veins near the heart.

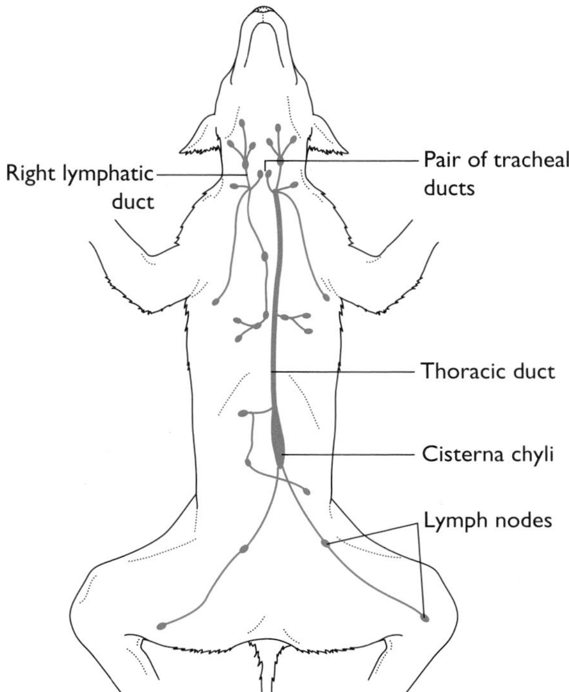

Fig. 7.8 Location of the lymphatic vessels and lymph nodes.

Chylothorax occurs when there is a leakage of lymphatic fluid (chyle) into the thoracic cavity. This can be due to the rupture of the thoracic duct (e.g., from trauma, tumour, or surgery) and the accumulation of fluid between the lungs and the pleura causes respiratory distress.

Lymph nodes

The lymph nodes (Fig. 7.9) are masses of lymphoid tissue situated at intervals along the lymphatic vessels (Fig. 7.8). They are bean-shaped and have an indented region, called the *hilus*, where the lymph vessels leave the node. A number of *afferent lymphatic vessels* carry lymph to each lymph node and enter the node on its convex surface. The lymph leaves the node at the hilus in the single *efferent vessel*.

Each node is surrounded by a fibrous connective tissue *capsule*. Inside, a network of tissue, called *trabeculae*, extends from the capsule and provides support for the entire node. The tissue of the node is divided into cortical and medullary regions. The cortex contains the germinal centres or *lymph nodules* that produce the *lymphocytes*, which play an important part in the immune system. The medulla is comprised of a reticular framework containing many phagocytic cells. Lymph flows through *spaces* or *sinuses* within the tissue of the node.

All lymph must pass through at least one lymph node before being returned to the circulation. Each node acts as a mechanical filter, trapping particles such as bacteria within the meshwork of tissue. The particles are then destroyed by phagocytic cells. Lymph nodes are distributed throughout the body and range in size. They can become enlarged during infection and are an indication of a disease process in the drainage region. In a generalised infection or disease all the lymph nodes may be enlarged; this is described as lymphadenopathy.

Some lymph nodes are superficial and can be palpated (Fig. 7.10). These include:

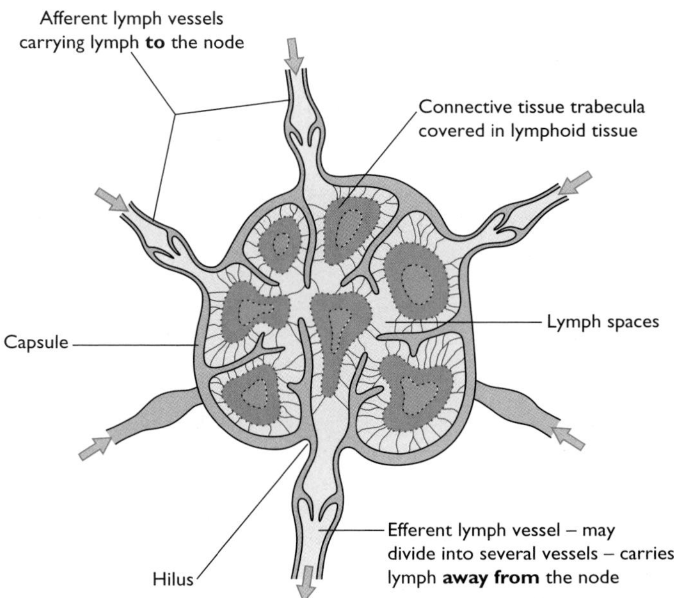

Fig. 7.9 Structure of a lymph node.

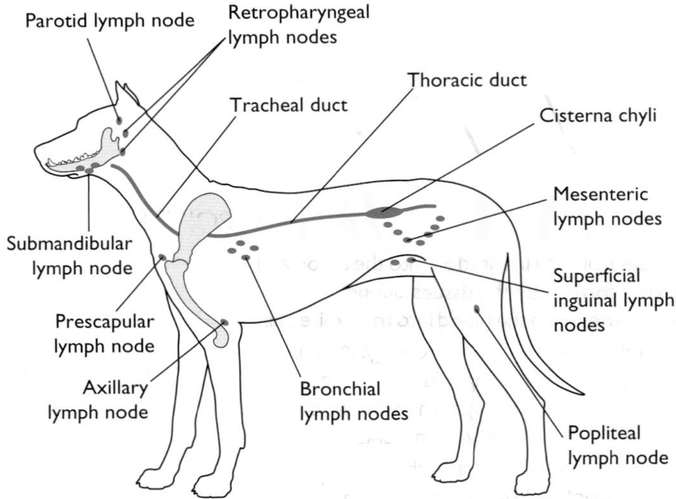

Fig. 7.10 Major lymph ducts and nodes. Some of the nodes are easily felt (see text).

- *Submandibular nodes*: two to five nodes in a group, lying at the edge of the angle of the jaw
- *Parotid node*: lies just caudal to the temporomandibular joint of the jaw
- *Superficial cervical nodes* also called the *prescapular nodes*: two on each side lying just in front of the shoulder joint, at the base of the neck on the cranial edge of the scapula
- *Superficial inguinal nodes*: two nodes on each side lying in the groin, between the thigh and the abdominal wall, dorsal to the mammary gland or penis
- *Popliteal node*: lies within the tissue of the gastrocnemius muscle, caudal to the stifle joint.

Lymphatic tissues

These include organs that contain lymphoid tissue and play an important part in the body's defence system.

Spleen

This is the largest of the lymphoid organs. The spleen is found within the greater omentum, closely attached to the greater curvature of the stomach. It is a dark red haemopoietic organ that is not essential for life, and therefore can be surgically removed if necessary, for example, if ruptured or if a tumour develops. The spleen has a number of functions:

1. Storage of blood: It acts as a reservoir for red blood cells and platelets.
2. Destruction of worn-out red blood cells: The phagocytic cells engulf and destroy the erythrocytes and preserve their iron content for re-use in haemoglobin synthesis.
3. Removal of particulate matter from the circulation: It 'filters' out foreign particles and bacteria and the phagocytic cells destroy them.
4. Production of lymphocytes: It produces lymphocytes for use in the immune system.

Thymus

This is of the greatest importance in the young animal. The thymus lies in the cranial thoracic inlet and cranial part of the thorax. It is active in late fetal and early postnatal life and is responsible for the production of T lymphocytes that give rise to the cell-mediated immune response. It begins to regress at the time of puberty and may eventually almost disappear.

Tonsils

These form a ring of lymphoid tissue around the junction of the pharynx with the oral cavity. They can be seen, especially when reddened and enlarged, on either side of the pharynx at the root of the tongue. They act as a 'first line' defence against micro-organisms that enter the mouth.

The immune system

The body has a number of natural defence systems such as the phagocytic blood cells that engulf and destroy invading bacteria, the inflammatory response, and the ability of the blood to form a clot, thus preventing blood loss and repairing damage. In addition to the phagocytic cells in the blood, there is a system of phagocytic cells distributed around the body in the tissues known as the *reticuloendothelial system*. These phagocytic cells are *macrophages* (agranular leucocytes) and are referred to by a number of names depending on where they are found; in connective tissue, for example, they are called *histiocytes*.

These defence mechanisms are all *non-specific* and the response is the same no matter what the stimulus, such as wounding, trauma or invading pathogen. However, the body also has a sophisticated immune system that provides a more *specific* response to a particular pathogen.

The main type of cell in the immune system is the *lymphocyte* and there are two types of specific immune response:

- *Humoral (antibody-mediated) immune response* involves the production of antibodies or immunoglobulins by the *B lymphocytes*. When a particular type of *antigen* (a foreign substance or invading organism that stimulates an immune response) enters the body, it stimulates the B lymphocytes to produce a corresponding protein called an *antibody*, which combines with the antigen and 'neutralises' it.
- *Cell-mediated immune response* involves the use of *T lymphocytes*, which recognise and help in the destruction of non-self cells (i.e., cells that do not belong to the body), or any of the body's own cells that have been altered by virus infections.

Vaccination is the introduction of antigenic material, such as a viral or bacterial element in an inactivated or harmless form, which will stimulate the body's immune response and prevent infection by developing an immunity to that specific pathogen.

Immune-mediated disease is a term that encompasses a range of inflammatory diseases whereby the body's immune system attacks its own organs and tissues. Examples include inflammatory bowel disease, keratoconjunctivitis sicca (KCS or 'dry eye') and non-regenerative haemolytic anaemia.

Respiratory system

KEY POINTS

- External respiration is the gaseous exchange between the air and the blood. Internal or tissue respiration is the gaseous exchange between the blood and the tissues.
- The function of most of the respiratory tract is to conduct inspired and expired gases into and out of the body.
- Air containing oxygen is inspired and expired by the respiratory muscles, which form the walls of the thorax and diaphragm and bring about changes in the volume and hence the internal pressure of the thoracic cavity.
- The pulmonary membrane within the alveoli is the only area where gaseous exchange takes place. Oxygen diffuses from the inspired air into the blood and carbon dioxide, formed by the tissues during metabolism, diffuses from the blood into the expired air.
- All tissues need oxygen to produce energy. As the needs of the body tissues change during their normal daily function, the respiratory system must be able to respond rapidly to supply varying amounts of oxygen.
- A complex control system exists within the hindbrain and within the peripheral blood system to monitor the status of respiratory gases and to maintain the body in a balanced state.

The function of the respiratory system is to conduct inspired air containing oxygen along the respiratory passages to the areas where gaseous exchange takes place and to conduct the expired air containing carbon dioxide out of the body.

Respiration is the gaseous exchange between an organism and its environment. All animals require oxygen to carry out the chemical processes that are essential for life: oxygen is needed by the cells to obtain energy from raw materials derived from food. This process involves the oxidation of glucose to yield energy in the form of adenosine triphosphate (ATP) (see Chapter 1). Water and carbon dioxide are produced as byproducts of this reaction. Respiration can be considered to occur in two stages:

1. *External respiration* is the gaseous exchange between the air and the blood; this occurs within the lungs.
2. *Internal* or *tissue respiration* is the gaseous exchange between the blood and the tissues; this occurs in the tissues.

The respiratory system consists of:

- Nose: the nasal cavity and the paranasal sinuses
- Pharynx
- Larynx
- Trachea
- Bronchi and bronchioles
- Alveoli

The upper respiratory tract comprises the nose, pharynx, larynx and the trachea; the lower respiratory tract comprises the bronchi, bronchioles and the alveoli. Clinical conditions are often defined as upper or lower respiratory tract diseases and it is important to understand the boundaries.

Structure and function

Nose

Inspired air enters the respiratory system through the nostrils or *external nares* leading into the *nasal cavity*, which is divided by a cartilaginous septum into the right and left *nasal chambers*. The entrance to the nasal cavity is protected by a hairless pad of epidermis consisting of a thick layer of stratified squamous epithelium, which is heavily pigmented and well supplied with mucous and sweat glands; this is known as the *rhinarium* and it is penetrated by the two curved nares (Fig. 8.1). The epidermis on a dog's nose has a unique patterning that is much like a human 'fingerprint'.

The right and left nasal chambers are filled with fine scrolls of bone called *turbinates* or *conchae* (Fig. 8.2). The chambers and the turbinates are covered by a ciliated mucous epithelium, which is well supplied with blood capillaries. The turbinates arising from the ventral part of the nasal cavity end rostrally in a small bulbous swelling visible through the nostril, the *alar fold.*

Epistaxis is defined as haemorrhage originating from the nose and may be bilateral or unilateral. It may be the result of trauma, infection, foreign bodies (e.g., grass seeds) or neoplasia.

Towards the back of the nasal chambers, the mucous epithelium covering the turbinates has a rich supply of sensory nerve endings that are responsive to smell; this is the *olfactory region.* These nerve fibres pass through the cribriform plate of the ethmoid bone to reach the olfactory bulbs of the forebrain (see Chapter 5). The remainder of the mucous membrane is the *respiratory region.*

The function of the turbinates and their ciliated mucous epithelium covering is to warm and moisten the incoming air as it passes over them. The cilia and mucus help to trap any particles that are present in the inspired air and waft them to the back of the nasal cavity, where they pass to the pharynx and are swallowed. The inspired air is therefore warm, damp and free from harmful particles, protecting the lungs from any form of damage.

Rhinitis is inflammation of the nasal cavity and may also involve the sinuses. A frequent cause is infection by *Aspergillus*, a common fungus found in materials such as dust, hay, straw and grass clippings. Clinical signs include sneezing, discharge and sometimes bleeding from the nose.

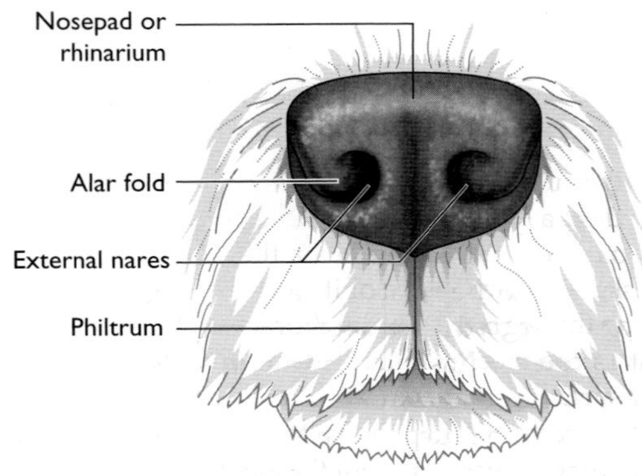

Fig. 8.1 The dog's nose – anatomical landmarks.

Paranasal sinuses

A sinus is an air-filled cavity within a bone. Within the respiratory system, they are referred to as the *paranasal sinuses* and lie within the facial bones of the skull (Fig. 8.2). They are lined with ciliated mucous epithelium and communicate with the nasal cavity through narrow openings.

- *Maxillary sinus* is not a true sinus in the dog but a recess at the caudal end of the nasal cavity.
- *Frontal sinus* lies within the frontal bone of the skull.

It is thought that the function of the paranasal sinuses is to lighten the weight of the skull, allowing the areas of the skull used for muscle attachment to be larger. This is evident in those species that have large, heavy skulls, such as the horse, which has numerous large paranasal sinuses. The paranasal sinuses also act as areas for heat exchange and as sites for mucus secretion.

Sinusitis, or inflammation of the sinuses, may be a complication of upper respiratory tract infections such as cat flu. This infectious disease is caused by several viruses (e.g., calicivirus) and presents as sneezing, coughing, ulceration of the tongue and conjunctivitis, accompanied by pyrexia and loss of appetite. Sinusitis is difficult to treat and may prolong the condition. In the worst-case scenario it may be necessary to drain the inflammatory exudate and introduce local antibiotics by trephination of the frontal sinus.

Pharynx

From the nasal cavity, the inspired air passes into the *pharynx*, a region at the back of the mouth that is shared by the respiratory and digestive systems. The pharynx is divided into the dorsal *nasopharynx* and the ventral *oropharynx* by a musculomembranous partition called the *soft palate* (Fig. 8.2). The soft palate extends caudally from the hard palate and prevents food from entering the nasal chambers when an animal swallows (see Chapter 9). The oropharynx conducts food from the oral cavity to the oesophagus; the nasopharynx conducts inspired air from the nasal cavity to the larynx, but air can also reach the respiratory passages from the mouth (e.g., during 'mouth breathing').

Mouth breathing, or orthopnoea, may occur during strenuous exercise to enable a greater volume of air to enter the lungs. It may also be seen in conditions that impair the flow of air through the nasal chambers (e.g., foreign bodies, tumours) or if the lung capacity is reduced (e.g., pneumothorax, haemothorax, pneumonia). The patient often lies in sternal recumbency with the neck and elbows extended.

A pair of Eustachian or auditory tubes also opens into the pharynx and connects the pharynx to each of the middle ears

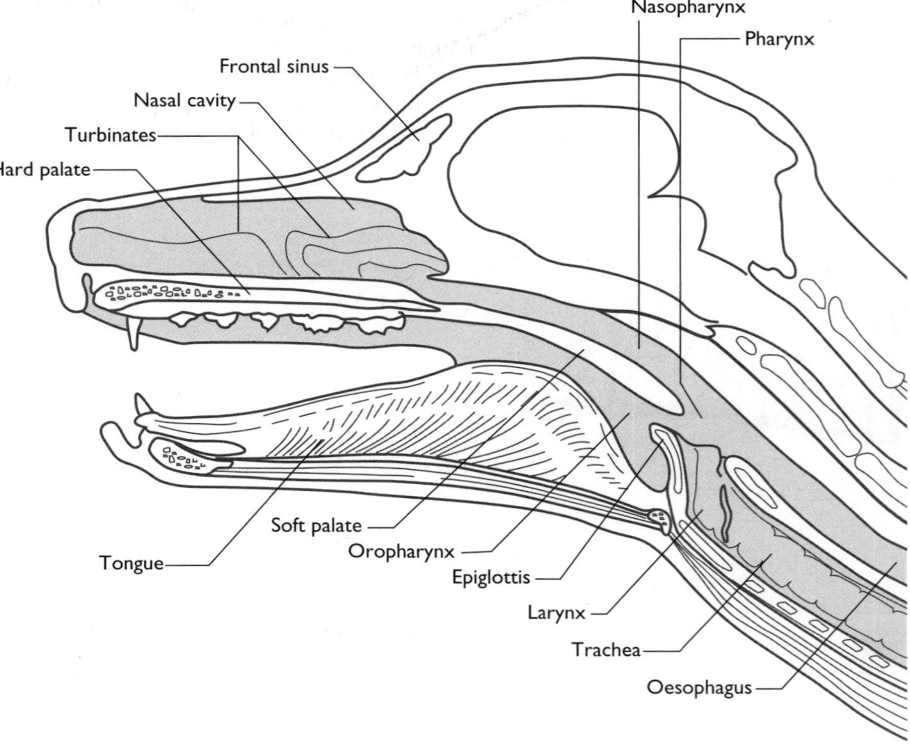

Fig. 8.2 Longitudinal section to illustrate the upper respiratory tract of the dog. (With permission from T Colville, JM Bassett, 2001. Clinical anatomy and physiology for veterinary technicians. St Louis, MO: Mosby, p 222.)

(see Chapter 5). The function of the Eustachian tubes is to equalise the air pressure on either side of the ear drum.

Larynx

The inspired air enters the *larynx*, which lies caudal to the pharynx in the space between the two halves of the mandible (Fig. 8.2). The function of the larynx is to regulate the flow of gases into the respiratory tract and to prevent anything other than gases from entering the respiratory tract.

The root of the tongue is attached to one side of the hyoid apparatus and the larynx to the other. When intubating a dog or cat, pulling the tongue forward will also pull the larynx forward and the epiglottis will fall downwards, opening the glottis so that the tube can be placed correctly.

The larynx is suspended from the skull by the *hyoid apparatus* (see Chapter 3), which allows it to swing backwards and forwards (Fig. 8.3). The hyoid apparatus is a hollow, box-like structure consisting of a number of cartilages connected by muscle and connective tissue. The most rostral of these cartilages, the *epiglottis*, is composed of elastic cartilage and is responsible for sealing off the entrance to the larynx or *glottis* when an animal swallows. This prevents saliva or food from entering the respiratory tract, causing the animal to choke. When the larynx returns to its resting position after swallowing the epiglottis falls forward, opening the glottis and thus allowing the passage of air to resume.

Laryngeal paralysis is a condition seen in older dogs, often of larger breeds (e.g., Labradors). The vocal folds hang within the lumen of the larynx and are unable to move out of the flow of air. This results in interference with the passage of air down the larynx and trachea, which could result in asphyxiation during exercise. It also causes a constant 'roaring' sound as the dog breathes.

Within the larynx is a pair of *vocal ligaments*. The mucous membrane covering the inner surface of the vocal ligaments forms the *vocal folds*, which project bilaterally into the lumen of the larynx. When air moves past the vocal folds they vibrate and sound is produced. These sounds can be modified by factors such as the size of the glottis and the tension of the vocal folds, resulting in a characteristic range of sounds (e.g., growling, barking, purring).

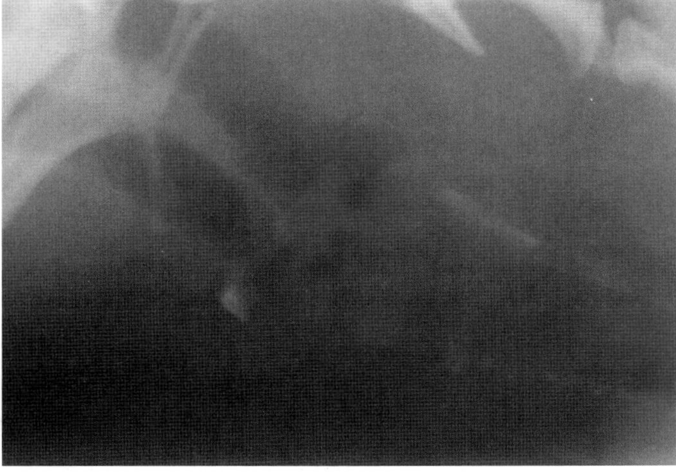

Fig. 8.3 Lateral view of dog's laryngeal area, showing the cartilages of the hyoid apparatus as they appear on X-ray.

Trachea

From the larynx, air enters the *trachea*. This is a permanently open tube attached to the caudal border of the laryngeal cartilages (Fig. 8.4). It lies on the ventral aspect of the neck, below the oesophagus and slightly to the right of it, and extends the length of the neck, passing through the cranial thoracic inlet. In the thoracic cavity it enters the mediastinum and terminates at a *bifurcation* above the heart.

The lumen of the trachea is kept open by a series of C-shaped rings of hyaline cartilage. These prevent the trachea from collapsing when the thoracic pressure falls and the incomplete rings allow food boluses to pass down the oesophagus unimpeded by the tracheal cartilages. The structure of the trachea is flexible to allow movement of the head and neck. The cartilage rings are connected by fibrous tissue and smooth muscle fibres.

The trachea is lined with *ciliated mucous epithelium*. The surface layer of mucus traps any foreign particles and the cilia 'sweep' the particles and mucus upwards to the pharynx, where they are spat out or swallowed. In some cases, such as in a dusty or smoky atmosphere, the production of mucus may increase. This mucus irritates the tracheal lining and causes the animal to cough. The *coughing reflex* serves to expel substances such as excess mucus and dust particles from the respiratory tract, preventing them from entering the lungs and is part of the animal's primary defence system.

Tracheal collapse may be seen in some small breeds of dog (e.g., Yorkshire Terriers), and causes a chronic 'honking' cough. There is a risk that during strenuous exercise the trachea may flatten, preventing the flow of inspired air. This causes the dog to collapse suddenly. During the period of unconsciousness, the trachea relaxes, air begins to flow again and the dog recovers.

Bronchi and bronchioles

The trachea divides (or bifurcates) into the right and left *bronchi* (sing. *bronchus*), entering each of the lungs respectively. As they enter the lung tissue the bronchi divide into smaller and smaller branches, like a tree. This arrangement is therefore known as the *bronchial tree*. The point at which each bronchus enters the lung is known as the *root* of the lung.

The bronchi are supported by complete rings of cartilage but, as the branches become smaller, the cartilaginous support gradually diminishes and then disappears completely, at which point the passages are called *bronchioles*. The bronchioles continue to branch into smaller passages throughout the lungs. Finally, the smallest diameter branches are known as the *alveolar ducts* and lead to the *alveoli*.

The walls of the bronchi and bronchioles contain smooth muscle, which is under the control of the autonomic nervous system. The respiratory passages are able to dilate to enable a greater volume of air to reach the lungs (e.g., during exercise), or constrict to their original size during 'normal' breathing.

Alveoli

The alveolar ducts end as the *alveolar sacs*, which resemble bunches of grapes. Each alveolar sac consists of a large number of alveoli, which are small, thin-walled sacs surrounded by capillary networks (Fig. 8.5). The epithelial lining of the alveolus is

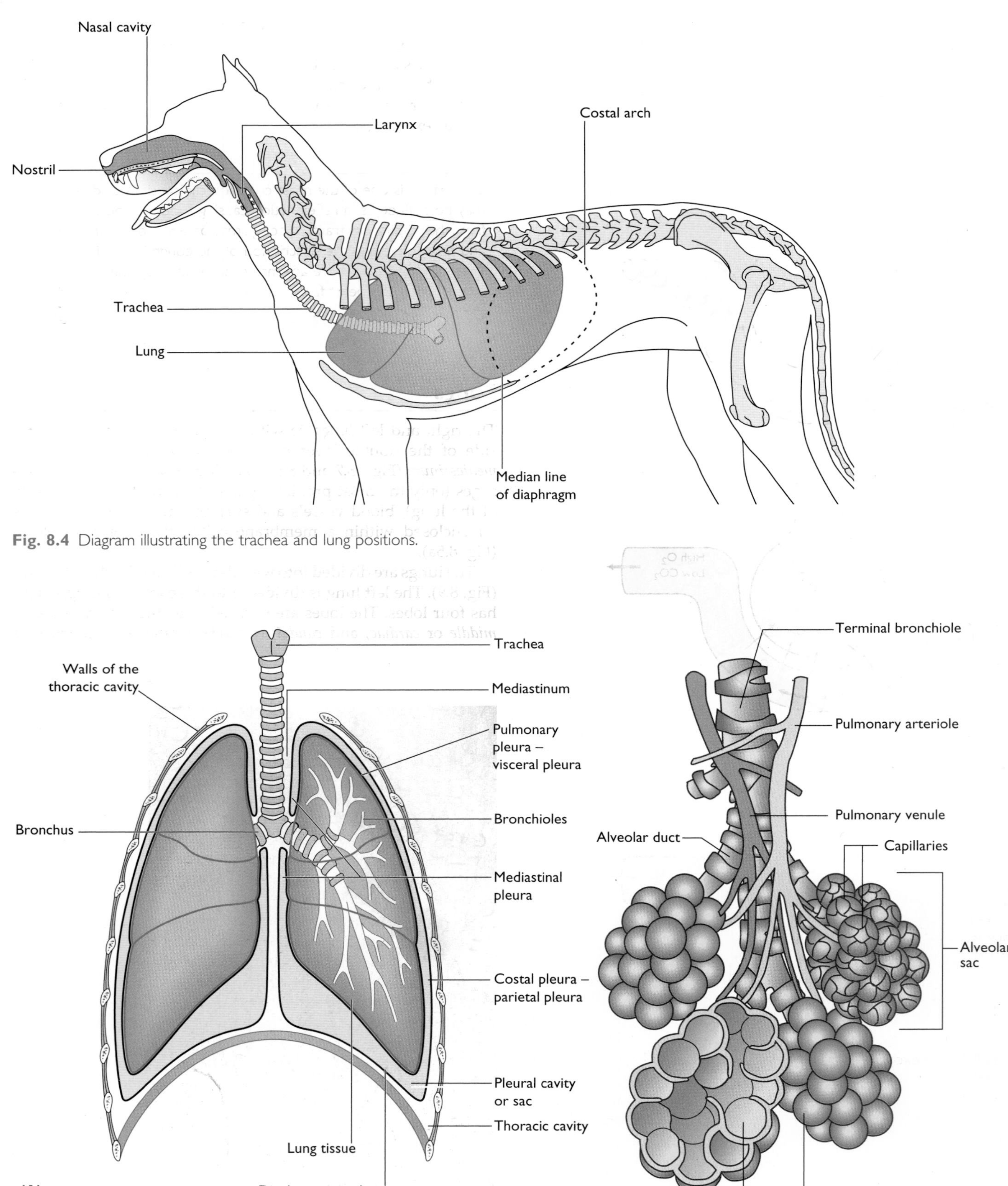

Fig. 8.4 Diagram illustrating the trachea and lung positions.

Fig. 8.5 The lungs within the thoracic cavity. **(A)** The pleural membranes. **(B)** The terminal air passages. (Part **B** with permission from T Colville, JM Bassett, 2001. Clinical anatomy and physiology for veterinary technicians. St Louis, MO: Mosby, p 227.)

called the *pulmonary membrane*, and is very thin to allow gaseous exchange with the blood to take place. Oxygen in the inspired air diffuses across the pulmonary membrane of the alveolus into the blood within the capillaries of the pulmonary circulation. Simultaneously, it is exchanged for carbon dioxide in the blood, which is to be excreted in the expired air from the lungs (Fig. 8.6). There are millions of alveoli in each lung, providing a large surface area for gaseous exchange.

The parts of the respiratory tract that are not involved in gaseous exchange (i.e., all but the alveoli) are referred to as the *dead space*. Their function is to conduct gases to and from the area of gaseous exchange.

Coughing is one of the most common clinical signs of disease and may be defined as 'a reflex action causing sudden expulsion of air from the respiratory tract'. A cough may be dry and hacking or moist and productive and the description of the cough is the first step towards diagnosis. There are many causes of coughing and they include left sided heart failure, foreign bodies, neoplasia, lungworm infection and pneumonia.

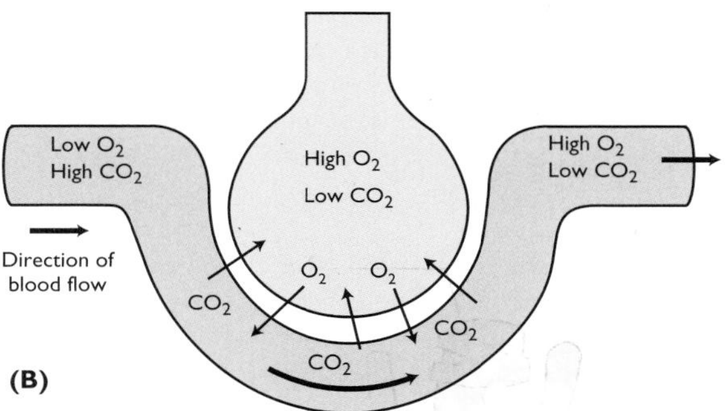

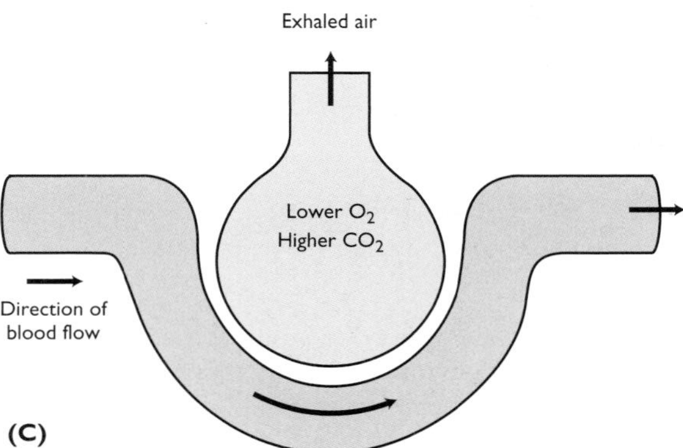

Fig. 8.6 The exchange of gases within the alveoli. **(A)** Inspiration: the air contains high levels of oxygen and low levels of carbon dioxide. Blood entering the alveolar capillary contains low levels of oxygen and high levels of carbon dioxide. **(B)** Gas exchange occurs: oxygen diffuses from air in the alveolus, where its level is high, into blood in the alveolar capillary, where its level is low. Carbon dioxide does the reverse, diffusing from alveolar capillaries into the alveolus. **(C)** Expiration: exhaled air contains less oxygen and more carbon dioxide than are present in room air. Next breath brings in a fresh supply of high oxygen air. (With permission from T Colville, JM Bassett, 2001. Clinical anatomy and physiology for veterinary technicians. St Louis, MO: Mosby, p 233.)

Lungs

The right and left *lungs* lie within the thoracic cavity on either side of the double layer of connective tissue known as the *mediastinum* (Figs. 8.7 and 8.8). Each lung consists of the air passages (only the most proximal parts of the bronchi are outside of the lung), blood vessels and surrounding connective tissue, all enclosed within a membrane called the *pulmonary pleura* (Fig. 8.5a).

The lungs are divided into well-defined lobes by deep fissures (Fig. 8.9). The left lung is divided into three lobes; the right lung has four lobes. The lobes are referred to as the *cranial* or *apical*, *middle* or *cardiac*, and *caudal* or *diaphragmatic*. The fourth lobe

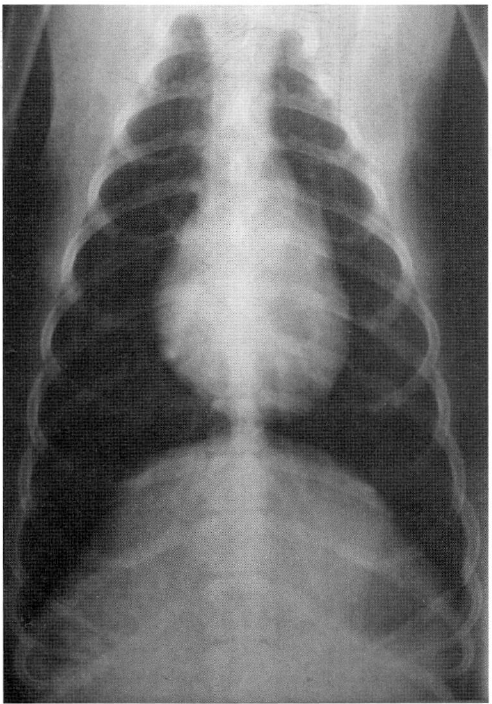

Fig. 8.7 Ventrodorsal radiograph of a dog's thorax. The lungs are full of air and appear dark on the X-ray.

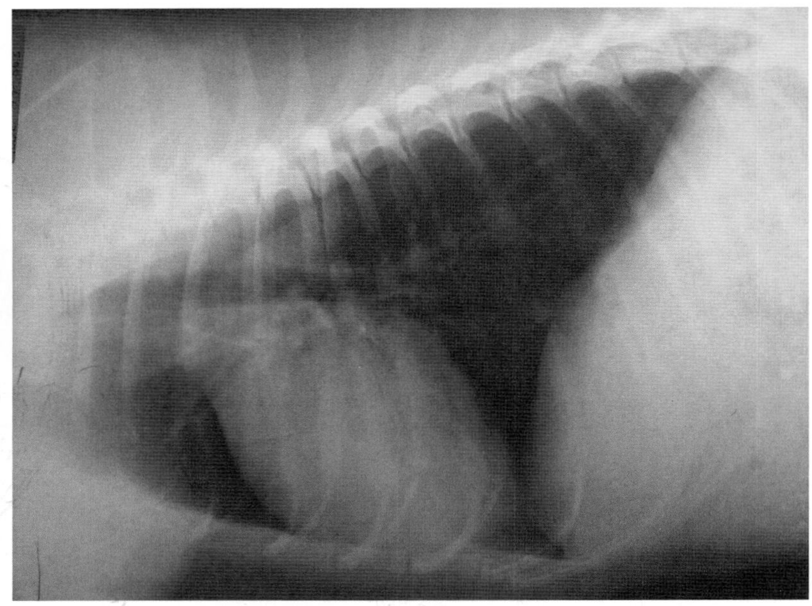

Fig. 8.8 Lateral radiograph of a dog's thorax. The lungs appear dark on the X-ray due to air, and allow the other structures to be visualised.

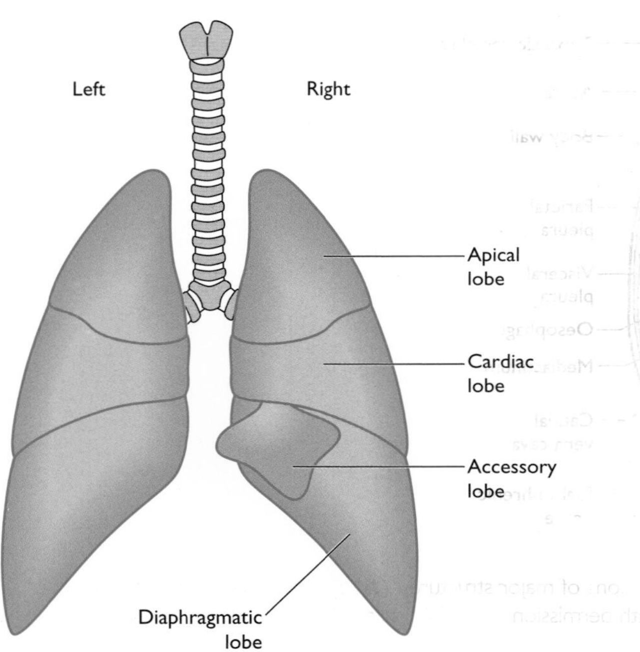

Fig. 8.9 The division of the lungs into lobes by deep fissures.

of the right lung is the *accessory lobe;* this is small and lies on the medial surface of the caudal lobe of the right lung.

Thoracic cavity

The thoracic cavity or *thorax* is divided into the *right* and *left pleural cavities* by a double layer of pleura known as the *mediastinum.* Each pleural cavity is lined by a single layer of serous membrane, the *pleural membrane* (Fig. 8.5). This secretes a small amount of serous or watery fluid, whose function is to reduce friction between the pleural surfaces as the lungs move during respiration.

Dyspnoea or difficulty in breathing may result from anything that replaces the normal vacuum of the pleural cavity, such as air (pneumothorax), blood (haemothorax) or pus (pyothorax). The ability of the lung to inflate fully will be impaired and the animal will show signs of respiratory distress.

All the structures lying in the pleural cavities are covered in the pleural membrane and it is named according to the structures it is covering. The *pleural cavity* lies between the two layers of pleural membranes and contains a vacuum and a small volume of pleural fluid (Fig. 8.5a).

Type of pleura	*Structures covered*
Diaphragmatic	Cranial aspect of the diaphragm
Pulmonary or visceral	Right and left lungs – outlines each lobe
Costal or parietal	Inner side of the ribs
Mediastinal	Mediastinum

Most of the organs in the thorax lie in the space between the two layers of mediastinal pleura; that is, the heart and its associated blood vessels, trachea and oesophagus (Fig. 8.10). The mediastinum of the dog and cat is quite tough and forms a complete barrier between the two pleural cavities. If one side is damaged or becomes infected then, providing that the mediastinum remains intact, the effect is limited to that side and the other lung can continue to function normally.

The mechanics of respiration

Respiration, which may also be referred to as breathing or pulmonary ventilation, is achieved by a coordinated series of actions carried out by muscles. This brings about the alternate expansion and reduction in the volume of the thoracic cavity.

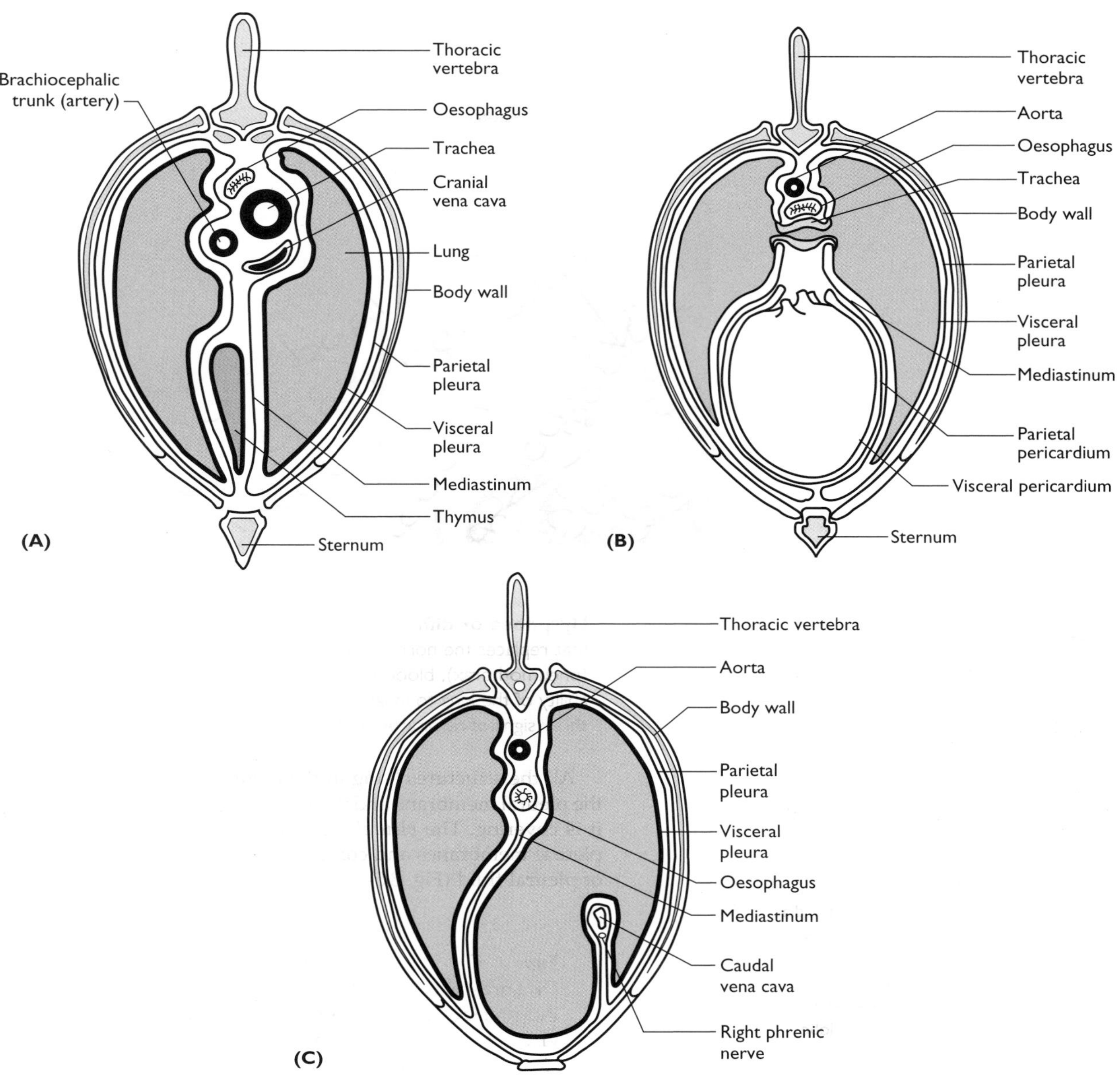

Fig. 8.10 Cross-section of the thorax at three different levels, showing the positions of major structures. **(A)** Section taken cranial to the heart. **(B)** Section taken through the heart. **(C)** Section taken caudal to the heart. (With permission from T Colville, JM Bassett, 2001. Clinical anatomy and physiology for veterinary technicians. St Louis, MO: Mosby, p 230.)

The lungs are suspended within the thoracic cavity, which is divided into the right and left pleural cavities by the pleural membranes. The pleural cavities contain a vacuum and, as they are totally enclosed, any increase in their volume will result in negative pressure and air will be sucked into the lung tissue. Conversely, if the volume of the pleural cavity decreases, the increase in pressure will push air out. This is the principle behind *inspiration* and *expiration*.

Three sets of muscles are responsible for respiration:

1. *Diaphragm* is a dome-shaped muscular structure that forms the boundary between the thoracic and abdominal cavities (see Chapter 4). It is innervated by the *phrenic nerve*, which arises from the cervical spine. When the diaphragm contracts, it flattens and increases the volume of the thoracic cavity.
2. *External intercostals* fill the intercostal spaces and are innervated by the *intercostal nerves* (see Chapter 4). As they contract, they lift the ribs upwards and outwards, thus increasing the volume of the thoracic cavity.
3. *Internal intercostals* fill the intercostal spaces and lie deep to the external intercostal muscles. They are also innervated by the intercostal nerves and their action is mainly passive, but during forced expiration they contract in conjunction with the abdominal muscles to force air out of the lungs.

- In *inspiration (or inhalation)* the diaphragm and external intercostal muscles contract and the volume of the thoracic cavity increases. The pressure in the pleural cavity falls, the lungs are pulled outwards and air is sucked down the trachea and into the lung tissue.
- *Expiration (or exhalation)* is a passive process. The diaphragm relaxes and regains its dome shape, the external intercostals relax and the ribs drop downwards. The volume of the thoracic cavity decreases, the pressure in the pleural cavity rises, the lungs collapse and air is pushed up and out of the trachea.

Control of respiration

During normal life, the changing metabolic needs of the body make demands on the respiratory system. As the tissues are remote from the organs involved in the intake and expulsion of gases, a complex system of control of respiration has evolved.

Within the pons and medulla of the hindbrain there are *respiratory centres* responsible for the control of inspiration and expiration. They are the *pneumotaxic* and *apneustic centres*, which control expiration, and the *inspiratory centre*, which controls inspiration. Impulses from the inspiratory centre travel to the diaphragm via the phrenic nerve and to the intercostal muscles via the intercostal nerves and bring about inspiration. Expiration is mainly passive but impulses from the expiratory centres may assist in expiration. These centres inhibit each other and cannot work simultaneously. They are responsible for the basic rhythm of respiration.

The rate and depth of respiration is controlled by receptors within the body:

- *Stretch receptors* lie within the walls of the bronchi and bronchioles and monitor the degree of stretching of the bronchial tree. When the lung is distended they send impulses via the vagus nerve to the inspiratory centre of the brain. Further inspiration is inhibited and expiration is stimulated via the apneustic centre. This is known as the Hering–Breuer reflex and prevents overinflation of the lungs.
- *Chemoreceptors:*
  - *Peripheral* are known as the *aortic bodies* (located in the walls of the aorta, close to the heart) and the *carotid bodies* (located in the walls of the carotid artery).
  - *Central* are found in the medulla of the brain. This is the major area for sensing carbon dioxide levels in the blood.

Both types of chemoreceptor monitor the levels of oxygen and the pH of the blood; for example, high levels of carbon dioxide in the blood lower the pH (i.e., the blood becomes more acidic). This change in pH is detected by the chemoreceptors, which stimulate an increase in the rate and depth of respiration. The carbon dioxide is expelled and the pH returns to normal.

The interrelationship between the control centres in the brain and the chemoreceptors in the peripheral circulation enable the respiratory system to respond rapidly to the changing state of the body.

Diaphragmatic paralysis. If this occurs, the lungs are unable to expand completely and the animal will experience respiratory distress. Causes include injury to the cervical spinal cord, surgery, phrenic nerve damage and severe head injuries. Some drugs may depress the respiratory centres and affected animals have to be placed on a ventilator.

Respiratory definitions

When an animal is breathing normally (at rest), the amount of air that passes into and out of the lungs during each respiration is called the *tidal volume*. However, this is only a fraction of the actual lung capacity and more air can be inhaled during forced inspiration; this is the *inspiratory reserve volume*. Conversely, it is possible to forcibly exhale more air than is expired during normal respiration; this additional amount of air is called the *expiratory reserve volume*. However, even after the most forced exhalation there is always some air left in the lungs and airways (otherwise they would collapse); this is called the *residual volume*.

The total amount of air that can be expired after a maximum inspiration is called the *vital capacity*. The amount of air that is left in the lungs after normal expiration is called the *functional residual capacity* and it is this that allows gaseous exchange to take place during expiration. The *total lung capacity* is the sum of the residual volume, expiratory reserve volume, tidal volume and inspiratory reserve volume. Much of the air drawn in at each breath is exhaled again before it reaches the alveoli (i.e., it is not involved in gaseous exchange); this is equal to the volume of the conducting system and is called the *dead space*.

The *respiratory rate* is the number of breaths per minute. In the dog the resting respiratory rate is 10–30 breaths per minute; in the cat it is 20–30 breaths per minute.

CHAPTER 9

Digestive system

KEY POINTS

- The digestive system of the carnivore is described as monogastric. The tract is relatively short, because meat is easy to digest and the stomach is simple.
- The teeth of the carnivore are sharp, pointed and powerful and the jaw has a scissor-like action. This enables meat to be cut and torn off the bones of prey.
- The majority of the tract is a long tube of varying diameter. Each part has a similar structure but shows functional adaptations.
- Food passes down the tract and is mixed with digestive juices by coordinated muscular movements known as peristalsis and rhythmic segmentation.
- Digestion occurs by the action of enzymes, each of which is specific to a particular food type.
- Digestive juices containing enzymes are secreted by intrinsic exocrine glands in the stomach and small intestine and by extrinsic glands such as the pancreas and gall bladder.
- Digestion results in the production of soluble molecules that can pass through the epithelium of the small intestine into the blood capillaries (amino acids and monosaccharides) or lacteals (fatty acids and glycerol).
- The products of digestion are carried around the body where they are metabolised and used by the tissues.
- Any unwanted or indigestible food remains are excreted in the faeces.

The maintenance of life depends on a constant supply of energy. Food provides energy and the digestive system has evolved to extract it from the nutrients taken into the body and then to excrete the indigestible remains. The digestive process occurs in several stages:

- *Ingestion* is the process of taking food into the body; this takes place in the mouth.
- *Digestion* is the process of breaking down the food into small chemical units; this occurs in the stomach and small intestine.
- *Absorption* is the process whereby the chemical units pass into the blood and are carried to the liver; this occurs in the small intestine.
- *Metabolism* is the process in which the chemical units are converted into energy for use by all the organs of the body; this takes place mainly in the liver.
- *Excretion* is the removal of any remaining indigestible material.

The digestive system (Figs. 9.1 and 9.2) consists of the following parts:

- Oral cavity or mouth, lips, tongue, teeth
- Pharynx
- Oesophagus
- Stomach
- Small intestine: duodenum, jejunum, ileum
- Large intestine: caecum, colon, rectum, anus

There are also several accessory glands, without which the digestive process cannot be completed:

- Salivary glands
- Pancreas
- Gall bladder
- Liver

The oral cavity

The oral cavity (Fig. 9.3), also known as the mouth or buccal cavity, contains the tongue, teeth and salivary glands. The function of the oral cavity is as follows:

1. To pick up the food: This is known as *prehension* and involves the use of the lips and tongue.
2. To break up the food into small boluses to aid swallowing: This is known as *mastication* or chewing and involves the use of the tongue, cheeks and teeth.
3. Lubrication of the food with mucus and saliva making it easier to swallow.
4. In omnivores and herbivores, digestion of carbohydrates begins in the mouth with the secretion of salivary enzymes. This does not occur in carnivores, such as dogs and cats, because food is held in the mouth for a very short time before it is swallowed.

The oral cavity is formed by the following bones of the skull (see Chapter 3):

- The *incisive* bone and the *maxilla* form the upper jaw.
- The *palatine* bone forms the roof of the mouth – the *hard palate.*
- The *mandible* forms the lower jaw; the paired mandibles join in the midline at the *mandibular symphysis.*

The mandibles articulate with the *temporal* bones of the skull, forming the *temporomandibular joint.* In carnivores the action of the joint is scissor-like to shear flesh off the bones of their prey.

The upper and lower jaws are linked by skin, forming the cheeks, under which lie the *muscles of mastication* (see Chapter 4). These muscles lie over the temporomandibular joint and give strength to the biting action. The entrance to the mouth is closed by the *lips*, composed of muscle covered in skin. The upper lip is split vertically by a division known as the *philtrum* (see Chapter 8, Fig. 8.1).

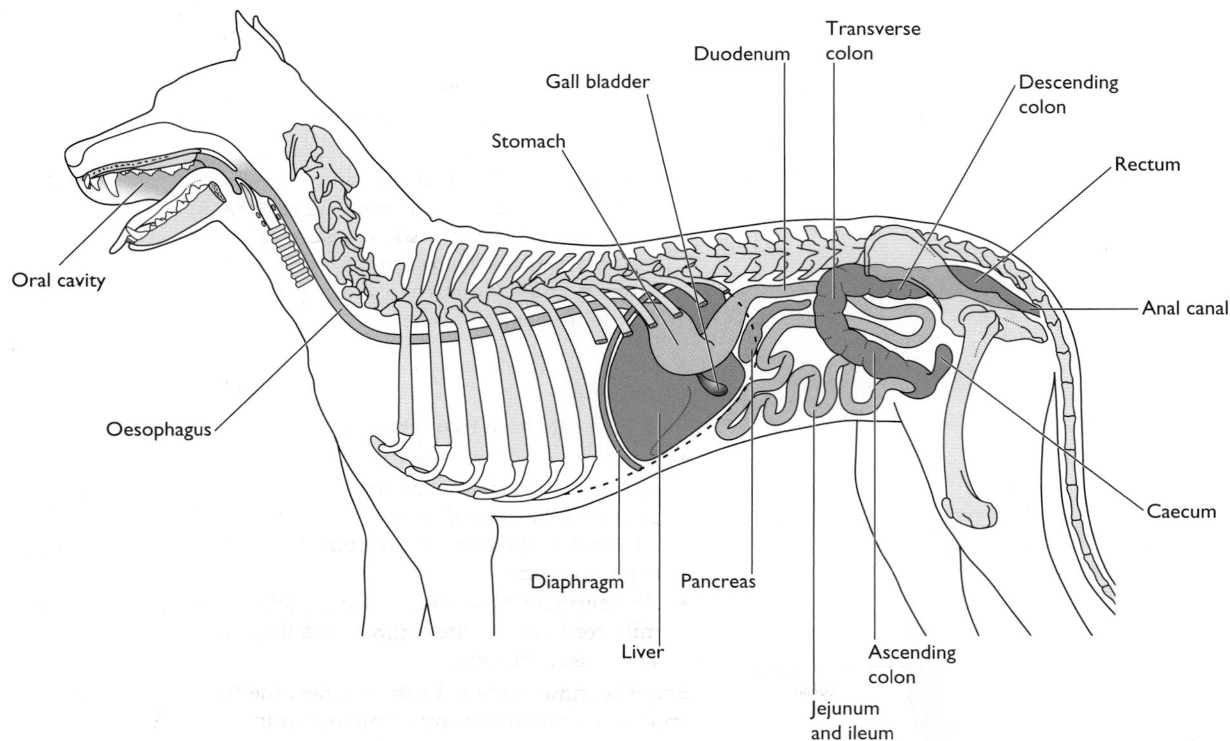

Fig. 9.1 Organs of the digestive system of the dog, left lateral view.

The entire oral cavity is lined by a layer of mucous membrane. It is reflected on to the jawbones, forming the *gums*. The mucous membrane covers the hard palate and extends over a flap of soft tissue at the back of the oral cavity; this is the *soft palate*, which extends caudally between the oral and nasal cavities and divides the pharynx into the *oropharynx* and *nasopharynx* (Fig. 9.3) (see also Chapter 8).

The tongue

The functions of the tongue are

1. To aid the ingestion of food.
2. To carry the receptors (taste buds) for the sensation of taste or *gustation* (see Chapter 5).
3. To help in the formation of a food bolus ready for swallowing.
4. To groom the fur, particularly in cats.
5. To assist thermoregulation: The tongue is used to apply saliva to the fur, which smoothes it down into a thinner and cooler layer; in dogs, panting, during which saliva evaporates from the tongue, helps to cool the body.
6. To produce vocalisation: Production of sound involves complicated movements of the tongue and lips.

The tongue lies on the floor of the oral cavity and is made of *striated muscle fibres* running in all directions. This enables the tongue to make delicate movements. The muscles are attached at the *root* of the tongue to the hyoid bone (see Chapter 8) and to the sides of the mandibles. The tip of the tongue is unattached and very mobile.

In an anaesthetised animal, the sublingual vein, running under the tongue, may be used for intravenous injections or for collecting blood samples, while the sublingual artery may be used for monitoring the pulse rate.

The tongue is covered in mucous membrane. The dorsal surface is thicker and arranged in rough *papillae*, which assist in control of the food bolus and in grooming. Some papillae are adapted to form taste buds, mainly found at the back of the tongue. Taste buds are well supplied with nerve fibres, which carry information about taste to the forebrain (see Chapter 5). Running along the underside of the tongue are the paired *sublingual veins* and *arteries.*

The teeth

The teeth are hard structures embedded in the upper and lower jaw and those of the dog and cat are described as being *brachydontic,* meaning that they are fairly low in profile and they cease to grow once they have reached their final size. Each jaw forms a *dental arch* or *dentary;* there are four dental arches in total. The teeth pierce the gums to sit in sockets or *alveoli.* The membrane covering the gums is known as the *gingival membrane* or *periodontal membrane.*

Structure

All teeth have a basic structure (Fig. 9.4). In the centre of each tooth is a *pulp cavity.* This contains blood capillaries and nerves, which supply the growing tooth. In young animals the cavity is relatively large but, once the tooth is fully developed, it shrivels and contains only a small blood and nerve supply. After a tooth has stopped growing the only changes occurring will be due to wear.

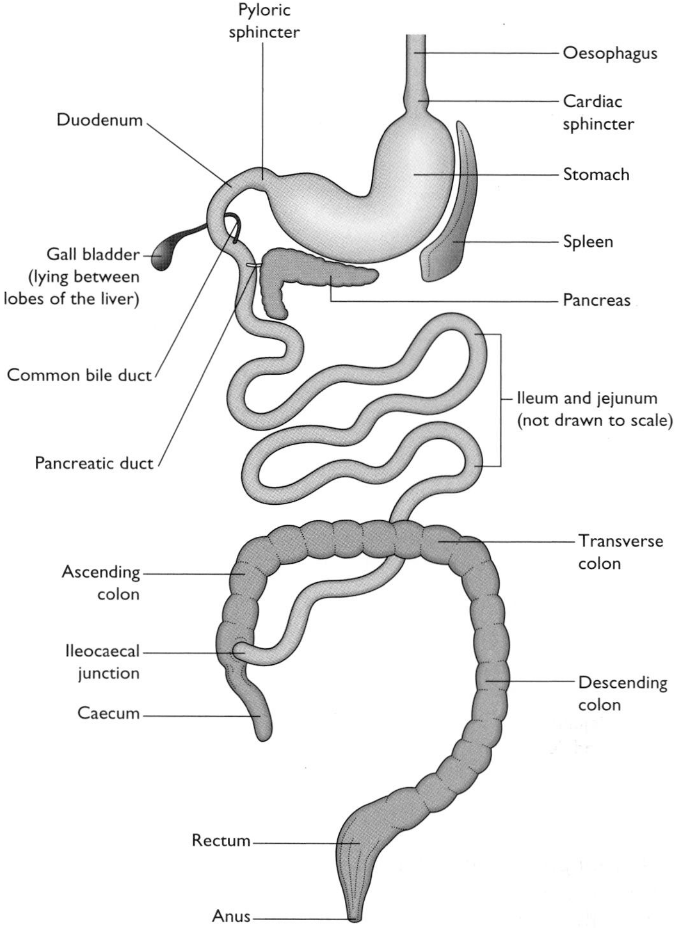

Fig. 9.2 The digestive tract removed from the body.

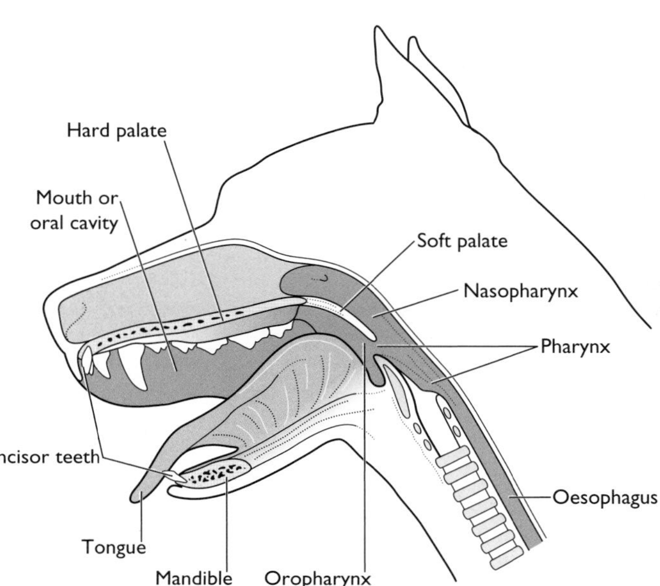

Fig. 9.3 Lateral view of the dog's head to show the oral cavity/digestive system.

Function

The teeth of a carnivore are adapted to shearing and tearing the flesh off the bones of their prey. There are four types of tooth, which are classified by their shape and position in the jaw (Fig. 9.5). This is summarised in Table 9.1.

Malar abscess. This is said to occur when the roots of the upper carnassial tooth become infected. The resulting abscess bursts through the bone and the skin to discharge pus just below the eye. Treatment requires removal of the tooth, which may be difficult because there are several roots and they may be deeply embedded in the maxillary bone.

Dentition

Dogs and cats have two sets of teeth in their lifetime:

- *Deciduous dentition,* also called the milk or temporary teeth, are present in the jaw at birth and erupt (push through the gums) as the animal grows. They are usually smaller and whiter than the permanent teeth and fall out as the adult teeth begin to erupt.
- *Permanent dentition,* also called the adult teeth, are larger than milk teeth and as the animal ages they show signs of wear. They last a lifetime.

Eruption times vary with the species, the type of tooth and the species of animal and are summarised in Table 9.2.

Dental formulae

Each species has a characteristic dental formula and this enables the veterinary surgeon to monitor the numbers of teeth lost as a result of disease or ageing. Each type of tooth is referred to by its initial letter: I is for incisor, for example. The following numbers show how many teeth of each type there are in the upper and lower jaws on one side of the head. The numbers are then multiplied by two to give the total number of teeth in the mouth.

Dog dental formula
Permanent: (**I**3/3, **C**1/1, **PM**4/4, **M**2/3) × 2 = 42 teeth
Deciduous: (**I**3/3, **C**1/1, **PM**3/3) × 2 = 28 teeth
Cat dental formula
Permanent: (**I**3/3, **C**1/1, **PM**3/2, **M**1/1) × 2 = 30 teeth
Deciduous: (**I**3/3, **C**1/1, **PM**3/2) × 2 = 26 teeth

Salivary glands

These are paired glands lying around the area of the oral cavity. Their secretions, known collectively as saliva, pour into the cavity via ducts. Saliva contains 99% water and 1% mucus; there are no enzymes in the saliva of the dog and the cat (Fig. 9.6).

The positions of the glands are

- *Zygomatic:* close to the eyeball within the orbit.
- *Sublingual:* medial to the mandible, under the mucosa covering the underside of the tongue.
- *Mandibular:* caudal to the angle of the jaw; can be palpated but may be mistaken for the mandibular lymph nodes, which are in this area.
- *Parotid:* between the base of the ear and the mandibular glands; can be palpated.

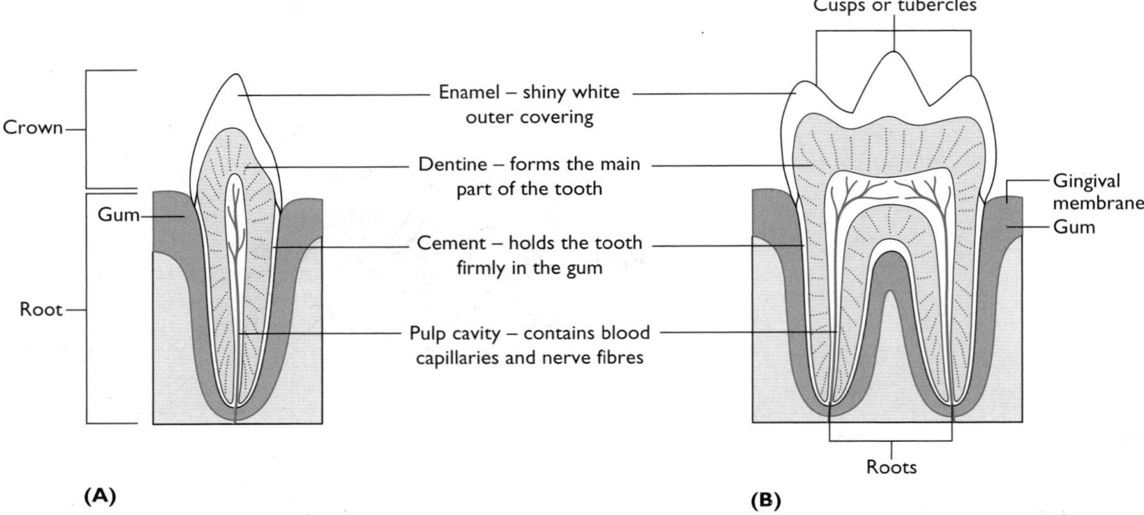

Fig. 9.4 **(A)** Shape and features of incisor and canine teeth. **(B)** Shape and features of premolar, molar and carnassial teeth.

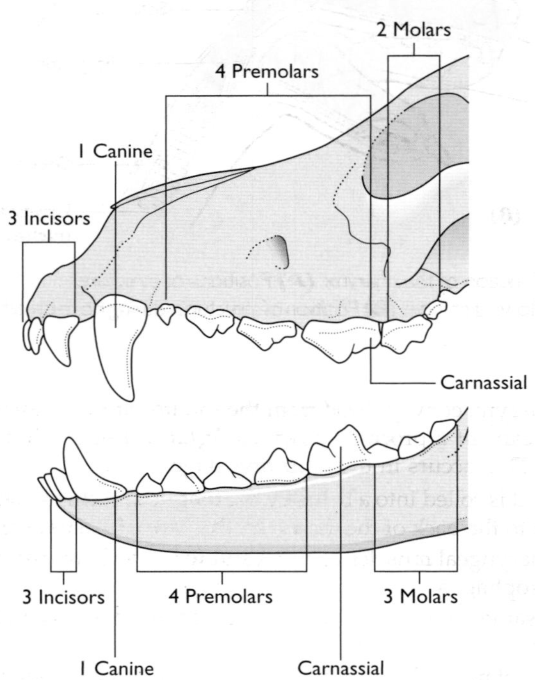

Fig. 9.5 Skull of an adult dog showing the permanent dentition.

Table 9.1 Tooth types and functions

Type	Position and shape	Function
Incisor (I)	Lie in the incisive bone of the upper jaw and in the mandible of the lower jaw; small, pointed with a single root	Fine nibbling and cutting meat; often used for delicate grooming
Canines (C) – 'eye teeth'	One on each corner of the upper and lower jaws; pointed, with a simple curved shape; single root deeply embedded in the bone	Holding prey firmly in the mouth
Premolars (PM) – 'cheek teeth'	Flatter surface with several points known as cusps or tubercles; usually have two or three roots arranged in a triangular position to give stability in the jawbone	Shearing flesh off the bone using a scissor-like action; flattened surface helps to grind up the flesh to facilitate swallowing and digestion
Molars (M) – 'cheek teeth'	Similar shape to premolars; usually larger with at least three roots	Shearing and grinding meat (NB: There are no molars in the deciduous dentition.)
Carnassials	Largest teeth in the jaw; similar shape to other cheek teeth; the first lower molar and the last upper premolar on each side	Very powerful teeth sited close to the angle of the lips; only found in carnivores

Production of saliva is continuous but may be increased by such factors as the sight and smell of food (particularly in dogs), fear, pain and irritant gases or other chemicals such as organophosphates. Salivation also often occurs just prior to vomiting and may be a warning sign to the owner!

The function of saliva is

1. To lubricate the food, making mastication and swallowing easier.
2. Thermoregulation: Evaporation of saliva from the tongue during panting or from the fur when applied during grooming causes cooling of blood in the underlying blood capillaries; this reduces the core temperature of the body.
3. In omnivores and herbivores, secretions from the parotid gland contain amylase, which begins carbohydrate digestion.

Table 9.2 Eruption times

Tooth type	Dog	Cat
Deciduous dentition		
Incisors	3–4 weeks	Entire dentition starts to erupt at 2 weeks and is complete by 4 weeks
Canines	5 weeks	
Premolars	4–8 weeks	
Molars	Absent	
Permanent dentition		
Incisors	3.5–4 months	12 weeks
Canines	5–6 months	
Premolars	1st premolars 4–5 months; remainder 5–7 months	Variable; full dentition present by 6 months
Molars	5–7 months	

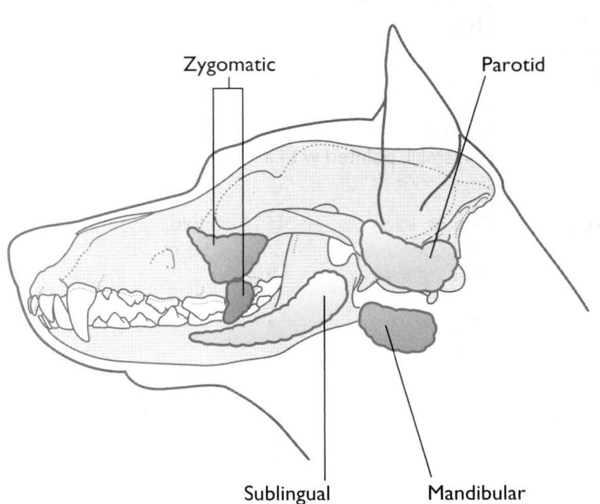

Fig. 9.6 Location of the salivary glands in the dog.

Pharynx

The pharynx forms a crossover point between the respiratory and digestive systems. It is a muscular tube lined with mucous membrane, connecting the back of the nasal and oral cavities with the oesophagus and the larynx and trachea. The soft palate extends caudally towards the epiglottis of the larynx and divides the pharynx into the nasopharynx and oropharynx (Fig. 9.3; see also Chapter 8). The walls of the pharynx contain diffuse areas of lymphoid tissue known as the *tonsils*. Their function is to protect the animal against disease (see Chapter 7). The most obvious are the palatine tonsils lying one on each side of the pharynx in a shallow recess. The *Eustachian* or *auditory tube* connects the pharynx to the middle ear. It enables the air pressure on either side of the tympanic membrane to equalise and thus maintains the flexibility and function of the ear drum (see Chapter 5).

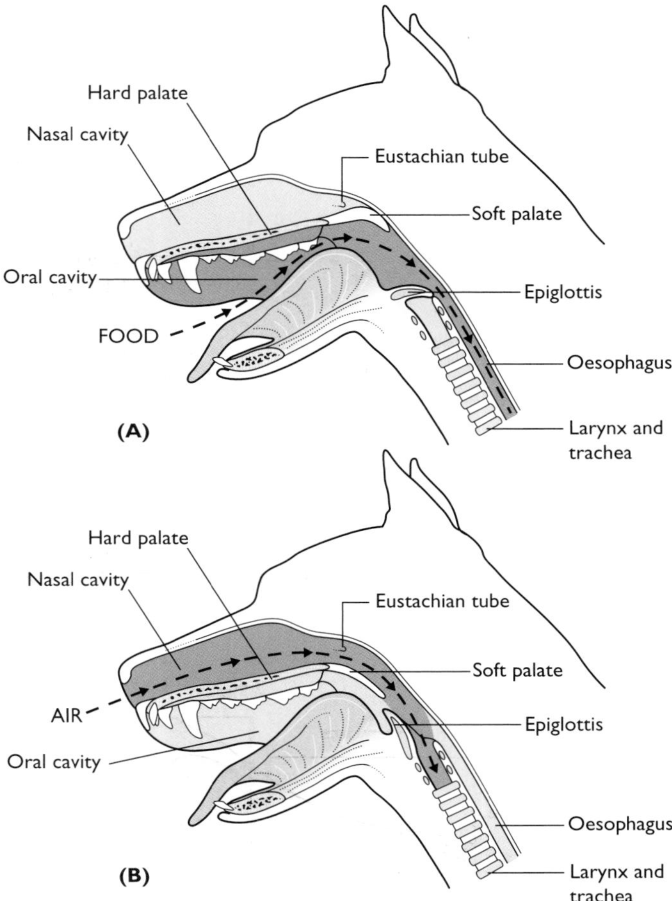

Fig. 9.7 Function of the pharynx. **(A)** Positions of structures during swallowing of food. **(B)** Position of structures during nose breathing.

The pharynx conveys food from the mouth into the oesophagus by means of a process known as *deglutition* or swallowing (Fig. 9.7). This occurs in the following stages:

1. The food is rolled into a bolus by the tongue and cheeks and is passed to the back of the mouth by the base of the tongue.
2. The pharyngeal muscles contract and force the bolus towards the oesophagus.
3. At the same time, the epiglottis closes to prevent food entering the larynx.
4. A wave of muscular contraction – *peristalsis* – pushes the food down the oesophagus.
5. When the food has passed through the pharynx, the epiglottis falls open and respiration starts again.

Oesophagus

This is a simple tube that carries food from the pharynx to the stomach (Figs. 9.1 and 9.2). In the neck, the oesophagus lies dorsal to the trachea and slightly to the left of it. It passes through the thoracic cavity, running within the mediastinum, dorsal to the heart base and between the two lungs. The oesophagus enters the abdominal cavity via the oesophageal hiatus of the diaphragm, which separates the thorax and abdomen.

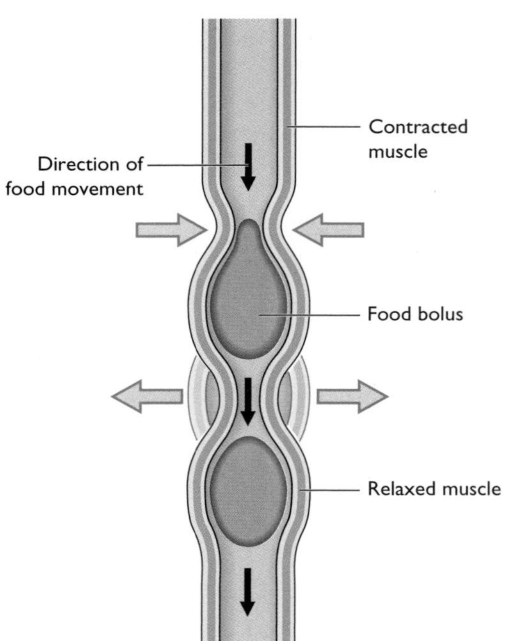

Fig. 9.8 Representation of peristalsis. Muscular contraction within the tube forces the food bolus along.

The walls of the oesophagus are lined with *stratified squamous epithelium* arranged in longitudinal folds. This protects against damage by food and allows for widthways expansion as the boluses pass down. Within the walls are circular and longitudinal bands of smooth muscle fibres. Contraction of these muscles brings about a series of *peristaltic waves* that force the food along the tube (Fig. 9.8). Food can pass in the reverse direction – *antiperistalsis* – seen during vomiting. The average time taken for food to pass down the oesophagus is 15–30 s but this depends on the type of food: liquids take a shorter time than dry foods.

Diagnosis of conditions of the digestive tract may be helped by the use of a 'barium meal' or barium series. Liquid barium sulphate is administered orally and a series of radiographs are taken over a period of several hours. Fig. 9.9 shows the result of the use of barium as a contrast medium and illustrates the anatomy of the canine digestive tract.

The abdominal part of the digestive system

The majority of the digestive tract lies within the abdominal cavity and can be divided into three parts:

- *Stomach:* used to store and mix ingested food
- *Small intestine:* the main site for enzymic digestion and the absorption of nutrients
- *Large intestine:* the site for absorption of water, electrolytes and water-soluble vitamins; any indigestible remains pass out of the anus as faeces.

Stomach

The stomach of the dog and cat is described as being *simple* (c.f. the compound stomach of ruminants; see Chapter 17) and digestion is said to be *monogastric*. The functions of the stomach are:

1. To act as a reservoir for food: Wild carnivores (particularly lions) may only eat every 3–4 days and then rest while food slowly digests.
2. To break up the food and mix it with gastric juices.
3. To begin the process of protein digestion.

The stomach is a C-shaped, sac-like organ lying on the left side of the cranial abdomen. Food enters from the oesophagus via the *cardiac sphincter* and leaves from the *pyloric sphincter* (Fig. 9.2). The inner curve of the sac is called the *lesser curvature* and the outer curve the *greater curvature*. The entire organ is covered in a layer of visceral peritoneum or *mesentery*, as are all the organs in the abdominal cavity. The mesentery attached to the inner curvature is called the *lesser omentum*, while that attached to the greater curvature is called the *greater omentum*. The *spleen* lies within the layers of the greater omentum. The walls of the stomach are thick and easily distended by food. When empty, the stomach lies under the ribs but when full the stomach may occupy a third of the abdomen.

Gastric dilatation and volvulus is a condition of large/deep-chested breeds of dog, such as the German Shepherd and the dachshund. It occurs when the stomach distends with gas and half-fermented food, becomes unstable and twists around on itself, preventing the escape of the gas. The dog suffers extreme discomfort and may rapidly go into shock and die if not treated to relieve the distension. In such cases, the stomach feels tight and drum-like and may fill half the abdomen.

Structure of the stomach wall

The stomach can be divided into three regions: the *cardia*, *fundus* and *pylorus*. Most of the gastric glands lie within the fundic region of the stomach. The walls of the stomach are lined with mucous membrane, the *gastric mucosa*. This is thrown into deep longitudinal folds known as *rugae*, which flatten out when the stomach fills with food. Within the mucosa are the *gastric pits* (Fig. 9.10), consisting of three types of cell responsible for the secretion of *gastric juices:*

- *Goblet cells* are found in all parts of the stomach. They secrete mucus to lubricate the food and to protect the stomach wall from damage by digestive enzymes (*autodigestion*).
- *Chief cells* are found within the fundus. They secrete *pepsinogen*, the precursor to the active enzyme pepsin; pepsin breaks down proteins to peptides.
- *Parietal cells* are found within the fundus. They secrete *hydrochloric acid* (HCl); this creates an acid pH which enables pepsin to work effectively.

Food enters the stomach via the cardiac sphincter. Distension of the stomach stimulates the secretion of the hormone *gastrin* from

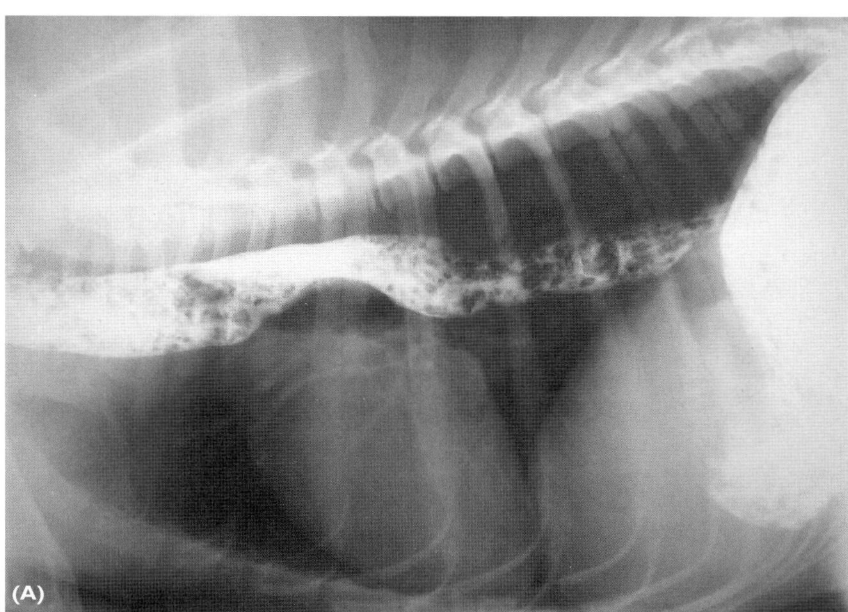

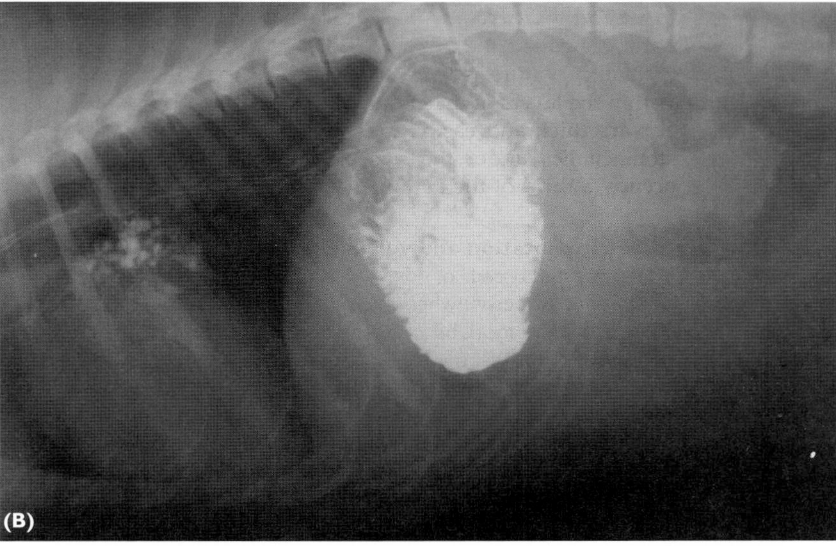

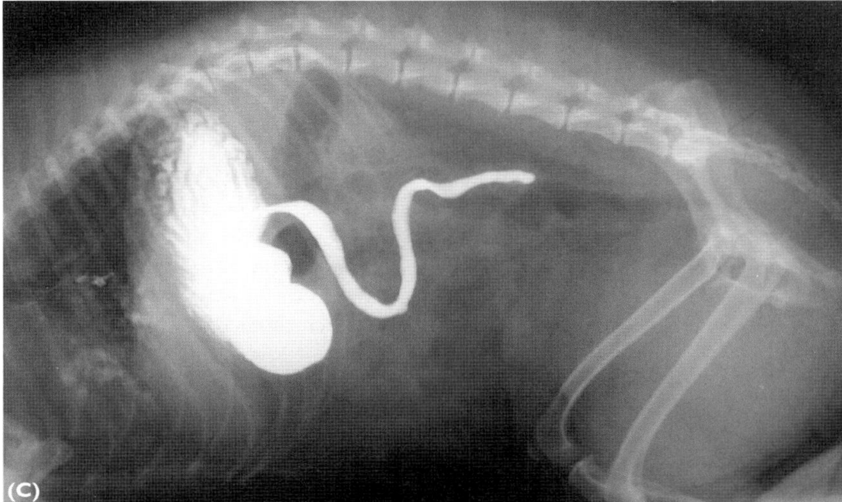

Fig. 9.9 Barium X-ray series illustrating the digestive tract. **(A)** The barium (radio-opaque white material) is in the oesophagus after being swallowed. **(B)** Barium enters the stomach. **(C)** Barium starts to leave the stomach and enter the duodenum.

Continued

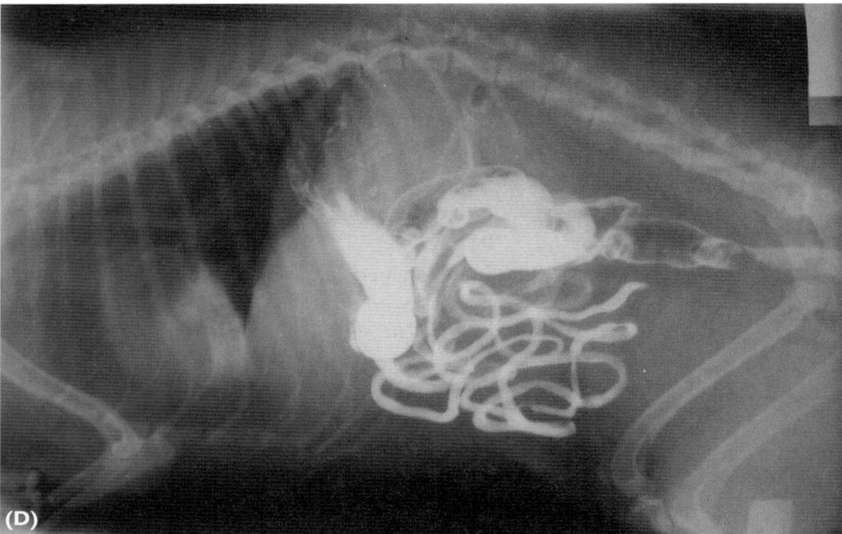

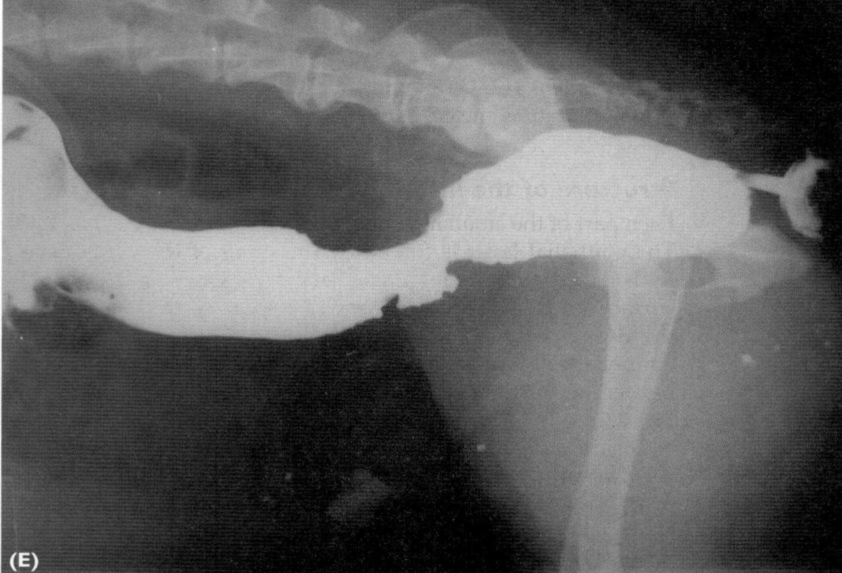

Fig. 9.9, cont'd **(D)** Most of the barium is now in the small intestine (a small amount remains in the stomach and some has entered the large intestine). **(E)** Barium in the colon and rectum applied by enema.

the stomach walls, which initiates the production of the gastric juices. Two types of muscular movement of the stomach break up and mix the food with the juices:

- *Peristalsis* pushes the food through the stomach (Fig. 9.8) and contributes to the rumbling of an empty stomach.
- *Rhythmic segmentation* breaks up and mixes the food boluses (Fig. 9.11).

Gastric emptying

Food in the stomach is broken up and partially digested, resulting in a soup-like liquid with an acid pH known as *chyme*. Chyme is released in spurts through the pyloric sphincter into the duodenum, where digestion continues. The time taken for food to pass through the stomach depends on the type of food. Liquids may take about half an hour, while more fatty or solid foods take about 3 h.

Vomiting is the 'return of ingesta and fluids against the normal direction of swallowing and peristalsis'. This is a very common presenting sign and there are three types:

- *True vomiting* is preceded by salivation and a feeling of nausea, followed by active abdominal contractions and expulsion of the vomitus. This may be caused by viral or bacterial infections, gastric irritation, foreign bodies, travel sickness, endoparasites, abdominal neoplasia and many metabolic diseases.
- *Passive vomiting or regurgitation* is caused by overflow of oesophageal contents (e.g., megaoesophagus or an oesophageal foreign body).
- *Projectile vomiting* is a violent ejection of stomach contents. This is characteristic of pyloric stenosis, a condition seen in neonates. It occurs when the muscle of the pyloric sphincter is overdeveloped and restricts the passage of chyme out into the duodenum.

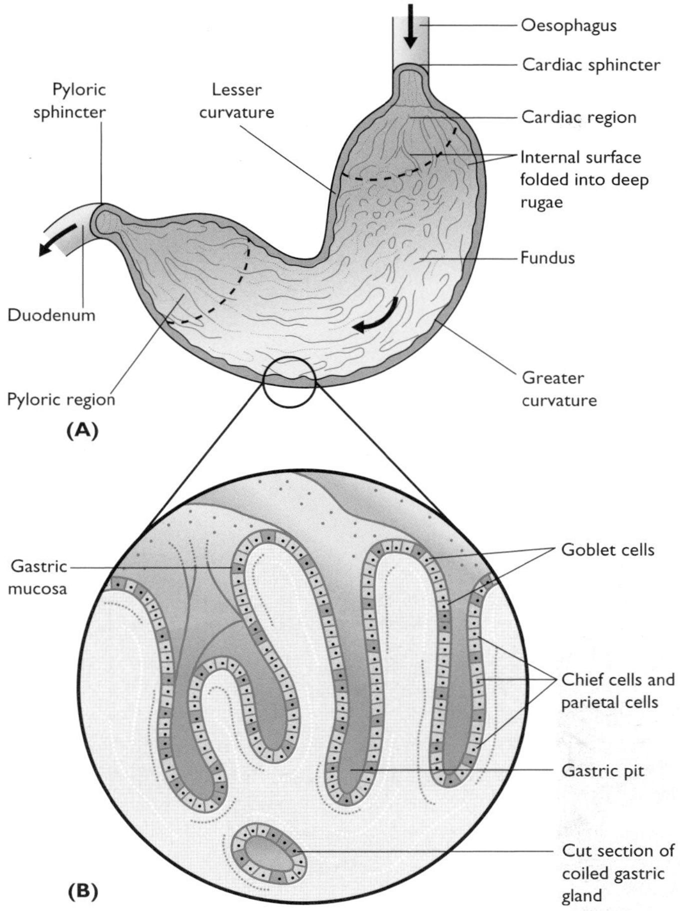

Fig. 9.10 **(A)** Structure of the stomach. **(B)** Enlargement to show a gastric pit.

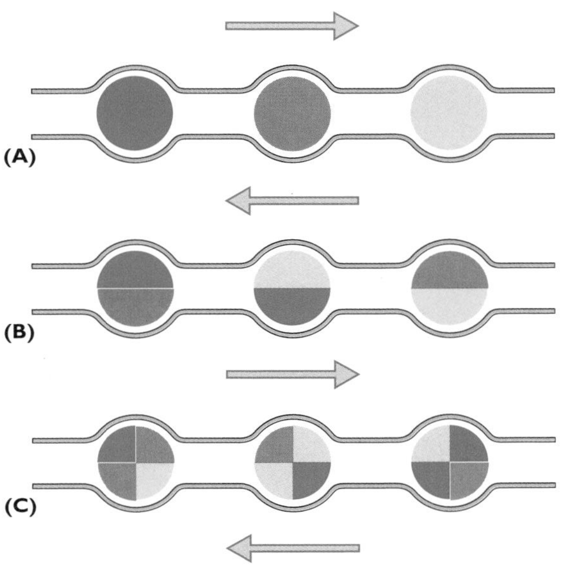

Fig. 9.11 Rhythmic segmentation within the gastrointestinal tract serves to break up and mix food boluses.

Small intestine

The small intestine is the major site of enzymic digestion and absorption. It is a long, relatively narrow tube and may be up to 3.5 times the body length. Food passes along the small intestine and is mixed with digestive juices by peristalsis and by rhythmic segmentation. It is divided into three parts, each of which has a similar structure but shows functional adaptations (Figs. 9.2 and 9.9):

- The *duodenum* is a U-shaped tube with the *pancreas* lying in the loop of the 'U'. The duodenum lies in a fixed position as the mesentery, the *mesoduodenum*, is short. The *pancreatic duct* leading from the pancreas and the *common bile duct* from the gall bladder open into it. Within the walls are glands, known as Brunner's glands, which secrete a mixture of digestive enzymes known as *succus entericus*. The duodenum leads into the jejunum.
- The *jejunum* and *ileum* are difficult to distinguish from each other. They constitute a long tube with no fixed position as the *mesojejunum* and *mesoileum* are long, allowing the tract to fill any available space in the peritoneal cavity. Within the walls are digestive glands known as the *crypts of Lieberkühn*. The ileum ends at the *ileocaecal junction*, where it joins the caecum.

Structure of the intestinal wall

Each part of the small intestine has a similar structure (Fig. 9.12). The epithelial layer is folded into millions of tiny, leaf-shaped folds called *villi* (sing. *villus*). Their function is to increase the surface area of the epithelium to maximise the efficiency of the digestive and absorptive processes. Extending from each epithelial cell is a border of tiny *microvilli*, which form a 'brush border' to further increase the surface area (see Chapter 2, Fig. 2.2).

Inside each villus is

- A network of blood capillaries that convey small molecules from the breakdown of carbohydrates and proteins to the liver via the hepatic portal vein.
- A lymphatic capillary known as a *lacteal*. Each lacteal carries *chyle*, a milky fluid resulting from fat digestion, from the small intestine to the cisterna chyli in the dorsal abdomen.

The pancreas

The pancreas is a pale pink, lobular gland lying in the 'U' of the duodenum, whose secretions are essential to the digestive process. It lies outside the digestive tract and is described as an *extrinsic gland*. The pancreas has an endocrine part (see Chapter 6) and an exocrine part and is classed as a mixed gland. The exocrine part secretes digestive enzymes and bicarbonate into the duodenum via the pancreatic duct (Fig. 9.2).

The gall bladder

The gall bladder lies within the lobes of the liver and is a reservoir for bile, produced by the liver. Bile contains bile salts needed for fat digestion and is stained yellow-green by bile pigment or *bilirubin* produced from the breakdown of old erythrocytes. It is secreted into the duodenum via the *common bile duct*.

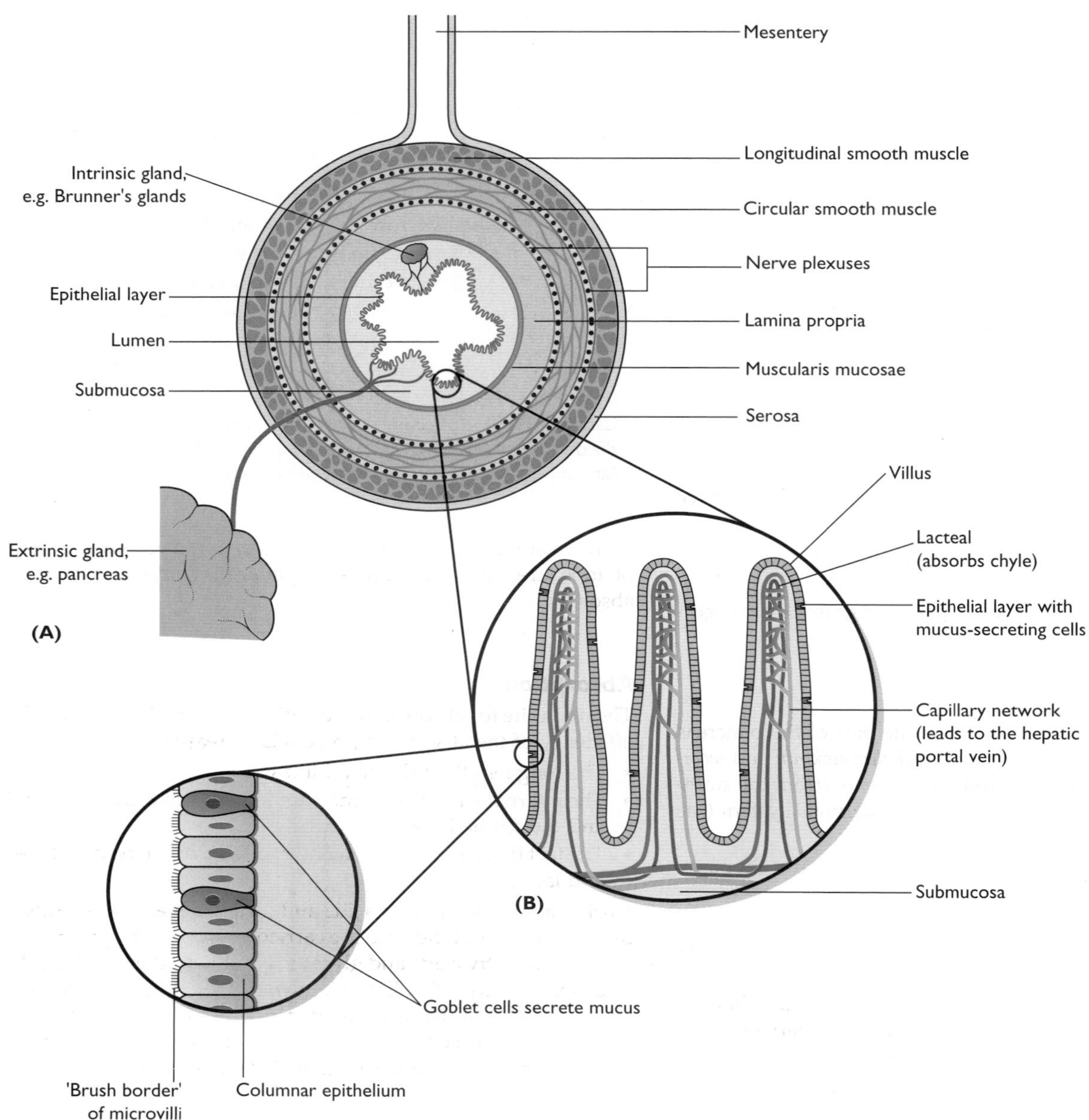

Fig. 9.12 **(A)** Cross-section through an area of intestine to show structure. **(B)** Enlargement to show the villi and absorptive epithelium.

Exocrine pancreatic insufficiency or EPI. This is a condition in which the pancreas fails to produce sufficient enzymes to digest the food. Levels of trypsin are the most significant because this enzyme activates the other enzyme precursors. The condition is particularly common in German Shepherd dogs. Affected dogs are thin, often lethargic, ravenously hungry and they produce large amounts of fatty (steatorrhoea) slightly runny faeces. Treatment is based on providing synthetic trypsin as a powder, which is added to the food, but feeding the dog on raw pig's pancreases has also proved successful.

Digestion

Food is ingested in the form of proteins (polypeptides), carbohydrates (polysaccharides) and fats (lipids). For food to be a useable source of energy, it must be broken down into soluble molecules that are small enough to be absorbed through the wall of the small intestine and into the bloodstream; this is digestion. In mammals this process occurs by the use of chemicals called *enzymes*. Each enzyme is designed to act on a specific material or substrate, and not on any other. They are usually named after the substrate on which they act; for example, lipase acts on lipids (fats) and maltase acts on maltose.

An enzyme is a protein that acts as a catalyst, increasing the speed of a reaction. Some enzymes may be produced in an inactive form, known as a precursor, which must be converted to the active form by another enzyme before they can work.

There are four sources of digestive juices containing the enzymes: gastric juices, pancreatic juices, bile salts and intestinal juices. Digestion in the carnivore begins in the stomach.

Gastric juice

This is secreted by the gastric pits in response to production of the hormone *gastrin* from the stomach wall (see Chapter 6). It contains:

- *Mucus* is secreted by goblet cells to lubricate the food and protect the gastric mucosa from autodigestion.
- *Hydrochloric acid* is secreted by parietal cells. This denatures or breaks down proteins, making digestion easier. It creates an acid pH of 1.3–5.0, which facilitates protein digestion.
- *Pepsinogen* is secreted by chief cells. It is converted to the active enzyme pepsin by HCl.
- *Pepsin* converts protein molecules to peptides (smaller molecules) by a process known as hydrolysis.

The liquid food resulting from this process of gastric juice digestion is known as *chyme.*

Pancreatic juice

This secretion is produced by the exocrine part of the pancreas and occurs in response to the hormones *cholecystokinin* and *secretin* (from the wall of the duodenum) and *gastrin* (from the stomach wall), and stimuli from the autonomic nervous system (see Chapter 6). It contains:

- *Bicarbonate* neutralises the effects of the acid in the chyme, allowing other enzymes to work.
- *Digestive enzymes,* many of which are inactive precursors, which prevents autodigestion and destruction of the pancreas:
  1. *Proteases* act on proteins and include:
     - *Trypsinogen*, converted to active trypsin by another enzyme, *enterokinase*, present in succus entericus.
     - *Trypsin*, which activates other enzyme precursors. It acts on peptides and other proteins to produce amino acids. A trypsin inhibitor within the pancreas prevents spontaneous conversion of trypsinogen to trypsin and autodigestion.
  2. *Lipases* are activated by bile salts. They convert fats to fatty acids and glycerol.
  3. *Amylases* act on starches, a form of plant carbohydrate, and convert them to maltose.

Bile salts

The presence of chyme in the duodenum causes the gall bladder to contract and produce bile. Bile emulsifies fat globules so that they have a larger surface area on which enzymes can act, and also activates lipases.

Intestinal juice

Secretion of intestinal juice is stimulated by the hormone *secretin* produced in response to the passage of chyme through the pyloric sphincter (see Chapter 6). The intestinal juices are produced by:

- Brunner's glands in the duodenum; the secretions are known as *succus entericus.*
- Crypts of Lieberkühn in the jejunum and ileum.

A number of enzymes are present, many of which are also produced by the pancreas:

- *Maltase* converts maltose to glucose.
- *Sucrase* converts sucrose to glucose and fructose.
- *Lactase* converts lactose to glucose and galactose.
- *Enterokinase* converts trypsinogen to trypsin.
- *Aminopeptidase* converts peptides to amino acids.
- *Lipase* converts fats to fatty acids and glycerol.

Protein (polypeptides) converted to amino acids
Carbohydrates (polysaccharides and disaccharides) converted to glucose and other simple sugars (monosaccharides)
Fats converted to fatty acid and glycerol (monoglycerides)

The result of the digestive process is that the basic constituents of food are converted into small molecules that can now be absorbed.

Absorption

The main site for absorption is the villi of the small intestine. The efficiency of the absorptive process is increased by:

- The long length of the small intestine
- The internal surface area increased by the presence of the villi and the epithelial 'brush border'
- The fact that each villus is well supplied with blood capillaries and lacteals

During absorption amino acids and simple sugars are absorbed by the blood capillaries and are carried by the hepatic portal vein to the liver. Fatty acids and glycerol are absorbed by the lacteals. They form a fatty milky liquid known as *chyle*, which is carried to the cisterna chyli, lying in the dorsal abdomen (see Chapter 7, Fig. 7.7). Here it is mixed with lymph and carried to the heart by the thoracic duct, where it joins the blood circulation.

Large intestine

This is a short tube of a wider diameter than the small intestine. Each part has a similar structure to that of the small intestine. However, in the lumen there are no villi and no digestive glands, but there are more goblet cells. These secrete mucus, which lubricates the faeces as it passes through. The large intestine is divided into:

- *Caecum* is a short, blind-ending tube joining the ileum at its junction with the ascending colon: this is the *ileocaecal junction* (Fig. 9.2). In carnivores it has no significant function.
- *Colon* is divided into the *ascending*, *transverse* and *descending colon* (Fig. 9.1) according to the relative position in the peritoneal cavity, but all are a continuation of the same organ. The descending colon is held close to the dorsal body wall by the *mesocolon.* Within the colon water, vitamins and electrolytes are absorbed, ensuring that the body does not lose excessive water and become dehydrated.

- *Rectum* is the part of the colon running through the pelvic cavity. It is held close to the dorsal body wall by connective tissue and muscle (Fig. 9.9).
- *Anal sphincter* marks the end of the digestive tract. It is a muscular ring that controls the passage of faeces out of the body. It has two parts:
  - *Internal anal sphincter*: Inner ring of smooth muscle; control is involuntary.
  - *External anal sphincter*: Outer ring of striated muscle; control is voluntary.

The lumen of the sphincter is constricted and lined with deep longitudinal folds of mucous membrane that stretch to allow the passage of bulky faeces.

Defaecation

The faecal mass passes through the large intestine by means of peristalsis, antiperistalsis, rhythmic segmentation and infrequent but strong contractions known as mass movements. These movements are involuntary but, as the faecal mass enters the pelvic cavity, stretching of the rectal wall stimulates voluntary straining brought about by abdominal contractions. The anal sphincter, which is normally held tightly closed, relaxes, the abdominal muscles contract and the mass is forced out.

Composition of faeces

Normal faeces have a colour and smell that is characteristic of the species. They are described as being 'formed' – the water content is such that the faeces keep their shape (watery faeces do not). Normal faeces contain:

- Water and fibre
- Dead and living bacteria – normal commensals of the large intestine, which may contribute to the smell
- Sloughed intestinal cells
- Mucus
- Contents of anal sacs
- Stercobilin – a pigment derived from bile that gives faeces their colour

Lying between the two anal rings, in the '20 to 4' position, are the *anal sacs*. These are modified sebaceous glands, which vary from pea to marble size depending on the species and breed of animal. Their secretions coat the faeces as it passes out and the characteristic smell is used by the animal for territorial scent marking, particularly in wild species. Impacted anal sacs may be a problem in dogs fed on softer diets.

The sequence of muscle contraction and nervous control involved in defaecation requires coordination by the nervous system. Any damage to the spinal cord (e.g., disc prolapse or severe trauma), may result in faecal incontinence or faecal retention.

Diarrhoea is 'frequent evacuation of watery faeces'. This is a common presenting sign. It may be acute or chronic and is an indication of some form of intestinal disturbance, such as maldigestion, malabsorption, increased peristalsis or gastrointestinal irritation. However, the most common cause of diarrhoea, in dogs especially, is dietary mismanagement. This can be easily corrected by starvation for 24 h followed by a light diet of fish or chicken and rice for a further 24 h.

The liver

The liver is the largest gland in the body and lies in the cranial abdomen. The cranial aspect is convex and is in contact with the diaphragm. The caudal aspect is concave and is in contact with the stomach, duodenum and right kidney (Fig. 9.1). The liver is deep red in colour because it has a large volume of blood flowing through it. It is divided into several large *lobes*, in the centre of which is the *falciform ligament*. This is the remains of fetal blood vessels from the umbilicus and is of little significance in the adult animal (see Chapter 7). The *gall bladder* lies between the lobes in the centre of the caudal aspect. It stores bile, which pours into the duodenum via the common bile duct.

Liver disease. Because the liver has so many functions the clinical signs of liver disease may be non-specific and include vomiting, diarrhoea, weight loss, anterior abdominal pain and pale faeces. More specific signs include jaundice (yellowing of mucous membranes), ascites (fluid in the abdomen), oedema (fluid under the skin) and cirrhosis (replacement of diseased liver tissue by fibrous tissue).

Histologically, the liver consists of thousands of cells known as *hepatocytes* (Fig. 9.13). These are responsible for all the many functions of the liver. The hepatocytes are arranged in hexagonal liver *lobules* surrounded by connective tissue. Running through the lobules between the hepatocytes are minute blood *sinusoids* carrying blood from the *hepatic portal vein*. Each hepatocyte is bathed in plasma, which percolates across the lobule to drain into the *central vein*. The central veins flow into the *hepatic vein* and so to the caudal vena cava. Thus the products of digestion are carried from the small intestine by the blood to every hepatocyte, where they are used for metabolism. The liver tissue receives arterial blood in the *hepatic artery*.

Between the hepatocytes are tiny channels known as *bile canaliculi*, into which bile is secreted. The canaliculi form an interconnecting network that eventually drains into the gall bladder. There is no direct connection between the sinusoids and the canaliculi.

The liver has many functions and is essential to normal health.

1. *Carbohydrate metabolism:* Glucose is a source of energy for the body but it can only be used by the cells in the presence of the hormone insulin, secreted by the pancreas. Excess glucose is stored as glycogen (glycogenesis) in the liver. This is broken down to release glucose (glycogenolysis) when blood glucose levels are low. In this way, the liver keeps blood glucose levels within a narrow range (see Chapter 6, Fig. 6.3).
2. *Protein metabolism:* The liver has several important roles here:
   - *Formation of plasma proteins: Albumin* maintains the balance of fluids in the body; *fibrinogen* and *prothrombin* are involved in the blood clotting mechanism; *globulins* form part of the immune mechanism.
   - *Regulation of amino acids*: There are 20 amino acids that are essential to form body protein. The liver cells use these amino acids to make new proteins and as the 'building blocks' of other organic compounds. Amino acids that are not essential may be converted into more useful ones by a process known as *transamination*.

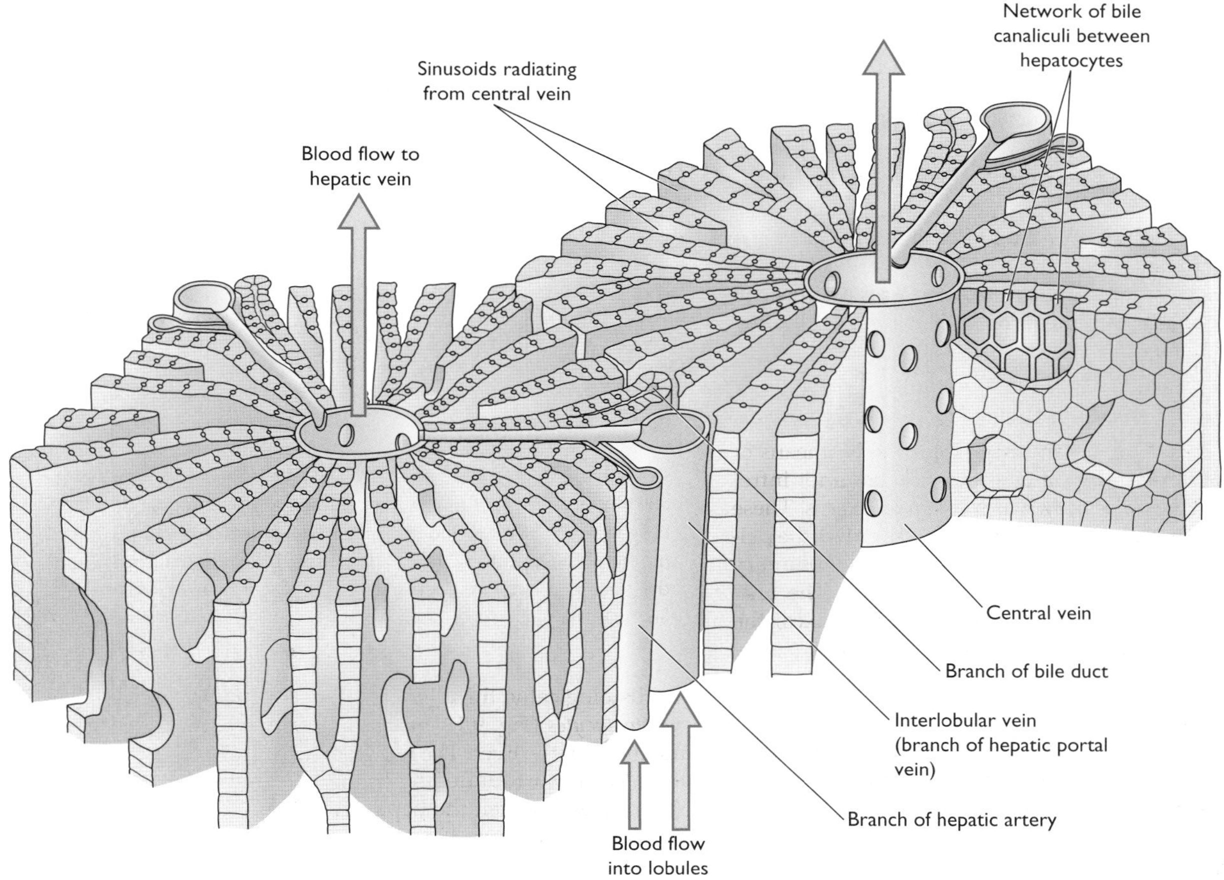

Fig. 9.13 Structural organisation of the liver.

- *Production of urea*: Surplus amino acids cannot be stored in the body and are converted by the liver to ammonia and then to urea. This process is known as *deamination.* Urea is excreted in the urine.

3. *Fat metabolism:* Fat is a source of energy for the body. The liver converts fatty acids and glycerol into phospholipids, for the formation of cell membranes, and to cholesterol for bile salts. Excess fat is stored in deposits around the body.
4. *Formation of bile:* Stored in the gall bladder.
5. *Destruction of old red blood cells:* Haemoglobin is excreted as bilirubin in the bile.
6. *Formation of new red blood cells:* The liver carries out this task only in the fetus.
7. *Storage of vitamins:* Mainly the fat-soluble vitamins A, D, E and K, but some water-soluble ones may also be stored.
8. *Storage of iron.*
9. *Regulation of body temperature and production of heat.*
10. *Detoxification of certain substances* (e.g., alcohol).
11. *Detoxification and conjugation of steroid hormones.* (See Fig. 9.13.)

CHAPTER 10

Urinary system

KEY POINTS

- The functional unit of the kidney is the nephron; each kidney contains many thousands of nephrons.
- Each nephron is made of several parts, each of which has a role in modifying the glomerular filtrate.
- Within the glomerular capsule of the nephrons, blood passes over a fine filter. Water and very small particles are removed. This is known as ultrafiltration and forms what is known as the glomerular filtrate.
- Large particles such as red blood cells and plasma proteins remain in the blood.
- The very dilute glomerular filtrate passes down the nephrons and undergoes a series of modifications, which result in the formation of urine. The final volume of urine is significantly reduced and reflects the status of the extracellular fluid (ECF) of the body.
- The function of the kidney is to regulate the volume and the osmotic concentration of the body fluids so that they remain constant. This is one of the homeostatic mechanisms of the body and is essential if the body is to function normally.
- The kidney is also responsible for the excretion of nitrogenous waste in the urine.
- Urine is stored in the bladder and removed from the body via the urethra.
- Urine samples can provide useful diagnostic information.

If the metabolic processes of the body are to function effectively, the chemical composition and volume of the tissue fluid must be kept constant. The most important function of the urinary system – and principally that of the kidney – is to maintain this constant internal environment, described as *homeostasis*.

The urinary system lies in the abdominal and pelvic cavities. It is anatomically linked with the genital or reproductive system and may be referred to as the *urogenital system*. Both systems share the urethra, which runs through the penis of the male and joins the vagina of the female.

The parts of the urinary system are:

- A pair of kidneys
- A pair of ureters
- Bladder
- Urethra

The functions of the urinary system are:

- To regulate the chemical composition and volume of the body fluids – *osmoregulation*
- To remove nitrogenous waste products and excess water from the body – *excretion*
- To act as an endocrine gland by the secretion of the hormone *erythropoietin* (see Chapter 6)

The kidney

There are two kidneys lying in the cranial abdominal cavity, one on each side of the midline ventral to the lumbar hypaxial muscles (Fig. 10.1). Each kidney is closely attached to the lumbar muscles by a covering of parietal peritoneum. There is no mesenteric attachment, as seen in other abdominal organs, and the kidney is described as being *retroperitoneal*. The right kidney lies slightly cranial to the left because the stomach has evolved to lie on the left side of the abdomen, pushing the left kidney out of position. Lying close to the cranial pole of each kidney are the ovaries of the female and the adrenal glands (Fig. 10.2).

Macroscopic structure

The kidneys of the cat and dog have a characteristic bean shape and the indented area is known as the *hilus*. This is the point at which blood vessels, nerves and the ureters enter and leave the kidney. The kidneys are normally a deep reddish-brown but the colour may be affected by any substance filtering through them. On a lateral radiograph of the abdomen, a normal kidney can be seen to be equivalent in size to approximately 2.5 vertebrae (Fig. 10.3). The smooth outer surface may be surrounded by a layer of fat, which acts as an energy reserve and protects the kidney from external damage.

When examining the cut surface of a normal kidney cut longitudinally, it is possible to see four layers (Fig. 10.4). From the outside inwards these are:

1. *Capsule*: This is the protective layer of irregular dense fibrous connective tissue closely attached to the cortex. It can be easily peeled away from a healthy kidney but any adhesions may indicate previous infection or damage.
2. *Cortex*: This dark red outermost layer of the kidney contains the renal corpuscles and convoluted tubules of the nephrons.
3. *Medulla*: This is slightly paler than the cortex and it may be possible to see the triangular-shaped *pyramids*, which contain the collecting ducts and, between them, tissue containing the *loops of Henle* of the nephrons.
4. *Pelvis*: This is basin-shaped and made of fibrous connective tissue, which gives it a whitish appearance. Urine formed by the nephrons drains into the pelvis and out of the kidney via a single ureter.

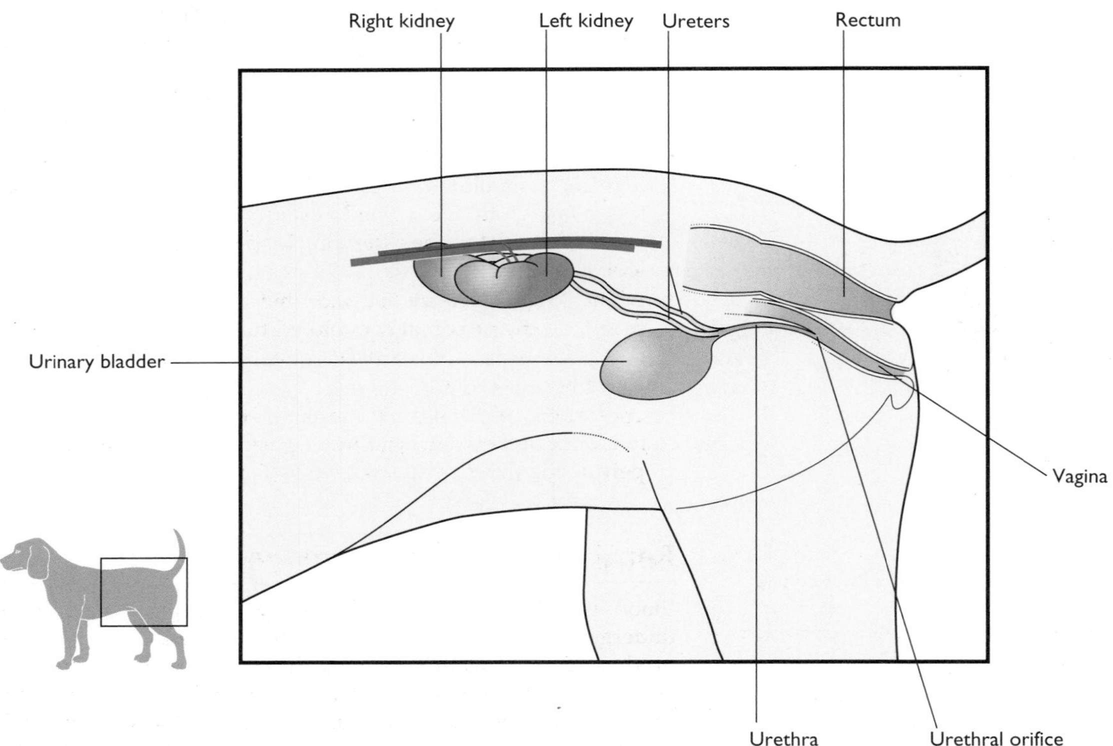

Fig. 10.1 The position of the urinary system in the bitch.

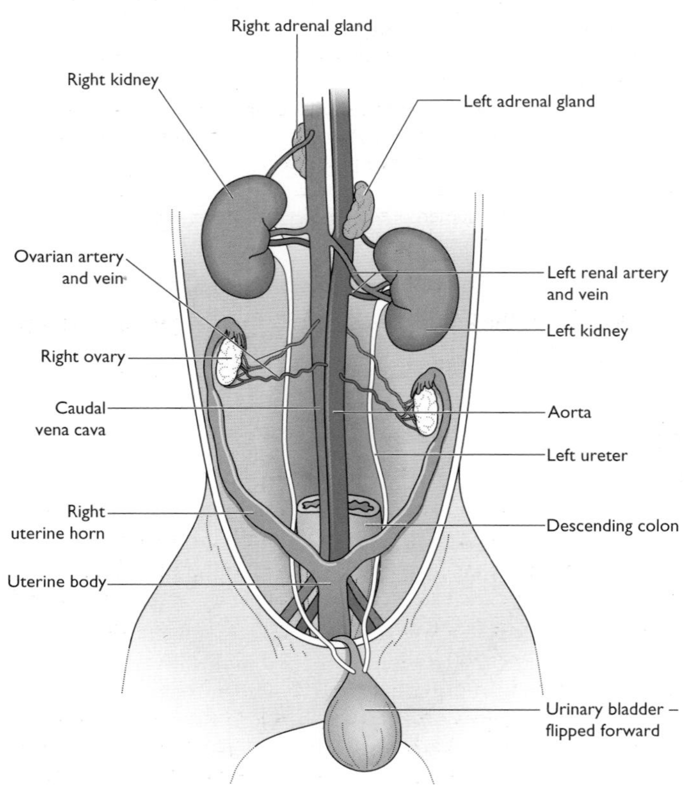

Fig. 10.2 Ventrodorsal view of the urogenital system of the bitch.

Renal failure: This may be acute or chronic and the condition affects the size of the kidney.

In acute renal failure the kidneys become swollen and painful to palpate.

In chronic renal failure the kidneys become shrunken, hard and do not cause pain when they are palpated.

Blood supply

Arterial blood is carried from the aorta in a single *renal artery* to each kidney (Fig. 10.4). This carries 20% of cardiac output. Within the tissue of the kidney, the renal artery divides into several *interlobar arteries*, which pass between the renal pyramids and into the cortex. Here capillaries supply the renal tubules and also give off numerous capillary networks known as *glomeruli* (sing. *glomerulus*) (Fig. 10.5). Each glomerulus supplies an individual nephron. The capillaries then recombine to form *interlobar veins*, which enter the single *renal vein*. This carries venous blood to the caudal vena cava.

Blood entering the kidney carries oxygen, nutrients and waste products from the tissues of the body; blood leaving the kidney carries carbon dioxide produced by the kidney tissues, but the nitrogenous waste products have been removed via the glomeruli.

Microscopic structure

The functional unit of the kidney is the *nephron* (Fig. 10.5). Each kidney contains about a million nephrons, which are closely

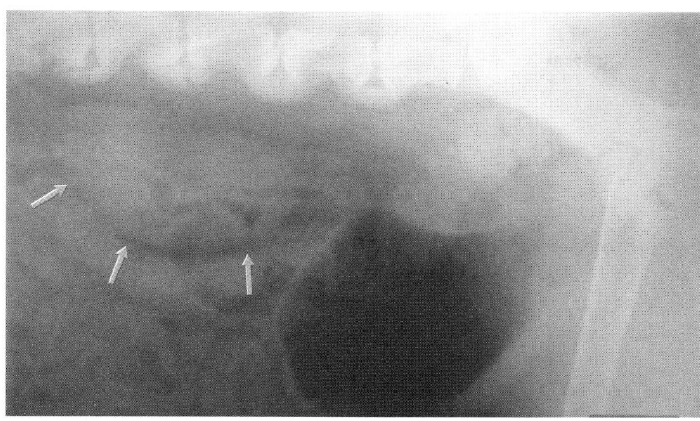

Fig. 10.3 Radiograph of the kidney area. The bladder has been inflated with air for contrast and the kidney (arrows) can be seen to measure about 2.5 times the length of the lumbar vertebrae.

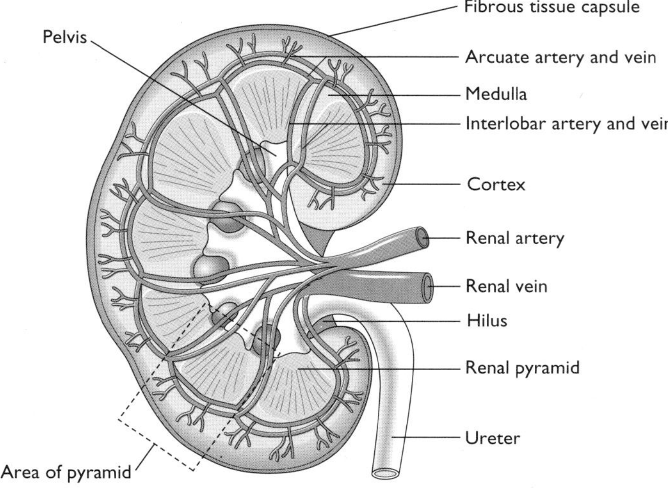

Fig. 10.4 Parasagittal section through the dog kidney.

packed together. They are responsible for the filtration of blood and the production of urine. Each nephron is a long tubule divided into several parts:

- *Glomerular capsule* is a cup-shaped structure enclosing a network of blood capillaries called the *glomerulus* (Fig. 10.6). The capsule may also be known as *Bowman's capsule*. The capsule and the glomerulus form the *renal corpuscle*. The basement membrane of the inner surface of the capsule, which is in close contact with the endothelium of the glomerular capillaries, is lined by podocyte cells between which are tiny pores (Fig. 10.6). These pores are of such a size that they will allow the passage of fluid and small molecules, but restrict the passage of larger molecules. The outer surface of the capsule is continuous with the epithelium of the proximal convoluted tubule. Fluid filtered by the capsule drains into the space between the two layers and continues into the next part of the nephron.
- *Proximal convoluted tubule* is a long, twisted tube leading from the neck of the capsule and lying in the renal cortex (Fig. 10.5). The tubules are lined in *simple cuboidal* or *columnar* epithelium. The side of the epithelium directed towards the lumen of the tubule is lined by fine *microvilli* forming a 'brush border'. This increases the surface area for the reabsorption of water and electrolytes.
- *Loop of Henle* is a U-shaped part of the tube leading from the proximal convoluted tubule and dipping down into the renal medulla. The tubule is lined in *simple squamous* epithelium, which is thicker in the ascending loop than in the descending loop (Fig. 10.5).
- *Distal convoluted tubule* is a short but less twisted part of the tube than the proximal convoluted tubule. It lies in the renal cortex and is lined in *cuboidal* epithelium without a brush border.
- *Collecting duct*: Each duct receives urine from several nephrons and conducts it through the pyramids into the renal pelvis. The ducts are lined in *columnar* epithelium.

Renal function: The formation of urine

Blood is filtered by the kidneys and the resulting filtrate undergoes a series of modifications within the renal tubules to produce urine. This urine is very different in composition and volume from the original filtrate. For every 100 L of fluid filtered from the blood only 1 L is produced as urine; 99% of the original filtrate is reabsorbed back into the blood. The changes made to the filtrate reflect the status of the ECF and in particular that of the blood plasma.

The physiological processes occurring in the renal nephrons are:

- *Osmosis* is the passage of water from a weaker to a stronger solution across a semi-permeable membrane.
- *Diffusion* is the passage of a substance from a high concentration to a low concentration.
- *Reabsorption* is the passage of a substance from the lumen of the renal tubules into the renal capillaries and so back into the circulation; this is an active process and requires energy.
- *Secretion* is the passage of chemical substances from the renal capillaries into the lumen of the tubules and out of the body in the urine; this is an active process and requires energy.

Blood enters the kidney and is carried to the capillaries forming the glomeruli.

Glomerulus

Blood pressure within each glomerulus is high because:

- The blood has come straight from the renal artery and the aorta, both of which carry blood under high pressure.
- The smooth muscle in the walls of the efferent arteriole leaving the glomerulus is able to constrict, under the control of the hormone *renin*, and thus regulate the pressure of blood in the glomerulus.

High pressure in the glomerulus forces fluid and small molecules out of the blood through the pores of the basement membrane into the capsular lumen. Larger-sized particles such as red blood cells, plasma proteins and any substance bound to protein molecules (e.g., hormones) are retained in the blood. This process is known as *ultrafiltration* and the filtrate is referred

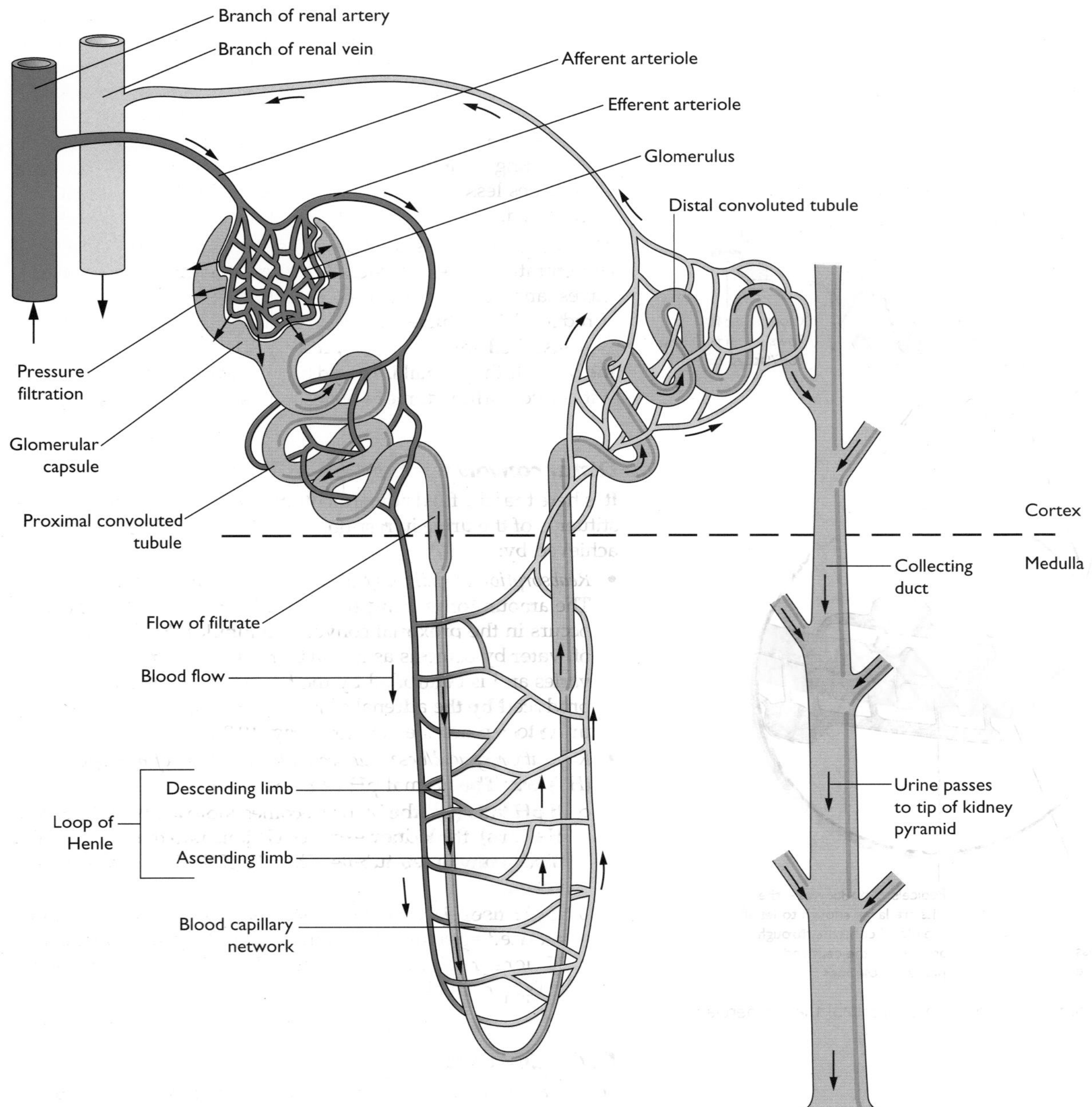

Fig. 10.5 A renal nephron.

to as the *glomerular filtrate* or *primitive urine*. The glomerular filtrate is very dilute and contains 99% water and 1% chemical solutes.

Proximal convoluted tubule

Approximately 65% of all the resorptive processes take place here (Fig. 10.7). These are:

- *Reabsorption of water and sodium*: Sodium (Na^+) and chloride (Cl^-) ions are actively reabsorbed from the filtrate into the blood. Water is reabsorbed by osmosis in response to the movement of Na^+ ions; 80% of all the Na^+ and Cl^- ions in the filtrate are reabsorbed at this point.
- *Reabsorption of glucose*: In the normal animal the glomerular filtrate contains glucose which is *all* reabsorbed back into the blood, so normal urine does not contain glucose. This reabsorption occurs up to a certain level referred to as the *renal threshold*.
- *Concentration of nitrogenous waste*: The main waste product is urea, produced as a result of protein metabolism by the liver. Water reabsorption concentrates the levels of urea in the tubules.
- *Secretion of toxins and certain drugs*: These are actively secreted into the filtrate. Penicillin and its more modern derivatives, given therapeutically, are secreted from the blood and carried to the bladder in the urine. It is therefore a useful antibiotic for the treatment of bladder infections.

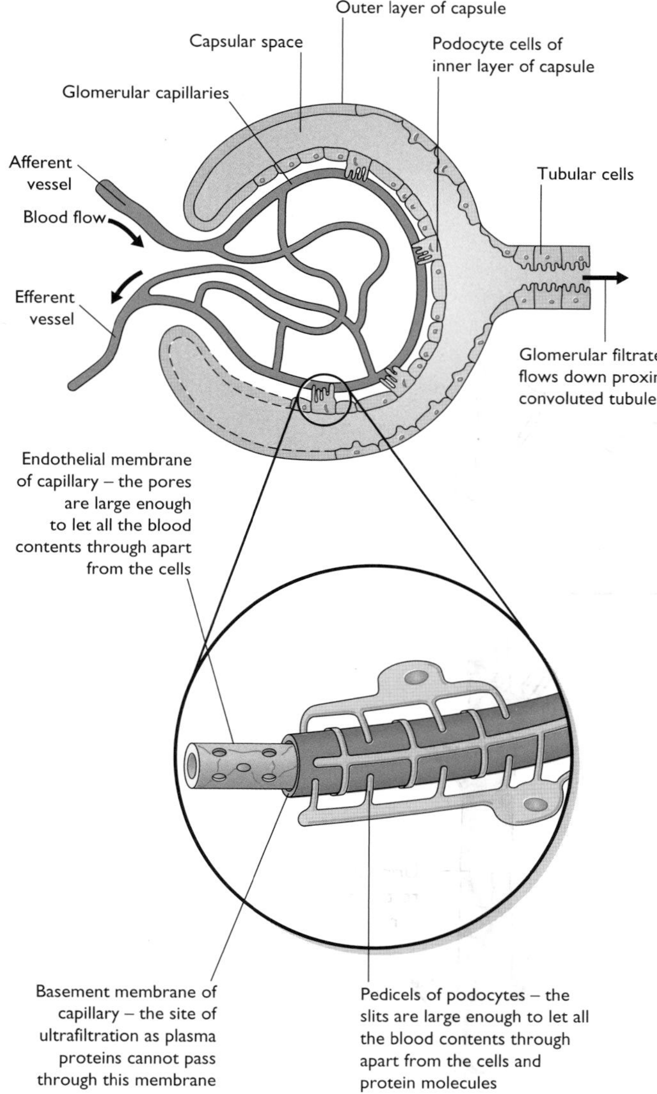

Fig. 10.6 Structure of the basement membrane of the glomerular capsule.

In cases of **diabetes mellitus**, there is too much glucose in the blood (*hyperglycaemia*). This overflows into the glomerular filtrate and the tubules reabsorb it up to the limit of the renal threshold. The excess passes on down the tubules and out in the urine: *glucosuria* is a diagnostic sign of diabetes mellitus.

Loop of Henle

The function of the loop of Henle is to regulate the concentration and volume of the urine according to the status of the ECF. The glomerular filtrate flows first into the descending loop and then into the ascending loop, both of which lie in the medulla (Fig. 10.7).

- *Descending loop of Henle*: The walls of the tubule are *permeable* to water but do not contain the mechanism to reabsorb Na^+. Water is drawn out of the tubule by osmosis, pulled by the concentration of Na^+ ions in the surrounding medullary tissue. The filtrate becomes more concentrated as it passes down the loop and reaches maximum concentration at the tip.
- *Ascending loop of Henle*: The walls are *impermeable* to water but contain sodium pumps that actively reabsorb Na^+ into the medullary tissue and capillaries. This draws water from the descending loop. Water cannot be drawn from the ascending loop because it is impermeable. The filtrate becomes less concentrated because the Na^+ ions have been removed.

The net result of this mechanism is that the filtrate is the same concentration when it enters the loop of Henle as it is when it leaves and passes into the distal convoluted tubule, but it is reduced in volume as water has been removed. This water is reabsorbed into the blood; it has been conserved for use by the body. If the animal is dehydrated, more water is reabsorbed; if it is overhydrated, more water will be lost in the filtrate.

Distal convoluted tubule

It is here that the final adjustments are made to the chemical constituents of the urine in response to the status of the ECF. This is achieved by:

- *Reabsorption of sodium (Na^+) and secretion of potassium (K^+)*: The amount of reabsorption of Na^+ is much smaller than occurs in the proximal convoluted tubules. Reabsorption of water by osmosis as a result of reabsorption of Na^+ varies and is controlled by the hormone *aldosterone* produced by the adrenal glands. K^+ is excreted into the urine to replace the Na^+ ions (Fig. 10.7).
- *Regulation of acid/base balance by the excretion of hydrogen (H^+) ions:* The normal pH of blood is 7.4.
  - If pH falls (i.e., the blood becomes more acid due to excess H+ ions), the kidney excretes H^+ ions into the urine via the distal convoluted tubule. The pH of the blood returns to normal.
  - If pH rises (i.e., the blood becomes more alkaline due to reduced amounts of H^+ ions), the kidney stops excreting H^+ ions, retaining them in the blood. The pH of the blood falls to normal.

Collecting duct

Here the final adjustments are made to the volume of water in the urine in response to the status of the ECF (Fig. 10.7). The hormone *antidiuretic hormone* (ADH), produced by the posterior pituitary gland, is able to change the permeability of the duct walls to water.

Diuretics are drugs used to increase the volume of urine produced and so reduce the volume of fluid in the body. One of the most commonly used – furosemide – is a 'loop diuretic', which acts on the loops of Henle. It prevents reabsorption of Na^+ so water is not reabsorbed by osmosis and remains in the urine as it flows through the tubules.

- If the animal is dehydrated, the volume of the plasma and ECF will be reduced. ADH will be produced and the permeability of the collecting ducts to water will be increased.

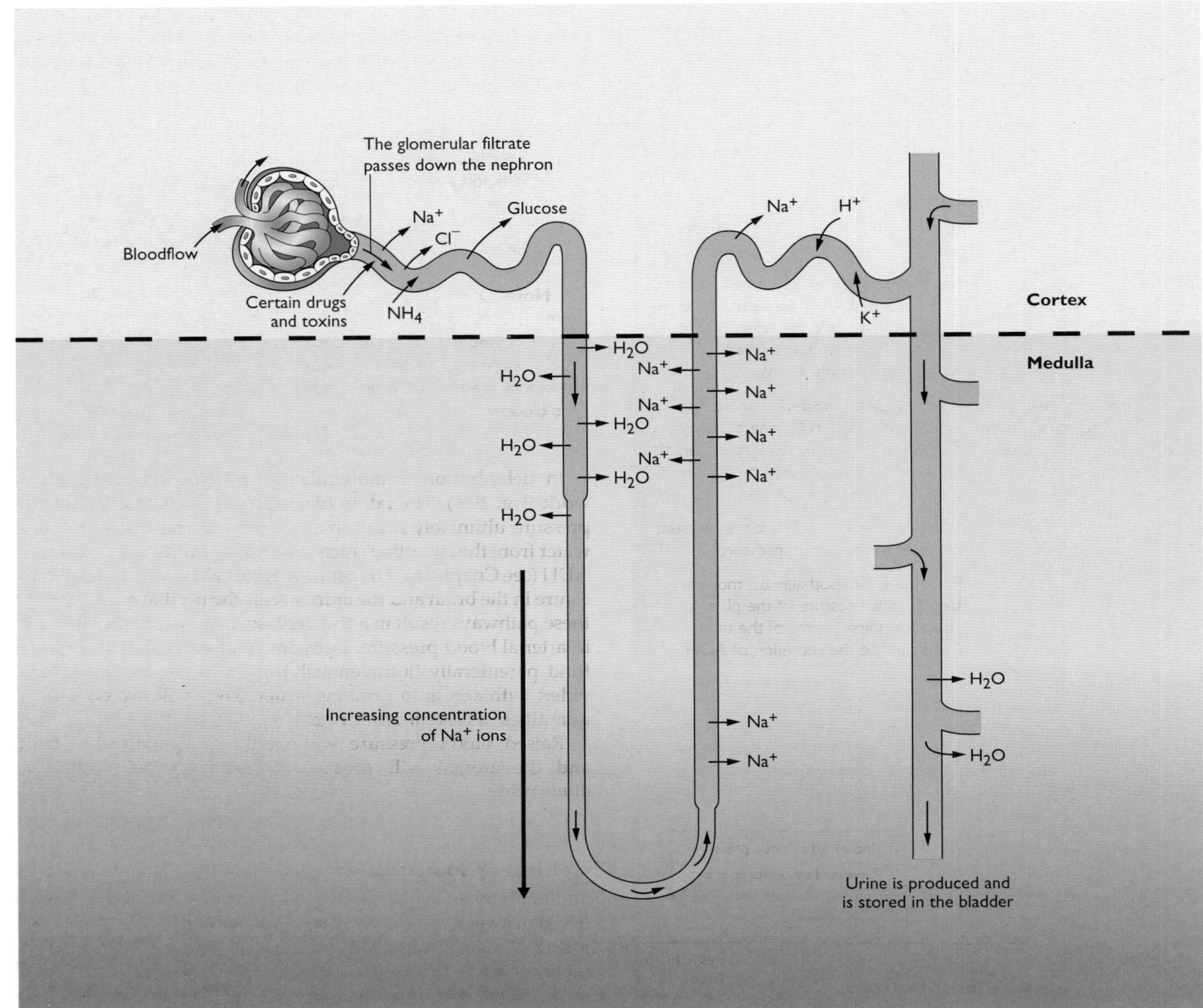

Fig. 10.7 Diagrammatic representation of the processes occurring in the different parts of the nephron.

Water will be drawn through the walls by the high concentration of Na^+ ions in the surrounding medullary tissue (secreted by the ascending loop of Henle), and into the plasma and ECF (Fig. 10.7).

As a result of the above processes, the ultrafiltrate that passed through the glomerular capsule has now become concentrated urine by the repeated effects of reabsorption and secretion.

Diabetes insipidus is caused by a lack of ADH, whose main function is to concentrate the urine as it flows through the collecting ducts in response to changes in the ECF. When this is lacking the urine has a very low specific gravity and is almost like water. The main clinical signs are of polydipsia and polyuria.

Osmoregulation: Control of renal function

Osmoregulation ensures that the volume of the plasma and the concentration of dissolved chemicals in the plasma and other tissue fluids remain constant. Homeostasis is maintained and the body can function normally. Several factors are involved in the control of osmoregulation (Table 10.1) and it is achieved in two ways:

- Control of the amount of water lost from the body
- Control of the amount of salt (NaCl) lost from the body

Control of water loss (*Fig. 10.8*)

Water is lost by the healthy animal in urine, faeces, sweat and respiration. Very small amounts may also be lost in vaginal

Table 10.1 Factors involved in osmoregulation

Controlling factor	Function
Renin (hormone)	Produced by the glomeruli of the kidney in response to low arterial pressure
Angiotensinogen (plasma protein)	Converted to angiotensin by the action of renin
Angiotensin (protein)	Causes vasoconstriction; stimulates the release of aldosterone from the adrenal cortex
Aldosterone (hormone – mineralocorticoid)	Secreted by the cortex of the adrenal gland; acts mainly on the distal convoluted tubules but has a lesser effect on the collecting ducts; regulates the reabsorption of Na^+ ions
Antidiuretic hormone (ADH or vasopressin)	Secreted by the posterior pituitary gland; mainly affects the collecting ducts by changing their permeability to water; also has an effect on the distal convoluted tubules
Baroreceptors	Found in the walls of the blood vessels; monitor arterial blood pressure
Osmoreceptors	Found in the hypothalamus; monitor the osmotic pressure of the plasma; affect the thirst centre of the brain and influence the secretion of ADH

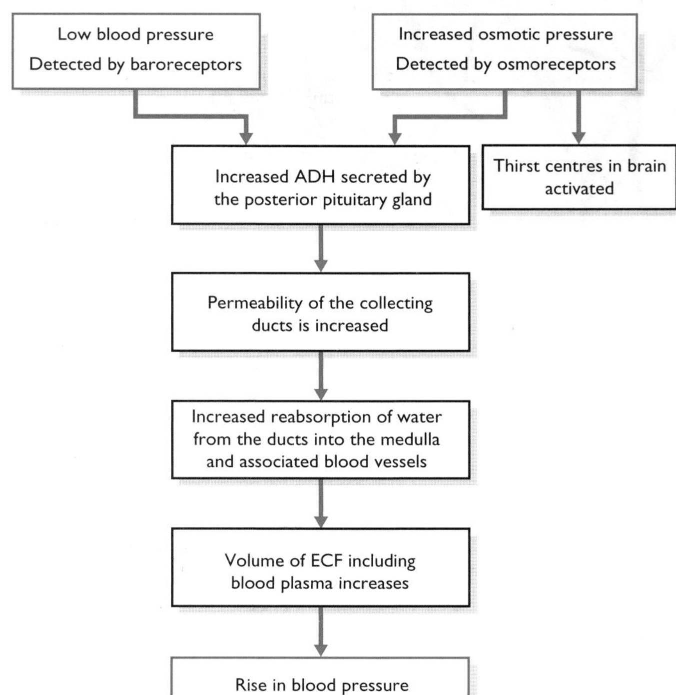

Fig. 10.8 Mechanism controlling the amount of water lost from the kidney.

secretions and tears. If this water loss is not replaced by food and drink, or if the water loss is excessive (e.g., in vomiting, diarrhoea or haemorrhage), the total volume of ECF falls and the animal is described as being *dehydrated*.

A dehydrated patient will show:

- *Lowered blood pressure*: A fall in the volume of ECF results in a fall in blood plasma volume and consequently a fall in blood pressure.
- *A rise in osmotic pressure*: A fall in plasma volume results in a rise in the concentration of Na^+ ions in the blood and as a result a rise in the osmotic pressure of the blood.

Note: **Osmotic pressure** is the pressure needed to prevent osmosis from occurring. It is dependent on the number of particles of undissolved molecules and ions in a solution. **Blood pressure** is the pressure exerted on the inside of the walls of the arterial blood vessels by the blood. It is detected by baroreceptors in the walls of the blood vessels.

In dehydration, osmoregulatory mechanisms will start to work (Fig. 10.8). The fall in blood pressure and rise in osmotic pressure ultimately result in an increase in the reabsorption of water from the collecting ducts, under the control of the hormone ADH (see Chapter 6). The osmoreceptors also stimulate the thirst centre in the brain and the animal feels the need to drink. Both of these pathways result in a rise in plasma volume and an increase in arterial blood pressure. Dehydrated animals should be given fluid parenterally (intravenously) or, in less severe cases, provided with access to drinking water. They will excrete *reduced* quantities of *concentrated* urine.

Raised blood pressure will result in the opposite effect, and the animal will produce *increased* quantities of more *dilute* urine.

Control of sodium levels

Sodium is taken into the body in the form of salt (NaCl) in food. It is lost in sweat, faeces and urine. Sodium is found in the ionised form Na^+ in all the body fluid compartments and plays a fundamental part in determining arterial blood pressure. High Na^+ levels in the diet draw water into the plasma by osmosis. This raises blood volume and blood pressure also rises. Conversely, if an animal has a low level of Na^+, less water is drawn into the plasma and blood volume falls; this lowers the arterial blood pressure. The osmoregulatory mechanisms take steps to correct this, resulting in a compensatory rise in blood pressure (Fig. 10.9).

Regulation of Na^+ in the plasma occurs mainly in the distal convoluted tubule and is controlled by the hormone *aldosterone*, secreted by the cortex of the adrenal gland (see Chapter 6).

Excretion

Excretion is the removal of waste products from the body. These are formed within the tissues as a result of metabolic processes and are useless, surplus to the requirements of the body or potentially harmful to the body tissues. Excretion by the kidneys removes:

- *Water*: In varying amounts dependent on the volume of the ECF and controlled by osmoregulatory processes

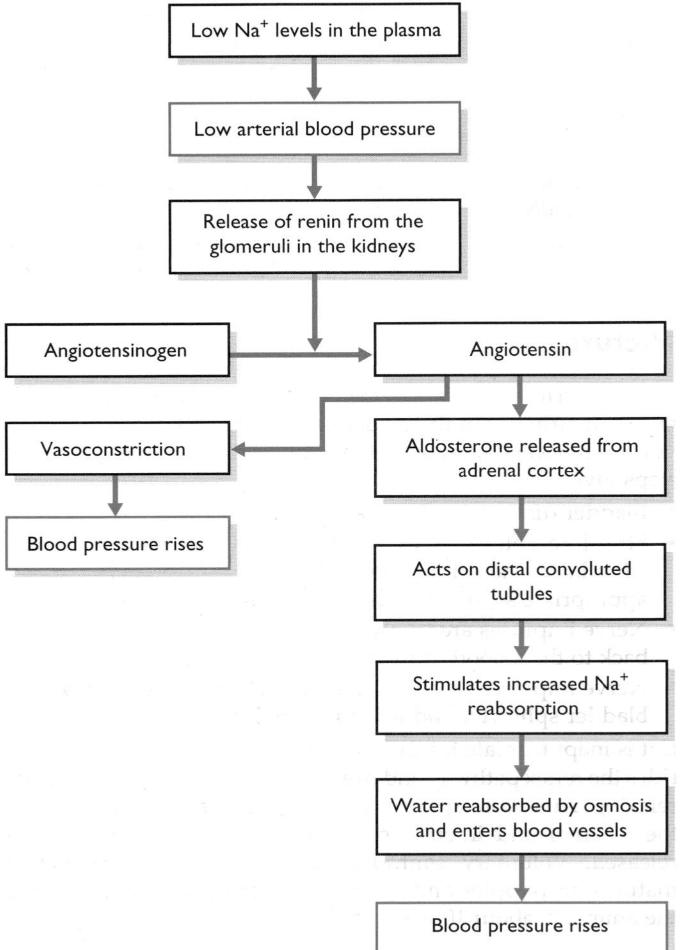

Fig. 10.9 Mechanism controlling sodium (and therefore blood pressure) in the kidney.

- *Inorganic ions*: The amount depends on the osmotic pressure of the blood and other body fluids and is controlled by osmoregulatory processes.
- *Nitrogenous waste products*: These result from the metabolism of protein taken into the body in food. Protein is broken down by the process of digestion into amino acids, which are carried to the liver by the blood and converted into body protein. Surplus amino acids cannot be stored by the body, so undergo a process of *deamination* in which they are broken down. Ammonia, which is extremely toxic to the cells, especially those of the nervous system, is formed as a by-product. Within the liver ammonia combines with carbon dioxide in a series of reactions known as the ornithine cycle and urea is formed:

$$CO_2 + 2NH_3 = \underset{\text{[urea]}}{CO(NH_2)_2} + H_2O$$

Urea passes into the circulation and is carried to the kidney, where it is excreted in the urine.

Kidney disease can present in many forms and the symptoms are related to the fact that all kidney functions are affected and the homeostatic mechanisms cease to work. Chronic renal failure commonly occurs in older cats and dogs and develops when the nephrons are gradually replaced by fibrous connective tissue as a normal 'old age' change. Clinical signs, many of which are related to rising levels of urea in the blood, develop when 75% of the nephrons have ceased to function. Acute renal failure is sudden, often catastrophic and may affect any age of animal. Potential causes include infection (e.g., leptospirosis), nephrotoxins (e.g., antifreeze) and urinary obstruction.

- *Products of detoxification*: Hormones, certain drugs and poisons are inactivated within the liver and excreted by the kidney.

Other parts of the urinary system

The ureters

Urine formed by the nephrons leaves each kidney by a single ureter at a point known as the *hilus* (Fig. 10.4). Each ureter is a narrow muscular tube running caudally towards the bladder, one on each side of the midline in the dorsal abdomen (Figs. 10.2 and 10.3). Each ureter is suspended from the dorsal body wall by a fold of visceral peritoneum, the *mesoureter*.

Urine is pushed along the tube towards the bladder by peristaltic waves brought about by contraction of the smooth muscle fibres forming the ureter walls. *Transitional epithelium* lines the ureters and allows for expansion as urine passes along.

The bladder

Each ureter enters the single bladder close to the neck. The ureters underrun the bladder mucosa for a short distance before opening into the lumen at an oblique angle. This arrangement acts as a valve preventing backflow of urine along the ureter. This area within which the two ureters enter the bladder is known as the *trigone* (Fig. 10.2) because there are three structures entering or exiting the bladder: two ureters and the urethra.

The bladder is a pear-shaped hollow organ. The rounded end points cranially, while the narrow end or *neck* points caudally and usually lies within the pelvic cavity. Its function is to collect and store urine. When full, the bladder extends into the abdomen, pulling the neck ventrally over the edge of the pelvic brim with the ventral surface of the bladder touching the abdominal floor; when empty most of the bladder lies in the pelvic cavity.

In cross-section, the bladder consists of an inner lining of *transitional epithelium*, which enables the walls to expand when filling with urine. A submucosal layer of *elastic tissue* and *smooth muscle* is arranged in folds to allow expansion. The smooth muscle fibres are continuous with those of the internal bladder sphincter. The bladder is surrounded by a layer of *peritoneum*, which covers only the cranial end lying in the abdomen. All organs in the pelvic cavity are surrounded by connective tissue and muscle and are not covered in peritoneum.

Urolithiasis is the formation of mineral 'stones' known as uroliths or calculi in the bladder. These may cause a blockage in the urinary tract. The most common site for blockage in the cat is at the tip of the penis; the most common sites in the male dog are as the urethra bends over the ischial arch and as it passes through the os penis. Blockage is rare in the female animal because the urethra is shorter and more distensible.

The neck of the bladder ends in the *bladder sphincter*, whose function is to control the flow of urine out of the bladder and down the urethra. It consists of two concentric parts:

- *Internal sphincter*: made of smooth muscle; under involuntary control
- *External sphincter*: ring of striated muscle; under voluntary control

The urethra

The urethra is a tube that conveys urine caudally from the bladder through the pelvic cavity to the outside. Its structure varies according to the sex of the animal, and in the case of the male animal, between cats and dogs.

- *Female*: The urethra is a short tube, opening into the floor of the reproductive tract at the junction of the vagina and vestibule. The opening is known as the *external urethral orifice* and is located in the centre of a small ridge, the *urethral tubercle*. This is a useful landmark when catheterising a bitch and can be seen when using a speculum.
- *Male*: The urethra is divided into two parts: the *pelvic urethra* and the *penile urethra*. There is a difference between the dog and the tomcat:
- *Dog* (see Chapter 11, Fig. 11.1): Close to the neck of the bladder, there are three openings into the urethra; one of these is from the *prostate gland* and two are from the *deferent ducts* or *vas deferens* (one from each testis). The urethra runs caudally through the pelvic cavity as the pelvic urethra, over the edge of the ischial arch where it is joined by erectile tissue to form the penis. The penile urethra opens to the outside at the tip of the penis.
- *Tomcat* (see Chapter 11, Fig. 11.2): There is a short length of urethra, cranial to the openings from the prostate gland and the deferent ducts, known as the *preprostatic urethra*, which is not found in the dog. The urethra continues caudally and opens to the outside in the perineal area, ventral to the anus. There is no penile urethra lying outside the pelvic cavity. Close to the end of the urethra are the openings from the paired *bulbourethral* glands.

From the point at which the deferent ducts join it, the urethra conveys both urine and sperm to the outside of the body.

Micturition

Micturition (often incorrectly referred to as urination) is the act of expelling urine from the bladder. It is normally a reflex activity but can be overridden by voluntary control from the brain. The steps involved are:

- Bladder distends with urine formed by the kidneys.
- Stretch receptors in the smooth muscle of the bladder wall are stimulated and send nerve impulses to centres in the appropriate segment of the spinal cord.
- Nerve impulses are transmitted via parasympathetic nerves back to the smooth muscle, and initiate contraction.
- Nerve impulses also stimulate relaxation in the internal bladder sphincter and urine is expelled.

If it is inappropriate for the animal to micturate, the brain overrides the reflex pathway and prevents the bladder sphincter from relaxing. At a more appropriate time, the brain stimulates both the external and internal sphincters: they relax and urine is released. Voluntary control develops as the young animal matures; in puppies and kittens it is not fully developed until the animal is about 10 weeks old.

Urinalysis

Urine is derived from the ultrafiltrate of plasma so it reflects the health status of the whole animal. The analysis of urine, or urinalysis, is a useful diagnostic tool. Normal urine contains only water, salts and urea. The clinical parameters used to evaluate a sample of urine are shown in Table 10.2.

Table 10.2 Normal values shown by the urine of the dog and cat

Clinical parameter	Normal value	Comments
Daily volume	Dog: 20–100 ml/kg body weight	*Polyuria*: increased volume of urine *Oliguria*: reduced volume of urine
	Cat: 10–12 ml/kg body weight	*Anuria*: absence of urine
Appearance	Clear, yellow, characteristic smell	Tomcat urine has an unpleasant strong smell; old samples smell ammoniacal
pH	5–7	Carnivorous diet produces acid urine; herbivorous diet produces alkaline urine
Specific gravity (SG)	Dog: 1.016–1.060 Cat: 1.020–1.040	Reflects the concentration of urine; exercise, high environmental temperatures and dehydration will cause a rise in specific gravity
Protein	None	*Proteinuria*: presence of protein May indicate damage to nephrons, chronic renal failure, inflammation of the urinary tract

Continued

Table 10.2 Normal values shown by the urine of the dog and cat—cont'd

Clinical parameter	Normal value	Comments
Blood	None	*Haematuria*: presence of blood *Haemoglobinuria*: presence of haemoglobin, due to rupture of red cells May indicate damage or infection to the urinary tract
Glucose	None	*Glucosuria*: presence of glucose May indicate diabetes mellitus or Cushing's disease; levels of glucose in the filtrate exceed the renal threshold and excess is excreted in the urine
Ketones	None	*Ketonuria*: presence of ketones May be accompanied by acid pH and smell of 'peardrops' in urine and on the breath
Bile	None	*Bilirubinuria*: presence of bile Indicator of some form of liver disease
Crystals and casts	In small quantities, these may be considered to be normal	Crystalline or colloidal material coalesces to form casts of the renal tubules, which are flushed out by the urine; in large quantities crystals may form larger calculi, uroliths or stones and block the tract

CHAPTER 11

Reproductive system

KEY POINTS

- The male gonad is the testis, responsible for spermatogenesis and the secretion of testosterone.
- The male reproductive tract conducts the sperm from the testis into the female reproductive tract during mating.
- The female gonad is the ovary, responsible for the production of ova and the secretion of oestrogen and progesterone.
- The release of ova from the ovary is associated with a regular cycle of interrelated hormonal changes in the ovary and the reproductive tract and in the animal's behavioural patterns; this is known as the oestrous cycle.
- Fertilisation of the ovum by one spermatozoon occurs in the uterine tube and the developing embryos implant in the wall of the uterine horns.
- The extra-embryonic membranes and the embryo develop from different parts of the rapidly dividing ball of cells derived from the original fertilised ovum.
- Genetics is the science of inheritance and is the method by which characteristics are passed from one generation to another.
- Information about these characteristics is carried on the genes within the nucleus of every cell.
- Genes pass from parent to offspring by means of germ cell division by meiosis, fertilisation to form a zygote and cell division by mitosis to form an embryo and then a fetus.
- The activity of genes within the individual follows Mendel's laws of inheritance, which enables the outcome of selective animal matings to be predicted.

Reproduction is the means by which a species is able to perpetuate itself. If animals lived for ever, there would be no need for another generation to take over from previous ones; in reality, all animals become old or 'worn out' and die and must be replaced if the species is not to become extinct.

All species of mammal have evolved separate sexes and they reproduce *sexually*. This is in contrast to less highly evolved species, which may reproduce *asexually* – producing offspring that are identical to the parent. Sexual reproduction involves the transfer of genetic material. After mating specialised germ cells – *spermatozoa* from the male and *ova* from the female – fuse to form a single-celled *zygote*. The zygote undergoes cell division to form the *embryo*. The offspring resulting from sexual reproduction are genetically different from one another and from their parents.

The reproductive system shares part of its structure with the urinary system and the combined systems may be referred to as the *urogenital system*.

Male reproductive system

The male dog is known as a dog; the male cat is known as a tomcat. The reproductive system of the dog and the tomcat are generally similar; any differences will be described where appropriate (Figs. 11.1 and 11.2). The parts of the male reproductive tract are:

- Testis
- Epididymis
- Deferent duct, also called the vas deferens
- Urethra
- Penis
- Prostate gland, an accessory gland
- Bulbourethral gland, an accessory gland seen only in the tomcat

The testis

The testis is the male gonad, with functions as follows:

1. To produce spermatozoa (sperm) by the process of spermatogenesis; these fertilise the ova produced by the female
2. To produce a little fluid to transport the sperm from the testes into the female tract and to aid their survival
3. To secrete the hormone testosterone, which influences spermatogenesis, the development of male secondary sexual characteristics and male behaviour patterns (see Chapter 6)

There is a pair of testes, which, in the adult animal, lie outside the body cavity in the *scrotum* – a sac of relatively hairless and often pigmented skin. Spermatogenesis occurs most efficiently at temperatures below that of the core body temperature, so the testes are carried outside the body cavity in a cooler environment. In the dog, the scrotum lies between the hind limbs; in the cat it is attached to the perineum, ventral to the anus. Internally, the sac is divided into two, each part containing one testis; the left testis often hangs lower than the right one. Within the wall of the scrotum is the *dartos muscle*. In cold weather this contracts and thickens the scrotal skin, raising the temperature; in warm weather, the muscle relaxes and the scrotum becomes thinner and thus cooler. A constant temperature for spermatogenesis is therefore maintained.

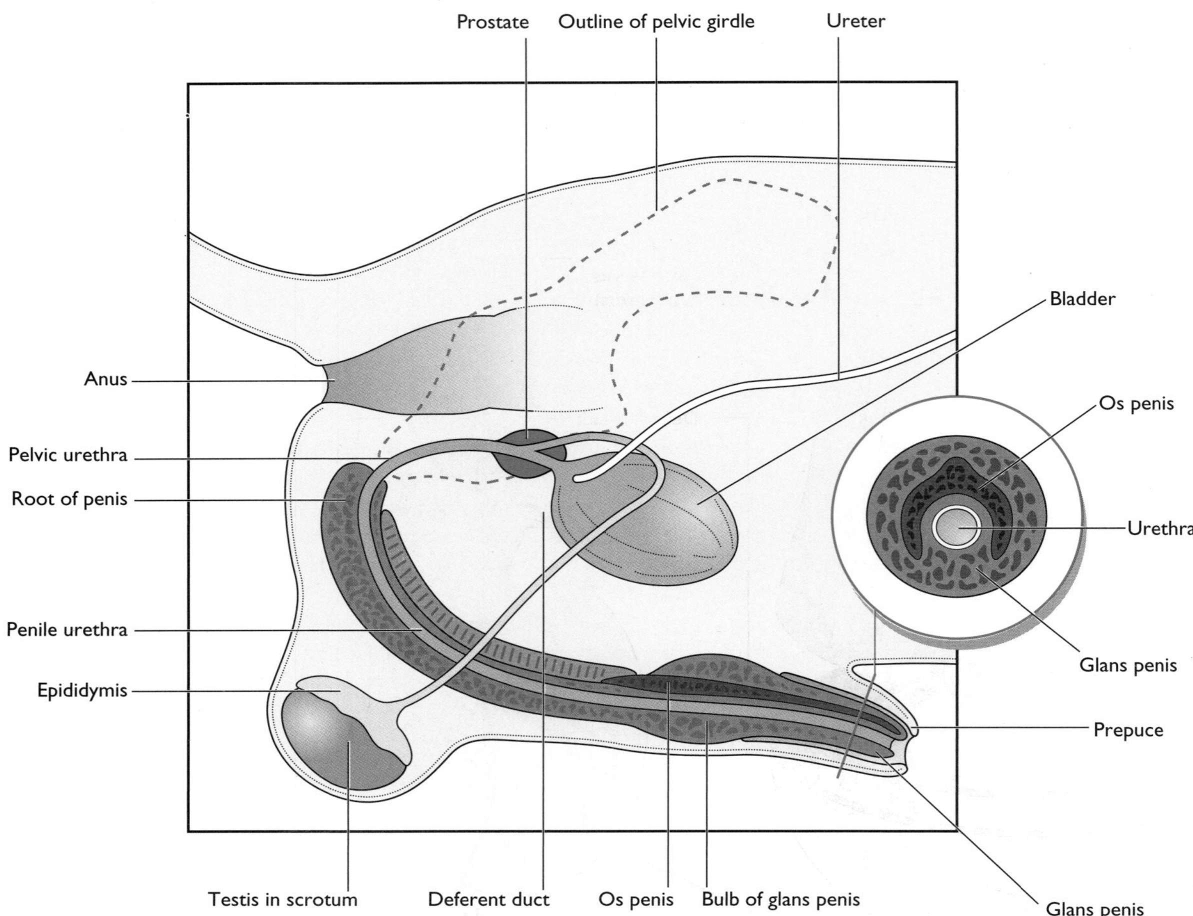

Fig. 11.1 Reproductive system of the dog.

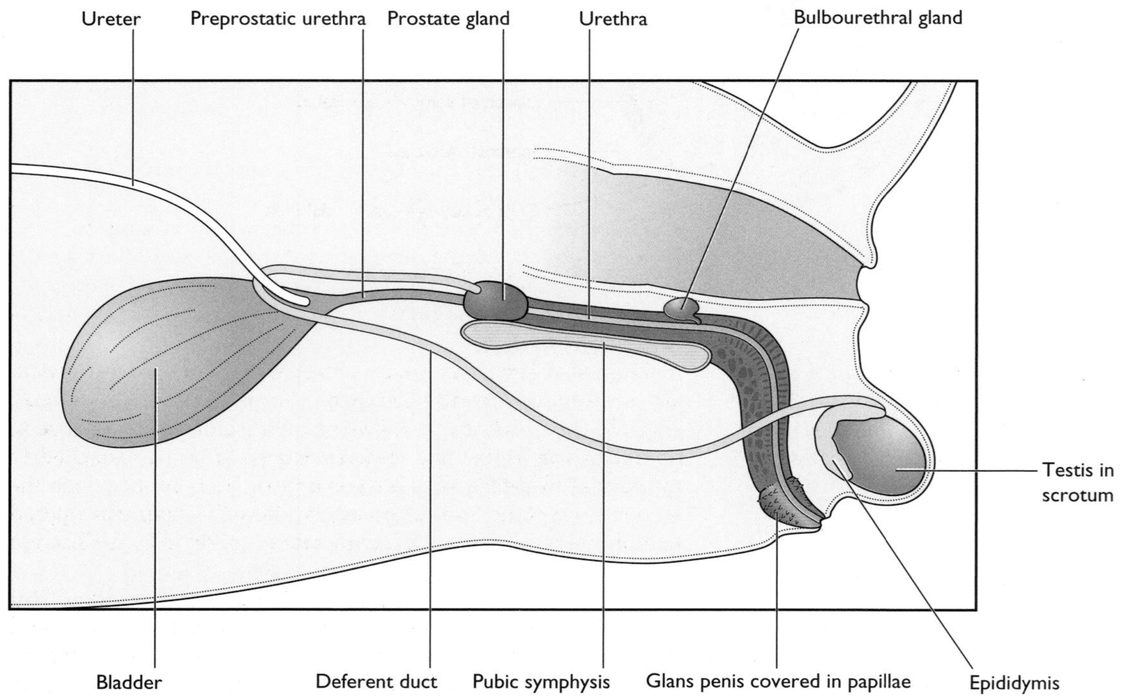

Fig. 11.2 Reproductive system of the tomcat.

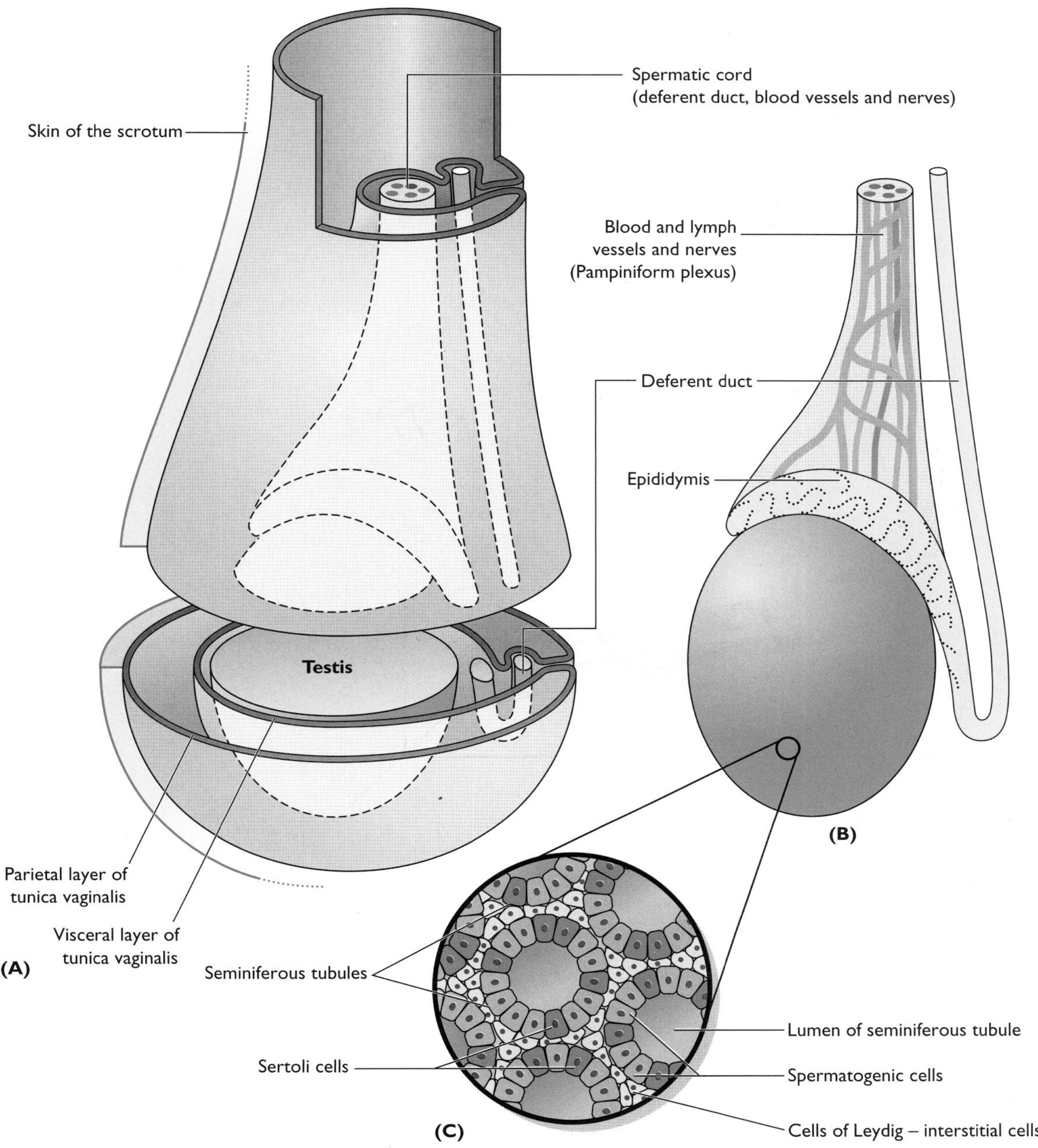

Fig. 11.3 **(A)** Testis within scrotum, **(B)** Scrotum removed, **(C)** Cross-section through the seminiferous tubules.

Each testis is an oval-shaped structure wrapped in a double layer of peritoneum known as the *tunica vaginalis* (Fig. 11.3). The testicular tissue consists of numerous blind-ending tubules known as *seminiferous tubules*, which are lined by two types of cells:

- *Spermatogenic cells* divide by *meiosis* to produce immature sperm or spermatids; each spermatid contains the haploid number of chromosomes (see Chapter 1).
- *Sertoli cells* secrete *oestrogen* and nutrients that prolong the survival of the sperm.

Lying between the tubules are the *cells of Leydig* or *interstitial cells*. They secrete *testosterone* and are under the control of *interstitial cell stimulating hormone* (ICSH) (see Chapter 6), produced by the anterior pituitary gland.

The coiled seminiferous tubules make up most of the testicular tissue and eventually combine to form slightly larger *efferent ducts*. These drain into the *epididymis*, lying along the dorsolateral border of the testis. The *cauda epididymis* or *tail* is attached to the caudal extremity of the testis and is the point at which the temperature of the testis is lowest. It is here that sperm are stored and undergo a period of maturation ready for fertilisation (Fig. 11.4).

The blood supply to the testis is via the *testicular artery*. This leaves the aorta in the abdomen, just caudal to the renal artery. As it enters the scrotum, the testicular artery runs alongside the epididymis and then divides to form the convoluted *pampiniform plexus*. This complicated capillary network ensures that the blood is cooled before it enters the testicular tissue.

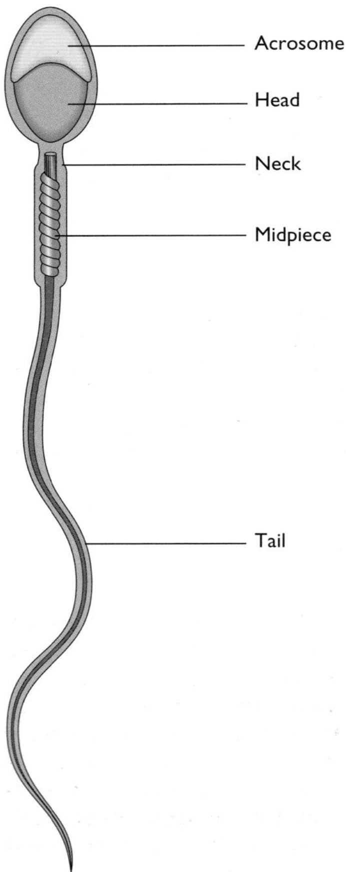

Fig. 11.4 A normal spermatozoon. The acrosome protects the head of the sperm and contains enzymes that aid penetration of the ovum. The head contains the haploid number of chromosomes. The midpiece contains enzymes and mitochondria to provide energy for movement. The tail produces a powerful propulsive force.

Testicular descent

In the early embryo, the undifferentiated gonads develop inside the abdomen close to the kidney. In the male, the gonad becomes the testis and a band of tissue known as the *gubernaculum* forms and runs from the caudal end of each testis to the inside of the developing scrotal sac. During late gestation, the testes are pulled caudally by the contraction of the gubernaculum and they migrate through the abdomen. The testes leave the abdominal cavity via the *inguinal canal*, a channel between the fibres of the external abdominal oblique muscle in the groin or inguinal area (see Chapter 4). As each testis with its associated blood capillaries, nerve and deferent duct passes through the inguinal canal into the scrotum, it becomes wrapped in a double fold of peritoneum, which forms the tunica vaginalis (Fig. 11.3).

The testes begin their descent into the scrotum during early neonatal life and should be palpable within the scrotum by 12 weeks of age in the puppy and 10–12 weeks in the kitten. Failure of the testes to descend is described as *cryptorchidism*; the testes may be retained in the abdomen or within the inguinal canal.

Cryptorchidism. Retention of the testis may be a hereditary condition and affected dogs should not be used for breeding. Bilaterally cryptorchid dogs are usually sterile but may have normal sexual libido (desire). As the dog grows older, the retained testis is more likely to develop a Sertoli cell tumour, the diagnostic signs of which may be bilateral symmetrical alopecia, enlarged mammary glands (gynaecomastia) and attractiveness to other male dogs.

- *Monorchid*: term used when one testis is retained.
- *Bilateral cryptorchid*: term used when both testes are retained.

Deferent duct

The epididymis continues as the *deferent duct* (also called the *vas deferens* or *ductus deferens*; Figs. 11.1 and 11.2), which passes out of the scrotum into the abdominal cavity via the inguinal canal within the *spermatic cord*. The spermatic cord is wrapped in the tunica vaginalis and also contains the testicular artery and vein and the testicular nerve. Lying within the cord is a strip of muscle derived from the internal abdominal oblique muscle and known as the *cremaster muscle*. Contraction of this muscle raises the testis closer to the body in response to cold and works in conjunction with the dartos muscle to maintain a constant temperature for the testes.

During ejaculation, the sperm and fluid produced in the seminiferous tubules are propelled along the epididymis and up the deferent duct, which joins the urethra. At this junction, the walls of the deferent ducts are thickened and glandular; the whole area is surrounded by the *prostate gland* (Figs. 11.1 and 11.2).

The penis

The functions of the penis are to:

- Convey sperm and fluids from the testis into the female reproductive tract during mating
- Convey urine from the bladder to the outside via the urethra

The urethra runs through the centre of the penis and extends from the bladder to the tip of the penis. It is shared by both the reproductive and urinary systems (see Chapter 10). The penis of the dog and the tomcat are anatomically different.

The dog

The penis runs from the ischial arch of the pelvis, passes cranioventrally along the perineum and between the hind limbs (Fig. 11.5). The urethra lies in the centre and is surrounded by a layer of cavernous erectile tissue known as the *corpus spongiosum penis*. This is expanded proximally into the *bulb of the penis* and, towards the tip, as the *glans penis*. Surrounding this and serving to attach the penis to the ischial arch is a pair of erectile tissue *crura* (sing. *crus*), known as the *corpus cavernosum penis*. These form the *root* of the penis at its attachment to the ischial arch. The urethra runs in a groove between the two crura.

Cavernous erectile tissue is made of connective tissue perforated by 'caverns' lined by endothelium. During sexual excitement these caverns fill with blood under pressure and the tissue becomes engorged and erect.

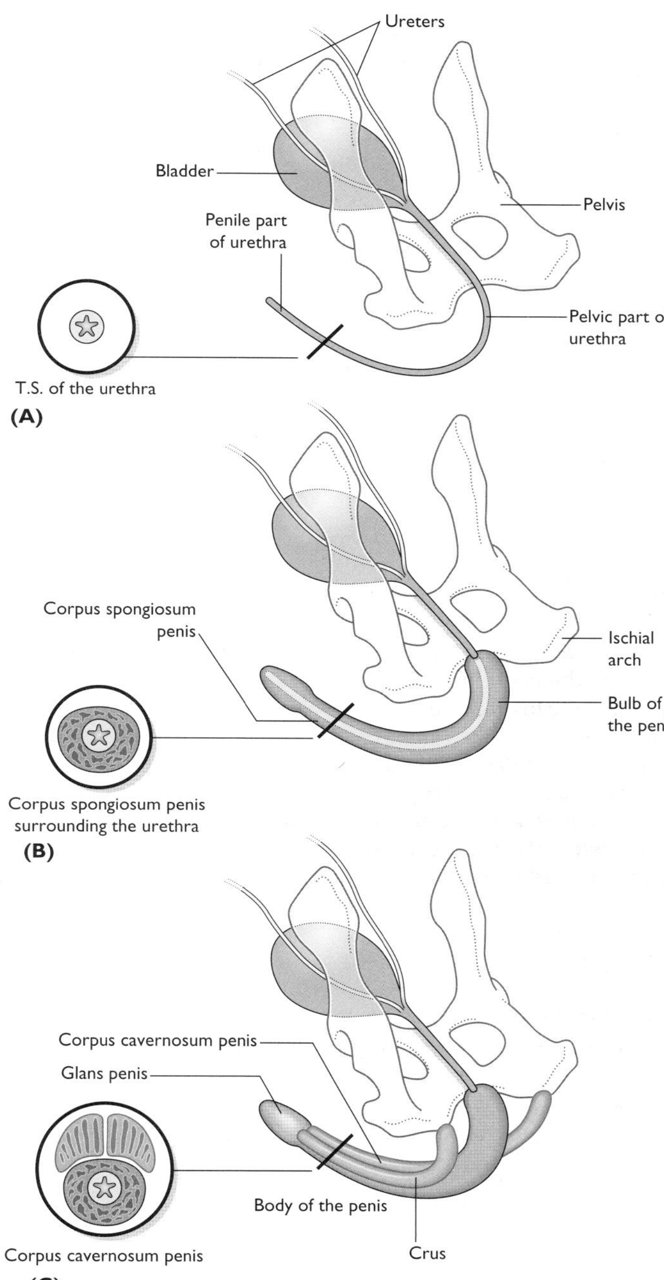

Fig. 11.5 Structure of the penis in three layers, with transverse sections through the urethra. **(A)** Shows the urethra only. **(B)** Shows the urethra with the layer of cavernous erectile tissue surrounding it: the corpus spongiosum penis. **(C)** Shows the corpus cavernosum penis, which forms the two crura and attaches the penis to the ischial arch.

Within the tissue of the glans penis is a tunnel-shaped bone, the *os penis*, whose function is to aid entry of the penis into the vagina of the bitch during the early stages of mating when erection is only partially complete. The canine os penis lies *dorsal* to the urethra, which runs through the 'tunnel' in the bone. At this point the urethra cannot expand and this can be a common site for urethral blockage with urinary calculi.

Balanitis or Balanoposthitis. Many dogs develop an infection of the lubricating glands of the prepuce, which results in a greenish-yellow discharge. The condition is so common that it is considered almost normal and is usually only treated if the mucous membrane becomes ulcerated and the discharge is blood-stained or smelly. The dog will usually lick the discharge away – a behavior common in many male dogs!

The distal part of the penis is contained within a sheath of hairy skin known as the *prepuce*. This is suspended from the ventral abdominal wall and covers and protects the penis. It is lined with mucous membrane and is well supplied with lubricating glands. During mating, the prepuce is pushed back to reveal the glans penis. Afterwards, the *retractor penis muscle* pulls the penis back into the prepuce.

The tomcat

The main parts of the penis are similar to those of the dog, except that the cat penis is shorter and points backwards – the external opening is ventral to the anus (Fig. 11.2). The glans penis is covered with tiny barbs, which elicit a pain reflex as the male withdraws from the female after mating. This stimulates the nerve pathway to the hypothalamus, resulting in ovulation approximately 36 hours later – known as *induced ovulation*. The *os penis* lies *ventral* to the urethra in the cat. During sexual excitement, the penis engorges and points cranioventrally so that the mating position in cats is similar to that seen in the dog.

Accessory glands

The function of the accessory glands is to secrete *seminal fluids*, which:

- Increase the volume of the ejaculate to aid the passage of sperm into the female tract
- Provide the correct environment for sperm survival
- Neutralise the acidity of the urine within the urethra

There are two types of gland (Figs. 11.1 and 11.2):

- *Prostate gland* is bilobed and lies on the floor of the pelvis, surrounding the urethra. In the dog, it is close to the neck of the bladder; in the cat, there is a short *preprostatic urethra* cranial to the gland (see Chapter 10).

Prostatic hypertrophy. This means that the prostate gland becomes enlarged and is not necessarily associated with cancer of the prostate, which is rare in dogs and cats. The condition is linked to levels of testosterone and hypertrophy is common in uncastrated older dogs. It may obstruct the passage of faeces as they pass down the rectum, which lies dorsal to the gland within the pelvic cavity leading to constipation. This is relieved in the short term with an enema, but in the long term castration will help to reduce the size of the gland.

- *Bulbourethral glands*, found only in the tomcat, lie on either side of the urethra, cranial to the ischial arch (Fig. 11.2).

Female reproductive system

The female dog is known as a bitch; the female cat is known as a queen. The parts of the female reproductive system are:

- Ovary
- Uterine tube, oviduct or Fallopian tube
- Uterus – uterine horns and body
- Cervix
- Vagina
- Vestibule
- Vulva

The reproductive tract of the bitch and queen are similar and vary only in size (Fig. 11.6). The tract is designed to carry several fetuses during a single pregnancy and is said to be *bicornuate* (two horns). The bitch and the queen bear litters of young: they are *multiparous.*

The ovary

The ovary is the female gonad. The functions of the ovary are:

- To produce ova or eggs ready for fertilisation by the sperm of the male
- To act as an endocrine gland, secreting the hormones oestrogen and progesterone

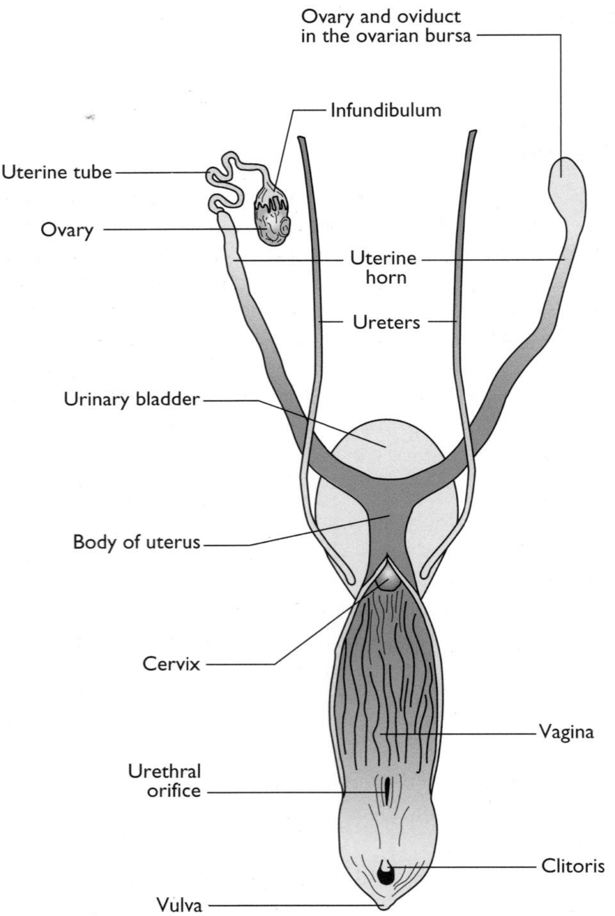

Fig. 11.6 Dorsal view of the reproductive system of the bitch. (With permission from T Colville, JM Bassett, 2001. Clinical anatomy and physiology for veterinary technicians. St Louis, MO: Mosby, p 330.)

There is a pair of ovaries, one lying on each side of the dorsal abdominal cavity, caudal to the kidney (see Chapter 10, Fig. 10.2). The ovary is held close to the kidney by the *ovarian* or *suspensory ligament* (Fig. 11.7), which contains a small amount of smooth muscle that allows the ligament to stretch in response to the weight of the fetuses during pregnancy. The ovary is suspended from the dorsal body wall by part of the visceral peritoneum called the *mesovarium,* which also encloses the infundibulum of the uterine tube. Part of the mesovarium forms a pocket-like structure known as the *ovarian bursa,* which completely covers the ovary. Within this is a small opening allowing ova to leave the ovary; this is a potential means of entry of infection into the peritoneal cavity.

The tissue of the ovary consists of a framework of connective tissue, smooth muscle and blood capillaries, within which are a large number of germ cells and developing follicles (Fig. 11.8). In an immature animal, each ovary is oval with a smooth outline but, as sexual maturity approaches, the ovary becomes nodular as the enlarging follicles protrude from the surface.

The uterine tube

This is also known as the *oviduct* or *Fallopian tube* (Fig. 11.6). The functions of the uterine tubes are:

- To collect ova as they are released from the Graafian follicles
- To convey the ova from the ovaries to the uterine horns
- To provide the correct environment for the survival of both the ova and sperm

Each uterine tube is a narrow convoluted structure lying close to the ovary (Fig. 11.7). The open end is funnel-shaped and known as the *infundibulum.* It is fringed with finger-like processes known as *fimbriae,* which spread over the surface of the ovary to capture ova as they are released. The ova pass down the lumen of the tube, which is lined with ciliated columnar epithelium. The cilia propel the ova along the tube towards the uterine horns. The uterine tube is suspended by part of the visceral peritoneum known as the *mesosalpinx,* which is continuous with both the mesovarium and the mesometrium.

The uterus

The uterus is a Y-shaped structure lying in the midline of the dorsal abdomen (Fig. 11.6). During pregnancy, the weight of the conceptuses pulls the uterus ventrally and at full term it occupies the greater part of the abdomen. The function of the uterus is:

- To provide a receptacle in which the embryos can develop into full-term fetuses
- To provide the correct environment for the survival of the embryos
- To provide the means whereby the developing embryos can receive nutrients from the dam; this is made possible by the *placenta*

The uterus consists of two parts. A pair of *uterine horns* lead from the uterine tubes. Each horn is about five times the length of the uterine body and, during pregnancy, contains the developing embryos. The two horns join to form a short central *body.*

The wall of the uterus has three layers:

1. *Endometrium*: is the lining of columnar mucous membrane, glandular tissue and blood vessels. During pregnancy this

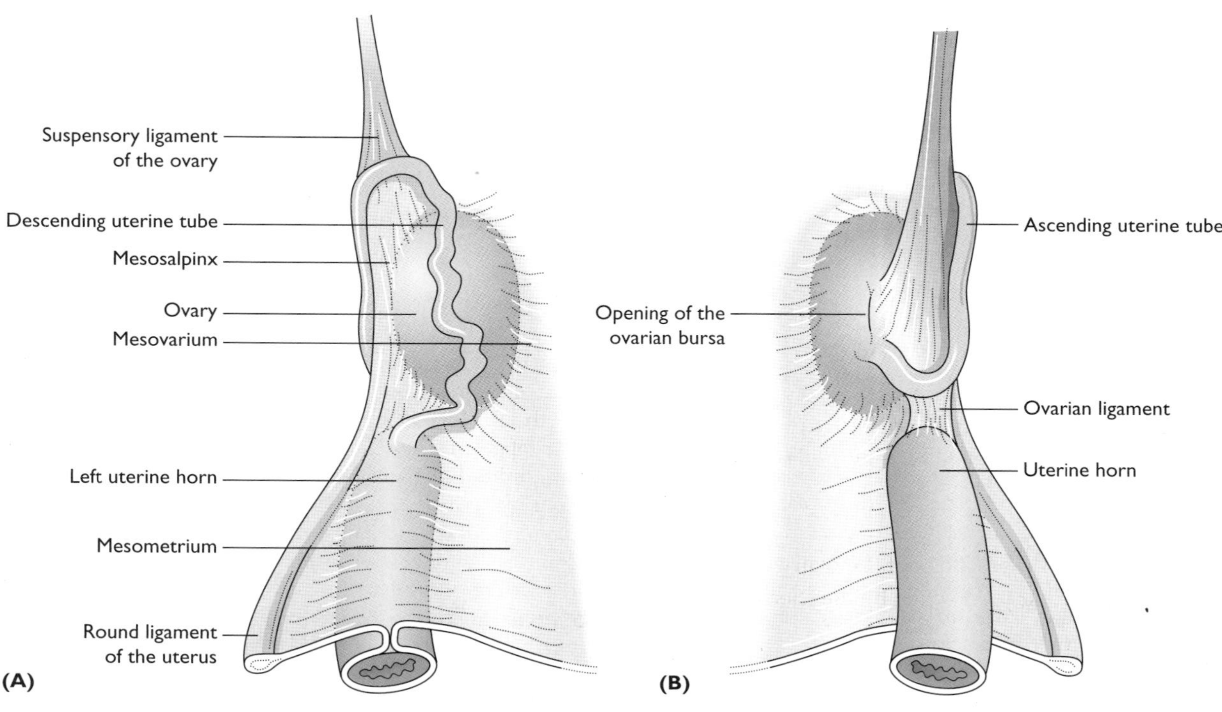

Fig. 11.7 Anatomy of the ovarian region of the bitch: **(A)** Lateral view, **(B)** Medial view.

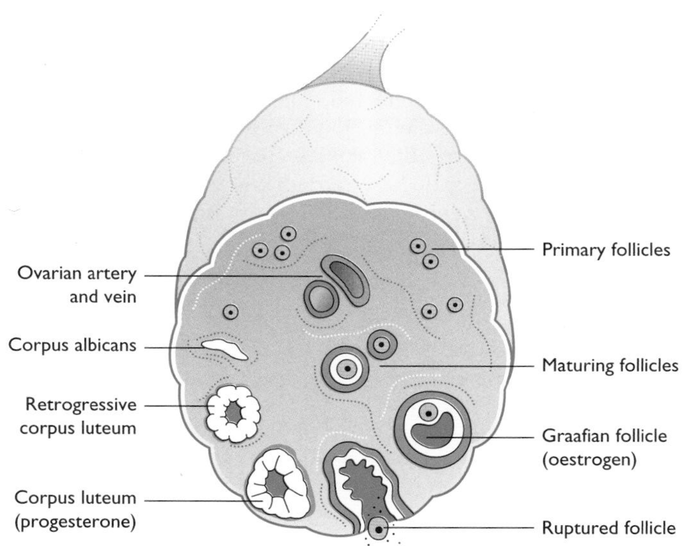

Fig. 11.8 Longitudinal section through an ovary to show ovarian activity.

thickens to provide nutrition for the embryo before implantation and to support the developing placenta.
2. *Myometrium*: comprises layers of smooth muscle that produces strong contractions during parturition.
3. *Mesometrium* or *broad ligament* is a fold of the visceral peritoneum that suspends the uterus from the dorsal body wall and is continuous with the mesovarium and mesosalpinx.

The cervix

The cervix is a short, thick-walled muscular sphincter that connects the uterine body with the vagina (Fig. 11.6). Running through the centre is a narrow *cervical canal*, which is normally tightly closed and relaxes only to allow the passage of sperm or fetuses. During pregnancy, the canal is blocked by a mucoid plug, which protects the conceptuses from infection. In the non-pregnant animal, the cervix lies in the pelvic cavity but during pregnancy the weight of the conceptuses pulls the cervix cranially and ventrally over the edge of the pelvic brim.

Ovariohysterectomy, more commonly called 'spaying', is performed by the veterinary surgeon to prevent unwanted pregnancies and oestrous cycles. The surgical procedure involves the complete removal of the reproductive tract from the ovaries to a point just cranial to the cervix. Ligation of the major blood vessels is essential, particularly if the procedure is performed during oestrus or pregnancy as the vessels may be extremely well developed.

Blood supply to the reproductive tract

The blood vessels run within the mesovarium, mesosalpinx and mesometrium. They are:

- *Ovarian artery* arises from the aorta just caudal to the renal artery and supplies the ovary, uterine tube and uterine horn.
- *Uterine artery* anastomoses with the ovarian artery and supplies the caudal part of the tract. It can be seen as a relatively large artery running on either side of the cervix.

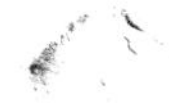

Pyometritis. This is a condition seen in older unspayed bitches, although it can occasionally occur in unspayed queens. As a result of the influence of progesterone the uterus becomes filled with pus. The condition is most often seen in bitches over 6 years of age who have never had puppies and may have had a season within the previous 6 weeks. The bitch presents with polydipsia, polyuria and a vaginal discharge that may be smelly. In some cases there is no discharge and the bitch is extremely unwell and may be anorexic and vomiting. There are many variations to the general pattern and the condition should always be considered in an elderly entire bitch who has been 'below par' for some time and has recently had a season. The treatment is immediate ovariohysterectomy, which should be performed before the bitch is too ill to tolerate a general anaesthetic.

The vagina and vestibule

The vagina and vestibule form a channel leading to the external opening of the reproductive tract – the *vulva*. The vagina leads from the cervix to the *external urethral orifice* – the point at which the urethra joins the reproductive tract (Fig. 11.6). The vestibule leads from the external urethral orifice to the vulva and is shared by both the urinary and reproductive tracts.

The lumen is lined by *stratified squamous epithelium*, which undergoes hormonal changes during the oestrous cycle. The lining epithelium is folded longitudinally to allow widthways expansion during parturition and is surrounded by layers of smooth muscle. These are very strong and during canine mating they tighten on the penis of the male and maintain the 'tie'.

The epithelial cells lining the vagina undergo hormonal changes during the oestrous cycle. These changes may be used as an aid to the correct timing of mating. The technique, known as *vaginal exfoliative cytology*, involves making smears from vaginal swabs taken every other day during pro-oestrus and early oestrus. The smears are then stained and examined microscopically looking for diagnostic changes in the cells that provide an indication of the stages of the cycle.

The vulva

The vulva marks the external opening of the urogenital tract. It consists of two parts:

- *The labia* comprise two vertical lips joined dorsally and ventrally; the vertical slit between them is known as the *vulval cleft*. They are normally held closed to prevent the entry of infection. During pro-oestrus and oestrus in the bitch, the labia enlarge, but this is not seen in the oestrous cycle of the queen.
- *The clitoris* is a knob-like structure of cavernous erectile tissue lying in the *clitoral fossa* just inside the ventral angle of the vulval cleft. It is the equivalent of the male penis.

The mammary glands

Although these are not strictly part of the reproductive tract, they are essential to reproduction in the mammal. The presence of mammary glands is the defining characteristic of the class Mammalia. All mammals feed their young on their secretions, known as *milk*, produced during a process known as *lactation*.

Mammary glands are modified cutaneous glands. In the dog and cat, they are present in both sexes but are rudimentary in the male. The glands lie externally on the ventral wall of the abdomen and thorax, on either side of the midline.

- The bitch has five pairs of mammary glands.
- The queen has four pairs of mammary glands.

Each gland consists of glandular tissue embedded in connective tissue and lined by a secretory epithelium (Fig. 11.9). The milk produced drains through a network of sinuses that eventually form *teat canals*. These open onto the surface of each teat, known as a *teat orifice*. Each gland has one teat but each teat has several orifices.

Mastitis. This inflammation of the mammary glands may result from infection or from failure to suckle the young puppies or kittens, such as may occur if the litter dies or if they are weaned too suddenly. Milk will continue to be secreted, building up in the glands, and acting as a focus for infection. The glands will feel hot, hard and painful to the touch. The dam will become anorexic and pyrexic and the milk may be watery or brown in colour, showing evidence of clots. The condition should respond to antibiotics but should be prevented by gradual weaning of the litter from 3–4 weeks onwards.

Lactation

This is the production of milk and normally occurs during pregnancy. It is influenced by three hormones:

- *Progesterone* is secreted by the corpus luteum within the ovary and causes enlargement of the mammary glands during pregnancy.
- *Prolactin* is secreted by the anterior pituitary gland in the last third of pregnancy and stimulates the production of milk.
- *Oxytocin* is secreted by the posterior pituitary gland during the last hours of pregnancy and enables the glands to release or 'let down' the milk in response to suckling by the neonate.

Composition of milk

This varies between different species and is an important consideration when feeding orphaned animals. The milk produced by

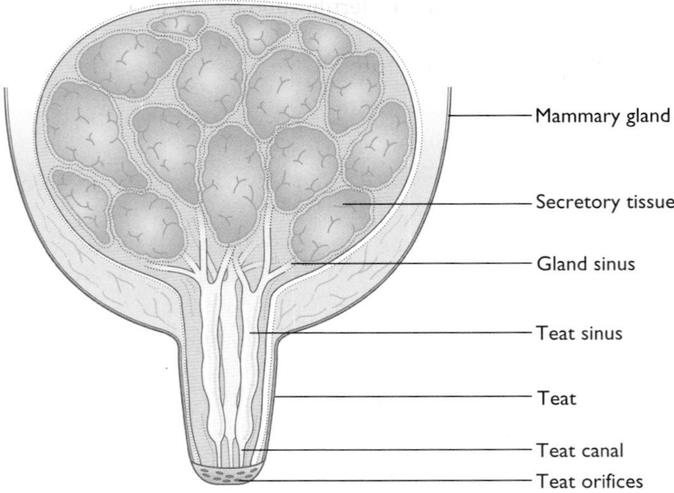

Fig. 11.9 Section through a mammary gland.

Table 11.1 Average composition of milk

Constituent	Quantity (%)
Water	70–90
Fat	0–30
Protein	1–15
Carbohydrate	3–7
Minerals	1.5–1: calcium phosphate, magnesium, sodium, potassium and chloride Milk is deficient in iron and copper; traces of iodine, cobalt, tin and silica are present
Vitamins	A, B_2, B_5, E, K Milk is low in vitamins C and D

NB. Milk from a cat contains the amino acid taurine, because cats have a specific requirement for this.

the bitch and the queen is more concentrated and contains more protein and twice as much fat as cow's milk. The average composition of milk is shown in Table 11.1.

The first milk secreted by the dam following parturition is known as *colostrum*. It is rich in maternal antibodies, which provide the neonate with immunity to diseases to which the dam has been exposed. It is essential that the neonate takes in colostrum within the first 24 hours of life. During this time, the protein antibodies can be absorbed by the small intestine without being digested. After 24 hours, normal protein digestion starts and the antibodies are broken down and destroyed. After a few days, production of colostrum stops and the composition of the milk remains constant.

The oestrous cycle

The oestrous cycle is the rhythmic cycle of events that occurs in sexually mature non-pregnant female mammals and includes limited periods of sexual receptivity known as *oestrus*. The function of the oestrous cycle is:

- To produce ova ready for fertilisation by the male spermatozoa
- To prepare the female reproductive tract to receive the fertilised ova
- To initiate behavioural patterns in the female that indicate to the male that she is receptive to mating
- To stimulate the female to stand still and allow the male to mate with her

For the oestrous cycle to achieve the aim of a fertile mating, the timing of all interrelated components must coincide. The pattern and timing of the oestrous cycle varies between species – the cycle shown by the bitch is different from that shown by the queen.

Each cycle is divided into phases of varying lengths. These are:

1. *Pro-oestrus*: period in which the reproductive tract is under the influence of oestrogen
2. *Oestrus*: period during which the female will allow herself to be mated
3. *Metoestrus*: also called dioestrus; period during which the tract is under the influence of progesterone
4. *Anoestrus*: period between cycles during which there is little or no ovarian activity

During the oestrous cycle simultaneous changes occur in:

- The ovary and reproductive tract; includes ovulation
- The endocrine system; interaction between the hormones oestrogen, progesterone, follicle stimulating hormone (FSH) and luteinising hormone (LH)
- The animal's behavioural patterns

Ovary and reproductive tract

At birth, the ovary contains all the germ cells that animals will ever need; these act as a reservoir from which the primary follicles develop. At the onset of puberty or sexual maturity, several primary follicles develop to form ripe Graafian follicles. In multiparous species, there will be many follicles, divided between the two ovaries, but not necessarily equally. Each Graafian follicle consists of an ovum formed by the process of meiosis and containing the haploid number of chromosomes (see Chapter 1). This is suspended in fluid and surrounded by an outer layer of follicular cells. The Graafian follicle secretes the hormone *oestrogen* (Fig. 11.8).

When the follicle has reached full size, it ruptures to release the ovum – the process of *ovulation*. The ovum passes down the uterine tube and the remaining follicular tissue becomes reorganised to form the *corpus luteum*. The corpus luteum secretes the hormone *progesterone*.

Within the reproductive tract, the uterine walls become thickened and more glandular to create a suitable environment for implantation of the fertilised ova. The vaginal epithelium also changes and the bloodstained discharge, seen in pro-oestrus in the bitch, comes from the lining of the vagina.

Hormonal changes

Ovulation and the oestrous cycle are associated with a cycle of interrelated hormonal changes in the ovary and anterior pituitary gland (Fig. 11.10) (see Chapter 6):

1. External stimuli such as increasing day length or a rise in environmental temperature stimulate the hypothalamus in the forebrain. This releases *gonadotrophin releasing hormone* (GRH), which acts on the anterior pituitary gland.
2. The anterior pituitary secretes *follicle stimulating hormone* (FSH), which stimulates a few primary follicles in the ovary to ripen into Graafian follicles.
3. The ripening follicles secrete increasing levels of *oestrogen*, which:
   - Produces the behaviour of the female seen during pro-oestrus
   - Prepares the reproductive tract for mating
   - Stimulates the secretion of *luteinising hormone* (LH) from the anterior pituitary gland
   - Inhibits further secretion of FSH
4. As a result of FSH inhibition, oestrogen levels begin to fall. LH acts on the ripe follicles and brings about ovulation. After the release of the ovum, the remaining follicular tissue becomes luteinised (i.e., converted into the corpus luteum).

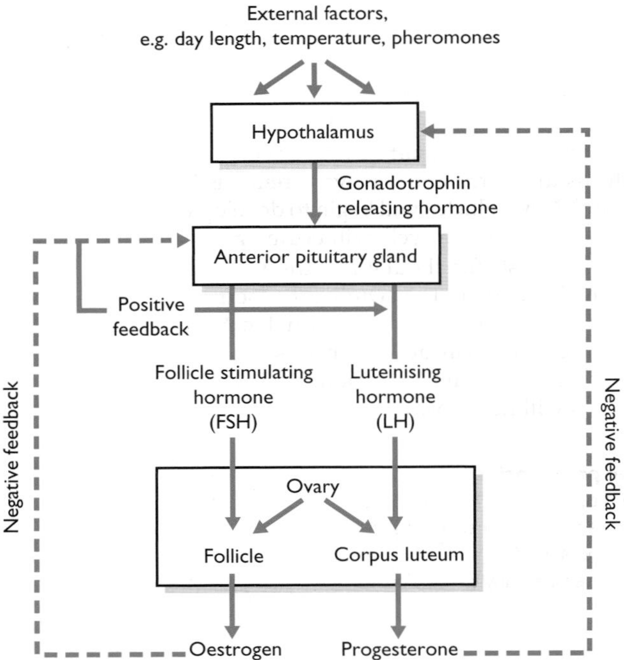

Fig 11.10 Inter-relationships between the female reproductive hormones.

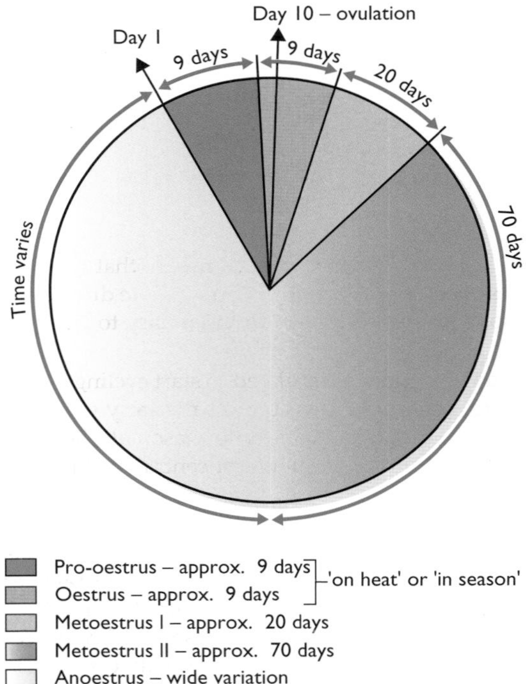

Fig. 11.11 Phases of the oestrous cycle of the bitch.

5. The corpus luteum begins to secrete *progesterone*. The increasing levels of progesterone and the decreasing levels of oestrogen stimulate mating behaviour in the bitch – she will allow the male to mount her.
6. Progesterone is the dominant hormone during pregnancy. It:
   - Prepares the reproductive tract to receive the fertilised ova
   - Causes enlargement of the mammary glands
   - Inhibits the secretion of GRH from the hypothalamus, which inhibits FSH output and prevents the development of any more follicles

If the animal has not conceived, the corpus luteum regresses and the cycle begins again. The hormonal cycle of the queen is slightly different. The queen is an *induced ovulator* so progesterone, secreted by the corpus luteum, will only be present if she is mated.

Behavioural changes and external signs

The bitch

- Bitches usually have one or two oestrous cycles a year and during the period of oestrus they are described as being 'in season' or 'on heat'.
- The bitch is *monoestrous*, meaning that during each period of ovarian activity there is only one period of oestrus, and there is no recognised breeding season; bitches may come into season at any time of the year.
- The bitch is a *spontaneous ovulator*, meaning that ovulation occurs without the stimulus of mating and takes place around the tenth day of the cycle (Fig. 11.11).
- Bitches reach sexual maturity or puberty at about 6 months but there is wide variation between breeds; larger breeds mature significantly later than smaller breeds. Puberty is marked by the onset of the first season.

The phases of the oestrous cycle (Fig. 11.11) are as follows:

- *Pro-oestrus* lasts for about 9 days. The vulva becomes enlarged and there may be a bloodstained vaginal discharge. The bitch may urinate more frequently, which serves to advertise the fact that she is in season. She will be excitable and flirtatious with males and may try to escape to find them. However, if a male tries to mount her she will growl and clamp her tail tightly to her rump to prevent mating.
- *Oestrus* lasts for about 9 days. The vulva remains enlarged but the discharge becomes straw-coloured. The 'flirty' excitable behaviour continues and if a male dog attempts to mount the bitch she will stand still, put her tail to one side and allow mating. *Ovulation* takes place on day 10 of the complete cycle (the first day of pro-oestrus is counted as day 1) but there is no external sign.
- *Metoestrus* can be divided into two phases:
  - *Metoestrus I* lasts for approximately 20 days, during which the vaginal discharge dries up, the swollen vulva shrinks and the bitch's behaviour returns to normal. At the end of this phase, the bitch appears to be back to normal, but internally the corpus luteum in the ovary continues to secrete progesterone.
  - *Metoestrus II* lasts for approximately 70 days. There are no external signs, but the corpus luteum secretes progesterone, which causes the body to remain in an almost pregnancy-like state. In some bitches this causes overt symptoms of a *false pregnancy* or *pseudocyesis*.
- *Anoestrus* lasts for 3–9 months. The behaviour and appearance of the bitch are normal and there is almost no ovarian activity. Towards the end of this period, some of the primary follicles will begin to develop and secrete oestrogen and the cycle begins again.

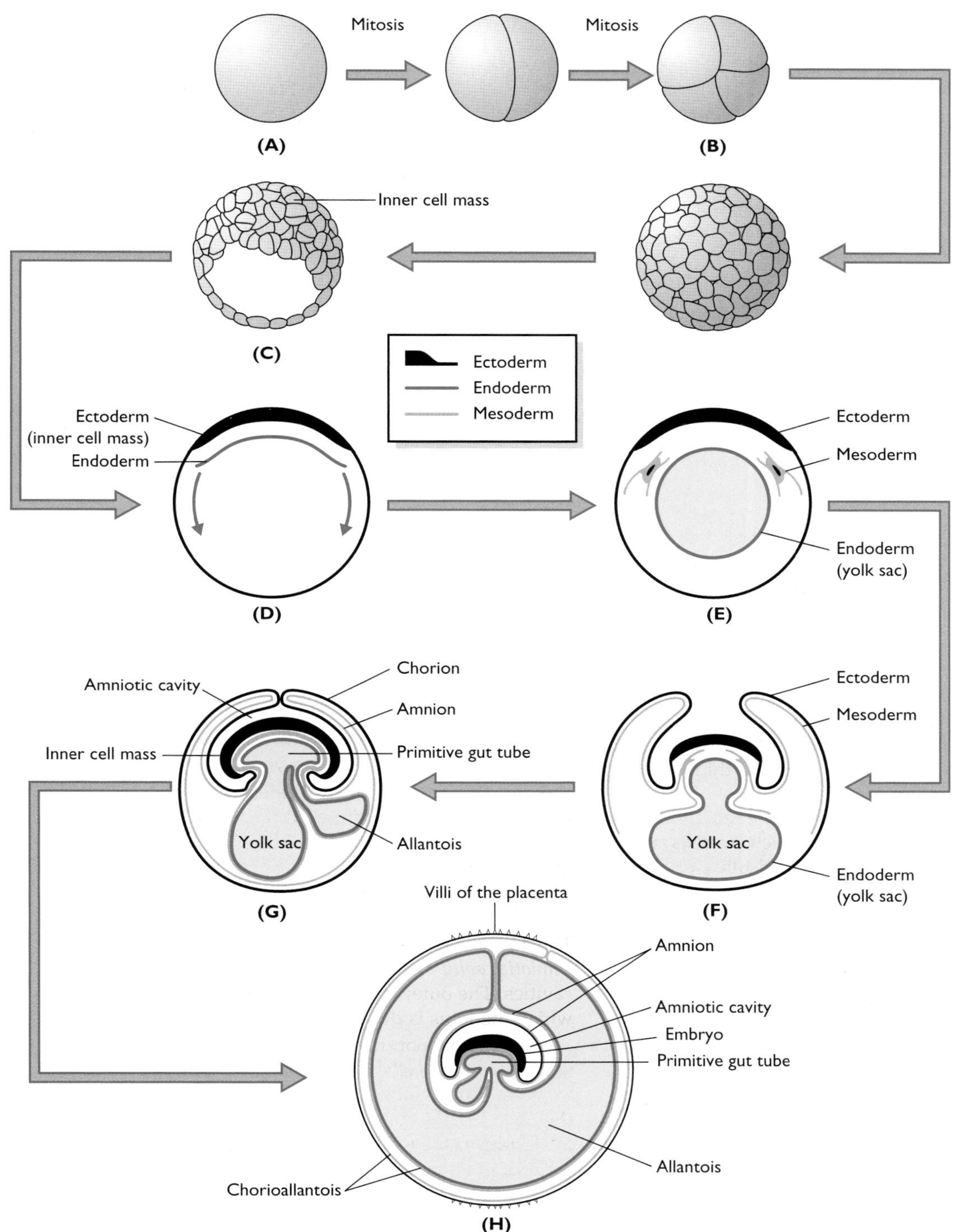

Fig. 11.14 Early embryonic development (see text also). **(A)** The fertilised cell divides by mitosis to form a ball of cells, the morula **(B)**. The morula develops a cavity and is known as the blastocyst **(C)**. A layer of endodermal cells starts to line the trophoblast **(D)** and forms the beginning of the yolk sac **(E)**. Blocks of mesoderm start to form as the inner cell mass starts to be pinched off to form the embryo mesoderm **(F)**. Another space forms from the primitive gut tube; this is the allantois **(G)** and the yolk sac begins to regress. Developing villi form a band around the extra-embryonic membranes **(H)**.

fetus goes through a period of rapid growth until it reaches its final size prior to birth.

The later stages of development in a medium-sized breed of dog are summarised in Table 11.2. Kittens are often slightly in advance of puppies of the same stage.

The placenta

The placenta is a thickened vascular band that develops from the allantochorion around the centre of the conceptus. The allanto-chorion produces small, finger-like villi that burrow into the

Table 11.2 The developmental stages of the canine embryo and fetus

Timescale	Stage of development
3 weeks	5 mm long; forelimbs and hind limbs are small buds sticking out from the trunk; amnion is complete and the allantois is formed
4 weeks	20 mm long; limbs are small cylinders with evidence of a paw shape; eyes are pigmented; external ear has a ridge of visible skin
5 weeks	35 mm long; ear flap is distinct; eyelids partly cover the eyes; digits can be seen on the paws; external genitalia are near to final positions; tactile (sinus) hairs are present on the upper lip; formation of internal organs (organogenesis) is complete
6 weeks	60 mm long; prominent scrotal or vulval tissues; digits widely spread; eyelids are fused; hair follicles and tactile follicles present on the body; claws present; ossification of skeleton at 45 days
7 weeks	100 mm long; body hair and colour markings are developing
8 weeks	150 mm long; hair covering is complete; pads have developed
9 weeks	Ready for birth

endometrium of the uterine horn. Blood capillaries covering the membrane extend into the villi and come into close apposition with the blood capillaries of the endometrium. These form the maternal and fetal parts of the placenta, which are *not* continuous with each other.

The villi develop into broad bands running around the 'waist' of the conceptus. Nutrients and oxygen pass from the dam across the placenta and into the fetus via the umbilical blood vessels; waste products pass in the opposite direction. The *umbilical cord* contains the umbilical artery and vein, the remnants of the yolk sac and the stalk of the allantois connected to the urachus, which leads from the bladder.

The placenta of the dog and cat is restricted to one zone and is therefore described as being a *zonary placenta* (Fig. 11.15). Other species have more diffuse types of placenta (see Chapter 17). Between the placenta and the membranes, at the edge of the placenta, is an area where blood has escaped from broken blood capillaries and become trapped. This is the *marginal haematoma* and it stains the parturient discharges green in bitches and brown in queens. This discolouration is normal!

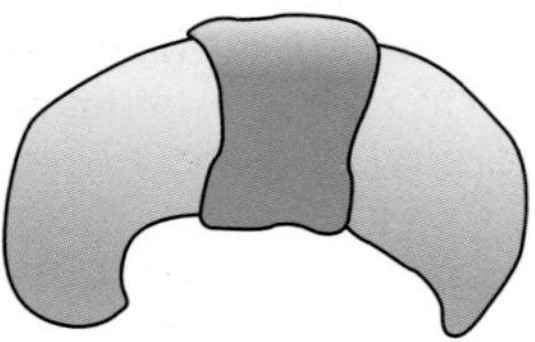

Fig. 11.15 The zonary placental attachment seen in dogs and cats. (With permission from T Colville, JM Bassett, 2001. Clinical anatomy and physiology for veterinary technicians. St Louis, MO: Mosby, p 338.)

Fundamental genetics

Genetics is the science of inheritance and is the method by which *characteristics* or *traits* are passed from one generation to another. These characteristics may be visible (e.g., eye or coat colour) but also may be the less obvious but vital characteristics such as blood grouping or metabolic pathways in the liver – the formation of every enzyme or protein in the body is controlled genetically. The information that determines these characteristics is carried by structures known as *genes*. Genes are arranged in long chains known as *chromosomes*, which are found within the nucleus of every cell in the body (see Chapter 1).

Chromosomes

Chromosomes are made of the protein *deoxyribonucleic acid (DNA)*, which consists of two parallel unbranched strands twisting around each other in a double helix. The strands are formed by a series of four *amino acids* – adenine, thymine, guanine and cytosine – arranged in a varying sequence. The amino acids, which are also called bases or nucleotides, form cross-links with the opposite strand to create a ladder-like structure (Fig. 11.16). Each base only forms a cross-link with a specific other base (i.e., adenine only links with thymine and cytosine only links with guanine). These are then referred to as *base pairs*. The sequence of bases on one strand determines the sequence of bases on the opposite strand and this sequence or genetic code determines the makeup of each gene along the chromosome. The genetic code within each gene determines the type of protein formed by the cells.

In a resting cell the helical structure of each chromosome is tightly coiled within the nucleus so that when the nucleus is seen under a light microscope it appears very dense. The chromosomes can be more easily differentiated when they uncoil prior to cell division by mitosis or meiosis (see Chapter 1).

Chromosomes are always considered in pairs – one of each pair is received from each parent. Each species of animal has a characteristic number of pairs of chromosomes within the

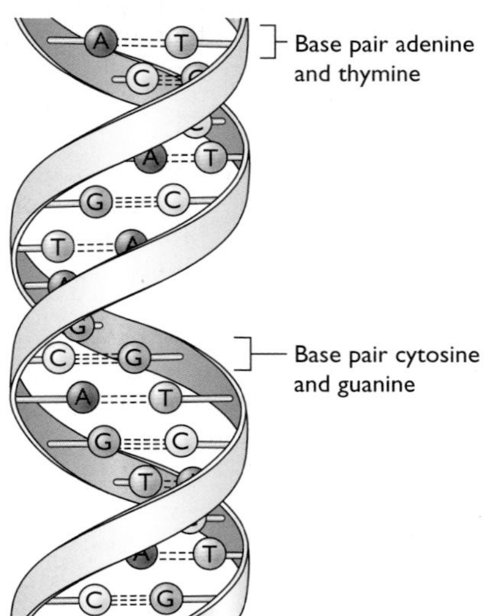

Fig. 11.16 The double-helical structure of DNA.

Table 11.3 Characteristic number of chromosomes in the nucleus of a range of species

Species	No. of pairs (diploid number)	Total number of chromosomes
Dog	39	78
Cat	19	38
Human	23	46
Horse	32	64
Sheep	27	54
Ox	30	60
Pig	19	38
Kangaroo	6	12

nucleus of every cell (Table 11.3). The total complement of chromosomes is known as the *diploid number*. This becomes halved to the *haploid number* during meiosis. Thus each *gamete* (ovum or spermatozoon) formed by meiosis contains the haploid number. After fertilisation, during which the nucleus of the ovum fuses with the nucleus of the sperm, the resulting *zygote* contains the diploid number of chromosomes and cell division to form the embryo begins.

Within the majority of chromosome pairs the chromosomes are identical to one another and they are described as being *homologous* (Fig. 11.17). Within each cell there is one pair of chromosomes that may not be homologous; these are the *sex chromosomes*. The other chromosomes in the cell are referred to as the *autosomes* and they influence all the characteristics that are not concerned with sex determination.

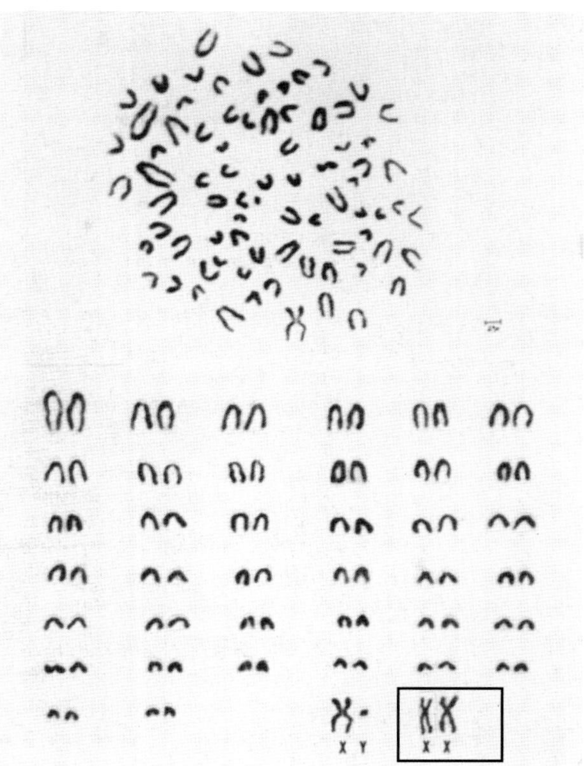

Fig. 11.17 Metaphase spread and karyotype of a dog. The dog has a total of 78 chromosomes in each cell. This chromosome spread is from a male. A female would have XX sex chromosomes (boxed) instead of the X and Y chromosomes. (With permission from S Long, 2006. Veterinary genetics and reproductive physiology. Edinburgh: Butterworth-Heinemann, p 27.)

Sex determination

Within each cell one pair of the total complement of chromosomes is the sex chromosomes, which are concerned with the determination of the sex of the animal. These are given the letters X and Y. The Y chromosome is small and carries the genes that determine male characteristics; there is very little room for any other genes. The X chromosome is larger and carries the genes that determine female characteristics, although it may carry other genes as well.

In the mammal the female has two X chromosomes while the male has an X and a Y, which means that the female has more space for genes than the male. To compensate for this, one of the X chromosomes of the female is inactivated and becomes contracted, forming a *Barr body*.

The male mammal is responsible for determining the sex of his offspring. During meiosis (see Chapter 1) within the ovary or testis four daughter cells are produced; these are either sperm or ova, known as the germ cells. The germ cells will be identical to one another but different from the parent cells. All the pairs of chromosomes split up and each *one* of a pair goes into the newly formed germ cells. Thus the sperm may contain either X or Y chromosomes while the ova will contain only X chromosomes. During fertilisation the sperm cell fuses with the ovum to produce a zygote, which will be either XY or XX (i.e., male or female).

Male × Female = XY × XX

	X	Y
X	X X	X Y
X	X X	X Y

This results in two male offspring (XY) and two female (XX) offspring, meaning that there is a 50% chance of producing either sex at each mating.

Genes

Genes are the units of inheritance. They are short sections of the base pairs making up the strands of DNA that are the chromosomes. The sequence of base pairs within the gene provides the code for each characteristic in the cell and hence the entire individual. Each gene influences *one* characteristic, although each characteristic may be influenced by several genes. These are known as *polygenic characteristics*.

In order to be able to describe genes and the way in which they function it is necessary to learn a new set of terms (Table 11.4). A particular gene will always be found at the same site on a particular chromosome; this site is referred to as its *locus* (*pl. loci*). The process of gene mapping is aimed at identifying the locus of every gene on every chromosome in the cell. As chromosomes

Table 11.4 Genetic terminology

Term	Definition
Diploid number	Number of chromosomes found in a normal cell
Haploid number	Number of chromosomes found in a germ cell (ovum or sperm); half the diploid number and results from meiosis
Gamete	Either the ovum or the spermatozoon; contains the haploid number of chromosomes
Zygote	Results from fusion of the ovum with the sperm and contains the diploid number of chromosomes
Mitosis	Method of cell division occurring in somatic cells (i.e., all the cells of the body except the germ cells)
Meiosis	Method of cell division occurring in the germ cells
Locus	The position of a gene on a chromosome
Allele	A gene on the same locus of a pair of homologous chromosomes
Homozygous gene	Identical genes on the same locus
Heterozygous gene	Non-identical genes on the same locus
Dominant gene	A gene that overrides its allele
Recessive gene	A gene whose characteristic is not expressed when paired with a dominant gene but will be expressed with an identical recessive gene
Phenotype	The outward appearance of an individual
Genotype	The genetic makeup of an individual

are thought of in homologous pairs it follows that there will be another gene at the identical locus; this gene is referred to as its *allele*.

Genes at the same locus affect the same characteristic but they need not produce the same effect. For example, both genes in a pair may affect eye colour but one may instruct the cells to make blue eye pigment while the other produces brown pigment. Genes at the same locus that produce the *same* effect (e.g., both brown eyes) are said to be *homozygous*; genes at the same locus that produce a *different* effect (e.g., one produces blue eyes and one brown eyes), are said to be *heterozygous*.

When a gene produces a characteristic effect it is said to be *expressed*. If only one of a pair of heterozygous genes is expressed the gene is described as being *dominant* and the gene that is not expressed is described as being *recessive*. Dominant genes override the effect of recessive genes and the recessive genes are only expressed when there is no dominant gene to override it (i.e., when they are homozygous). Occasionally there are cases where alleles giving different instructions for the same characteristic are both expressed (e.g., blood groups in humans). Such genes are described as being *co-dominant*.

The majority of genes act independently of one another but some genes can suppress the activity of genes at the same loci. These genes are said to exhibit *epistasis*. Epistasis is seen in albino animals and occurs when the albino gene suppresses all other genes associated with coat colour, resulting in a colourless or white coat.

An animal may have an external appearance that is different from what would be predicted by its genetic makeup. The external appearance of an animal is known as the *phenotype*. The genetic makeup is known as the *genotype* and this can only be accurately appreciated by examination of the DNA. The phenotype of an animal is influenced not only by the genes but also by environmental factors such as diet, disease and exercise. This can be expressed as 'phenotype = genotype + environment'. An example of this might be a fat whippet; this breed is naturally (genetically) very thin but can become fat (phenotype) by overeating (environment).

Mutations

It is important to understand that genes cannot normally be altered and will pass unchanged from generation to generation. The only reason that they may or may not be expressed in the phenotype is because they are dominant or recessive when mixed with the genes from another germ cell (i.e., after division by meiosis followed by fertilisation). Occasionally a genetic change or *mutation* does occur but this is usually a random chance mutation or the result of chemical change or damage (e.g., by radiation). These changes will then pass into the next generation. Mutations may result in a harmful condition that could kill the affected individual (e.g., development of cancer cells), and then the gene will die out on the death of the affected individual. However, it might produce a characteristic that gives the animal an advantage that could enhance its chances of survival, such as a change of coat colour, which might provide camouflage). The affected animal would then reproduce and pass its beneficial gene on to the next generation.

Genetic nomenclature

The language of genetics can be expressed using a system of letters, which can then be used to predict the outcome of mating or crossing one animal with a particular genotype to another animal with a different genotype.

- Genes are always expressed in pairs, one of which comes from the male parent and the other from the female parent.
- The individual genetic characteristics are given a relevant letter of the alphabet.
- The dominant characteristic is written as a capital letter and the recessive characteristic is given as a lowercase letter.
- Thus, for coat colour in the Labrador, where black colour is dominant over chocolate, one could use the letters B (Black) and b (Chocolate).
- A dog with the genotype BB is homozygous for that gene and would have the phenotype of a black coat.
- A dog with the genotype Bb is heterozygous for that gene and would have the phenotype of a black coat.
- A dog with the genotype bb is homozygous for that gene and would have the phenotype of a chocolate coat.

Mendel's laws of inheritance

For many years scientists were unaware of the method by which characteristics were passed from one generation to another, although they recognised that children bore a certain resemblance to their parents. In the mid-19th century an Austrian monk called Gregor Mendel (1822–1884), while working in the gardens of his monastery, developed an interest in plant and animal breeding. From his observations over many years he developed his laws of inheritance, which led him to be able to predict the outcome of various crosses.

- *Mendel's first law of inheritance* states, 'There are factors that control development and these factors retain their individuality from generation to generation'. This is known as the *law of segregation* and it may also be expressed as 'alleles separate to different gametes'. The factors are the structures that we now know as genes and the law means that genes at the same locus on homologous chromosomes separate at meiosis to go into different germ cells.
- *Mendel's second law of inheritance* states, 'Each pair of genes is inherited without being influenced by the presence of other genes'. This is known as the *law of independent assortment* and it means that at meiosis each gene behaves independently as the cell splits into two gametes. The arrangement of the genes in the gametes is further influenced by the process of crossing over (see Chapter 1). This law is true in most instances but there are examples of linked genes that do not behave independently. These genes have loci that are next to each other on the same chromosome so at meiosis they are likely to pass into the germ cells attached to each other. An example of this are the genes for blue eyes and white coat colour – white animals often have blue eyes.

Specialised types of gene

Most genes follow Mendel's laws and are passed on predictably; however, there are some types of gene that may have effects that are less predictable.

Sex-linked genes

Genes that are located on one of the sex chromosomes (i.e., X or Y) are therefore most commonly associated with one or other of the sexes. Most sex-linked genes are found on the X chromosome because it is larger than the Y chromosome and has more space to carry genes. Sex-linked genes are usually recessive; examples include the genes for haemophilia, colour-blindness and orange coat colour in cats. These characteristics are almost always associated with males, although they may occasionally affect females.

The mechanism of inheritance is:

- If a male animal carries a sex-linked gene on his X chromosome it will be expressed because the Y chromosome has no effect on it.
- If a female animal carries a sex-linked gene on *one* of her X chromosomes but not on the other (i.e., she is heterozygous for the gene), it will *not* be expressed because the gene is recessive and requires two genes to be expressed. However she may pass it on to her offspring and she is described as being a *carrier*.
- If a female animal has a sex-linked gene on *both* of her X chromosomes (i.e., she is homozygous for the gene), it will be expressed.

Sex-limited genes

These are genes that influence a characteristic that is seen in only one sex. These genes are switched on by reproductive hormones produced by the animal at the onset of puberty (i.e., oestrogen or testosterone). Examples of sex-limited genes include breast size in women and milk yield in cows.

Lethal genes

These are genes that are incompatible with life. An animal that expresses a lethal gene will die from its effects sooner or later. They are usually recessive genes so affected individuals must be homozygous for the gene. There are three types of lethal gene:

- *Classical lethal*: Affected individuals may die in the uterus or very soon after birth. An example is absence of a tail – a form of spina bifida in cats. Manx cats are heterozygous for the gene and only lack a tail.
- *Delayed lethal*: Affected individuals will die from a progressive condition later in life. Examples include polycystic kidneys in Persian cats and hypoplastic kidneys in a range of species.
- *Semi-lethal*: These produce mild abnormalities that may not necessarily kill the animal. An example is haemophilia, which may be treated by blood transfusions or synthetic clotting factors.

Selective breeding

Selective breeding is the term used to describe the selection of certain individuals as stud animals for breeding rather than allowing all animals to breed randomly. In theory this means that beneficial or desirable characteristics will be passed on to the next generation while harmful or deleterious characteristics will be bred out, but in fact if selective breeding is carried out incorrectly it can create even more problems. Using one's knowledge of genetics it is possible to predict the outcome of crossing one animal with another and so create an individual that is a perfect representation of its breed and is not afflicted by any inherited conditions.

Monohybrid crosses

Matings in which only *one* characteristic is identified and followed through the generations are described as *monohybrid crosses*.

An example is spot colour in Dalmatian dogs. There are two variations in the spot colour – black, which is more common, and liver. The gene for black spots is dominant while the gene for liver spots is recessive.

Let the gene for black spots be represented as the letter B.

Let the gene for liver spots be represented as the letter b.

Example I

Mate a homozygous black-spotted dog to a homozygous liver-spotted bitch.

(i.e., BB × bb)

Using a grid known as a Punnett square, we can work out the genotypes for the first filial generation, referred to as the F1 generation.

Genes from the male (*in the sperm*)

	B	**B**
b	**Bb**	**Bb**
b	**Bb**	**Bb**

Genes from the female (*in the ova*)

The F1 generation will consist entirely of puppies with the Bb genotype and their phenotype will be black-spotted.

Example 2

Mate a heterozygous black-spotted dog to a heterozygous black-spotted bitch.
(i.e., Bb × Bb)
The F1 generation will be:

	B	b
B	BB	Bb
b	Bb	bb

- The genotypes will be 1BB:2Bb:1bb.
- The phenotypes will be three black-spotted puppies to one liver-spotted puppy.

There is a 1 in 4 chance of producing the double-recessive individual when you use a monohybrid cross. When crossing two animals that are heterozygous for any characteristic you will always get the same ratio of genotypes of 1:2:1. Statistically, if you use a large sample of animals you are more likely to achieve this ratio. In a litter of four puppies you might not breed the liver-spotted puppy; however, if you produced 100 puppies you significantly improve the chances of breeding a liver-spotted puppy.

Example 3

Mate a homozygous liver-spotted dog to a heterozygous black-spotted bitch.
(i.e., bb × Bb)
The F1 generation will be:

	b	b
B	Bb	Bb
b	bb	bb

- The genotypes will be 2Bb:2bb.
- The phenotypes will be two black-spotted puppies to two liver-spotted puppies – there is an equal chance of producing black- or liver-spotted puppies.

Back-crossing to the recessive

This is a technique using test matings to ascertain whether an animal is carrying a particular recessive gene. This may be a gene that causes a harmful condition such as the eye disease progressive retinal atrophy or, in more minor cases, an unwanted coat colour. A recessive gene will only be expressed if an animal is homozygous for that gene. If the animal is heterozygous, the gene will not be expressed but the animal will carry the gene and may pass it on to its offspring.

For example: progressive retinal atrophy (PRA) is a condition seen in breeds such as Labradors, Golden Retrievers, Collies and Spaniels. It causes gradual deterioration of the retinal blood vessels and results in blindness by the time the dog is about 18 months old. It is important to identify carriers of the gene so that they do not pass it on to their puppies.

Let the gene for normal sight be S.
Let the gene for PRA be s.
Thus dogs with:

- the genotype SS will have normal sight
- the genotype ss will have PRA and go blind by 18 months old
- the genotype Ss will have normal sight but will be carriers of this recessive gene

The suspect bitch under investigation could have the genotype Ss or SS.

1. Suppose the suspect bitch is Ss.
   Mate her to a dog who is known to have PRA and will therefore have the genotype ss.
   The F1 generation will be:

	s	s
S	Ss	Ss
s	ss	ss

The puppies will be 2Ss – carriers of the gene but unaffected; 2ss – affected by the condition.

2. Suppose the suspect bitch is SS.
   Mate her to the known affected dog ss.
   The F1 generation will be:

	s	s
S	Ss	Ss
S	Ss	Ss

All the puppies will have the genotype Ss, meaning they will be unaffected by PRA but because they will be carriers of the gene they would have to be neutered and not used for breeding. In this example if a bitch produces puppies that are not affected you can be sure that she is homozygous for normal sight; if she produces puppies that are affected by PRA she must be heterozygous. If the heterozygous bitch was mated to an unidentified heterozygous dog the F1 generation would produce genotypes in the ratio of 1SS:2Ss:1ss, which means there is a 1 in 4 chance of producing an affected puppy.

It is essential to identify carriers of harmful genes but in practice test matings are expensive and take time. Analysis of pedigrees may be helpful, assuming they are correct, but nowadays DNA analysis may be much quicker and much more accurate.

Dihybrid crosses

A dihybrid cross is one in which *two* characteristics are identified. Each gene obeys Mendel's second law of independent assortment and will move independently. It may be paired with any other gene, resulting in a wide variation of genotypes and phenotypes. This can appear very complicated but, as in the previous monohybrid cross, if you cross two animals that are heterozygous for both characteristics you end up with a predictable ratio of genotypes, in this case of 9:3:3:1 (compared to 1:2:1 for a monohybrid cross) and the chances of producing an animal that is recessive for both characteristics is 15:1 (compared to 3:1 for a monohybrid cross).

If you expand this idea to crossing individuals with *three* characteristics it is known as a *trihybrid cross*. When you cross two animals that are heterozygous for all three characteristics the predicted ratios of the genotypes are 27:9:9:9:3:3:3:1 and the chances of producing the one individual that is homozygous for all three recessive characteristics is 63:1.

This theory is extremely important when attempting to breed the perfect example of a particular species or breed or just a perfectly healthy animal. The aim is to achieve homozygosity for beneficial characteristics without achieving homozygosity for harmful characteristics. It is important to understand the reducing chances of producing an individual that is homozygous for large numbers of characteristics.

Breeding strategies

Hundreds of years of selective breeding of cats and dogs have led to the development of distinct breeds. A *breed* may be defined as 'a group of animals of the same species linked by a set of common characteristics'. When an animal of one breed is crossed with another animal of another breed the result is a *crossbreed* or *mongrel*, which is a normal fertile animal that is capable of reproducing and passing on the characteristics of both breeds to the next generation but will bear very little resemblance to its parents, such as the Labradoodle, which results from crossing a Labrador with a Poodle. The appearance of the Labradoodle is totally unpredictable and individuals in the same litter will differ markedly from each other. The advantage of crossing two animals of the *same* breed is that you can predict what the offspring will look like. When crossing two mongrels the assortment of the genes may be completely random and the outcome unpredictable. The skill of breeding lies in understanding Mendel's laws and in selecting the correct animals to be mated to each other. Random selection could result in a Crufts champion but it would be very, very lucky.

The aim of selective breeding is to achieve homozygosity for all the genes which control the desirable characteristics.

For example, suppose an animal that is homozygous for gene Z is mated to an animal that is heterozygous for gene Z.
(i.e., ZZ × Zz)
Then the F1 generation will be:

	Z	Z
Z	ZZ	ZZ
z	Zz	Zz

If one of the homozygous individuals is then crossed back to one of the parents (i.e., ZZ × ZZ), then the offspring of the F2 generation will all be homozygous. The parents of the F2 generation are described as breeding 'true' for that characteristic and the outcome is predictable. When homozygosity is achieved the characteristic is described as being *fixed* in the breed. In attempting to reach this situation breeders will use a range of breeding strategies.

- *Inbreeding* is the mating of two individuals that are *more* closely related than the population as a whole (e.g., brother to sister or mother to son). The aim is to get closer and closer to homozygosity to fix the characteristic in as few generations as possible. If the inbreeding strategy is followed for too many generations, harmful genes may be fixed as well as the desirable genes, resulting in a condition known as *inbreeding depression*. This produces weak, unhealthy examples of the breed, so inbreeding is not recommended.
- *Outbreeding* is the mating of two individuals that are *less* closely related than the population as a whole (e.g., father to great-granddaughter or to fifth cousin). This strategy may be used to counteract the effect of inbreeding depression. As the animals used are only distantly related, the offspring are likely to be heterozygous for both desirable and harmful genes. Any recessive genes will not be expressed in the genotype, producing a healthier stronger individual, a condition known as *hybrid vigour* or *heterosis*. This breeding strategy leads to much slower fixing of genes and it is less easy to accurately predict the outcome of a mating. An extreme version of outbreeding is seen when two unrelated breeds are crossed, such as a German Shepherd with a Dachshund. The appearance of the resulting mongrel puppies cannot be predicted, although they will be perfectly healthy and will all be different from one another and from their parents. Mongrels are often assumed to be free from inherited abnormalities.
- *Line breeding* is the mating of two individuals that are more closely related than those in outbreeding but less closely related than in those in inbreeding (e.g., mother to grandson or mating second cousins). This strategy is the most commonly used in selective breeding because, although it fixes the characteristics more slowly and the offspring are less predictable, it has none of the problems associated with inbreeding depression.

Congenital and inherited defects

Selective breeding aims to fix desirable characteristics but it can also result in the fixing of harmful genes. These are associated with poor health and in some cases eventual death. Animals may be born with a variety of harmful conditions but these need not necessarily be caused genetically.

- *Congenital defects* are present in the animal at the time of its birth. They may be caused by damage to the embryo or fetus during the gestation period or during parturition, such as brain damage due to oxygen starvation during birth, or cerebellar hypoplasia caused by exposure to the feline infectious enteritis virus during gestation. Because congenital conditions are not carried by the genes, an affected animal may produce healthy offspring.
- *Inherited defects* are carried on the genes. They are inherited from the parents and may be passed from generation to generation. Most inherited defects are caused by recessive genes and will only be expressed when the animal is homozygous for that gene. Breeders of any species have a responsibility to know which inherited defects exist in their chosen breed or species. They should be able to identify affected individuals and prevent them from breeding so that the genes are not passed to their offspring.

Examples of inherited defects in dogs and cats include:

- *Hip dysplasia* is seen in larger breeds of dog (e.g., Labradors, Golden Retrievers and German Shepherds). Malformation of the acetabulum or femoral head that form the hip joint causes laxity in the joint, which eventually causes osteoarthritis. The Kennel Club (KC) and the British Veterinary Association (BVA) have a monitoring scheme to identify affected animals. Dogs with a high hip score should not be used for breeding.
- *Elbow dysplasia* is seen in a range of dog breeds (e.g., Bassett Hounds, Golden Retrievers, Labradors and Newfoundlands). Various anomalies affect the elbow joint, resulting in instability when weight-bearing. This causes lameness, osteoarthritis and pain. A KC/BVA monitoring scheme identifies affected individuals.
- *Eye defects* can be present in a large range of anomalies (e.g., progressive retinal atrophy, collie eye anomaly and hereditary cataracts). The KC/BVA/International Sheepdog Society run a monitoring scheme to identify affected individuals.
- *Entropion*, in which in-turning eyelashes scratch the cornea and cause conjunctivitis and keratitis, has to be treated surgically. This is a polygenic characteristic occurring in breeds such as Sharpeis, Rottweilers and Labradors.

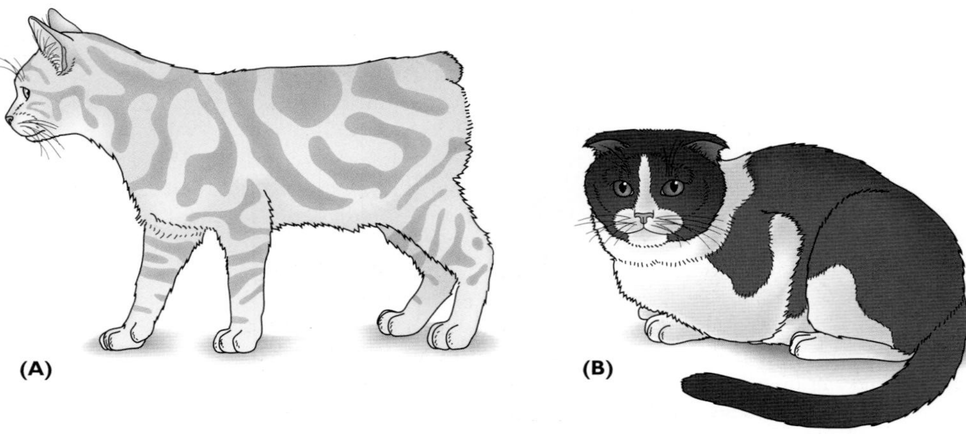

Fig 11.18 Two breeds of cat that originally resulted from a genetic abnormality: **(A)** Manx cats, **(B)** Scottish fold.

- *Ectropion* means the lower eyelids droop downwards, exposing the conjunctiva below the eye, which becomes dry and inflamed and must be treated surgically. This is a polygenic characteristic seen in breeds characterised by their soft, droopy eyes (e.g., Bloodhounds, Bassett Hounds and St Bernards).
- *Cryptorchidism* – retained testes – may be bilateral or unilateral. The retained testis will be infertile and may be more likely to develop a Sertoli cell tumour in later life.
- *Deafness* is linked to blue eyes and a white coat and is often seen in white cats and Dalmatians.
- *Haemophilia* is a defective clotting mechanism associated mainly with male animals. It is known as von Willebrand's disease in dogs.
- *Taillessness in cats* is a recessive gene. Homozygous form causes a form of spina bifida and results in the death of fetal kittens. Heterozygous form results in varying degrees of taillessness, which is the basis of the Manx breed of cat (Fig. 11.18A).
- *Flat-chested kittens* result from an autosomal recessive gene and is seen in Burmese kittens. Affected animals have difficulty breathing and do not thrive.
- *Folded ears in cats* result from an incomplete dominant gene. Heterozygous form has folded ears and this is the basis of the Scottish Fold breed of cat. Homozygous form has painful swollen joints and pain on movement (Fig. 11.18B).
- *Polydactyly* is multiple toes, seen in cats. Such cats are often referred to as 'witches' cats'. It causes few problems but affected cats have very large feet.

CHAPTER 12

Common integument

KEY POINTS

- The common integument is the outer covering of the body and includes the skin, hair, pads and claws.
- The skin covers the entire body and provides a protective layer.
- The skin consists of two layers: the epidermis and dermis, under which is the hypodermis or subcuticular layer. This basic structure is also seen in footpads and claws.
- Within the skin are a range of glands, the secretions of which contribute to the overall function of the skin.
- Other glands in the body (e.g., mammary glands and anal glands), are also modified skin glands.
- The skin of the dog and cat is covered in hair, which is derived from epidermal cells. The function of hair is to protect, to insulate and to communicate.
- The underside of the foot is hairless and protected by the footpads, also derived from modified epidermis.
- The ends of the digits are protected by hard epidermal structures known as claws.

The term *common integument* refers to the outer covering of the body. It is said to be the largest organ of the body and, because it has a variety of component parts, it has a range of functions. The integument includes:

- Skin
- Hair
- Footpads
- Claws

The skin

The skin covers the external surface of the body, forming a complete barrier against the external environment. It is perforated by various natural openings (e.g., the mouth and the anus), and at these points it blends with the mucous membranes lining the openings. The functions of the skin are:

1. *Protection*: It protects the underlying structures of the body and, in specialised thickened regions of the skin (e.g., pads of the feet), it gives added protection against physical trauma. It also acts as a physical barrier to protect against invasion by microorganisms, and sebaceous glands secrete an antiseptic sebum onto the surface. The skin also acts as a waterproof barrier; it is almost impermeable to water, preventing the body from drying out or from becoming waterlogged (e.g., when swimming). Pigmented areas in the skin and hair protect against damage from ultraviolet radiation.
2. *Sensory*: The surface of the skin is well supplied with many types of sensory nerve ending to detect temperature, pressure, touch and pain. This assists the body in monitoring its external environment.
3. *Secretion*: A range of glands within the skin produce secretions directly onto the skin's surface. These include *sebum* – produced by sebaceous glands; *sweat* – in the cat and dog sweating only occurs from active sweat glands of the footpads and nose; *pheromones* – produced by specialised skin glands.
4. *Production*: Ultraviolet light from the sun converts 7-dihydrocholesterol present in sebum into vitamin D. This is activated within the kidney and liver and increases the uptake and metabolism of dietary calcium.

Dogs, cats and other species of animal that are kept indoors without access to sunlight may suffer from skeletal problems caused by the lack of vitamin D in their bodies. This is then reflected in the levels of calcium in the bones and tissues.

5. *Storage*: Fat is stored under the skin as adipose tissue or subcutaneous fat. Fat is an energy store and also acts as a thermal insulating layer.
6. *Thermoregulation*: The skin prevents heat loss by diverting blood away from the surface by vasoconstriction, by erecting the hairs to trap a layer of insulating air, and by having an insulating layer of fat. Heat can be lost from the body when required (e.g., by the production of sweat). However, the skin only plays a minor role in heat loss in the dog and cat because they only have active sweat glands in their footpads and nose. Most of the dissipation of excessive body heat in dogs and cats occurs via panting, which may also be associated with anxiety, pain and respiratory distress.
7. *Communication*: Production of pheromones, which are natural scents used for intraspecific communication. Other 'scents' produced for communication are those of the circumanal glands and glands of the anal sacs. The integument also provides a means of visual communication, such as when a dog raises its hackles when threatened, which is seen as a warning of possible aggression.

Skin structure

The skin is composed of two layers: the *epidermis* or superficial layer, and the underlying *dermis* (Fig. 12.1). The *hypodermis* lies beneath the skin.

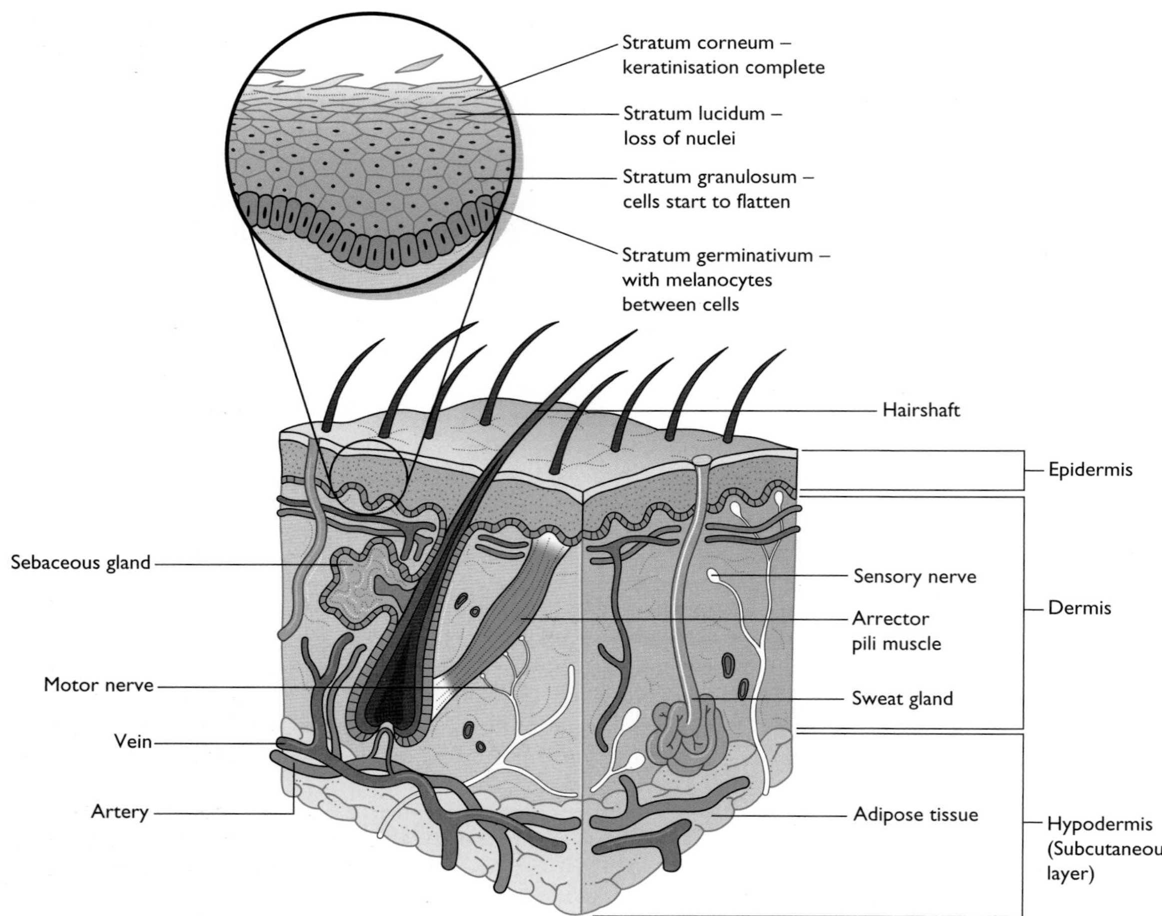

Fig. 12.1 Structure of the skin.

Epidermis

The epidermis is composed of *stratified squamous epithelium* and has multiple layers of cells that are continually renewed. New cells are produced in the deepest layers of the epidermis and are pushed upwards to the surface as a result of mitosis below (see Chapter 1). The surface cells are continually lost and these dead cells or *squames* are seen as scurf in the animal's coat. This process replaces the cells that are lost due to friction and wear. The layers, or *strata*, of the epidermis are, from deep to superficial:

> The colour of the skin and overlying hair may not necessarily be the same and this may be noticed when clipping an area for a surgical operation. It is interesting to note that the skin of polar bears is black but the fur is white!

1. *Stratum basale* or *germinativum*: Consists of a single layer of dividing cells (i.e., where the new cells are 'manufactured'). Pigmented cells or *melanocytes*, which contain granules of the pigment melanin, may also be present in areas such as the nose pad or footpad or in coloured areas of the body.
2. *Stratum granulosum*: The cells are flattened and the process of infiltration of the cells by the structural protein *keratin* (known as *keratinisation*) begins in this layer. Keratin provides protection in layers that get extra wear (e.g., footpads).
3. *Stratum lucidum*: The cells lose their nuclei and become clearer.
4. *Stratum corneum*: The most superficial of the epidermal layers. The cells have no nuclei and are dead; they are fully keratinised and flattened in shape.

The whole of the epidermis is avascular and receives its supply of nutrients from blood vessels within the dermis.

> In areas of the body that are covered in hair, the epidermis of the skin may only be a few cells thick (e.g., the skin over the abdomen). However, in areas unprotected by hair (e.g., the footpads), the epidermis is much thicker. This can easily be seen when examining a cut pad.

Dermis

The dermis is the deep layer of the skin, upon which the epidermis sits (Fig. 12.1). It is composed of dense connective tissue with irregularly arranged collagen and elastic fibres. The dermis has a generous supply of blood vessels, nerves and sensory nerve endings. The hair follicles, sebaceous glands and sweat glands also lie within the dermis but are formed from epidermal cells.

Hypodermis

The hypodermis, or subcutis or subcuticular layer, is not actually part of the skin, but is a layer of loose connective tissue and fat lying beneath the dermis. It also contains elastic fibres, which gives the skin its flexibility. This is evident when we grasp a fold of skin on the neck of a dog or cat to 'scruff' them. It is the hypodermis into which subcutaneous injections are given.

Dermatitis is inflammation of the skin. It is a common complaint in dogs and cats and may be caused by a number of things, but it is sometimes extremely difficult to ascertain exactly what is causing the problem. Allergic (atopic) dermatitis may be caused by food allergies, fleas, dust mites and pollen. Contact dermatitis is caused by an irritant or chemical with which the patient has been in contact. Affected animals are often itchy and may rub, lick or chew the affected area.

Skin glands

Within the dermis are a range of glands producing secretions directly onto the skin surface:

Sebaceous glands

These are alveolar or saccular glands whose ducts open into the base of the hair follicles. They secrete an oily substance called *sebum*, which forms a waterproof layer on the skin and coat, giving the coat's 'sheen' and making the skin supple. Sebum has an antiseptic quality that controls bacterial growth on the skin surface. Some of the modified sebaceous glands produce secretions that influence the behaviour of another animal. These are known as pheromones and are the 'scents' that dogs and cats produce as a means of communicating with other members of their own species.

Modified sebaceous glands include the following:

- *Tail glands* are found on the dorsal surface of the base of the tail. Their function is believed to be concerned with individual recognition and identification.
- *Circumanal glands* are located around the entire circumference of the anus. They drain into special sweat glands and their secretion is thought to contribute to the individual smell of a dog.
- *Anal glands* lie within the walls of the paired spherical anal sacs, located on either side and just below the anus. They produce a foul-smelling secretion that is expressed during defecation, coating the faeces and serving as a territorial marker (see Chapter 9).
- *Circumoral glands* are found on the lips of cats and their secretion is used for territorial marking. This can be observed when a cat rubs its face on objects such as furniture and its owner's legs!
- *Ceruminous glands* are found in the external ear canal and secrete cerumen (ear wax).
- *Meibomian* or *tarsal glands* open on to the eyelids and produce the fatty component of the tear film that moistens the eye.

Sebaceous cysts may develop when a hair follicle or skin gland gets blocked by dirt, scar tissue or as a result of infection. They may be confused with other 'lumps' such as skin tumours; however, they are benign and rarely problematic. If they burst they will release a grey/brown 'cottage cheese'-like substance.

Sweat glands

Also called *sudoriferous* glands. These are coiled glands found in the dermis, which are only active on the nose and footpads of dogs and cats.

You may notice when a cat or dog is stressed in the consulting room, it may leave 'sweaty' footprints on the consulting room table!

Mammary glands

These are greatly modified, enlarged sweat glands, which secrete milk for nourishment of the young (see Chapter 11).

Mammary gland tumours are the most common tumours in dogs. Most occur in unspayed bitches over 6 years of age. About half of mammary gland tumours are cancerous, but even benign tumours can cause discomfort as they enlarge, and may become ulcerated; therefore, removal of the tumour(s) is recommended.

Hair

The possession of hair or fur is a distinctive characteristic of mammals. It covers the entire body of the dog and cat except in areas such as the nose and footpads. In other areas, such as the scrotum and around the nipples, the hair covering is much sparser.

A hair is a keratinised structure and is produced by a *hair follicle*. The visible part of the hair, above the skin's surface, is called the *hair shaft* and the part of the hair that lies within the follicle is called the *hair root*.

The hair follicle originates from a peg of epidermal cells that grows down into the underlying dermis, where it forms a *hair cone* over a piece of dermis called the *dermal papilla* (Fig. 12.2). The papilla provides the blood and nerve supply for the growing hair. From the hair cone, the cells keratinise and form a hair. As the hair grows up through the epidermis to the skin's surface, the cells at the point of the cone die, forming a channel – the hair follicle. The hair continues to grow until it eventually dies and becomes detached from the follicle. Hair growth is cyclical and once the hair is shed a new hair follicle develops and a new hair will start to grow.

Moulting

The shedding of hair, or *moulting*, is influenced by the annual seasons, particularly the environmental temperature and day length. Most dogs moult more heavily in the spring and autumn, while cats only moult heavily in spring, followed by a lighter loss of hair throughout the summer and autumn. However, pet cats and dogs are usually kept inside centrally heated houses with electric lighting and this confuses the natural seasonal triggers. Moulting can therefore occur to some extent all year round.

Alopecia is the 'abnormal' loss of hair. It may be the result of allergies, endocrine disorders, an infestation of a skin mite such as *Demodex* or a fungal infection such as ringworm.

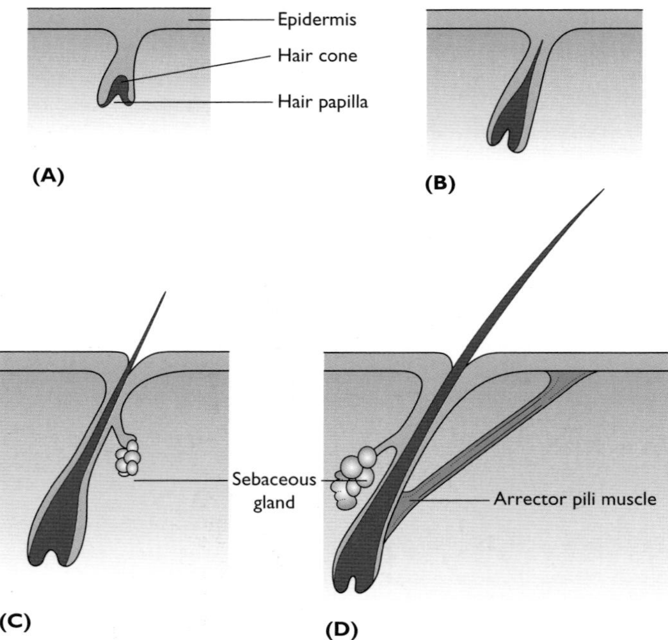

Fig. 12.2 The formation of hair: **(A)** Development of the hair papilla and hair cone. **(B)** The follicle starts to develop. **(C)** Sebaceous gland develops and the developing hair breaks through the skin. **(D)** A mature hair follicle with arrector pili muscle.

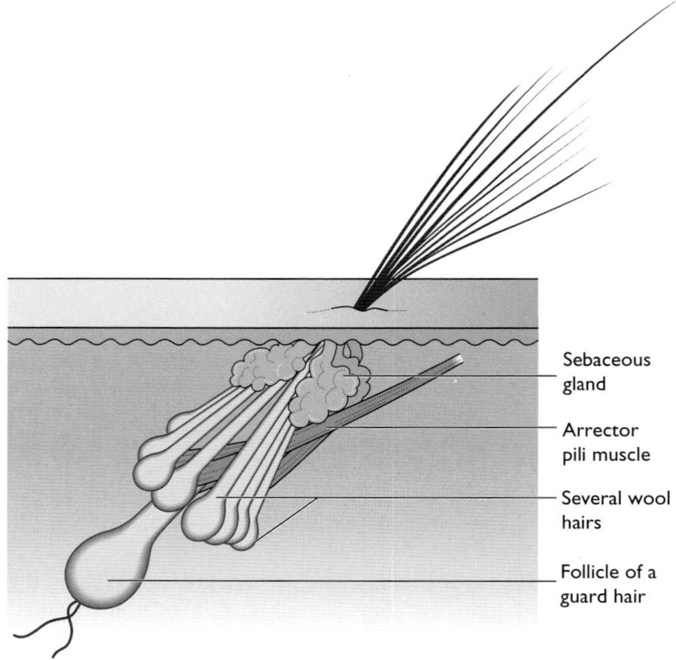

Fig. 12.3 A guard hair and wool hairs in a hair follicle.

Hair types

There are three major types of hair:

- *Guard hairs* are the thick, long and stiff hairs that form the outer protective coat of the animal. They lie closely against the skin and sweep uniformly in broad tracts, giving the coat of a dog or cat its smooth appearance. The nature of the guard hairs gives the coat its waterproof quality. Water 'runs off' the coat unless the animal is submerged in water for a long time. This prevents water from penetrating the coat and making the animal cold.

  One guard hair grows from each follicle and associated with it is a strand of smooth muscle called the *arrector pili* muscle (Fig. 12.3). The function of this muscle is to raise the hair from its resting position, trapping a layer of insulating air. The muscle is stimulated to contract by cold temperatures, but the hairs of the neck and back (hackles) in the dog, or those of the tail in the cat, can be raised in response to threat. (In humans, the effect of the arrector pili muscle is seen as 'goosebumps' on the skin.)
- *Wool hairs* form the innermost, soft undercoat. They are thinner, softer and shorter than guard hairs and more numerous. Their number fluctuates, especially in winter, as they serve to keep the body warm by providing an insulating layer. The thickness of the wool hairs varies between breeds. For example, Huskies have a very thick undercoat and are well adapted to extremely cold temperatures; Dobermans have a very short outer coat and no undercoat and have poor tolerance of cold weather. There may be a number of wool hairs growing from one follicle and these are associated with one guard hair (Fig. 12.3).
- *Tactile hairs* or *vibrissae* are the 'whiskers'. Also called sinus hairs, they are much thicker than guard hairs and protrude outwards beyond the rest of the coat. They are specialised hairs that grow from follicles found deep in the hypodermis. The follicle is surrounded by nerve endings that are responsive to mechanical stimuli such as touch or movement and provide sensory information from the environment. Tactile hairs are mostly found on the face, principally on the upper lip and near the eyes. However, they are also found in other areas, which vary between species, such as the cluster of tactile hairs on the carpus of the cat and the tuft of whiskers on a dog's cheek.

Footpads

The function of the footpads or digital pads is to protect the underlying joints and to act as shock absorbers as the animal walks or runs. They are covered by thick, pigmented, keratinised, hairless epidermis. The surface of the dog's footpads is roughened by conical papillae, which provide traction during walking. The pads of the cat are much smoother. Inside the pad, a digital cushion formed from thickened dermis and fatty vascular tissue absorbs the impact of the foot hitting the ground at speed. Sweat glands open to the surface of the pad.

The dog and the cat have seven pads on each forepaw (Fig. 12.4). These are:

- *Five digital pads*: One covers each distal *interphalangeal joint*, including one associated with the dew claw.
- *Metacarpal pad* covers the *phalangeal–metacarpal joint*; this is heart-shaped in the dog and round in the cat.

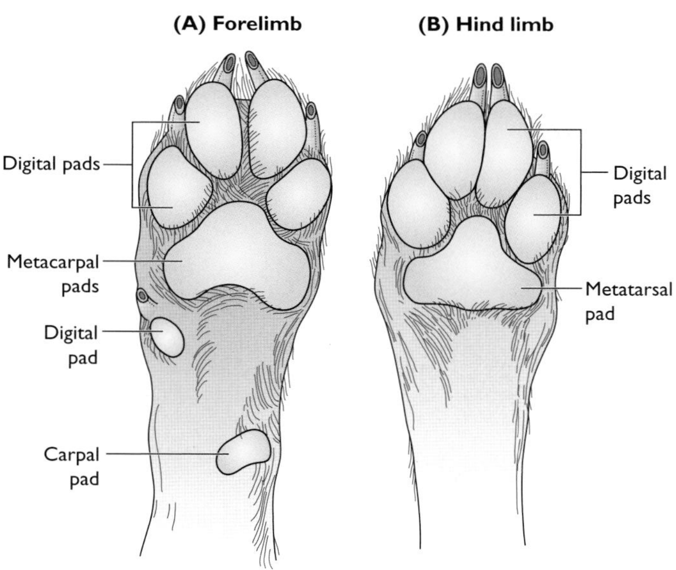

Fig. 12.4 Footpads on the fore **(A)** and hind limb **(B)** of the dog. There is no tarsal equivalent of the carpal pad.

- *Carpal pad*, or stop pad, lies just distal to the *carpal bones* and protects this area when an animal is running at high speed.

The hind paw has only five pads: one main metatarsal pad and four digital pads (Fig. 12.4).

Distemper, a disease of dogs, causes thickening of the footpads and the nosepad, and used to be called 'Hardpad'. It is poorly understood why the causative virus has this effect on the pads, but the distemper virus also affects the respiratory, central nervous and gastrointestinal systems. In the UK, thanks to widespread vaccination, this serious disease is uncommon.

Claws

Claws are composed of modified keratinised epidermis and form the horny outer covering of the distal or third phalanx of each digit, including the dew claw, where they cover the *ungual process* (Fig. 12.5). Their function is to protect the distal phalanges during walking and weight bearing and to provide grip. The claws of the dog are thick and strong while those of the cat are finer but much sharper and are used as weapons of offence. At rest, the claws of a cat are retracted into pockets of skin by elastic ligaments that run from the second and third phalanges. When the cat unsheathes its claws the action of the *digital flexor muscle* overcomes the tension in the elastic ligaments.

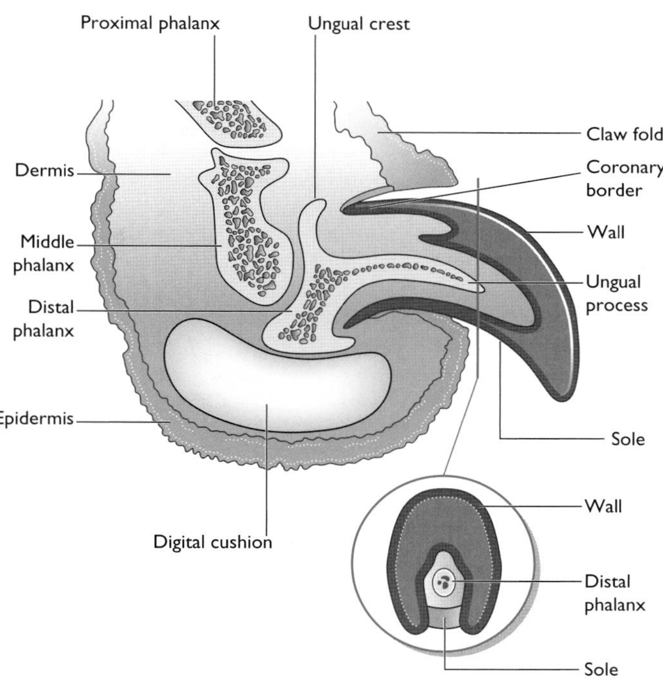

Fig. 12.5 Structure of the claw.

Each claw grows from a specialised region of epidermis called the *coronary border*, which lies underneath a fold of skin called the *claw fold*. The claw consists of two hard, laterally compressed *walls* with a ventral groove between them filled with softer horn known as the *sole*. The vascular dermis or *quick* lies at the base of the claw and bleeds if you cut the claws too short.

The claw grows continuously and normal 'wear and tear' usually prevents them from growing too long. However, in many dogs the claws can become overgrown and, if left, they can curl round and penetrate the pads. Special care should be taken with dew claws, if present, because they are not in contact with the ground and do not get worn down by walking.

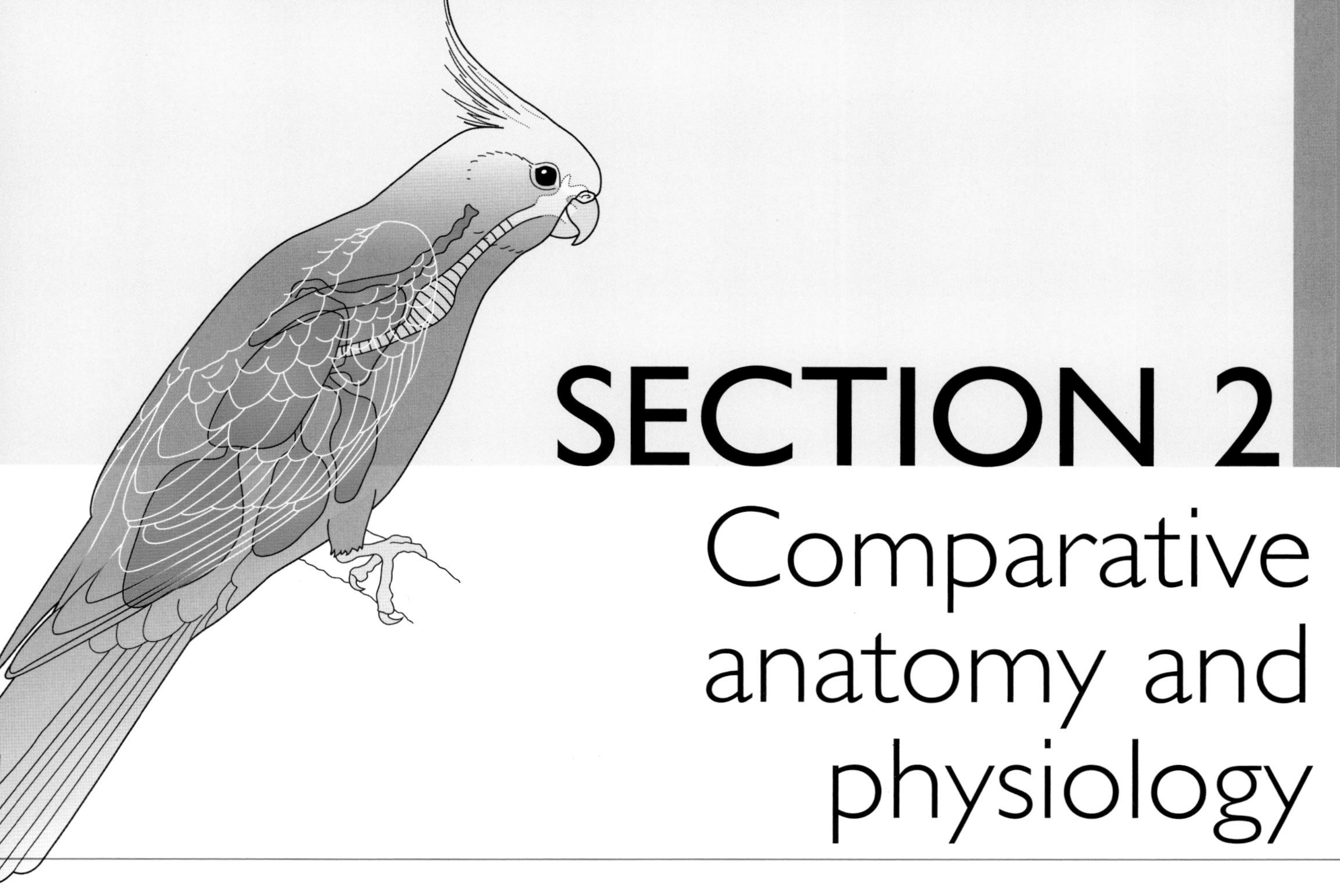

SECTION 2
Comparative anatomy and physiology

This section describes the anatomy and physiology of some of the less common species of pets, horses and the common species of farm animal. In some cases there may be less detail than in Section 1. It is assumed that, having studied the anatomy and physiology of the dog and cat in detail, the student will be able to apply this knowledge and appreciate both the similarities and the differences between the various species.

CHAPTER 13 Birds

The birds are a unique group of vertebrates. There are about 8500 known species in the world, all belonging to the class Aves. They are considered to have evolved about 150 million years ago from the thickly feathered *Archaeopteryx*, which links reptiles to birds. Birds and reptiles have much in common, such as the ability to lay eggs, but no other class of animal has feathers. The possession of feathers, and in the majority of species the ability to fly, is the reason for their success. Flight allows them to colonise new habitats, find new sources of food and escape predators. Much of their anatomy and physiology has evolved to facilitate life in the air.

Musculoskeletal system

The skeleton of the bird (Fig. 13.1) is unlike that of any other group of animals and it has developed from the evolution of powered flight. A combination of a reduction in the total number of bones and the fusion of many joints has resulted in a skeleton that provides a strong base for the attachment of the flight muscles. Although the skeleton must be light enough to enable the downward force of the wing to lift the bird into the air and to keep it airborne, when compared to mammals of a similar size birds are not exceptionally light.

Main features

Bone structure

- To lighten the skeleton the cortex of the bone is much thinner than in mammalian bones and many long bones are hollow. Internally, lightweight struts create a honeycombed interior and reinforce the bones (Fig. 13.2).
- Many of the larger bones are *pneumatic*: they are filled with air contained in membranous air sacs that connect with the respiratory system. These cut down the weight of the skeleton and so aid flight. The number of pneumatic bones is reduced in diving birds as they restrict the ability to stay under water.

Skeletal modifications

- The sternum is extended into a laterally flattened *keel* (Fig. 13.1), which provides a large surface area for the attachment of the major flight muscles. These are the *pectoral* muscles responsible for the powerful down stroke and the *supracoracoid* muscle responsible for the upstroke. Flightless birds (e.g., ostriches and emus) do not have a keel.
- To counteract the action of the flight muscles and to support the wings a large bone, the *coracoid*, lies between the keel and each shoulder joint (Fig. 13.1).
- The *number of joints* in the body is reduced. This is particularly seen in the vertebral column and results in a rigid trunk to support the action of the flight muscles.
- The *neck* is long and mobile and contains more cervical vertebrae than the 7 seen in all mammals; there may be as many as 25 in the swan. A long neck makes up for the lack of flexibility in the body and enables the bird to turn its head right round, creating the wide range of vision necessary for survival, to catch food and to preen all parts of its body.
- The number of caudal vertebrae are reduced and fused forming the *tail* or *pygostyle*. Some flight feathers are attached to the tail and play an important part in flight, balance and display. At the base of the tail is the *uropygial* or *preen gland*, which is essential for keeping feathers oiled and healthy.
- There is a *single body cavity*; birds have no diaphragm dividing the thorax and abdomen.
- There is no floor to the *pelvic cavity*, which makes the pelvis more distensible to facilitate the passage of eggs to the outside. Egg laying enables birds to reproduce without the need to carry the developing fetus around internally. This would increase the body weight and severely restrict the ability to fly.

Head *(Fig. 13.3)*

- A lightweight *beak* covering the mandible replaces the teeth and reduces the weight of the skeleton. Each species has a characteristic beak shape, which is adapted to its eating habits.
- Between the mandible and skull is the *quadrate bone*, which allows the bird to open its mouth wide and makes dislocation of the jaw very unlikely.
- Many birds also have a joint known as the *craniofacial hinge* between the upper beak and the skull. This increases the mobility of the beak during feeding.
- The *orbit* is large and thin-walled to lighten the skull and to house the large eyes (Fig. 13.3). Because much of the bird's brain is concerned with visual information, the eyes connect with large optic lobes in the brain.

Leg and foot

- Some of the bones are fused, forming a *tibiotarsus* and a *tarsometatarsus*, but the stifle joint is similar to that seen in mammals.
- Most of the muscles of the leg lie high up on the leg or on the body itself and control movements by means of long tendons.
- A *digital flexor tendon* (Fig. 13.4) runs in a tunnel behind the intertarsal joint and supplies each of the digits. It is responsible for bringing about the *perching reflex*, seen when a bird lands on a branch: the toes automatically flex and tighten on the branch, preventing the bird from falling off.
- Most birds have three toes pointing forwards and one pointing backwards, which is an adaptation for perching and

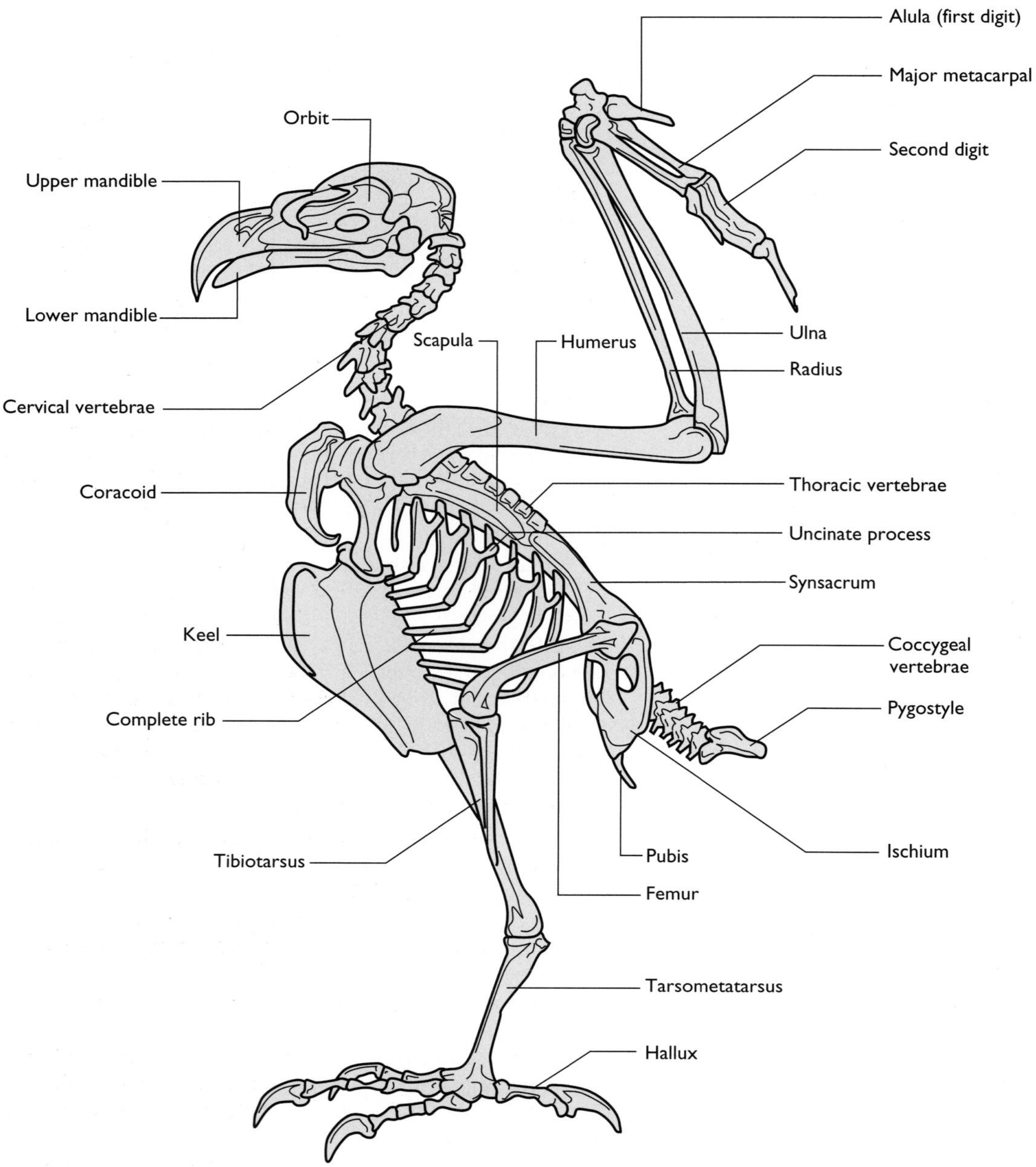

Fig. 13.1 Skeleton of a typical bird (hawk). (With permission from T Colville, JM Bassett, 2001. Clinical anatomy and physiology for veterinary technicians. St Louis, MO: Mosby, p 355.)

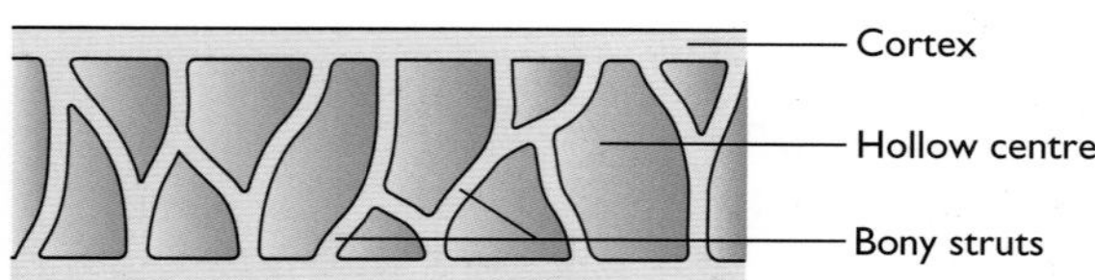

Fig. 13.2 Longitudinal section through an avian long bone. The bony struts serve to strengthen the bone.

holding prey, however, parrots have two toes pointing forwards and two backwards.

- The shape of the feet reflects the lifestyle of the species: ducks have webbed feet for swimming; raptors have strong talons for catching and killing their prey.

Wing

- The bones of each forelimb (Fig. 13.5) are reduced to a humerus, a separate radius and ulna, fused carpal and metacarpal bones and two digits:
  - *Digit 3*: The main digit is attached to the fused metacarpal bones and carries the primary feathers.
  - *Digit 1*: This forms the *alula* or bastard wing and carries a few feathers. It is essential for controlling take-off and landing.
- Most of the wing muscles are found on the body or at the proximal end of the wing and long tendons attached lower down the wing control movement. If the flight muscles were located on the wings, the extra weight would impede flapping flight.

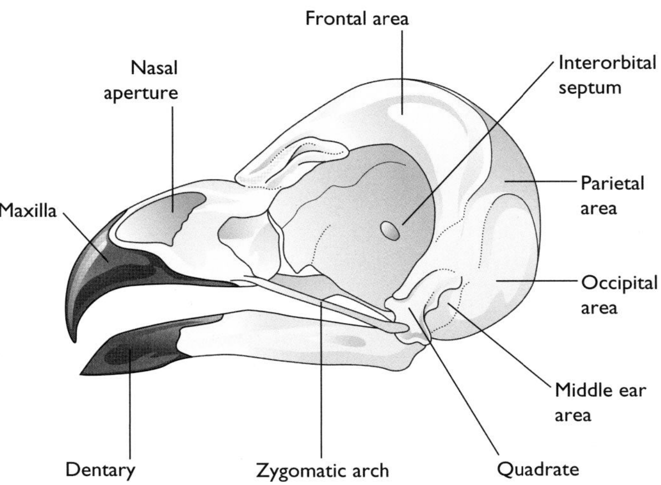

Fig. 13.3 The anatomy of the bird skull (barn owl).

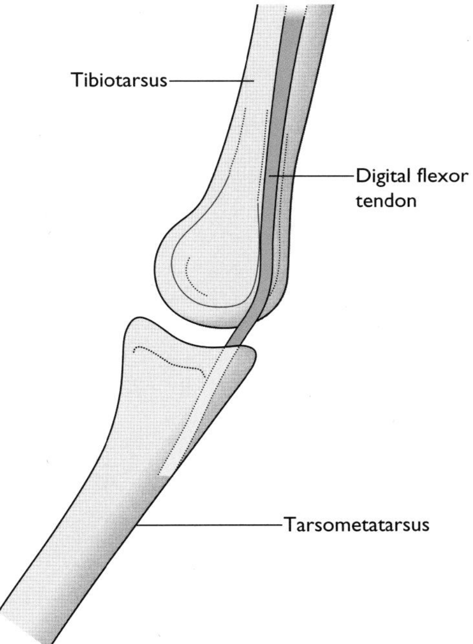

Fig. 13.4 Intertarsal joint in the avian leg. The digital flexor tendon runs in a tunnel within the metatarsal bone. It attaches to the caudal aspect of the digits and is important in the perching reflex.

- In cross-section the wing is slightly curved from front to back forming an 'aerofoil' shape. This creates lift as the bird flaps its wings.

Intraosseus catheterisation. This is a method of providing fluid therapy to birds via a bone.

The optimum site is the ulna or the proximal tibiotarsus because both these bones have a medullary cavity from which fluid can be rapidly absorbed. The advantage of using a bone is that the catheter is less likely to pull out and if it does, haemorrhage is less likely to occur.

Prevention of flight. It is sometimes necessary to restrict a captive bird's ability to fly and this may be done in one of two ways:

1. **Pinioning**: The end of the wing is cut off at the carpus (i.e., the 'hand' is cut off). This is usually done when the chick is 4–10 days old and is permanent because the bones do not grow back.
2. **Wing clipping**: Primary feathers 5–10 are clipped using a pair of sharp scissors; avoid cutting into the quick of the feather. One wing may be clipped, which destabilises the bird when it flies, or both may be clipped. Clipping does not prevent flying completely and the feathers will grow back at the next moult.

Feathers

Feathers are the distinctive feature of members of the class Aves. They develop from epidermal cells in a similar way to the hairs of mammals and the scales of reptiles. Feathers are made of keratin and create a strong but lightweight covering over the wing and the body.

All feathers have a similar structure (Fig. 13.6). The central *shaft* or *rachis* is filled with blood capillaries during growth but later, as the feather matures, it becomes hollow. On either side of the shaft, the *vane* consists of *barbs* and interlocking *barbules*. These hook together to form a flattened, wind-resistant surface.

The feathers must be kept clean in order to function effectively. Birds constantly groom themselves to 'zip up' the barbules and to apply the secretions from the preen gland at the base of the tail, which keeps the feathers waterproof.

There are several types of feather (Fig. 13.6):

- *Flight feathers*: long rigid feathers attached to the wing and the tail:
  - *Primaries*: attached to digit 3 and to the fused metacarpal bones (Fig. 13.5); usually 11 feathers but number varies with species; provide the major thrust during flight
  - *Secondaries*: attached to the ulna; shorter than the primaries
- *Contour or covert feathers*: cover the rest of the wing and the outermost layer of the body to produce a smooth outline; shorter and more flexible; the lower part of the vane (closest to the skin) is fluffy
- *Filoplume* and *down feathers*: lie close to the body underneath the contour feathers, forming an insulating layer; they have no barbs so they are fluffy. Filoplume is designed to break up, creating dust that absorbs sweat and dirt and keeps the bird clean.

Birds always shed dust from their feathers and this may be a source of pathogens. The zoonotic respiratory disease psittacosis is caused by the microorganism *Chlamydophila* (formerly *Chlamydia*) *psittaci* and is spread by feather and faecal dust. Avoid inhaling dust from suspected cases.

Moulting

Adult birds moult once a year, usually after the breeding season. The old feathers are lost over a period and during this time the birds are vulnerable: flight is affected and processes such as egg laying in domestic hens may cease. Production of new feathers requires energy so food intake, particularly the protein requirement, increases. Any nutritional deficiency may result in stunted

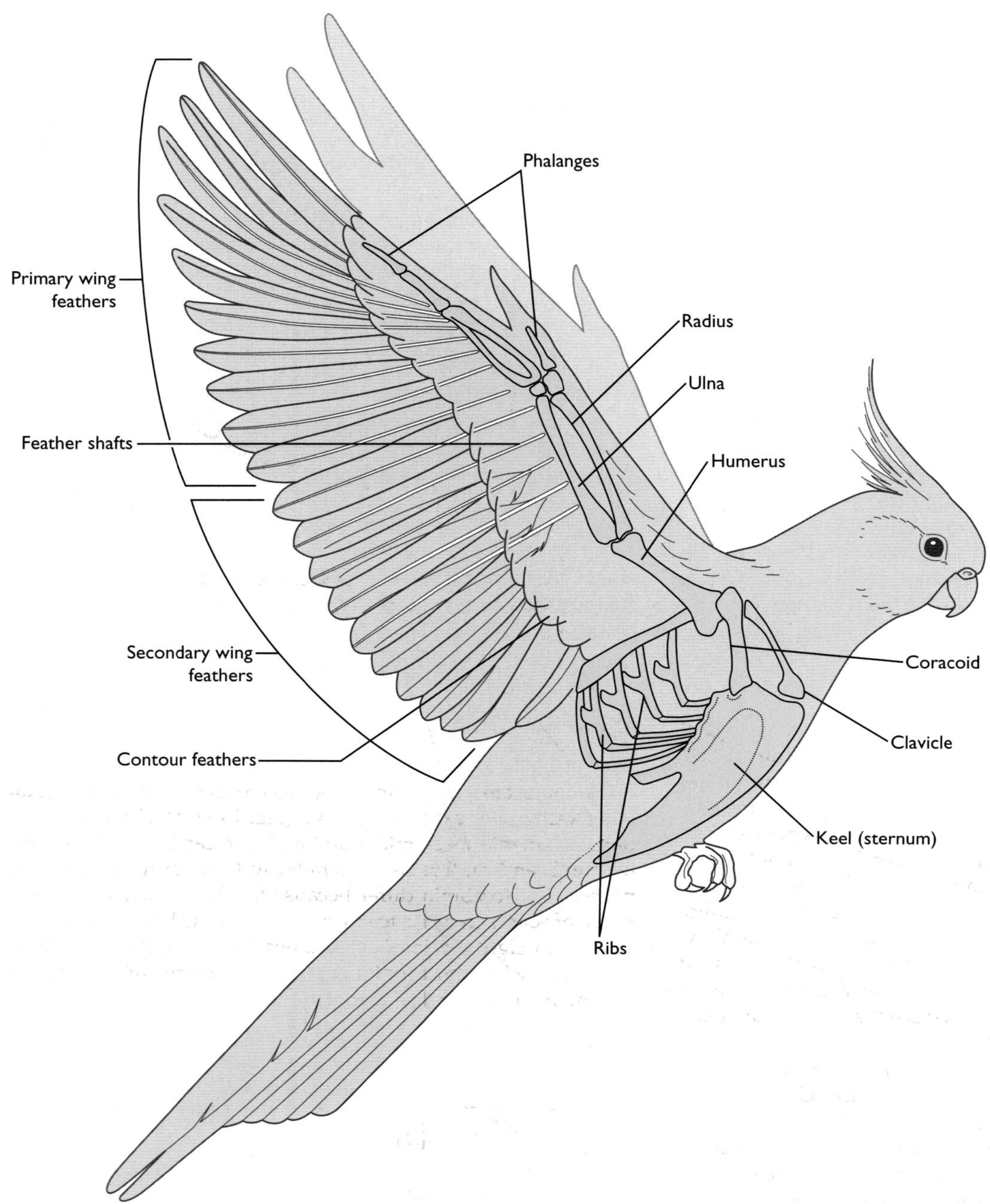

Fig. 13.5 Bird in flight showing the structure of the wing (forelimb).

feather growth or poor colouration. Feathers are used for flight, for insulation and, in some species, for display. Captive birds may be kept for their beauty and for showing.

When handling birds it is essential that the feathers are not damaged. They are only replaced at the next moult so the ability to fly may be seriously impaired, whilst the owner may be annoyed that their appearance has been affected.

When preparing birds for surgery, avoid plucking the feathers as this will affect the bird's ability to keep warm until the next moult. Damp the feathers with water or spirit and part them to reveal the skin.

Flight

Most of the surface of the wing is covered with flight feathers, forming a light but strong structure. It is slightly curved, the dorsal surface being longer and convex and the ventral surface shorter and more concave. This aerofoil shape generates maximum lift and minimum drag as the wing moves through the air. Air passing over the dorsal surface has to travel faster than the air passing under the wing, resulting in lower pressure over the dorsal surface, which generates lift. The lift force must equal the weight of the bird if flight is to occur.

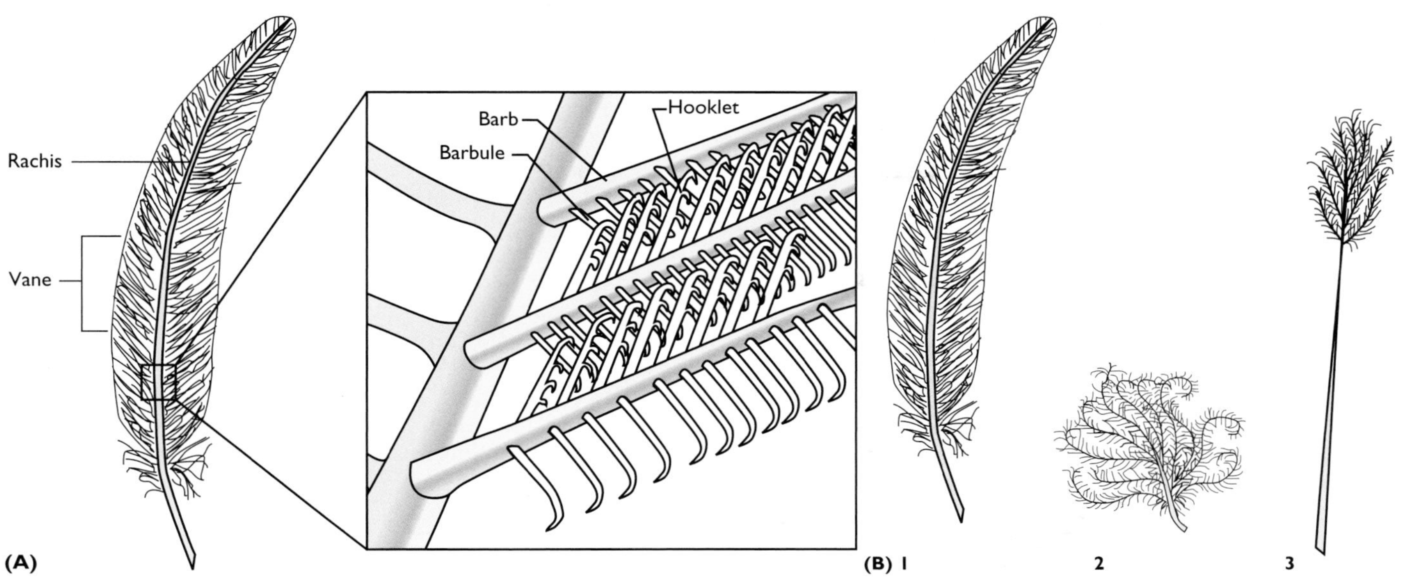

Fig. 13.6 **(A)** General structure of a feather. **(B)** Four types of feather: 1, Primary and contour; 2, Down; 3, Filoplume. (Adapted with permission from T Colville, JM Bassett, 2001. Clinical anatomy and physiology for veterinary technicians. St Louis, MO: Mosby, p 347.)

Control of flight is brought about by tilting the leading edge of the wing and the formation of slots between the feathers; for example, separation of the primary feathers and the alula allows some air through, which maintains a smooth air flow on the dorsal surface, thus increasing lift. If the angle of tilt is greater than 15° then lift is reduced and the bird stalls or falls out of the sky.

Wing shape affects the type and speed of flight. Soaring birds such as the albatross or buzzard have broad wings that maximise lift while the wings of many garden birds are short and allow rapid bursts of flapping flight. The wing tips of the buzzard are slotted to reduce turbulence while the feathers on the edge of a barn owl's wing are fringed to reduce the noise of the wing beat as the bird approaches its prey.

In gliding flight the wing is held still and at a low angle so that the bird gradually loses height. Birds such as the albatross actually lose very little height because of the size and shape of the wing and because they make constant adjustments to the angle of the leading edge. Species such as the vulture and the buzzard make use of thermals or upwards warm air currents, which allow them to soar and gain height.

In flapping or powered flight the bird's body is held almost stationary and the wings are moved rhythmically up and down to generate forward thrust as well as lift. The main power is provided by the large pectoral muscles, which extend from the keel to the humerus and make up to 20% of the body mass. In strong fliers such as the pigeon the muscles are deep red because of their high myoglobin content and their good blood supply. In species such as the domestic fowl and the turkey the muscles are almost white and are capable of producing powerful bursts of flight that only last for a short time.

At take-off maximum lift is helped by running or by launching from a branch. To land, the tail is used as a brake and the wings are extended into the stall position. The legs are extended to absorb the force of the impact and in perching birds the flexor tendons contract as the foot grasps the branch.

Special senses

The avian brain is larger in proportion to its body than that of all other vertebrates except mammals (Fig. 13.7). The basic division of the brain into fore-, mid- and hindbrain can be identified and the hind- and midbrains are similar to those of mammals. The parts of the forebrain differ because the bird needs a different range of senses in order to survive. Within the brain, the control centres for sight (optic lobes) and hearing (cerebellum) are well developed while those for touch, smell (olfactory bulbs) and taste are small and underdeveloped.

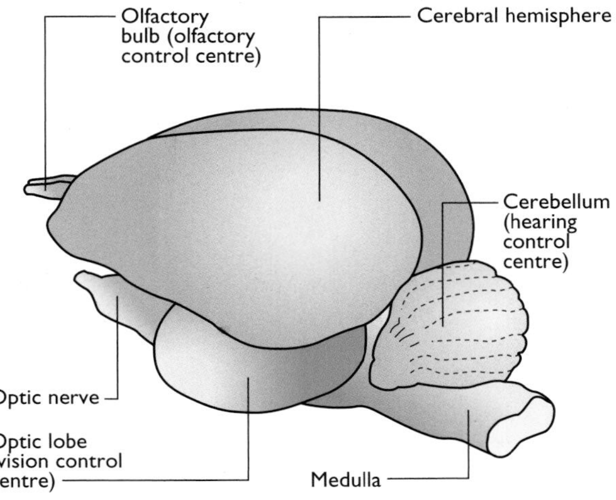

Fig. 13.7 Lateral view of a bird's brain. (With permission from T Colville, JM Bassett, 2001. Clinical anatomy and physiology for veterinary technicians. St Louis, MO: Mosby, p 359.)

Main features

Sight

This is a highly developed sense and is essential if the bird is going to be able to fly at high speed and/or altitude, search for food, escape from predators and find a mate. The *optic lobes* are large and occupy the majority of the midbrain (Fig. 13.7) and much of the skull is adapted to housing and protecting the large eyes. The orbits determine the shape of the eye, which in diurnal species can be round (e.g., in hawks), or flat (e.g., in swans). In nocturnal species, the eye may be tubular and the pupil is larger in relation to the retina, enabling more light to be gathered at night.

The eyes fill the orbits, leaving room for few eye muscles associated with movement. Birds have to move their heads rather than their eyes to pick up an image. The position of the eyes on the head varies according to feeding habits: predators such as owls and hawks have forward-pointing eyes producing binocular vision but a reduced size of visual field, while seed-eaters have laterally placed eyes that provide monocular vision but a wide visual field in which to locate predators.

The structure of the eye (Fig. 13.8) is similar to that of mammals but with a few differences:

1. The sclera forms the outermost protective layer and continues in the front of the eye as the transparent cornea. At the junction of the cornea and sclera is a ring of small bones known as the *sclerotic ring*, which reinforces the relatively large circumference of the eye.
2. The cornea is protected by an upper and lower eyelid and a *nictitating membrane*, similar to the third eyelid seen in the dog and cat. This is thin and transparent and washes moisture over the cornea to keep it clean. It is supplied with striated muscle so the bird is able to move the membrane voluntarily.
3. The iris is formed by *striated* muscle in contrast to the smooth muscle of the mammalian iris. This enables the bird to control the size of the pupil voluntarily.
4. The vitreous humour in the posterior chamber of the eye is similar to that of mammals but contains a ribbon-like structure attached to the retina known as the *pecten* (Fig. 13.8). This is thought to provide nutrition for the inner structures of the eye.
5. The retina contains photoreceptor cells – rods for night vision and cones for day and colour vision. Nocturnal birds have more rods than diurnal birds. Avian vision is superior to that of mammals for several reasons:
   - The photoreceptor cells are much thicker than those of any other vertebrate and result in a much more highly defined image.
   - In mammals, each nerve cell is connected to several photoreceptors but in the bird each photoreceptor cell is connected to an individual bipolar nerve cell so that each rod or cone is represented individually in the brain.
   - The retina has a relatively poor blood supply, because blood vessels interfere with the passage of light to the retina.

In some species of diving bird, the nictitating membrane has a clear 'window' in its centre. This is thought to act as a form of 'contact lens' to aid vision under water.

As birds can control the size of the pupil voluntarily, the pupillary light response or pupillary reflex is not a good diagnostic indicator of brain or eye function.

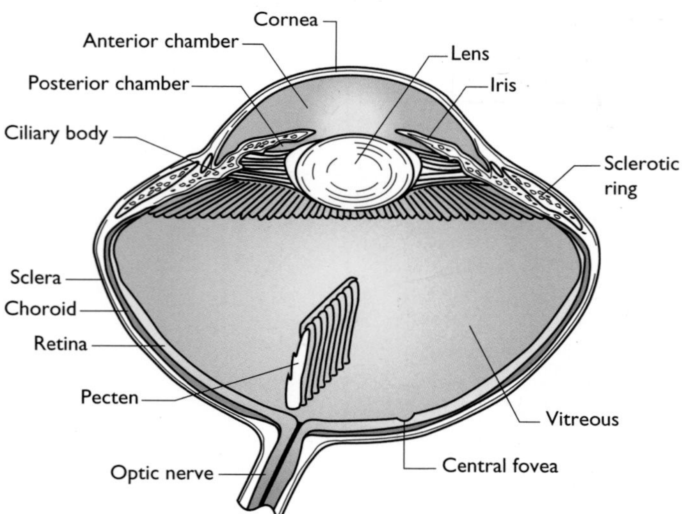

Fig. 13.8 Structure of the avian eye. (With permission from T Colville, JM Bassett, 2001. Clinical anatomy and physiology for veterinary technicians. St Louis, MO: Mosby, p 360.)

Hearing

The structure of the ear is simpler than in the mammal. The ears are found on the sides of the head just behind and slightly below the eyes. There are no external ear pinnae in any species – birds such as the eagle owl that appear to have ears actually only have tufts of feathers.

The ear consists of the external ear, which collects sound and carries it to the middle ear. This is a single bone, the *columella*, which transmits sound to the inner ear. The inner ear is similar to that of mammals and comprises the membranous canals responsible for balance and the cochlea responsible for hearing.

Nocturnal species have an extremely well-developed sense of hearing, which enables them to locate and catch prey in darkness. Barn owls, *Tyto alba*, in particular, have asymmetrical external ear openings (which help in the vertical location of sound), large eardrums, columellae and cochleae and a large acoustic centre in the hindbrain.

Taste

This is a poorly developed sense in birds and experiments have shown that the perception of tastes such as bitter, salty and sour is species-specific. There are relatively few taste buds and they are distributed around the sides of the tongue and soft palate.

Smell

Little is known about the avian sense of smell but it is thought to vary between species. In passerines and birds of prey it is very poor but the females of some species (e.g., mallards) secrete an odour that stimulates the males to breed. Other species (e.g., quail and albatross) use the sense of smell to locate food.

Touch

The skin is supplied with sensory nerve endings that are sensitive to heat, cold, pain and touch. Touch may be used to find food and touch-sensitive endings are found around the beak and mouth. Others are found at the base of the feathers and enable the bird to respond to the smallest movement of its feathers.

Respiratory system

The respiratory system of birds (Fig. 13.9) is very different from that of mammals and is thought to be 10 times more efficient. It is adapted to meet the needs of the bird when flying at speed and at high altitudes, where oxygen levels are low, without the bird losing consciousness. There are three main features:

- There is no diaphragm dividing the body cavity into thorax and abdomen.

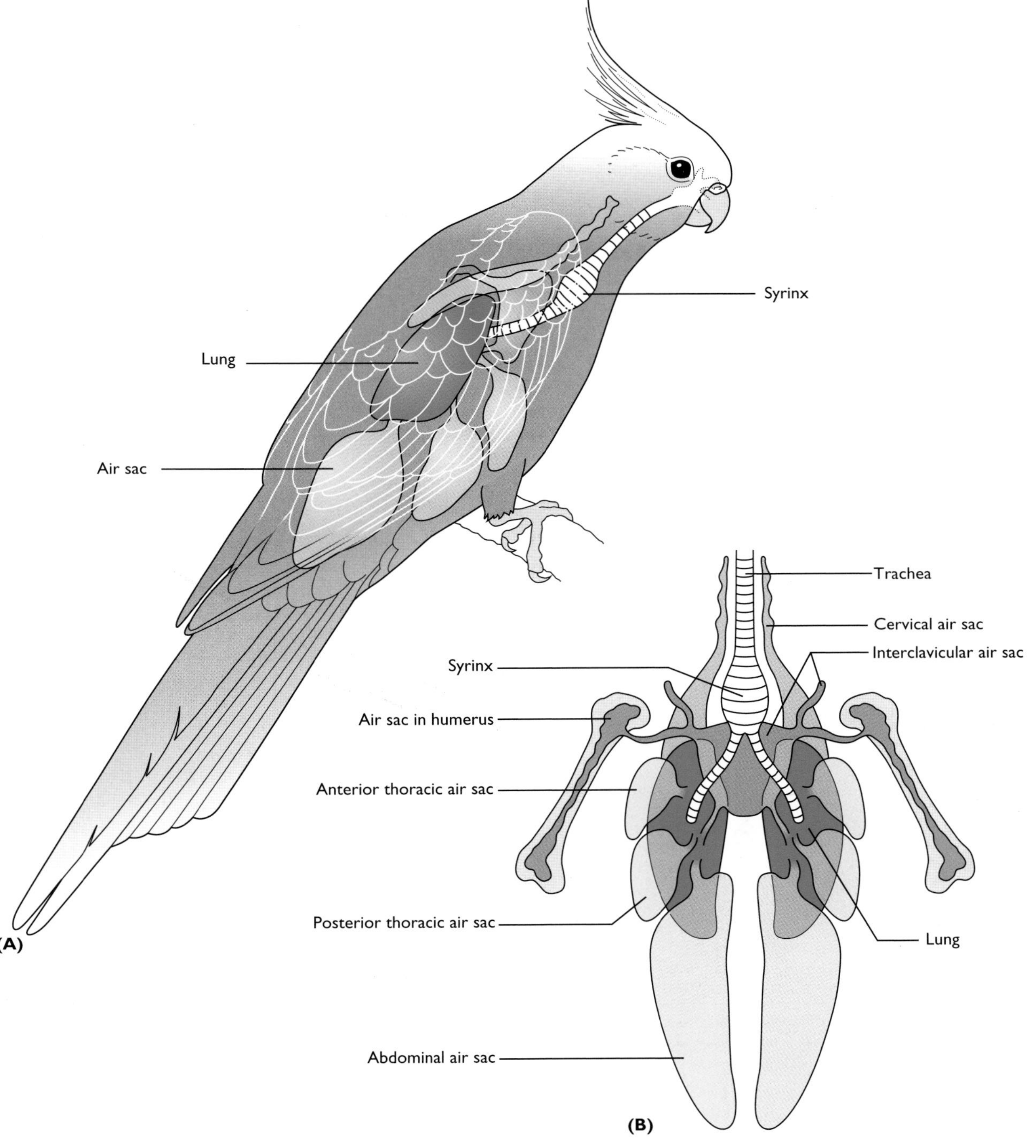

Fig. 13.9 The respiratory system of the bird *in situ* **(A)** and removed from the body **(B)**.

- The lungs are fairly rigid and do not expand as they fill with air.
- All free spaces in the body cavity and within the major bones (e.g., femur and humerus) are filled with membranous air sacs connected to the respiratory system.

Air enters the system via a pair of nostrils or *nares* leading into the nasal cavity, and also through the mouth. Some birds have a cleft in the hard palate known as the *choana* connecting the oral and nasal cavities. The nasal cavities contain several mucosa-covered *conchae*, which help to warm and filter the inspired air.

> Some diving birds do not have external nares because this would allow water to enter the airways during diving. They normally rely on mouth breathing. If the beak is tied to prevent the bird from pecking during treatment, there is a risk of asphyxiation.

Air passes through the *glottis* on the floor of the oral cavity and into a complex *larynx*, which does not possess vocal cords. The *trachea* is made of rigid interlocking rings and is relatively long; in some species it forms coils. Air travels down the trachea to the point where the trachea divides into right and left primary *bronchi*. At this point there is a swelling known as the *syrinx*, whose size and shape varies with the species. The combined effect of air passing through the larynx and the syrinx produces the characteristic sounds associated with the species.

> **Intubation**. Birds are easily intubated for anaesthesia because the glottis at the base of the tongue is easy to see. Always use an *uncuffed tube* to prevent rupture of the complete tracheal rings. The caudal air sacs may also be intubated after induction by injection or by mask, in cases where oral or beak surgery is to be performed.

The primary bronchi lead into the relatively dense lungs, closely applied to the dorsal body wall. Within the lung tissue the bronchi divide into further smaller bronchi and into cylindrical parallel tubes known as *parabronchi*. Air capillaries surrounded by pulmonary blood capillaries perforate the walls of the parabronchi and it is here that gaseous exchange takes place. This process is the same as occurs in mammals.

Leading from various bronchi within the lungs are thin-walled *air sacs*. Most birds have nine air sacs, which penetrate the spaces of the body cavity and the inside of many bones (Fig. 13.9). They are not involved in gaseous exchange and they are thought to act as a reservoir of air and to have a bellows effect, pushing air back through the lungs. They also lighten the weight of the skeleton and so aid flight.

> Never administer medication to a bird via an intraperitoneal injection because there is a risk that an air sac will be penetrated and it may rupture. Rupture of an air sac will impair respiration and may affect the bird's ability to fly.

> **Air sacculitis**. This is an infection of the thin-walled air sacs of the bird and is often caused by the common fungus *Aspergillus fumigatus*. Fungal spores are found within the inspired air and may come from substances such as mouldy hay. The fungus forms plaques on the air sacs and eventually they rupture, resulting in respiratory distress and ultimately death. Do not provide avian patients with hay; it is better to keep them on newspaper even though this may seem less comfortable.

Respiration

During respiration air circulates continuously and passes through the lungs twice (Fig. 13.10). Most gaseous exchange occurs during the second passage. This system ensures that the removal of oxygen from the inspired air occurs with maximum efficiency.

> As their respiratory system is so efficient, birds react rapidly to inhalation anaesthetics and anaesthesia may lighten or deepen much more quickly than is expected.

- *Inspiration*: Air passes through the lungs and either enters:
  - The caudal air sacs and inflates them, or
  - The parabronchi, where gaseous exchange takes place; this air then passes into the cranial air sacs and inflates them.
- Expiration
  - The abdominal muscles contract, squeezing air from the caudal air sacs back into the parabronchi, where further gaseous exchange takes place.
  - Air in the cranial air sacs passes straight through the lungs and out.

Circulatory system

The circulatory system follows a similar plan to that of the mammal. In order to provide for the high metabolic rate of the bird, the heart in particular must be able to pump the blood to deliver oxygen and nutrients to the tissues quickly and efficiently. In a resting chicken blood takes only 6 seconds to travel around the body.

Main features

Heart

This is a four-chambered pump lying in the cranial part of the thoraco-abdominal cavity and it is quite similar to the heart of the mammal. It is covered in a pericardial sac that sticks to some of the internal surfaces to hold the heart in place. The right atrio-ventricular valve has no chordae tendinae and is merely a thick muscular flap of the myocardium.

Circulation

The arrangement of the arteries, veins and capillaries (Fig. 13.11) is similar to that of mammals with the following differences:

- *Renal portal system*: Valves at the junction of the iliac veins with the caudal vena cava can divert blood returning from the caudal end of the body either into the kidneys, so excreting waste products, or into the caudal vena cava and so to the heart.
- There is a large blood supply to the flight muscles and wings via the *pectoral* and *brachial arteries*.
- Heat loss from the legs and feet of many terrestrial and aquatic species is reduced by a counter-current system of blood vessels in the lower limbs. Body heat in the arteries of the limbs is transferred to the blood returning to the heart in the

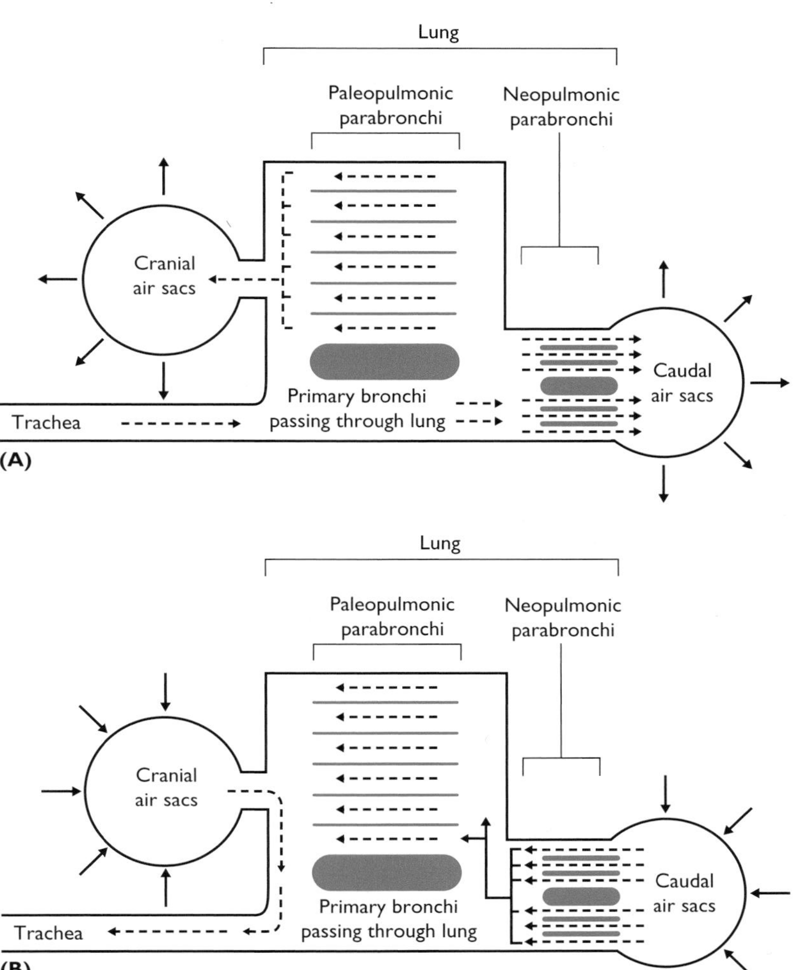

Fig. 13.10 Diagram to show the passage of air through the lungs and air sacs during respiration: **(A)** Inspiration, **(B)** Expiration.

veins, which lie parallel to the arteries. This means that the legs and feet are kept cool, reducing the temperature gradient between the blood and the external air, so less heat is lost from areas that are not insulated by feathers.

Intravenous injections or blood sampling can be carried out using the *brachial or basilic vein* on the medial side of the wing (Fig. 13.12) close to the elbow joint, the jugular vein in the neck and the medial metatarsal vein on the caudal aspect of the leg.

Blood

The erythrocytes or red blood cells are oval and nucleated, which is different from those of mammals but similar to those of reptiles.

Digestive system

The basic pattern of the digestive tract is much the same between species of birds and the upper part shows adaptations for flight (Fig. 13.13). The majority of the tract is suspended between the wings in the body cavity to centralise the weight, enabling the bird to keep its balance and remain stable in flight without the use of a long tail.

In-patient nutrition. It is vital to understand that the shape of a bird's beak is adapted to the type of food on which it normally feeds. When feeding in-patients there is no benefit in offering a bird the incorrect food because it will not be able to ingest it (e.g., a buzzard will not be able to eat peanuts). A well-stocked avian practice should have a range of species-friendly food types.

Main features

Oral cavity

The teeth, heavy jaw bones and muscles have been replaced by a beak and lighter bones and muscles. Birds are unable to chew their food but can manipulate it and break it into small pieces using the *beak* and the *tongue*. The shape of the beak varies according to species and is suited to the particular food type (Fig. 13.14). *Salivary glands* are present in most species and the saliva contains mucus. In some species, such as the sparrow,

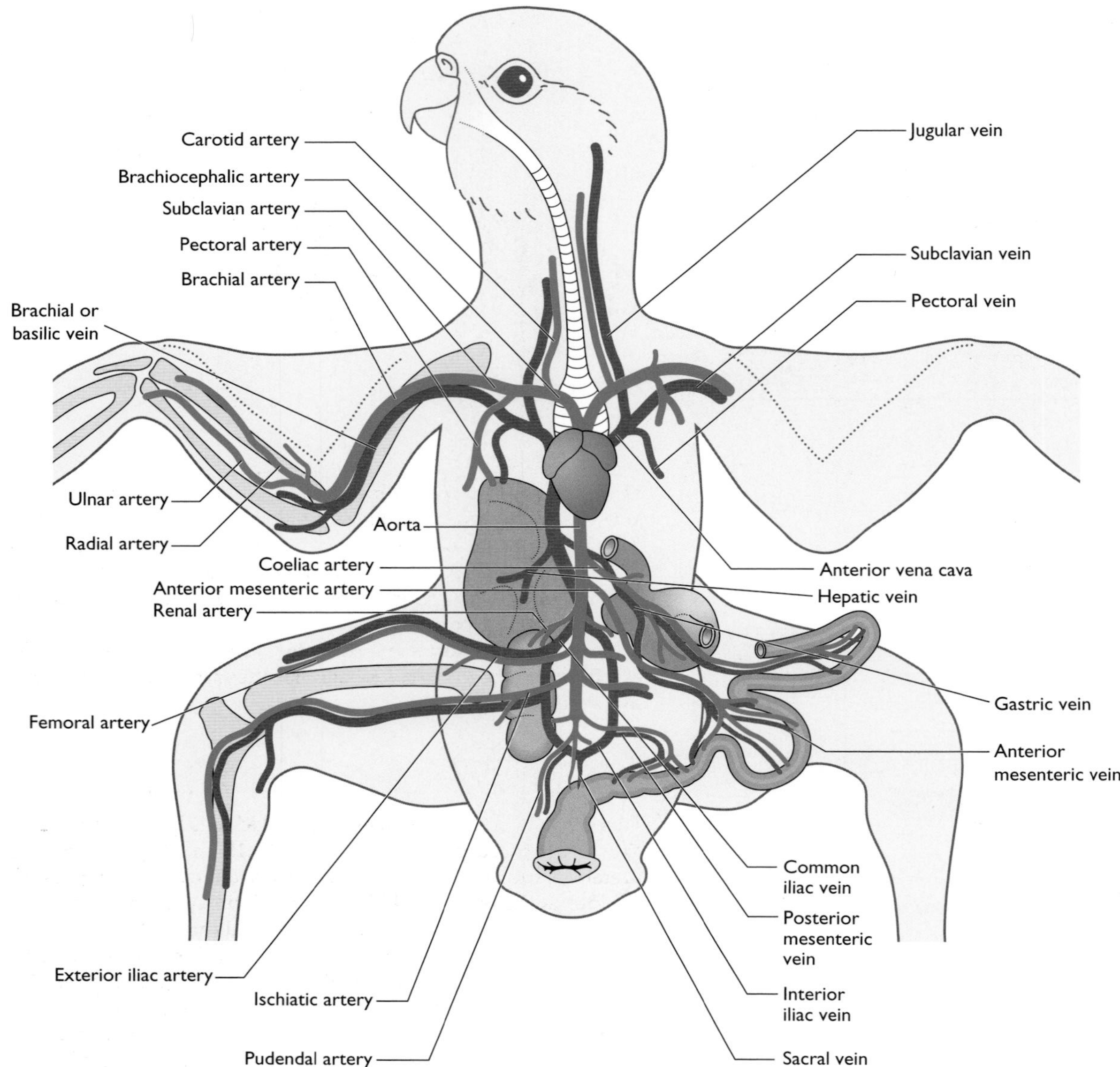

Fig. 13.11 The avian circulatory system.

the saliva is also rich in the enzyme amylase. *Taste buds* are found towards the back of the oral cavity and their structure is similar to those in other species.

Oesophagus and crop

Food passes down the oesophagus on the right side of the neck into the *crop* (Fig. 13.13). The oesophagus is thin-walled and distensible to allow the passage of relatively large pieces of food. The crop is a diverticulum of the oesophagus, lying outside the body cavity on the right side of the cranial thoracic inlet. It varies in size and shape according to the diet of the species – grain-eating birds have large bilobed crops while in owls and insectivores the crop may be rudimentary or absent.

The crop is principally a storage organ but in some species (e.g., doves and pigeons), the epithelial lining proliferates and sloughs under the influence of the hormone prolactin to produce 'crop milk'. This is rich in proteins and fat and is used to feed the young for the first few days after hatching.

Stomach

Food passes into the stomach, which has two parts:

1. *Proventriculus* is lined by gastric glands that secrete pepsin, hydrochloric acid and mucus. Here food is stored and mixed with these digestive juices.
2. *Gizzard* (*ventriculus*) is a thick-walled muscular organ in which mechanical digestion occurs. By means of powerful contractions the food is ground up and mixed with the digestive juices. The presence of grit in the diet helps the physical break-up of the food. In species that feed on softer or liquid foods, the gizzard is mainly a storage organ.

Small intestine

Food leaves the gizzard by the pylorus and enters the small intestine, which consists of a duodenum and ileum (Fig. 13.13). Beyond this there is no clear delineation into different parts. The pancreas, consisting of three lobes, lies in the duodenal loop and pours its secretions into the duodenum via three ducts. The

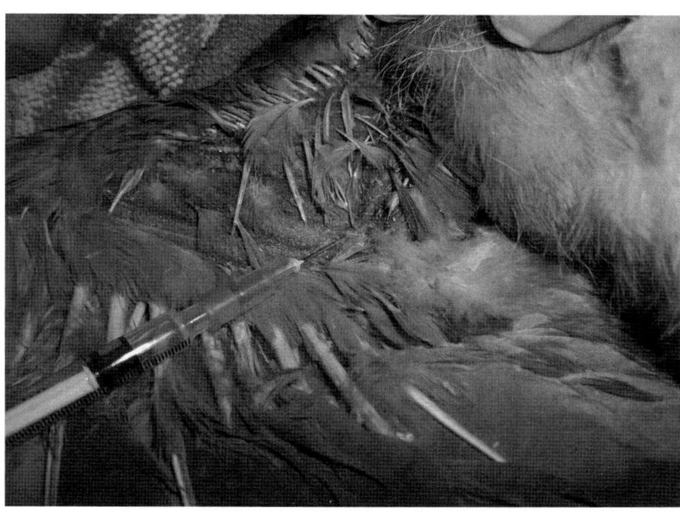

Fig. 13.12 Extended wing of a bird showing the brachial or basilic vein on the medial side of the wing.

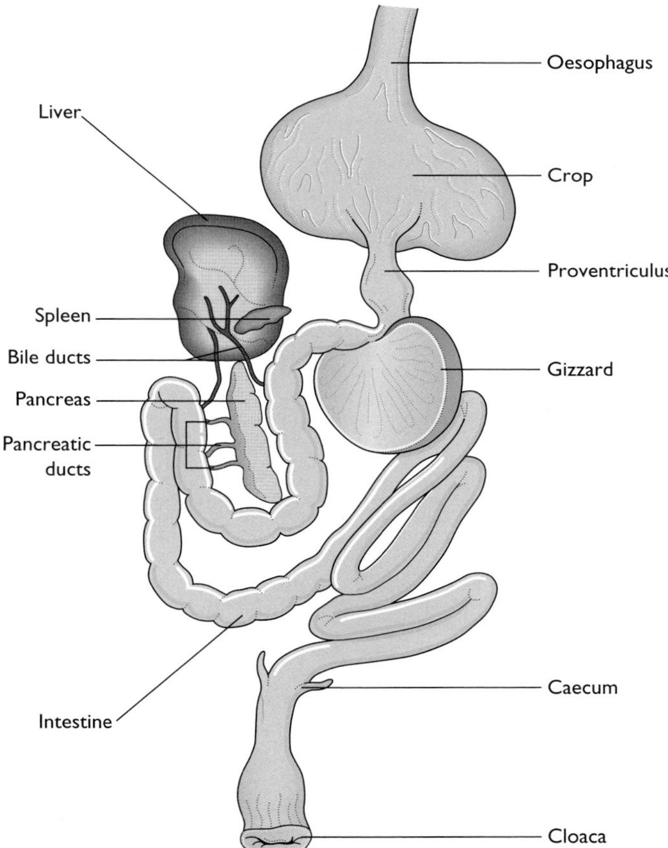

Fig. 13.13 Digestive system of the pigeon.

liver is bilobular and relatively large and some species (e.g., chickens, ducks and geese), have a gallbladder.

Aquatic species of bird that ingest slippery fish have relatively poorly developed salivary glands while those species eating a dry diet have well-developed glands.

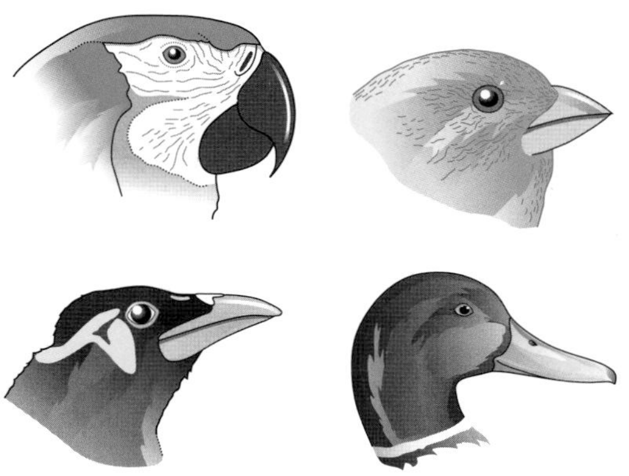

Fig. 13.14 Differences in beak shape between species.

Large intestine

This consists of a pair of blind-ending *caeca*, originating at the junction of the small and large intestines, a *rectum* and a *cloaca*. Bacterial digestion occurs in the caeca, which are large and prominent in herbivorous and granivorous species and owls but are rudimentary or absent in carnivorous and nectivorous species (e.g., hawks and parrots).

The rectum is short and terminates at the cloaca – the common exit from the body cavity shared with the urinary and reproductive systems.

Urinary system

This consists of a pair of symmetrical kidneys lying in a depression of the fused pelvic bones (Figs. 13.15 and 13.16). A pair of ureters carries urine to the outside via the cloaca. There is no bladder in the bird. The kidneys are relatively larger than those of mammals and occupy about 2% of body weight.

Birds excrete nitrogenous waste resulting from protein metabolism in the form of uric acid and urates. This is similar to reptiles but different from mammals, which excrete nitrogenous waste as urea. The waste materials are suspended in urinary water resulting from glomerular filtration and the resulting semi-solid urine leaves the kidneys via the ureters. In the cloaca it mixes with faecal material from the digestive tract. The material then moves by retroperistalsis into the rectum, where further reabsorption of water takes place, eventually producing a small volume of 'droppings'. Normal bird droppings (Fig. 13.17) consist of white urates and greeny-brown faeces surrounded by clear urine.

Many species of marine bird have a *salt gland* that enables them to deal with a salt water environment. In most birds it is located above the eye and secretes large quantities of sodium chloride. In this way the osmotic concentration of the body fluids is maintained within normal limits. Terrestrial species rely on the kidneys to regulate salt levels.

Reproductive system

Female

The tract comprises a pair of ovaries and oviducts leading to the cloaca (Fig. 13.15). However, in many species it is only the left side that is fully developed and functional, the right side being

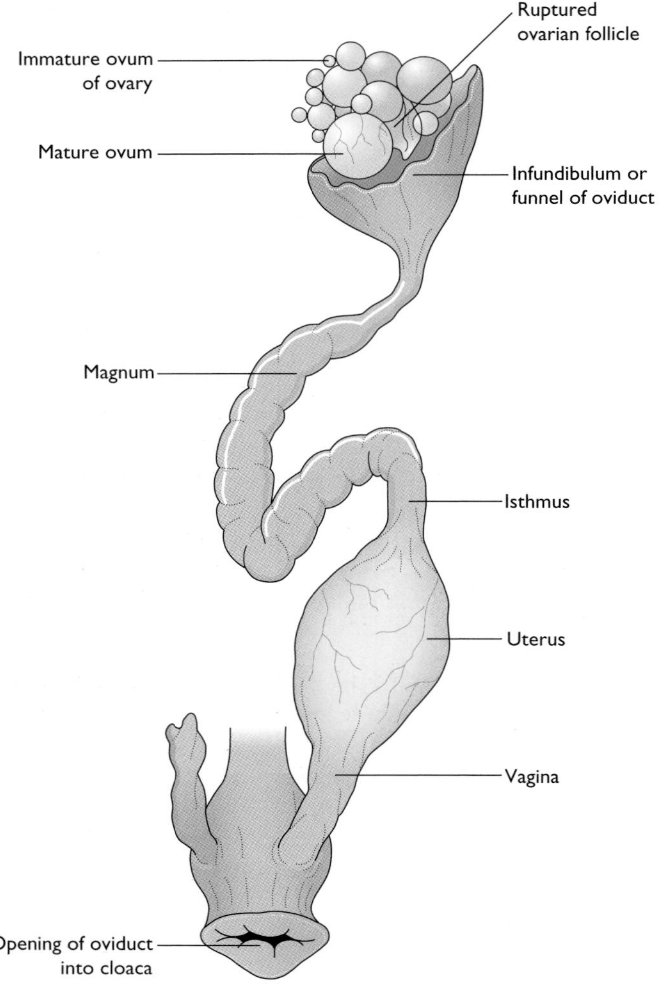

Fig. 13.15 Reproductive tract of the hen.

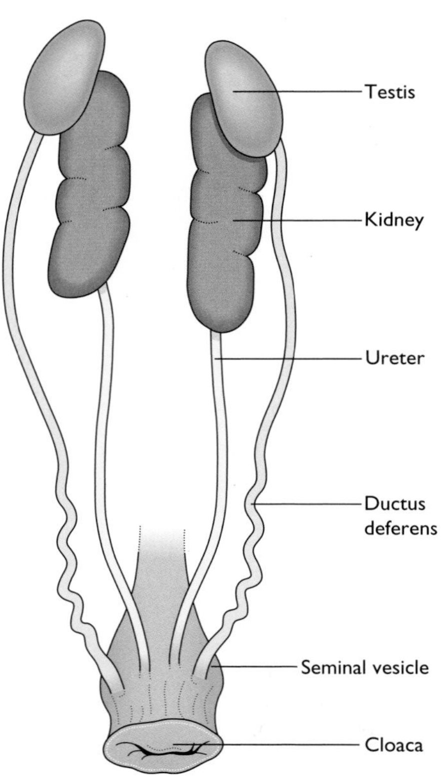

Fig. 13.16 Urogenital system of the male bird.

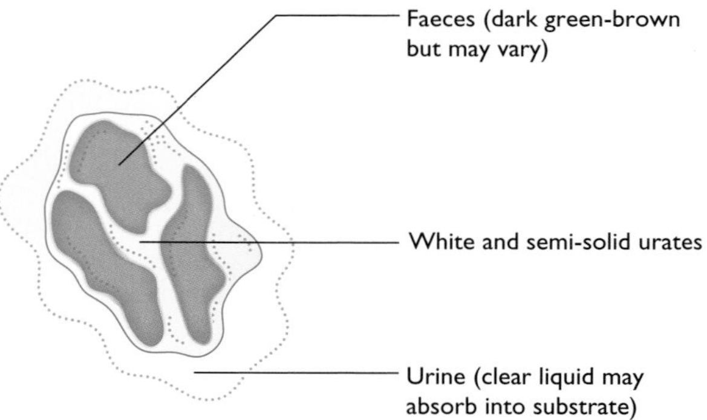

Fig. 13.17 Components of bird droppings.

vestigial. Ova develop within the ovarian tissue and consist of an oocyte and a yolk surrounded by several layers of cells. During the breeding season one ovum is released at approximately 24 h intervals until the clutch is complete.

Domestic poultry, derived from the Red Jungle Fowl, have been selectively bred to lay eggs over long periods – usually for 40 weeks per year. Wild birds will lay a clutch of eggs of a size appropriate to their species and then begin incubation. Some species may lay several clutches a year and their success is largely dependent on the weather and nutrition.

> The domestic hen takes approximately 24 h to produce an egg and having laid it she then starts again. The average hen lays 300–325 eggs a year. Hens lay fewer eggs in the darker months of the year but production increases as the day length increases.

The ovum is carried away down the left oviduct by peristaltic contractions. The oviduct is divided into distinct regions, each one of which contributes to the final egg:

1. *Infundibulum* is the funnel-shaped end of the oviduct that engulfs the ovum, preventing it from falling into the body cavity. Fertilisation takes place here and the first layer of albumen is added.
2. *Magnum* is the largest and most glandular part of the oviduct. The majority of the albumen is added here.
3. *Isthmus*: The walls consist of a thick layer of circular muscle. Inner and outer shell membranes are formed here.
4. *Shell gland* or *uterus*: The walls consist of longitudinal muscle lined with goblet cells. The egg takes up salts and water into the albumen and the shell membranes become calcified. Calcification occurs over about 15 h and pigmentation is added during the final 5 h.

The completed egg passes through a sphincter muscle into the *vagina* and then to the outside via the *cloaca*.

Male

The tract comprises a pair of *testes*, each one connected to the cloaca by a *vas deferens* (Fig. 13.16). The testes lie inside the body cavity and are attached to the body wall cranial to the kidneys. In seasonal breeders, the size and weight of the testes may increase during the active breeding season.

Spermatozoa are produced within the *seminiferous tubules* of the testes and pass through a series of convoluted tubules to the *ductus deferens*, where they are stored. Mature sperm are transported to the cloaca by a *vas deferens* leading from each testis.

Within the cloaca is a modified area of tissue forming a *phallus* or rudimentary penis, which becomes engorged with lymph during mating. In many species semen is transferred into the vagina of the female by positioning the engorged phallus against the everted cloaca of the female. Species such as ducks, geese, ostrich and rhea have a well-developed phallus that is capable of erection to introduce sperm directly into the female cloaca.

Sexual differentiation

It is not always easy to differentiate between the sexes of birds but in some cases, such as captive breeding programmes for endangered species, it may be important to be able to do this. The value of some species (e.g., large parrots) may be increased by knowing the sex of an individual.

There are several methods available, which depend on the species:

- *Sexual dimorphism*: The two sexes exhibit a different coloured plumage. This differentiation is only possible in some species:
  - Sexually mature female budgerigars have a pinky-brown *cere* above their beaks while the cere of the male is blue.
  - Female cockatiels have horizontal bars on the underside of the tail; the male loses these at about 1 year old.
  - Mallard drakes have an iridescent blue-green head and a maroon breast; the female's head is brown and her feathers are a speckled brown with a blue wing patch.
  - The adult male pheasant has a red face, green head and a long pointed tail; the female is smaller with mottled brown plumage.
- *DNA testing*: using a blood sample or cells taken from a growing feather
- *Surgical sexing*: The gonads within the body cavity are examined endoscopically under a general anaesthetic. As this technique is invasive and requires experience and a general anaesthetic, it is less frequently performed than DNA testing.

It is the female bird that determines the sex of the offspring rather than the male as in mammals.

CHAPTER 14

Small exotic mammals

For the benefit of this book, small exotic mammals are taken to include any small mammal that is not a dog or cat. These 'small furries' may not always seem to be exotic but in most first-opinion veterinary practices they are at least 'out of the ordinary'.

The rabbit (*Oryctolagus cunniculus*)

Rabbits belong to the mammalian order Lagomorpha. They were originally classified with species such as rats, mice and hamsters as members of the order Rodentia because they all have chisel-shaped incisors that are open-rooted and continue to grow throughout the animal's life. However, rabbits have two pairs of upper incisors while rodents have only one pair, leading to the reclassification of rabbits (and the related hare, *Lepus europaeus* and pika *Ochotona princeps*) as *lagomorphs*. Rabbits are burrowing herbivorous animals that live in large social groups. They are readily preyed upon by carnivores and much of their anatomy is adapted to sensing danger and making a rapid escape.

Tables 14.1 and 14.2 give physiological and reproductive parameters for rabbits.

Morphology

The wild European rabbit, *Oryctolagus cuniculus*, from which all our modern breeds are derived, weighs about 2.5 kg and is covered in brown ticked fur, often described as agouti-coloured. This colouration creates a dappled effect, which breaks up the outline and helps camouflage the individual. Selective breeding has led to the development of about 50 breeds of domestic rabbit in the weight range of 1–8 kg, with a variety of fur textures and colours, many of which would be unsuitable for life in the wild.

The *head* is rounded, with long, black-tipped upright *ear pinnae* set high on either side. They are large, representing approximately 12% of the body surface, and very vascular, which enables them to be used as a means of thermoregulation. The pinnae are extremely mobile and are designed to pick up sounds of danger. The lop breeds of rabbit have been developed to have ears that hang downwards.

The *eyes* are protuberant and set on either side of the head, providing a wide range of monocular vision to detect predators. Rabbits are crepuscular (active at dawn and dusk), and their sight is adapted to lower light intensities. The *lips* are soft and covered in sensitive hairs. The upper lip is divided by a deep *philtrum*, which enables the rabbit to nibble grass very short.

Mature female rabbits develop a large fold of skin under the chin known as the *dewlap* from which they pull fur to line their nests before giving birth. The skin of the rabbit is well supplied with *scent glands*, which are used for territorial marking. They can be found under the chin, at the anus and on either side of the perineum.

The *forelegs* are relatively short and used for digging, while the *hind legs* are longer and provide the propulsive force for the characteristic hopping method of locomotion. They also kick the earth away when the rabbit is digging its burrow. There are five toes on each forepaw and four on each hind foot. Each toe ends in a sharp claw, those of the hind feet being long and straight. The feet are entirely covered in fur and there are no footpads.

When the rabbit is at rest, the entire plantar surface of the hind limb from toes to hock rests on the ground. When grazing, among a group of rabbits there will always be one or two standing upright on their hind legs, watching for predators. If danger threatens they will thump their hind legs on the ground to warn the others. Both of these behavioural patterns can be seen in pet rabbits. Rabbits have short fluffy *tails* with white undersides. As the rabbit runs the white colouration 'flashes' to warn the rest of the group of possible danger.

Musculoskeletal system

The skeleton of the rabbit (Fig. 14.1) is delicate and makes up only 7–8% of the body weight. This is in contrast to the skeleton of the cat, which makes up 12–13% of body weight. The cortex of the long bones is normally thinner than those of the cat and older caged rabbits may additionally develop osteoporosis from lack of exercise and low calcium intake.

> When handling all rabbits, particular care must be taken to prevent struggling, which may result in fractured limbs or spine.

The number of vertebrae in each part of the vertebral column is: C7, T12–13, L7, S4, Cd16.

There are a few differences between the skeleton of the rabbit and that of the cat:

- The *scapula* is more sharply triangular and has a pronounced hook-shaped suprahamate process on the acromion (Fig. 14.2).
- The *acetabulum* or socket of the hip joint comprises the ilium, ischium and an accessory bone, the os acetabuli. The pubis is not involved in the formation of this socket, as is seen in the cat.
- In the *forelimb* the radius and ulna are completely fused; in the cat they are separate bones.
- In the *hind limb* the fibula is half the length of the tibia and is fused with it; in the cat they are separate bones.
- Rabbit muscle is also a much paler pink than the muscle of cats.

Table 14.1 Physiological and behavioural parameters of rabbits and small rodents

	Rabbit	Chinchilla	Chipmunk	Gerbil	Guinea pig	Golden hamster	Mouse	Rat
Average lifespan (years)	6–8	10	2–6	3–5	4–8	2–3	2–3	3–4
Adult weight (g)	1000–8000	400–600	70–120	50–60	750–1000	100	20–40	400–800
Body temp. (°C)	38.3	38.0–39.0	38.0	37.4–39.0	38.6	36.2–37.5	37.5	38.0
Respiratory rate (breaths/min)	35–60	40–80	70	90–140	90–150	74	100–250	70–150
Pulse rate (beats/min)	220	100–150	120	250–500	130–190	280–412	500–600	260–450
Dietary habits	Herbivorous; coprophagic	Herbivorous; coprophagic	Omnivorous; coprophagic	Omnivorous; coprophagic	Herbivorous; needs vitamin C; coprophagic	Omnivorous; coprophagic	Omnivorous; coprophagic	Omnivorous; coprophagic
Natural behaviour	Social; crepuscular	Social; nocturnal	Social; diurnal	Social; nocturnal	Social; diurnal	Solitary; nocturnal	Social; nocturnal	Social; nocturnal

Table 14.2 Reproductive data relating to rabbits and small rodents

	Rabbit	Chinchilla	Chipmunk	Gerbil	Guinea pig	Golden hamster	Mouse	Rat
Reproductive pattern	No true oestrous cycle	Seasonally polyoestrous: breeds from November to March	Seasonally polyoestrous: breeds from March to September	Polyoestrous	Polyoestrous	Polyoestrous	Polyoestrous	Polyoestrous
Length of oestrous cycle	Every 4 days	30–35 days	14 days	4–6 days	15–16 days	Every 4 days	4–5 days	4–5 days
Type of ovulation	Induced: occurs within 10 h of mating	Spontaneous	Spontaneous	Spontaneous	Spontaneous	Spontaneous	Spontaneous	Spontaneous
Gestation period (days)	28–32	111	28–32	24–26	63	15–18	19–21	20–22
Average litter size	2–7	2–3	2–6	3–6	2–6	3–7	6–12	6–12
Type of young at birth	Altricial	Precocial	Altricial	Altricial	Precocial	Altricial	Altricial	Altricial
Weaning age (weeks)	4–6	6–8	6–7	3–4	3–4	3–4	18 days	3
Age of sexual maturity	5–8 months	8 months	12 months	10–12 weeks	6–10 weeks	6–10 weeks	3–4 weeks	5–6 weeks

Digestive system

Rabbits are herbivorous and have been likened to 'little horses' in that both the rabbit and the horse are hindgut fermenters: the main chamber for the breakdown of plant material is part of the large intestine. Unlike the horse, however, the digestive system of the rabbit allows for rapid passage of food through the tract and rapid elimination of fibre. This has enabled the body size and weight of the rabbit to remain small, which allows the animal to show the speed and agility necessary to escape predators. By contrast, in the horse, fibre remains in the gut for some time, necessitating the evolution of a large-volumed fermentation chamber and consequently a large body size (see Chapter 16). The digestive tract of the rabbit (Fig. 14.3) is relatively long and makes up 10–20% of body weight.

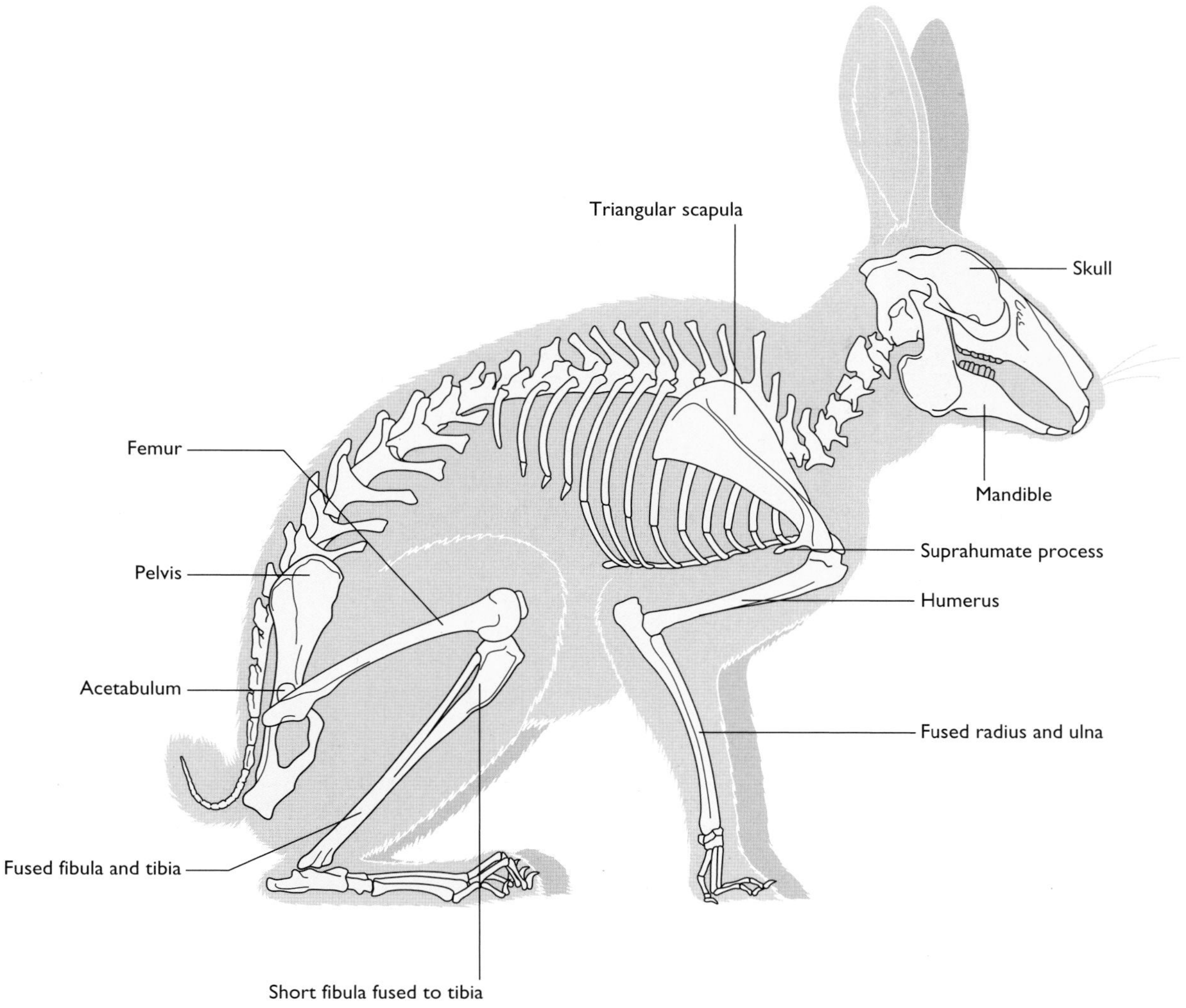

Fig. 14.1 Skeleton of the rabbit showing main features.

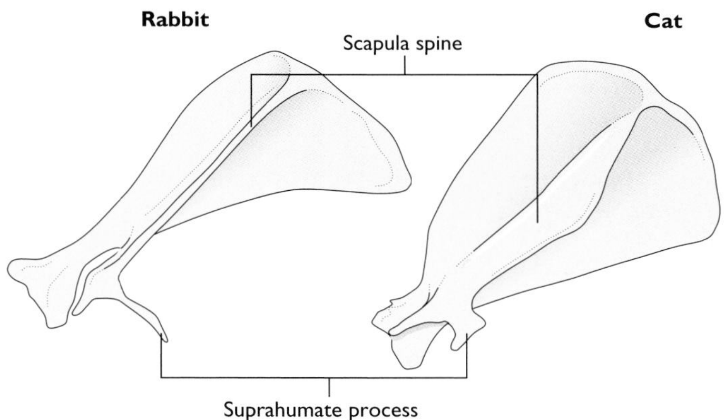

Fig. 14.2 The scapula of the rabbit compared to that of the cat.

Oral cavity

The opening of the mouth is small and is designed for nibbling grass, the tongue is relatively large and the oral cavity is long and curved, making examination of the cheek teeth and intubation for anaesthesia difficult. All the teeth (Fig. 14.4) are open-rooted and grow continuously throughout life. They must be kept worn down by hard or fibrous food materials.

The dental formula is:

[**I**2/1, **C**0/0, **PM**3/2, **M**3/3] $\times$ 2 = 28 total.

Malocclusion. If the teeth are misaligned or the diet does not include sufficient fibrous material, the teeth will not wear properly and the rabbit will suffer from a range of problems associated with difficulty in eating and in closing the mouth (Fig. 14.5). Malocclusion is one of the most common reasons for rabbits being presented to vets but it can be prevented by including large quantities of good-quality hay in the diet. Treatment of the overgrown incisors includes burring them off with a special type of circular burr or clipping them by using strong nail clippers. This latter is not recommended because the teeth may split lengthways leaving them open to infection.

The *incisors* have enamel only on the outer surface, which wears more slowly than the inner surface, creating the characteristic chisel shape needed for nibbling plant material. In the upper jaw the second pair of incisors are vestigial pegs and lie behind the first pair. There are no canine teeth and the space between the

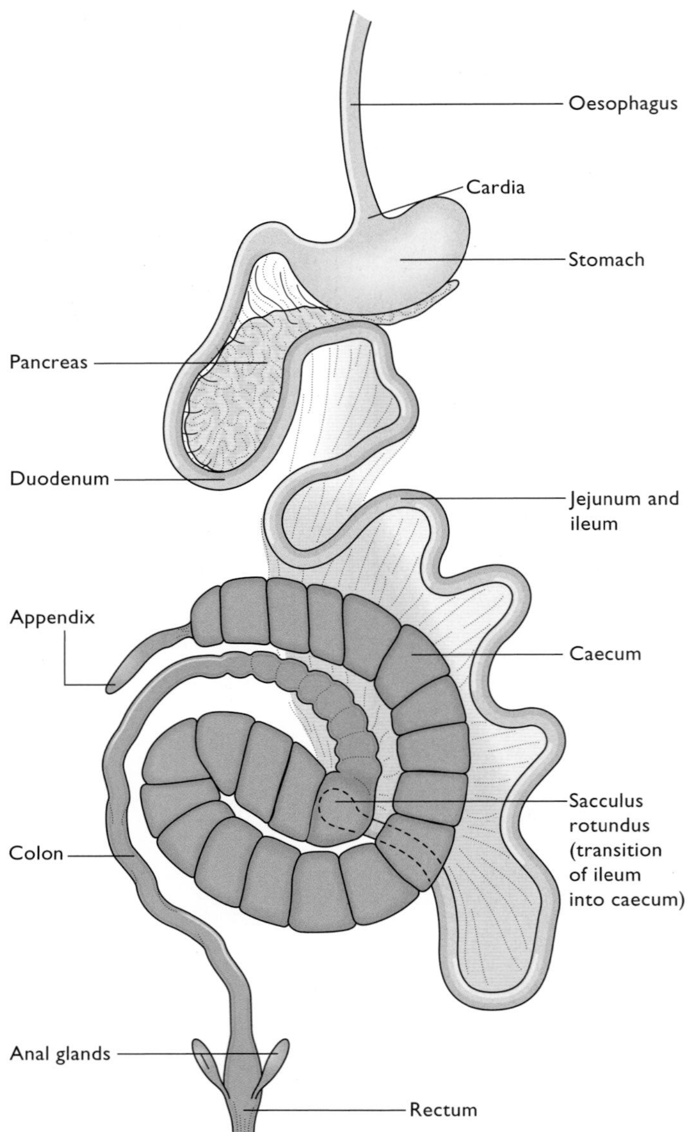

Fig. 14.3 Digestive system of the rabbit.

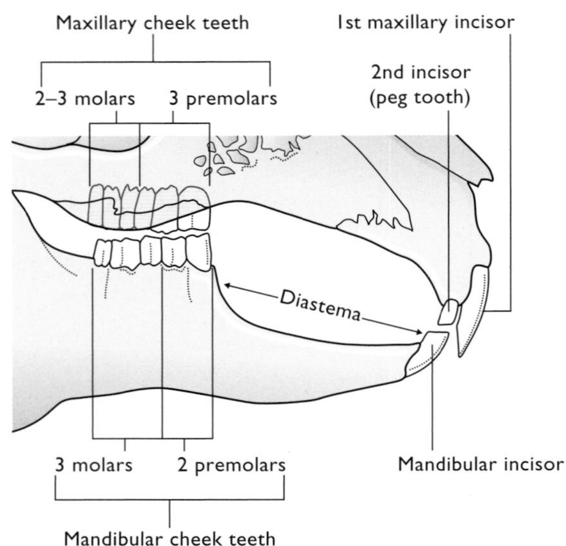

Fig. 14.4 Normal dentition of the rabbit.

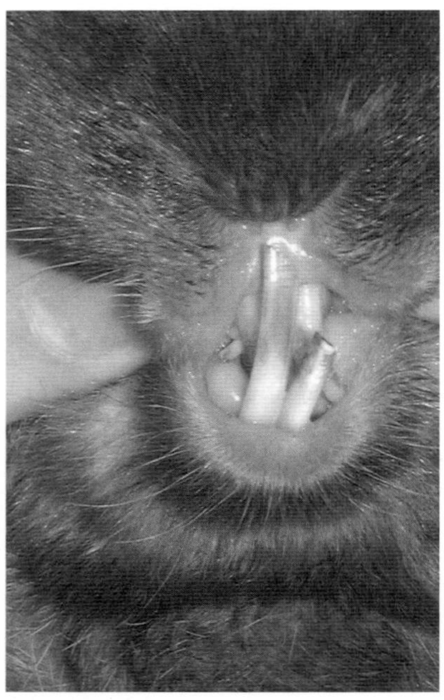

Fig. 14.5 Incisor malocclusion in a rabbit.

incisors and the cheek teeth is known as the *diastema.* The *premolars* and *molars* – cheek teeth – are flattened table teeth for grinding food. The jaw moves in a circular fashion to force the food against their roughened surfaces. The lower teeth grow at a faster rate than the upper teeth.

Stomach

This is a simple, thin-walled chamber that acts as a reservoir for food and is never truly empty. There are well developed *cardiac* and *pyloric sphincters.* Rabbits are unable to vomit because of the arrangement of the cardia in relation to the stomach.

Small intestine

The *duodenum* and *ileum* are long and have a relatively small lumen. The ileum terminates at the caecum, where there is a rounded structure, the *sacculus rotundus.* Inside this the mucosa is arranged in a network of lymph follicles and this area is often known as the *ileocaecal tonsil.*

Large intestine

The *caecum* is the largest organ in the abdominal cavity and lies on the right side. It is blind-ending, thin-walled and sacculated and coils around the other organs, folding in on itself three times. It terminates in a vermiform *appendix,* which contains abundant lymphoid tissue. Food passes on into the *colon*, which is also sacculated but shorter, with a smaller-diameter lumen.

Digestion

Rabbits are herbivorous, monogastric, hindgut fermenters. The ingested plant material passes down the tract by peristaltic contractions and undergoes enzymic digestion in the stomach and small intestine. The partially digested material enters the caecum, where it mixes with colonies of microorganisms responsible for the fermentation and breakdown of cellulose found within plant cell walls.

The now semi-liquid material passes into the colon. Contractions here pass fluid back into the caecum for re-use in the fermentation process and also separate fibrous from non-fibrous material, resulting in the production of two types of faeces:

- *Hard fibrous pellets* are produced within 4 h of eating. Fibre passes rapidly through the digestive tract and is essential for the stimulation of gut function but has no nutritive value.
- *Soft pellets* or *caecotrophs* are produced within 3–8 h of eating, often at night. They are covered in mucus, greener, low in fibre and high in protein, vitamins B and K and volatile fatty acids. Caecotrophs are eaten directly from the anus – a process known as *caecotrophy* or *coprophagia*. They are swallowed without chewing. The mucoid covering protects them from the stomach acid and facilitates absorption of the nutrients in the small intestine.

In this way, nutrients produced by microbial fermentation are made available to the rabbit. Food material passes through the digestive system twice in 24 h.

Respiratory system

The rabbit is an obligate nose breather, meaning that it *must* breathe through its nose. (Mouth breathing is often a poor prognostic sign.) The nose twitches 20–120 times per minute but ceases under general anaesthesia. The glottis is small and difficult to see because the view is impaired by the relatively large tongue. This can make intubation difficult and precautions must be taken to avoid reflex laryngospasm.

The thymus gland remains a considerable size into adult life. It lies ventral to the heart and runs cranially to the thoracic inlet. The thoracic cavity is quite small and breathing mainly involves the diaphragm. The lungs have three lobes on each side; the cranial lobes are small.

Urinary system

The kidneys are unipapillate, meaning that a single medullary pyramid drains into the renal pelvis and ureter. In the doe the ureters drain into the bladder, which is tough but thin-walled, and the urethra empties into the ventral wall of the vagina; in the buck the ureters drain low down on the neck of the bladder.

Urine

In the normal healthy rabbit this can vary in colour from deep red to yellow or white. It may also vary in turbidity from clear to cloudy (this is due to the presence of calcium). The kidneys are the main route for the excretion of calcium, and serum levels depend on dietary intake – excessive intake may cause calcification of the aorta and kidneys.

Reproductive system

Male

The male rabbit is known as a *buck*. There are two testes, which in the adult male lie in two almost hairless scrotal sacs cranial to the penis (Fig. 14.6). The testes descend at about 12 weeks of age but the inguinal canal remains open; there is no os penis. The buck has no nipples.

Female

The female rabbit is known as a *doe*. The reproductive tract of the doe is *bicornuate*, meaning that it has two separate uterine horns designed to hold litters of young (Fig. 14.7). There is no uterine body and each horn has its own *cervix* opening into the *vagina*. The mesometrium is a major fat storage organ. The doe has four or five pairs of nipples.

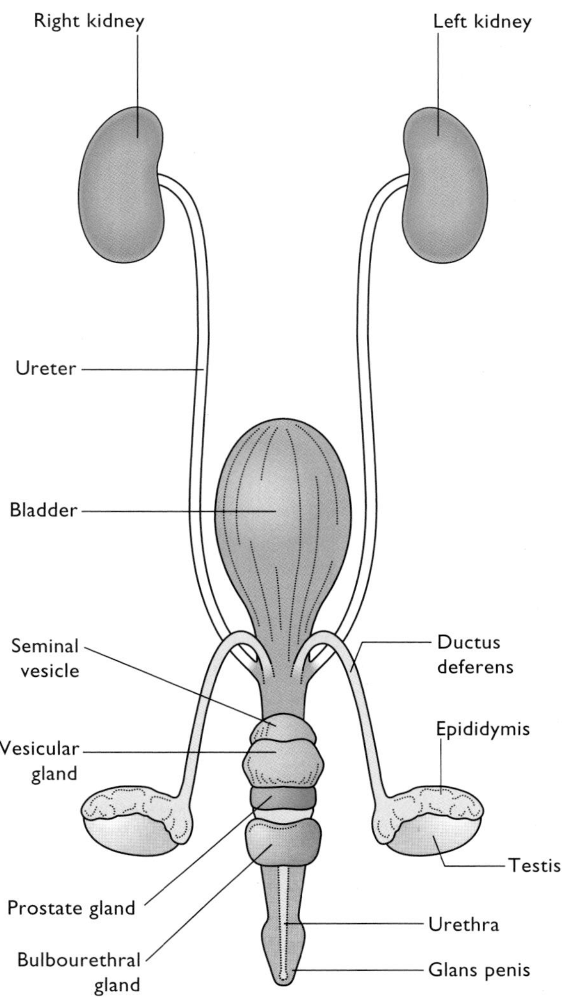

Fig. 14.6 Urogenital system of the male rabbit.

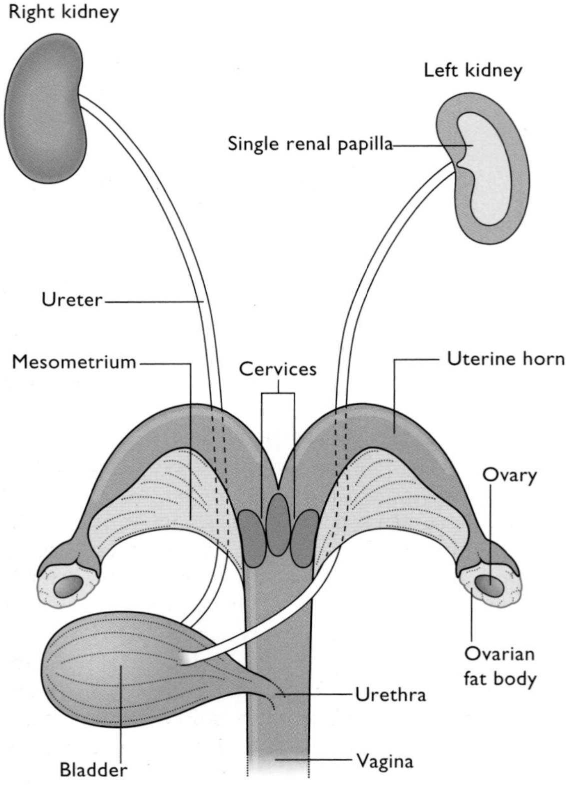

Fig. 14.7 Urogenital system of the female rabbit.

The female rabbit is an *induced ovulator* and does not have a well-defined oestrous cycle. There are periods of sexual receptivity every 4–6 days. Ovulation occurs within 10 h of coitus. The age of sexual maturity varies with the breed: small breeds are mature at about 5 months while larger ones mature as late as 8 months. The young are *altricial*: they are born hairless, deaf and blind and are totally dependent on their mother for the first few weeks of life. They are protected from the environment and predators by a warm, fur-lined nest but if disturbed the dam may eat them.

Wild rabbit does only feed their young once or twice a day, leaving them safe in their underground nest. When they return the individual kits feed only for few minutes and this period gets shorter as the kits mature. This pattern is also seen in pet rabbits and owners may be concerned that the dam is neglecting her young. If the kits are apparently thriving there is not a problem.

Sexual differentiation

This can be difficult in young rabbits and is easier after the testes of the male descend into the scrotum (Fig. 14.8).

- *Male:* The penis can be easily extruded and has a pointed end. Bucks over about 5 weeks have large relatively hairless scrotal sacs containing the retractable testes. They lie lateral and cranial to the penis.
- *Female:* The opening to the vulva is slit-like. Only the doe has teats, usually eight pairs, which lie along the ventral thoracic and abdominal body wall.

In the majority of placental mammals the scrotum lies caudal to the penis. However, in marsupials and in the rabbit the scrotum lies cranial to the penis.

Caesarian section. When a caesarean section is performed on a doe, a separate incision must be made in each uterine horn. The conceptuses cannot be pushed from one horn into another because the presence of a cervix at the base of each horn blocks their passage.

Small rodents

This group includes the small animals that are among the most popular children's pets: rats, mice, gerbils, hamsters, guinea pigs, chinchillas and chipmunks. They all belong to the order Rodentia – derived from the Latin *rodere*, meaning to gnaw – the common characteristic of which is that they have prominent, yellow-coloured incisor teeth with an open pulp cavity. This means that the teeth continue to grow throughout the animal's life and to maintain them at a normal length the animal must gnaw on hard or fibrous food material.

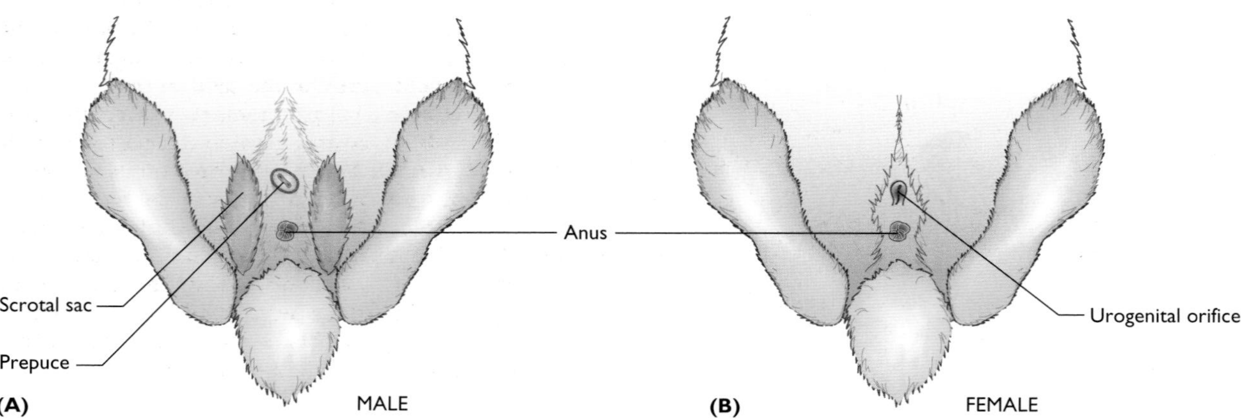

Fig. 14.8 Sexing a rabbit. (With permission from B O'Malley, 2005. Clinical anatomy and physiology of exotic species. Edinburgh: Elsevier Saunders.)

The Rodentia is one of the largest orders and comprises 40% of all mammals. They can be divided into three main groups:

- *Myomorphs* are the mouse-like rodents. They are all omnivorous and can be further subdivided into:
  - Mouse and rat: surface-living rodents
  - Gerbil and hamster: burrowing rodents
- *Sciuromorphs* are the squirrel-like rodents. They are omnivorous and the group includes the chipmunks.
- *Hystricomorphs* is a term related to the mode of reproduction. This group includes guinea pigs and chinchillas. They both have a long gestation period and produce precocial young; they are herbivorous.

Tables 14.1 and 14.2 give physiological and reproductive parameters for small rodents.

Myomorph group

Morphology

Mouse (Mus musculus)

The mouse is the most familiar and widely distributed rodent in the world. It is sociable and may be kept in small groups. The house mouse is about 6–8 cm in length, excluding its long tail, which is usually the same length as the body, and weighs about 20–40 g. It has a small head with a pointed nose and a split upper lip. Arranged around the area of the upper lips are several long, thin whiskers, which help the mouse to find its way around in the dark. The ears are very delicate, short and rounded. The eyes are large, dark and protuberant and provide a wide range of monocular vision. Their sight is poorly developed and they are photophobic. The long prehensile tail is almost hairless and covered in visible scales. Mice have four toes on the front feet and five on the hind feet; each toe ends in a small claw. Female mice have seven pairs of teats but they are absent in the male.

The natural colour of the mouse is greyish brown with a lighter underside. However, as a result of selective breeding, pet mice, known as fancy mice, can be found in a wide range of coat lengths and textures, colours, colour combinations, and with red or black eyes.

Rat (Rattus norvegicus)

The genus *Rattus* contains about 80 species of rat but it is the brown rat that has been developed into the pet or laboratory rat. It is a sociable animal and benefits from the company of its own species. They weigh 400–800 g, adult males being much larger than the females. The body shape of the rat is similar to that of the mouse but rats are considerably larger. The prehensile tail is thick and rasp-like and covered in scales. As in mice, rats have four toes on the forefeet and five on the hind feet, each ending in a small claw. Female rats have five pairs of teats but they are absent in males.

Rattus norvegicus is naturally brown but selective breeding has produced fancy rats with a wide range of coat colours, patterns and eye colours.

Hamster (Mesocricetus auratus)

The most common type of hamster kept in captivity is the golden or Syrian hamster which is a strictly solitary species and is also nocturnal. In the wild individuals only come together to mate and the young leave the nest as soon as they are independent. If kept in groups there will almost certainly be bloodshed.

Adult hamsters measure 12–15 cm in length and weigh about 100 g. The head and body merge into one another, creating a rounded, stocky shape. The nose is pointed with a divided upper lip. The eyes are dark and protuberant and the delicate ears are large, rounded and erect. Sight is poor in bright light and is adapted to the low light levels associated with their nocturnal behaviour. Hamsters have large cheek pouches extending from the oral cavity and reaching as far as the scapula in which they carry food to their larders. The tail is short and insignificant. There are four toes on the forefeet and five on the hind feet, each ending in a small claw. The female hamster has six pairs of teats but they are absent in the male.

The natural colour of the golden hamster is a rich golden-brown or orange on the back and white or cream on the underside. There is often a darker patch on the cheeks. The fur is short and thick and is designed to keep the hamster warm in the cold nights of the Syrian desert. There is a scent gland on each flank, which is most prominent in the male and is used to mark territory. Pet hamsters can be found in a variety of coat colours, textures and lengths and a variety of eye colours.

Other species of hamster may also be kept as pets. They are the Chinese hamster, *Cricetulus griseus*, and the Russian hamster, *Phodopus sungorus*. They are smaller, often sold as 'dwarf' hamsters, and have a light grey back with a black stripe along the spine and a white underside. Both these species are social animals and may be kept in groups. Mixed-sex groups will breed well and single-sex groups, particularly males, are likely to fight.

Gerbil (Meriones unguiculatus)

The gerbil belongs to a family of burrowing rodents often called sand rats. They are sociable animals, living in groups in the wild and in captivity they are happier if kept in small colonies.

The most common species kept as a pet is the Mongolian gerbil. When adult it can reach 8–10 cm from nose to the base of the tail. The tail is long and covered in fur with a tufted end and is usually about the same length as the body. An adult gerbil will weigh 50–60 g. The body is short and thick and at rest the gerbil sits upright with its forelegs off the ground. The head is broad with black protruding eyes and the ears are small, rounded and covered in fur. The forelegs are short with five-clawed toes and used to hold food. The hind legs and large furry feet with four-clawed toes resemble those of a small kangaroo. They enable the gerbil to stand firmly in the sand of the desert and to move with a characteristic jumping motion. The female gerbil has four pairs of teats but they are absent in the male. The male has a scent gland surrounded by a bald patch on its abdomen, which is rubbed on the ground to mark territorial boundaries.

The natural colour is reddish brown with dark guard hairs. This agouti colouration breaks up the animal's outline and camouflages it in the desert environment. The gerbil's underside is a lighter brown or cream, which serves to reflect heat from the hot sand. Pet gerbils can now be obtained in varying coat and eye colours, although patterned gerbils are less common.

The different species of small rodent should never be kept in the same cage, although it is sometimes possible to keep guinea pigs and rabbits together – opinions vary!

Digestive system of myomorphs

All these rodents are omnivorous and their teeth and digestive tract reflect their ability to eat a wide range of food material. In particular it is the ability of the mouse and the rat to eat almost anything that has enabled them to adapt to and survive in most of the world's habitats.

Dentition

The myomorphs have a common dental formula:

[**I**1/1, **C**0/0, **PM**0/0, **M**3/3] × 2 = 16 total.

The *incisors* are yellow–orange-stained, with the chisel shape necessary for gnawing and nibbling hard food materials. They are open-rooted, which enables them to grow continuously throughout the animal's life. The *molars* are flattened table teeth used for grinding food material. Once the permanent dentition is in wear the pulp cavity closes over so the molars do not continue to grow. The space between the incisors and the molar teeth is the *diastema* and is occupied by the cheek tissue.

Digestive tract

The *stomach* is simple and digestion is monogastric. The lining epithelium is mainly non-glandular in rats, mice and gerbils. There is a ridge between the oesophagus and the cardiac region of the stomach, which makes regurgitation of food material almost impossible. The *intestine* is relatively long, which allows time for the digestion of plant material. In most species there is no specifically adapted organ for the microbial breakdown of cellulose, as is seen in herbivores. However, the hamster has a distinct fore-stomach similar to the rumen of the cow and sheep for this purpose; the contents of this chamber have a high pH and are rich in microorganisms. There is no *gall bladder* in the rat.

Problems with overgrown incisors are the most common reason for small rodents to be presented to the vet. Symptoms include excessive salivation, clawing at the mouth and difficulty in eating. The treatment is to clip the incisors or reduce them with a surgical burr. The condition can be prevented by providing food that must be gnawed.

It is unnecessary to starve small rodents prior to anaesthesia – the stomach is impossible to empty as it usually contains ingested faecal pellets. Regurgitation and choking is unlikely to be a significant risk. Rodents have a high metabolic rate so starvation may result in a fatal hypoglycaemia.

All the myomorphs show varying degrees of *coprophagia* (eating their own faeces), which is a natural behaviour pattern. The faecal pellets may contribute a significant proportion of nutrients to the diet and are rich in vitamin B, produced by microorganisms living in the colon.

Reproductive system of myomorphs

Male

The adult male of this group has two testes in an external scrotum. In many species the inguinal canal remains open, allowing the testes to shrink and return to the abdomen during the non-breeding season. The testes of the Chinese hamster, *Cricetulus griseus*, remain internal. The reproductive tract is complex and comprises several large accessory glands. An os penis lies within the tissue of the penis.

Female

Females in this group have a *bicornuate* uterus, with a pair of long uterine horns and little or no uterine body. This arrangement has evolved to contain large numbers of developing embryos. The stages of the rodent oestrous cycle can be ascertained by microscopic examination of vaginal smears (exfoliative vaginal cytology). The female hamster may produce copious amounts of vaginal discharge, particularly around day 2 of the oestrous cycle. Mating may be confirmed by the presence of a 'copulatory plug'. This is a creamy gelatinous plug formed from the secretions of the male accessory glands; it remains in the vagina or may fall onto the cage floor.

The females of all these species of rodent are *polyoestrous* and *spontaneous ovulators*. Specific details are mentioned in Table 14.2. Myomorphs are sexually mature at a young age (the mouse reaches sexual maturity at 3–4 weeks, for example), and produce large litters of young. Both of these features contribute to the success of rodents in creating 'population explosions' over a short period. The neonates are *altricial:* they are totally dependent on the mother for several weeks and are born hairless, blind and deaf. At this stage they are very vulnerable and are kept hidden in some form of nest. If disturbed, the mother may exhibit cannibalism.

Sexual differentiation of myomorphs

As a general rule, the anogenital distance – the distance between the opening of the anus and the opening of the genital tract (penis or vulva) – is longer in the male than in the female (Fig. 14.9).

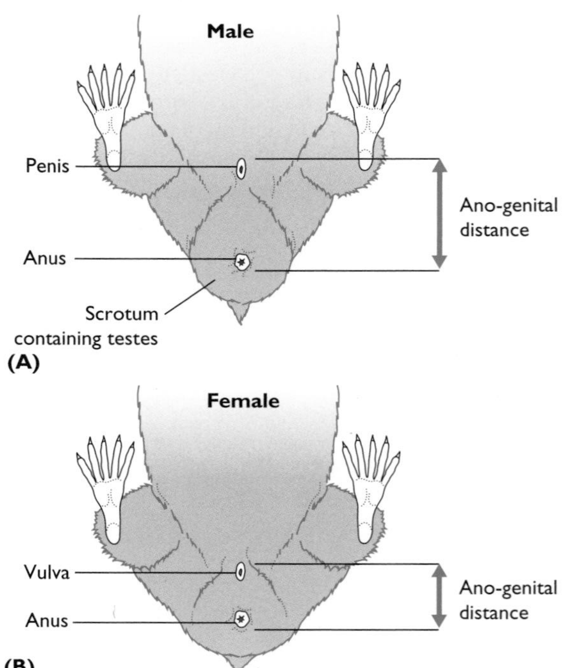

Fig. 14.9 General method of sexing rodents. The anogenital distance is larger in males than in females.

There are no teats in the male. There are also some species-specific indicators of sex:

1. Adult male hamsters have large external testes, which are retained in the scrotum by a pad of fat in the inguinal canal. This makes the rear outline of the male conical when viewed from above. The female has no scrotum so the rear outline is more rounded.
2. Newly weaned male gerbils have a pigmented scrotum.
3. Sexually mature male gerbils have a prominent ventral abdominal scent gland.
4. The testes of male hamsters shrink in the winter when temperatures and light levels may be lower; this may cause a male to be incorrectly identified as a female.

Hibernation. At temperatures of lower than 5°C hamsters may enter temporary hibernation and appear to be dead; the heart beat and respiration fall to almost undetectable rates. Never bury a hamster unless you are certain it is dead! There have been many reported cases of hamsters digging their way out of a grave.

Sciuromorph group

Chipmunk (*Tamias sibiricus*)

Morphology

The most common of the 24 species of chipmunk to be kept as a pet is the Siberian chipmunk. Adults reach 12–19 cm in length with a long bushy tail of approximately 11 cm and weigh 70–120 g. The fur varies from deep brown to greyish light chestnut. The dark prominent eyes are set on either side of the head and are outlined by a white stripe with an inner dark stripe running towards the ear. The small, furry ears have rounded tips and are set high on the head. Running along the back from the nape of the neck to the base of the tail are five dark stripes with four lighter ones in between. The tail is covered in chestnut grey hairs tipped with white. At rest the chipmunk sits upright supported by the hind feet and uses the forelimbs for holding food, similar to the familiar 'squirrel' position. Chipmunks have cheek pouches extending from the oral cavity that are used to carry food gathered from the woodland floor to storage chambers within their nests. The female has four pairs of teats but these are absent in the male.

Digestive system

The chipmunk is an omnivore and has a similar dentition and type of digestive tract to that seen in the myomorphs.

Reproductive system

Female chipmunks are *seasonally polyoestrous* and *spontaneous ovulators*. The breeding season is between March and September. The testes of the male descend into the scrotum in January and begin spermatogenesis. The female advertises her willingness to mate by a persistent chipping noise on the second day of her 3-day oestrous cycle. The reproductive tract of both sexes follows a similar pattern to that of the myomorphs (Table 14.2).

Hystricomorph group

Guinea pig (*Cavia porcellus*)

Morphology

The guinea pig, also called the *cavy*, originated from South America, where it is still used for food. They are a sociable species, living in large herds, and they are diurnal. Adults measure 20–35 cm, the males being larger than the females, and weigh 750–1200 g. The body is short and stocky with short legs and no tail. There are four toes on each forefoot and three on the hind feet, each ending in a short, sharp claw. The nose is rounded and the mouth is small with a split upper lip on which there are long, sensitive whiskers. The ears are small, very delicate and virtually hairless. Guinea pigs have a good sense of hearing and can detect frequencies higher than are detectable by the human ear. The eyes are prominent and situated on either side of the head. They have keen eyesight with the excellent peripheral vision necessary to spot predators. They also have an excellent sense of smell.

The natural coat of the guinea pig is short and smooth with dark brown ticked or agouti-coloured hairs providing the camouflage needed for life on open plains. Selective breeding has resulted in a variety of coat lengths, colours and patterns. The skin has an abundant supply of sebaceous glands along the dorsal surface and around the anus. The rump may be rubbed against the ground as a means of marking the territory. Both male and female guinea pigs have a pair of long inguinal nipples.

Skeletal system

Guinea pigs have large *tympanic bullae*, which can be palpated at the base of each ear. They have 32–36 vertebrae: C7, T13–14, L6, S2–3, Cd4–6. There are 13–14 *ribs*, of which the last two are cartilaginous. A small *clavicle* attaches between the scapula and the manubrium. In the female the *pubic symphysis* remains fibrocartilaginous until about 1 year old. After this time it becomes ossified, making normal parturition difficult in an elderly primigravid (first litter) sow. In younger sows the symphysis relaxes and a gap can be palpated just before parturition.

Digestive system

The guinea pig is a monogastric herbivore with a large caecum for microbial fermentation of plant material. The dental formula is:

$$[\mathbf{I}1/1, \mathbf{C}0/0, \mathbf{PM}1/1, \mathbf{M}3/3] \times 2 = 20 \text{ total.}$$

Both the *incisors* and the cheek teeth (*premolars* and *molars*) are open-rooted and continue to grow throughout the animal's life (Fig. 14.10). This can lead to dental problems if they are not worn down by the appropriate fibrous food. The incisors are normally white. The space between the incisors and the cheek teeth is called the *diastema* and is filled with the cheek tissue.

In guinea pigs with malocclusion, the molars in the lower jaw tend to grow medially and lacerate the side of the tongue, while those in the upper jaw grow laterally and lacerate the inside of the cheek. Both result in excessive salivation and dysphagia.

The *oral cavity* is small and narrow and contains the relatively large *tongue*. There are four pairs of *salivary glands*, which empty into the oral cavity near the molars. The *soft palate* is continuous

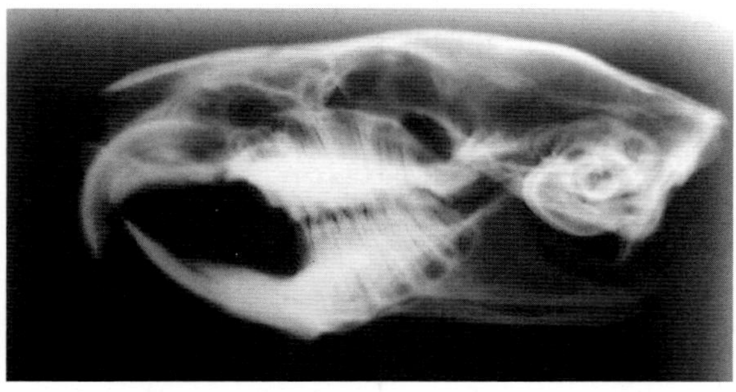

Fig. 14.10 Radiograph of a guinea pig's skull showing dentition.

with the base of the tongue and the *oropharynx* connects with the rest of the *pharynx* via a hole in the soft palate known as the *palatal ostium*.

The *stomach* (Fig. 14.11) is simple and is lined by a glandular epithelium. Gastric emptying takes about 2 h. The intestinal tract measures approximately 2 m. The *small intestine* lies mainly on the right side of the abdominal cavity while the much longer *large intestine* fills the central and left parts of the abdomen. The most significant organ is the *caecum*, measuring 15–20 cm, which is thin walled and sacculated with many lateral pouches created by thick bands of smooth muscle. At any one time it may contain 65% of the gut contents. The caecum contains microorganisms that are responsible for the breakdown of cellulose in the plant cell walls and for the addition of certain nutrients such as vitamin B.

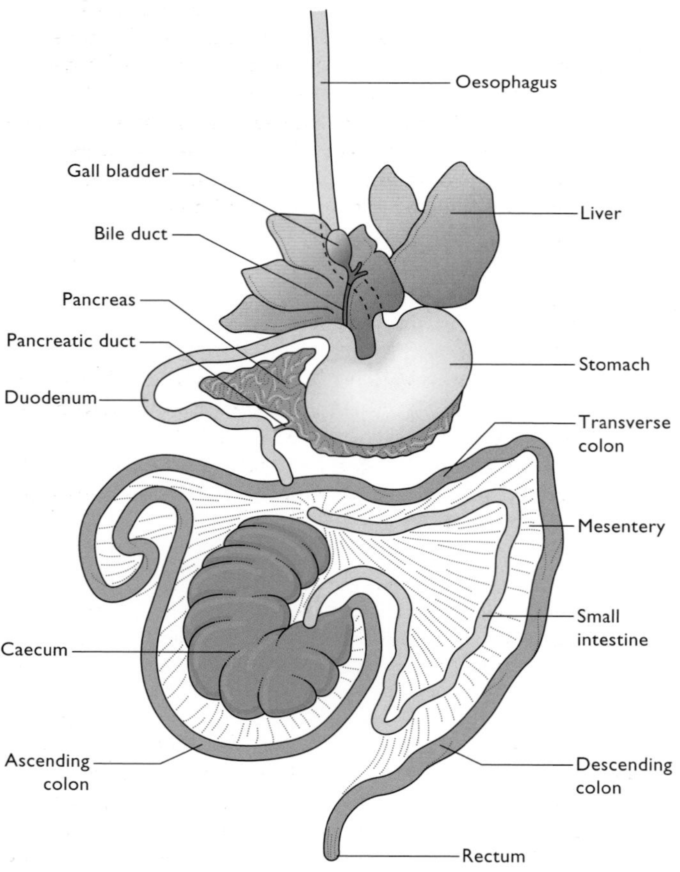

Fig. 14.11 The digestive system of the guinea pig.

When attempting to pass a feeding tube through the palatal ostium into the oesophagus of the guinea pig, make sure it does not slip to one side and damage the surrounding vascular soft palate.

The total time taken for food to pass through the digestive tract is approximately 20 h but it may take as long as 66 h if coprophagia is taken into account. Guinea pigs exhibit *coprophagia* or *caecotrophy* and may be seen to eat softer, more mucoid caecotrophs direct from the anus between 150 and 200 times a day. The liver has six lobes and there is a well-developed gall bladder.

The liver of the guinea pig is unable to synthesise vitamin C and deficiencies may occur if the animal does not receive a daily dietary source in the form of fresh greenery or synthetic supplements. Symptoms include a dull rough coat, stiff gait and lameness, pain on movement, diarrhoea, anorexia and general lethargy.

Urinary system

Each *kidney* has a relatively large renal pelvis with a single papilla. The *urine* produced by the guinea pig is alkaline, thick and often a cloudy white or yellow. The presence of crystals in urine is a normal finding.

Reproductive system

- *Male:* known as a *boar*. The two *testes* are able to be retracted through the inguinal canal, which remains open throughout life. In mature breeding boars the large testes lie in the scrotum on either side of the genital opening. Internally there are several *accessory glands* – the long, coiled vesicular glands, prostate, coagulating glands and the bulbourethral glands. There is an *os penis* and caudoventral to the urethral opening is a pouch containing two horny *styles* or projections, which evert externally during erection of the penis.
- *Female:* known as a *sow*. The uterus is *bicornuate* and consists of two long uterine horns, a short body and a cervix leading into the vagina.

The female guinea pig is *polyoestrous* and a *spontaneous ovulator*. Details can be found in Table 14.2. The gestation period is 63 days, which is long compared to that of other rodents, and the young are *precocial*, meaning they are born fully furred with their eyes open and can be independent of their mothers. This enables them to eat solid food almost immediately after birth, although for the first few weeks they also suckle from the mother. They are born in the open, unprotected by a nest, and have to move around to escape predators if necessary.

Sexual differentiation

Guinea pigs are easy to sex and this can be done almost from birth.

- *Male:* Mature boars have clearly defined testes. The penis can be prolapsed by applying gentle pressure at its base, cranial to the urethral opening.
- *Female:* The perineal tissues form a Y-shaped depression. The vulval opening lies at the intersection of the Y, with the anus at the base of the Y. If pressure is applied cranial to the vulval opening, there will be no penile prolapse.

Both sexes of guinea pig have a pair of inguinal nipples.

Chinchilla (*Chinchilla lanigera*)

Morphology

Chinchillas originate in the mountains of South America and were imported into the UK to be bred for their fur. Nowadays, with a change in attitude towards the wearing of fur, chinchillas are mainly kept as pets. Chinchillas are almost extinct in the wild and the only species likely to be found in captivity is *C. lanigera*. They have a compact body with short limbs and a short, bushy tail. They weigh 400–500 g and the females are larger than the males. The nose is pointed and there are long, sensitive whiskers on the divided upper lip. They have dark, prominent eyes on either side of the head that are adapted to seeing in poor light and large, round, delicate ears. At rest the chinchilla sits upright supported by its large hind feet and uses its forepaws for holding food. They have four clawed toes on each fore and hind paw and the palmar and plantar surfaces of the feet are hairless.

The natural colour of the fur is blue-grey. The fur is soft and very dense, which is due to the fact that as many as 60 hairs may grow from a single follicle. When fluffed up, the chinchilla appears to be quite large but under the fur the skeleton is relatively small. Selective breeding has produced a range of other colours.

Digestive system

Like the guinea pig, chinchillas are *monogastric herbivores* with a large caecum for the breakdown of cellulose. The dental formula is:

[**I** 1/1, **C** 0/0, **PM** 1/1, **M** 3/3] × 2 = 20 total.

Teeth are present in the jaw at birth. Both the *incisors* and the cheek teeth (*premolars* and *molars*) are open-rooted and grow continuously throughout the chinchilla's life. The chisel-shaped incisors, which are yellower than those of the guinea pig, have been reported as growing as much as 6 cm in a year. The cheek teeth are flattened table teeth for grinding fibrous plant material. The space between the incisors and the cheek teeth is known as the *diastema*. As with all species of rodent, dental problems are one of the most common conditions seen by veterinary surgeons.

The *oral cavity* is small and narrow. Like guinea pigs, the base of the tongue is continuous with the soft palate and the entrance to the pharynx is via a small hole, the *palatal ostium*.

The stomach is relatively large and simple. The intestine is long and has evolved to digest plant material. The caecum is long and coiled and holds a smaller percentage of the total intestinal contents than in the guinea pig or rabbit. The colon is sacculated. Microbial fermentation occurs within the caecum, resulting in the formation of caecotrophs, which are rich in nutrients such as vitamin B. The chinchilla exhibits coprophagia but digestive studies show that, while the guinea pig ingests both caecotrophs and faecal pellets at intervals throughout the day, the chinchilla only consumes faecal pellets at night and caecotrophs between 8 am and 2 pm.

> The chinchilla has evolved to survive on the relatively poor but highly fibrous diet of grasses found high up in the Andes. A healthy diet for a chinchilla should therefore include high levels of fibre and protein. Treats such as apples, figs and sultanas must be given in moderation. It is not uncommon for chinchillas to die from constipation or diarrhoea caused by an over-indulgent owner.

Reproductive system

- *Male:* There is no true scrotum. The *testes* remain in the open inguinal canal or in the abdomen. On either side of the anus are two *postanal sacs* in which the caudal epididymis can lie. In the presence of a female the testes swell and become very obvious. The *penis*, which may be 1.5 cm long in the adult, is easily visible below the anus, from which it is separated by a small area of hairless skin. It is supported by the presence of a small bone known as the *baculum*.
- *Female:* The uterus consists of two long *uterine horns*, each of which terminates in a *cervix*. This is similar to the rabbit but different from the structure seen in the guinea pig. The two cervices then lead into the single *vagina*. Both male and female chinchillas have three pairs of *mammary glands:* one inguinal pair and two lateral thoracic ones. The teats tend to protrude sideways, allowing the young to sit beside the dam and suckle.

The female chinchilla is *seasonally polyoestrous* and a *spontaneous ovulator*. Details can be found in Table 14.2. The gestation period is 111 days, which is exceptionally long for a member of the rodent family. The young are *precocial* (born fully furred and capable of living an independent life); however, they continue to suckle from the dam until they are weaned at about 6–8 weeks.

Sexual differentiation

Chinchillas are quite easy to sex and this can be done at birth.

- *Male:* As with many rodent species, the anogenital distance is longer in the male than it is in the female (Fig. 14.8). There is a hairless band between the penis and the anus. The penis can be extruded by gentle pressure at its base.
- *Female:* The anogenital distance is shorter. A relatively large urinary papilla lies close to the anus and can be mistaken for a penis; however, there is no hairless band between it and the anus. The opening to the urethra is on the tip of this papilla and the opening to the slit-like vulva is immediately caudal to it.

The ferret

The domestic ferret, *Mustela putorius furo*, is a member of the order Carnivora and the family Mustelidae. Other related species include badgers, otters, stoats and weasels, all of which are long-bodied, agile creatures capable of producing a characteristic pungent smell from their anal glands and from numerous sebaceous glands distributed within the skin.

> Many people suggest that removing the anal glands of the ferret will help to reduce the 'ferrety' smell; however, because the smell is also produced by its sebaceous glands, 'descenting', as it is known, will not help the problem.

Ferrets are most closely related to the European polecat, *Mustela putorius*, found in parts of the UK and northern Europe. It is almost certain that the Egyptians domesticated the polecat to produce the modern ferret. Although working ferrets are still used for hunting rabbits and rats, nowadays ferrets are becoming more popular as pets and in the USA there may be as many as 7 million pet ferrets!

Morphology

The ferret has a flexible, tubular body with short legs and a long, thick tail. This shape enables it to go down rabbit holes and to squeeze through openings in a cage or in the house, so steps must be taken to prevent escape! The *neck* is long and muscular and of approximately the same diameter as the rest of the body. The *head* is relatively small with small ears set wide apart on the crown. The eyes point forward and are also set wide apart, providing binocular vision; however, ferrets' eyesight is poor and adapted to the low light levels found in tunnels.

The *legs* are short and used for digging and traction, but the ferret is also able to climb and may scale great heights. There are five toes on each *foot*, ending in non-retractable claws; in working ferrets these are kept long. The first digit on each foot has only two phalanges while the other digits have three.

The *skin* of the ferret is thick, especially over the neck and shoulders where it provides protection against bites. It is well supplied with *sebaceous glands*, which are the main source of the ferret's body odour. Ferrets also have a pair of well-developed *anal glands*, which produce a yellow serous secretion with a strong smell. The *fur* is thick and in the past this has led to ferrets being used in the fur trade. The natural colour is a cream undercoat with black guard hairs, black feet and tail and a black mask on the face. This is the colouration of the polecat and in the ferret is known as 'fitch'. Other naturally occurring colours are albino and sandy or cinnamon. Selective breeding of pet ferrets has led to the development of about 30 other colour variations. Ferrets moult in the spring and autumn and the fur may vary between the seasons: it may be shorter and darker in the summer months and longer and lighter in the winter.

Musculoskeletal system

The general pattern of the skeleton is shown in Figs. 14.12 and 14.13. The vertebral formula is C7, T15, L5–6, S3, Cd18. The spine is extremely flexible and allows the ferret to bend at an angle of at

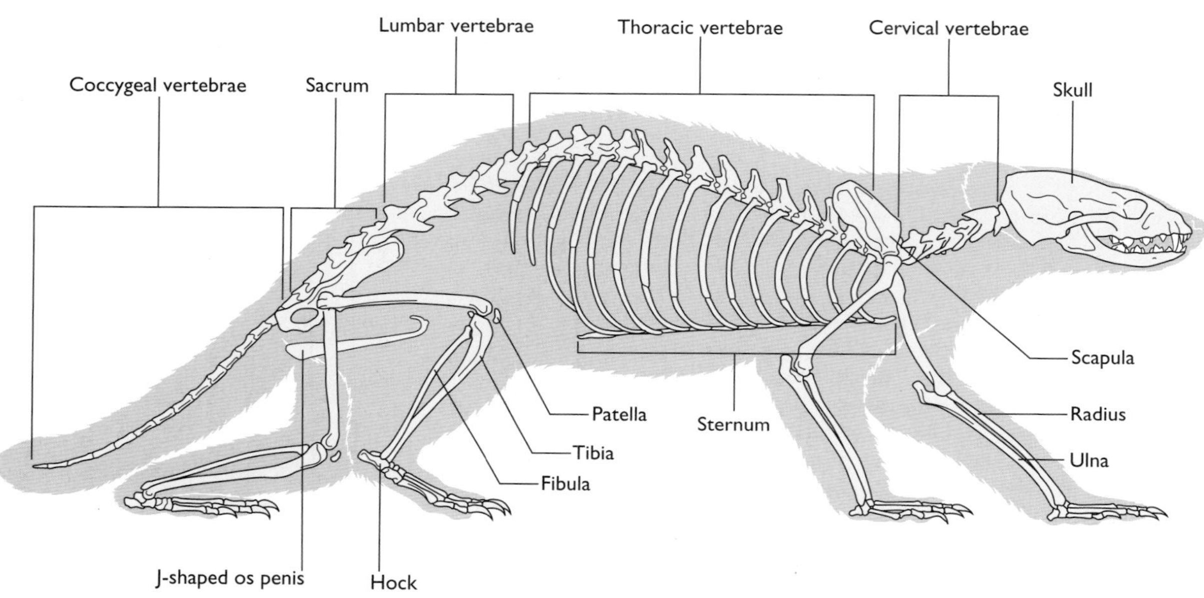

Fig. 14.12 The skeleton of the ferret.

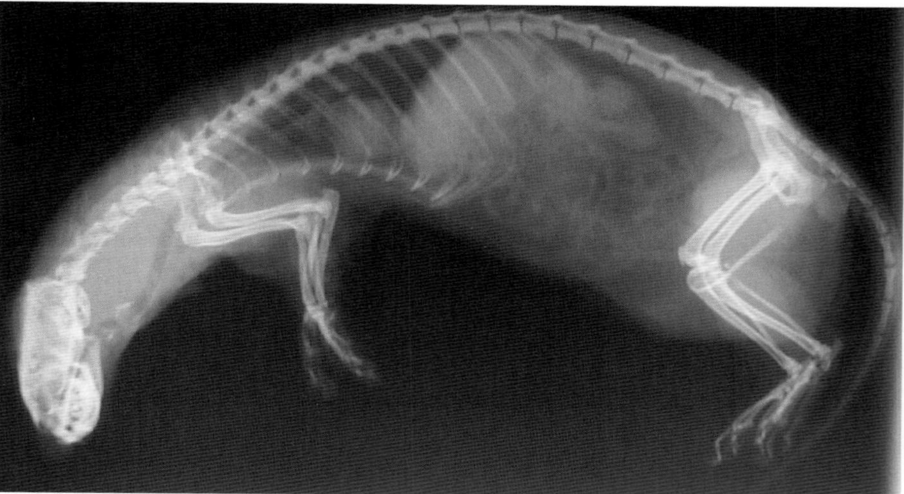

Fig. 14.13 Whole body radiograph of a male ferret.

least 180°. Ribs 1–10 attach to the sternum and the remainder form the costal arch. The thoracic inlet is very small and the presence of any abnormal mass here may interfere with swallowing and respiration (Fig. 14.13).

Digestive system

The ferret is a true carnivore and this is reflected in the anatomy of its dentition and digestive tract (Fig. 14.14). As in other carnivores, the teeth are very sharp and are adapted for shearing flesh off bone. The dental formula is:

[**I**3/3, **C**1/1, **PM**3/3, **M**1/2] × 2 = 34 total.

The *incisors* are prominent, the upper incisors being slightly longer and covering the lower ones. The *canines* are large and the roots are longer than the crown – they may be visible when the mouth is closed. The third upper premolars are the largest cheek teeth and are known as the *carnassials*. The deciduous teeth erupt at 20–28 days and the permanent teeth at 50–74 days.

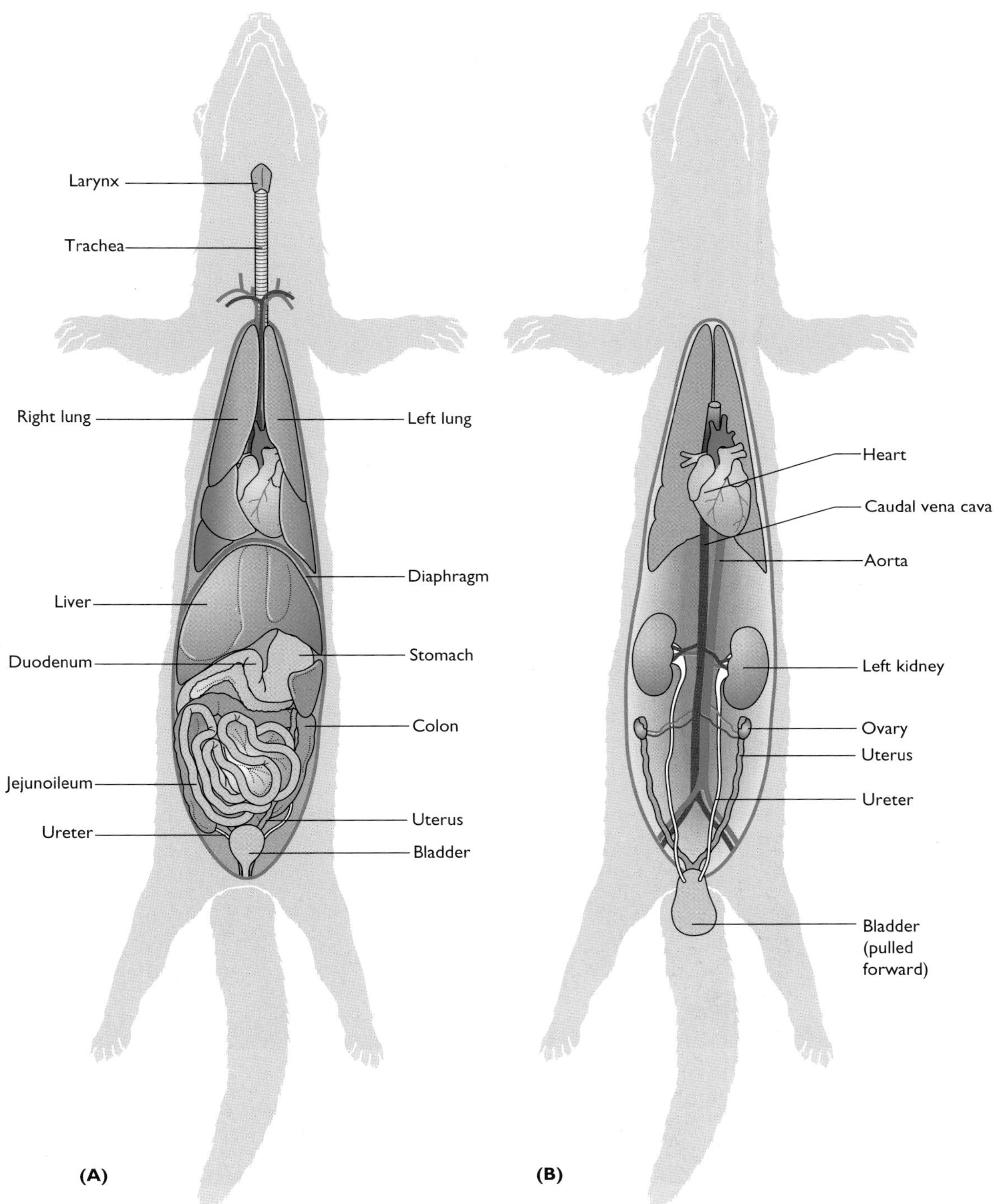

Fig. 14.14 (A) Internal anatomy of the female ferret. **(B)** Digestive tract removed.

In common with other carnivores, the length of the digestive tract (Fig. 14.14) is short; this results in a short gastrointestinal transit time of 3–4 h in the adult animal. The *stomach* is simple and small but capable of enormous distension to hold a large amount of food prior to its digestion. The pylorus is well developed. The stomach lies within a curve of the six-lobed *liver* in the anterior abdomen. The ferret has a pear-shaped *gall bladder* and its *pancreas* has two limbs that are connected close to the pylorus. Ferrets are able to vomit.

The *small intestine* is approximately 190 cm in length and consists of a duodenum, ileum and jejunum, which are almost indistinguishable on gross examination. The large intestine is approximately 10 cm in length. There is no caecum or ileocaecal valve.

Urinary system

The left kidney lies caudal to the right and both lie within the retroperitoneal fat. The cranial end of the left kidney is covered by the caudate lobe of the liver. The bladder is small and in the male the base of the bladder and the adjacent urethra are surrounded by the prostate gland.

Reproductive system

- *Male:* known as a *hob*. The male ferret has a J-shaped *os penis* lying within the caudal section of the penis and dorsal to the penile urethra (Fig. 14.12). The two *testes* are carried externally in the scrotum. Sexual maturity is usually reached during the first spring after birth, at about 4–8 months of age. Once the testes have descended the inguinal ring closes and they are not able to be retracted. Spermatogenic activity increases within the seminiferous tubules of the testes from December to July and the testes become noticeably enlarged in preparation for the breeding season from March to August. The opening of the prepuce is on the ventral abdomen in a similar position to that seen in the dog. The male ferret has teats. A castrated male ferret is known as a *hobble*.
- *Female:* known as a *jill*. The uterus consists of a pair of long uterine horns with no uterine body, a typical *bicornuate uterus*, adapted to produce litters of young. The average litter size is 8–10 kits but litters as large as 18 have been reported. The *vulva* lies on the perineum, ventral to the anus. During the non-breeding season, it is small and slit-like, but during oestrus it becomes swollen and resembles a small doughnut.

The female ferret is *seasonally polyoestrous* and an *induced ovulator*. If the jill is mated, ovulation occurs within 30–40 h of coitus. The gestation period is 42 days.

Postoestrous anaemia. Because the jill is an induced ovulator, if she is not mated, she will remain in oestrus for the entire breeding season and the associated high oestrogen levels may result in bone marrow depression and anaemia. This usually corrects itself at the end of the breeding season but if it recurs for several years in succession it may result in death. Treatment includes immediate spaying and if very severe, a blood transfusion and intensive care.

CHAPTER 15

Reptiles and fish

Reptiles

The Class Reptilia includes about 6500 species, all of which breed on land. The Class is divided into four Orders of which only two are significant as far as exotic pets are concerned. The four Orders are as follows:

- *Rhynchocephalia* includes the tuatara; very rare and unlikely to be kept in captivity.
- *Crocodilia* includes the crocodiles and alligators; rarely kept as pets.
- *Chelonia* includes tortoises, terrapins and turtles.
- *Squamata* includes Suborder Sauria (19 families of lizards), Suborder Serpentes (11 families of snakes) and Suborder Amphisbaena (one family, not kept in captivity).

These animals share many anatomical and physiological features so general reptilian anatomy and physiology will be discussed first, and any specific adaptations will be mentioned in the subsequent sections on lizards, snakes and the shelled reptiles.

General anatomy

Skeletal system

Reptiles are vertebrates and have an internal bony skeleton that, to some extent, shares the basic skeletal plan exhibited by members of the class Mammalia. However, there are distinctive modifications in the skeleton of the snakes, tortoises and turtles that will be discussed later.

Cardiovascular system

The *heart* has three chambers rather than four. There is a right and left atrium but only one ventricle. The ventricle is functionally, but not anatomically, divided into three subchambers and receives blood from both the right and left atria. Deoxygenated blood from the right atrium is directed towards the pulmonary artery, but the oxygenated blood returning from the lungs to the ventricle may pass either to the aortic arches or to the pulmonary circulation again.

A significant feature of a reptile's peripheral circulation is the *renal portal system*, which transports blood from the hind limbs and tail directly to the kidneys. This has clinical implications when injecting into the caudal half of the body, as some of the drug may be excreted in the urine before reaching the systemic circulation.

Respiratory system

Gaseous exchange occurs in the same way as it does in mammals but the most significant difference in the anatomy of the respiratory system of reptiles compared to that of mammals is that reptiles lack a *diaphragm*. As in the bird, the body cavity is not divided into two. Respiratory infections are common in reptiles but because they lack a diaphragm they lack an active, expulsive cough reflex and these infections can be severe or even fatal.

Digestive system

The more specific features of the digestive system of lizards, snakes and chelonians are covered separately. However, in general, the digestive system terminates in a common exit, the *cloaca*, consisting of three parts: the *coprodeum* collects the faeces, the *urodeum* collects urinary waste and the *proctodeum* is the final chamber that acts as a collecting area prior to the elimination of the waste.

Urinary system

The paired *kidneys* consist of nephrons without loops of Henle. This means that they are unable to produce concentrated urine. Chelonians have large bladders, which may occupy up to 25% of their body weight. Not all lizards have bladders, although a bladder is present in the green iguana (*Iguana iguana*). Snakes do not have bladders. The urine may change within the bladder so urinalysis in reptiles may not be an indication of kidney function, as it is in mammals.

Reproduction

Reptiles are *oviparous*, meaning they lay eggs. The yolk of the egg provides the nourishment for the developing young, in contrast to mammals, where the young are nourished directly by the mother via the placenta. Some reptiles are *ovoviviparous* or 'live-bearing': they retain the developing young within the egg, which remains in the oviducts, and appear to give birth to live individuals. However, the nutrients are still obtained from the yolk of the egg inside which the young develop.

Dystocia or 'egg-binding' is commonly seen in reptiles. It can occur for a number of reasons, such as lack of a suitable nesting place, stress, calcium deficiency and infection.

For a few days before and after ecdysis, reptiles can be easily damaged and handling should be kept to a minimum. Changes in the normal shedding pattern may be an indication of poor health in some species.

The integument

The skin of reptiles is thick and keratinised and is protected by scales or horny plates. Reptiles grow by a process known as *ecdysis*, during which they shed or slough the old skin. Beneath this is a new layer, which, to start with, is quite soft and easily damaged. Ecdysis varies with species and may be partial shedding, as seen in lizards, or entire, as seen in snakes.

Thermoregulation

Reptiles are *ectothermic*, meaning they are unable to regulate their internal temperature and are dependent on the external environment to raise the body temperature and increase their metabolic rate. To do this they employ a number of behavioural patterns, such as basking in sunlight or spreading themselves as flat as possible in order to increase the surface area exposed to the sun. Each species has a preferred body temperature (PBT) or preferred optimum temperature zone (POTZ). This is the body temperature at which the reptile functions most efficiently. Below the PBT digestion and reproduction are impaired and the immune system does not function so that reptiles kept at low temperatures are more likely to become ill. The advantage of being ectothermic is that a reptile does not waste energy on maintaining its body temperature and therefore requires less food. Mammals require a constant supply of food while some reptiles can fast for several weeks at a time. This fact has enabled reptiles to colonise niche environments such as hot arid deserts and also enables them to survive hibernation and cold temperatures much better than mammals.

Tortoises, terrapins and turtles

Tortoises, turtles and terrapins are members of the Order Chelonia. (N.B.: In the USA all shelled reptiles are referred to as turtles.) They are characterised by a hard outer shell consisting of a domed upper part called the *carapace* and a flatter ventral part called the *plastron* (Fig. 15.1). The shell forms a bony 'box' that protects the soft internal parts of the body. The shell is covered with horny plates or *scutes*, which are named according to the most adjacent part of the body. The scutes grow from the outside so that an annual ring develops along the periphery of each one, making the overall shell larger. In some species these 'growth rings' can be used to estimate age but as new shell growth may be interrupted by reduced nutrition, seasonal change and hibernation, it is not a reliable method.

Anatomical features

Skeleton

Chelonians are vertebrates and their skeleton resembles that of other vertebrates. However, the pectoral and pelvic girdles are within the rib cage and are orientated vertically to buttress the shell (Fig. 15.1). The ten vertebrae form part of the under surface of the carapace.

When handling reptiles you should be aware that the slow, sluggish creature that you take out of the cage will soon warm up in your hands and may suddenly have the energy to make a dash for freedom!

Cardiovascular system

Chelonians possess the normal reptilian three-chambered heart and renal portal system. The outer shell of chelonians makes auscultation of the heart difficult, but it may be aided by putting a damp towel around the shell.

Intravenous injection or blood sampling may be carried out by using the jugular vein in the neck or the dorsal venous sinus, which is in the midline of the tail on the dorsal surface.

Respiratory system

The rigid outer shell of chelonians prevents the body wall from expanding during breathing. Respiration is accomplished with the aid of limb and head movements, which move in and out and alter the internal pressure in the body cavity. Chelonians breathe through their external nares or nostrils, so mouth breathing may indicate a respiratory problem. The glottis lies at the base of the tongue, and the trachea is short, which allows the tortoise to breathe when the neck is withdrawn. The lungs are positioned dorsally, below the carapace, and aid buoyancy in aquatic species (Fig. 15.1).

Digestive system

Chelonians do not have teeth and depend on their horny beak to cut off pieces of food. They have large, fleshy tongues that cannot protrude from the mouth. The oesophagus runs down the left side of the neck and joins the stomach, which lies transversely across the body (Fig. 15.2). The small intestine is relatively short (compared to mammals) and the colon ends in the *cloaca*, which is the common chamber into which the urogenital and digestive systems empty.

Stomatitis or 'mouth rot' is an infection of the oral cavity and is a very common condition of chelonians and snakes. This condition is often triggered by factors such as stress, trauma, malnourishment and poor husbandry. It is commonly seen in chelonians following hibernation and is often the cause of post-hibernation anorexia syndrome.

Urogenital system

In chelonians the ureters conduct relatively unconcentrated urine from the kidneys into a thin-walled urinary bladder (Fig. 15.2). Male chelonians possess a single, large penis that protrudes from the floor of the cloaca.

Sexual differentiation

Most species of Chelonia are sexually dimorphic: there are visible differences in external features such as colouration, tail length, shell size and shape. Features include:

- Male tortoises have longer tails than females (Fig. 15.3).
- The plastron of the male is concave to enable him to mount the domed carapace of the female.
- The caudal scute of the female may be curved upwards to allow her to elevate her tail during mating.
- The male terrapin has longer front claws than those of the female.

Lizards

Lizards belong to the Suborder Sauria, which includes about 3750 different species classified into 19 families.

Anatomical features

Skeleton

The skeleton of the lizard follows the basic vertebrate plan, but there is no sternum (Fig. 15.4). Most lizards have four legs and most species take their weight on all their legs; however, some species, such as the basilisk, can run on two legs. The anatomy of the limbs indicates the mode of locomotion.

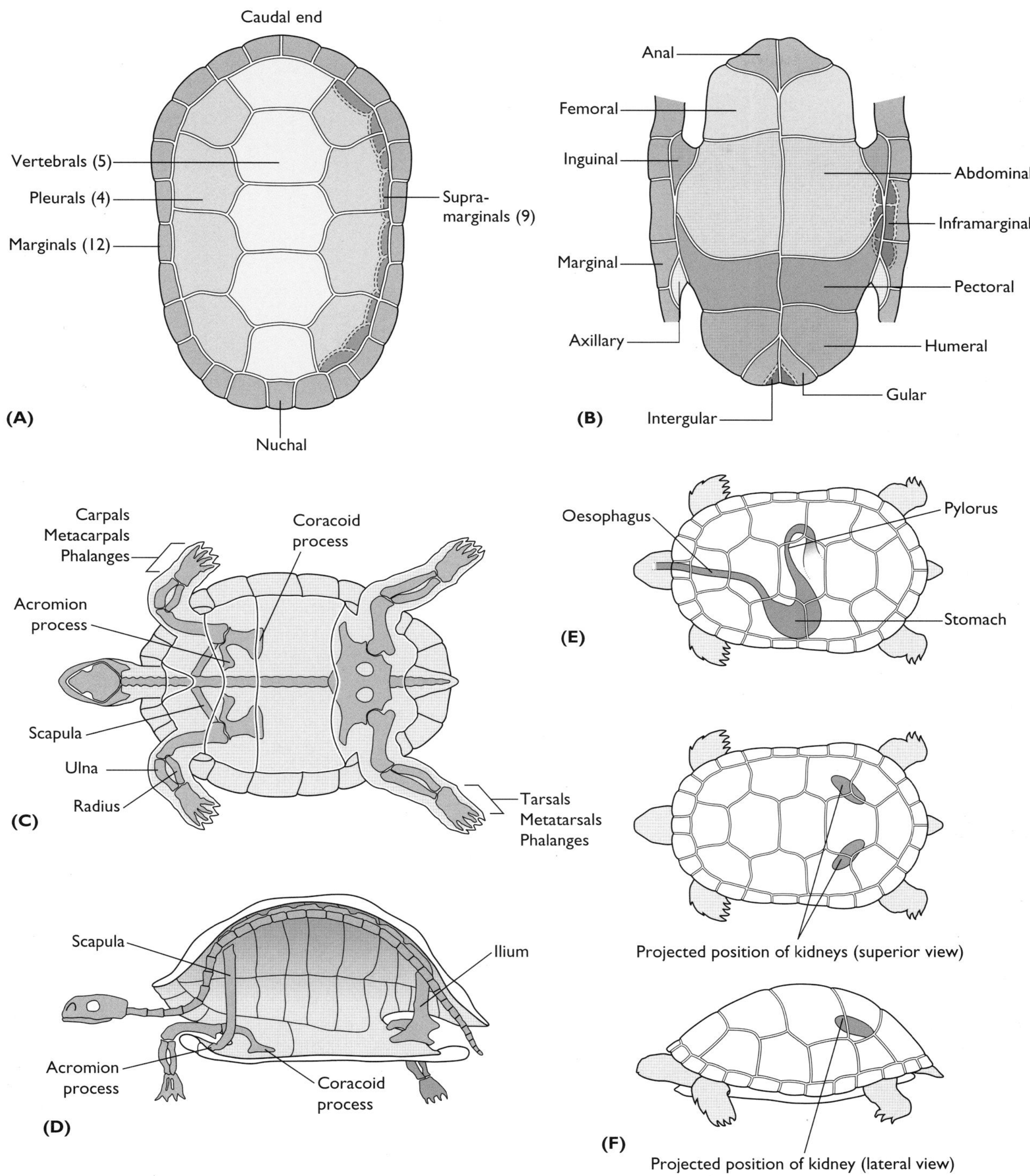

Fig. 15.1 Anatomy of the tortoise (*Testudo* spp.). **(A)** Carapace. **(B)** Plastron. **(C)** Ventral view of skeleton. **(D)** Left side view of skeleton. **(E)** First part of intestinal tract. **(F)** Position of the kidneys.

Many species of lizard show *autotomy*. This is the ability to shed their tail as a defence against predators. Once shed, the tail keeps squirming and distracts the predator while the lizard runs away! A replacement tail may grow but it is often a different colour and may be shrunken; internally the replacement vertebrae are cartilaginous rather than bony. If a lizard is stressed or if the tail is damaged it may fall off; this must be considered when handling or injecting into the tail muscle. As a result of autotomy the tail muscles go into spasm and prevent excessive blood loss.

Integument

Lizards have thick, scaly skin and grow by shedding the skin (*ecdysis*). In lizards the skin comes off in pieces and some species will eat the sloughed pieces. The family Skinkidae – the skinks – shed their skin in one piece; they are covered in scales that fit tightly together, producing a smooth streamlined outline. Some species of lizard, such as chameleons, are able to change the colour of their skin. This is due to the presence of *chromatophores* in the skin and helps to camouflage the lizard. Members of the

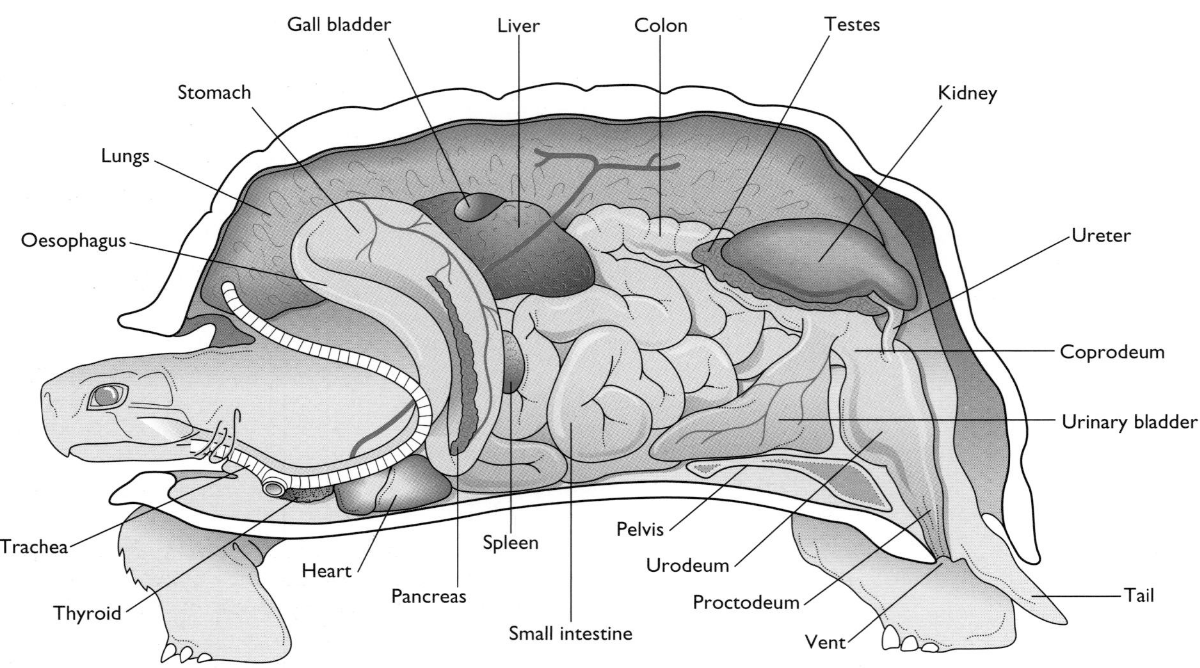

Fig. 15.2 Internal anatomy of the tortoise.

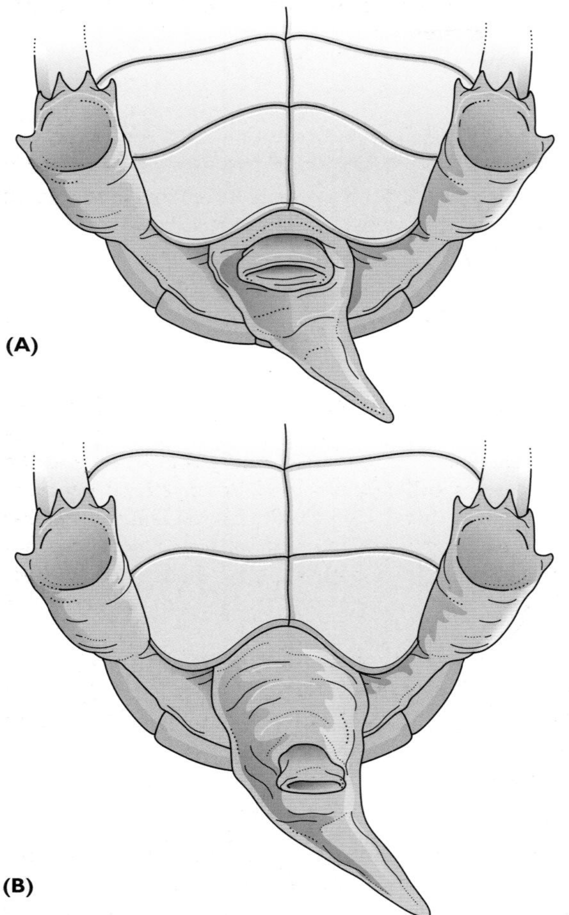

Fig. 15.3 Determining the sex of chelonians. **(A)** Female. **(B)** Male. The tail of the male is longer, the plastron is concave and the cloacal opening is further down on the tail.

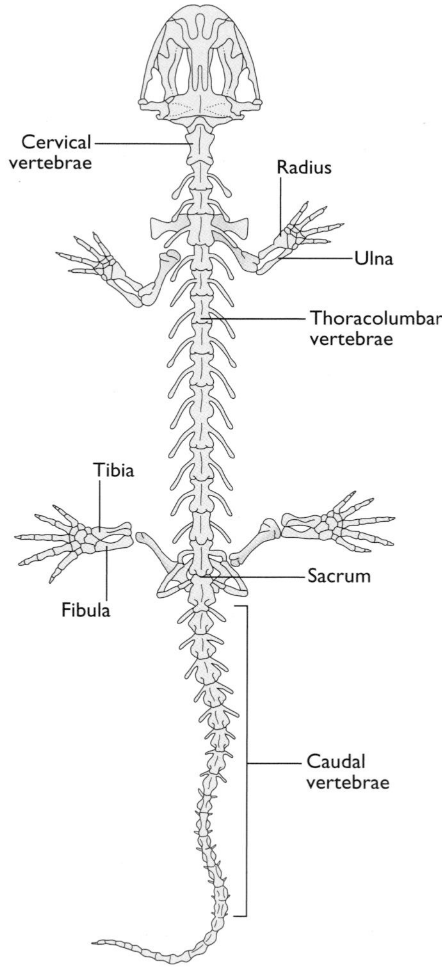

Fig. 15.4 Skeleton of a lizard.

family Gekkonidae – the geckos – are characterised by having layers of overlapping scales or *lamellae* on the underside of their feet. This enables them to grip on to apparently smooth surfaces such as glass.

Special senses

The *ear* is responsible for both hearing and balance. The tympanic membrane is easily visible in a shallow depression on the side of the head and is covered by a thin layer of skin that is shed periodically with the rest of the skin. The *eye* is protected by an eyelid in most species of lizard and in some species the lower lid is transparent to allow vision even when the lids are closed.

Cardiovascular system

Lizards possess the typical reptilian *three-chambered heart* and the *renal portal system* as previously described. They have a large ventral abdominal vein and care must be taken when making a midline incision.

Intravenous injection or blood sampling may be carried out by using the ventral venous sinus, which lies in the midline of the ventral surface of the tail but it should not be used in species that are able to shed their tail. In larger species the cephalic vein on the forelimb may be used; in smaller species enough blood for a blood smear may be collected by clipping a toe nail.

Respiratory system

The diaphragm is absent and breathing is accomplished by expansion and contraction of the ribs. In addition various species of lizard also use their lungs, which are highly flexible, for display, threat, buoyancy and vocalization.

Digestive system

Lizards do not chew their food but tear it off in pieces that are of a swallowable size. Most lizards possess simple conical *teeth*, which do not sit in sockets as they do in mammals and which may be pleurodontic or acrodontic:

- *Pleurodonts*: The teeth that are attached to the inner sides of the mandible. Species include the Iguanidae. These teeth are regularly shed and then replaced.
- *Acrodonts*: The teeth are attached to the biting edges of the mandible. Species include chameleons and agamids. These teeth are not shed but wear with age.

The *tongue* is used to 'taste' the environment in conjunction with *Jacobsen's organ* in the roof of the mouth.

The digestive tract of lizards varies depending on the type of diet, which may be insectivorous, carnivorous, herbivorous or omnivorous depending on the species (Fig. 15.5). The *stomach* is simple and elongated, and a *caecum* is present in herbivorous species. The digestive tract terminates in the typical reptilian *cloaca*.

Urogenital system

Most species of lizard possess a urinary bladder (Fig. 15.5). *Male* lizards possess paired copulatory organs called *hemipenes* (Fig. 15.6). Each hemipenis is a hollow structure with a closed end that lies invaginated in the base of the tail, posterior to the cloaca. The hemipenes are stored in an inverted position in the base of the tail. Only one hemipenis is used during copulation and is erected by filling with blood. It is then inserted into the cloaca of the female. The shape of the hemipenes varies with the species. *Female* lizards lay eggs. They have a pair of ovaries and oviducts but there is no uterus. The eggs pass out of the body via the cloaca (Fig. 15.7).

Some species of lizard consist entirely of females and reproduction is by means of *parthenogenesis* in which the young develop from an unfertilised egg; they are all female.

Sexual differentiation

The method of determining the sex of a lizard is dependent on the species.

- *Sexual dimorphism*: Many species show differences in shape and colour between the two sexes. Males may also show display patterns such as flashing colours or the use of erectable crests to attract the female.
- *Base of the tail*: Males may have a more swollen base to their tail, inside which lie the hemipenes.
- *Presence of femoral or preanal pores* (Fig. 15.8): Different species show various patterns of pores on the inner surface of the inguinal region.

Snakes

Snakes belong to the Suborder Serpentes, which includes around 2400 species divided between 11 different families.

Anatomical features

Skeleton

Snakes are legless and have an elongated body (Fig. 15.9). They have a complex skull, which is described as being *kinetic*; this means that the bones of the jaw are loosely connected and the two halves of the mandible are joined by an elastic ligament to allow wide separation (Fig. 15.10). These features enable the snake to ingest large items of prey. Snakes do not have thoracic limbs but a few possess vestigial pelvic limbs, seen as external spurs in the pelvic region of species such as boas and pythons.

The snake has many *vertebrae* – numbers vary from 150 to over 400 – all with a similar shape. Each vertebra gives off a pair of ribs, which are fused to the vertebra but are not joined in the ventral midline; there is no sternum.

Integument

The epidermal scales of the integument show differences according to the region of the body. In the dorsal and lateral parts of the body the scales are small and on the ventral surface they are larger and thicker. The tough, smooth skin of the snake does not grow with the snake but is shed periodically, usually in one piece to reveal a new skin underneath (*ecdysis*). At the time

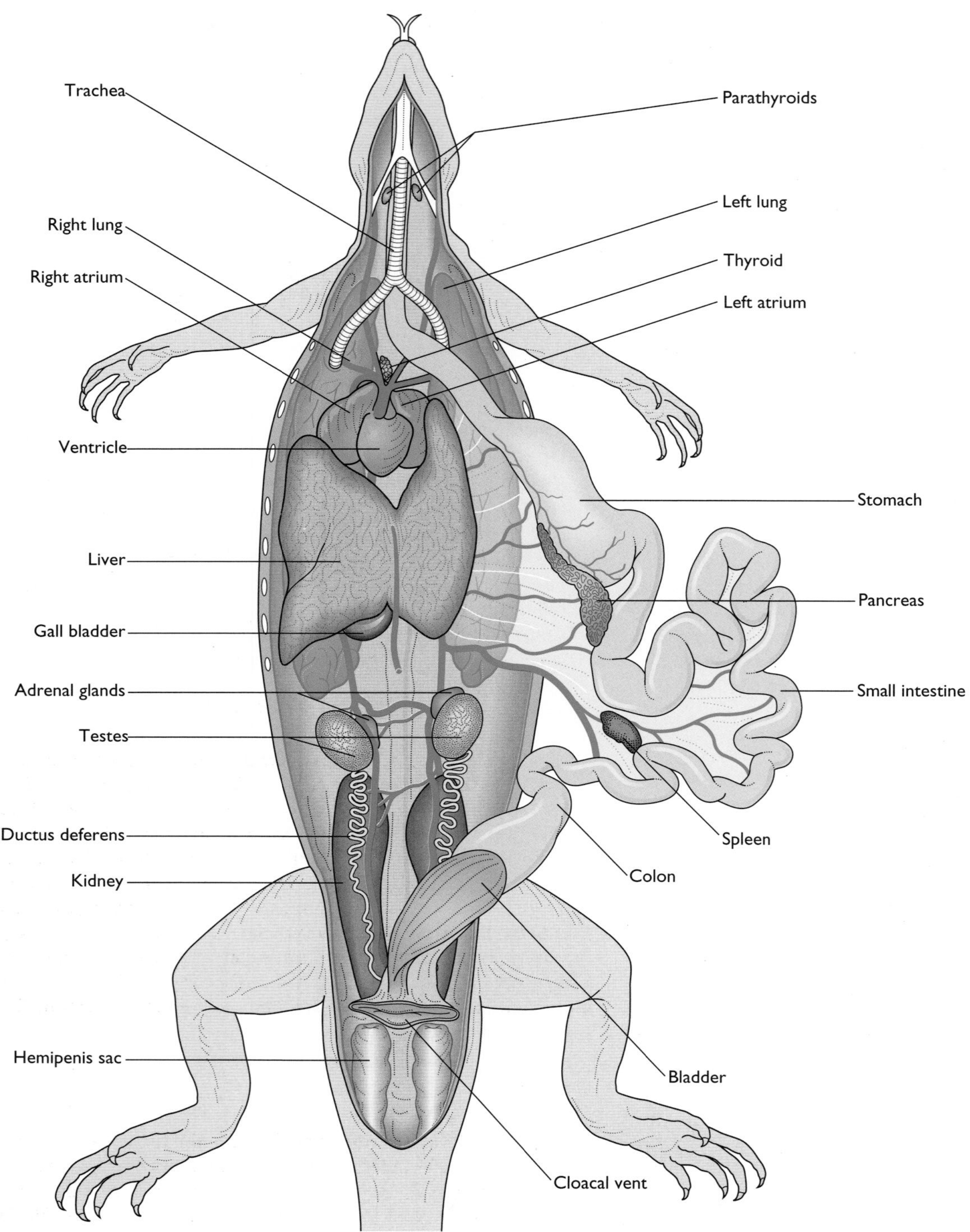

Fig. 15.5 Internal anatomy of a lizard.

of shedding the snake skin may have a dull appearance caused by the lifting of the old outer layer of skin. Snakes do not have moveable eyelids, as are seen in mammals, but the upper and lower eyelids are fused together to form a transparent *spectacle* over the cornea. During ecdysis the spectacle becomes cloudy prior to being shed along with the rest of the skin. Just before shedding the snake may be withdrawn and anorexic and handling should be kept to a minimum.

Special senses

The eyes are protected by the spectacle lying over the surface of the cornea. Tear-like secretions are produced between the cornea and spectacle. The ear of the snake has no tympanic membrane and no middle ear cavity. Some species of snake, such as members of the family *Boidae* – the boas – have heat-sensitive pits on the upper jaw that are used to detect their prey. These are so sensitive that they can pick up heat changes of 0.001°C.

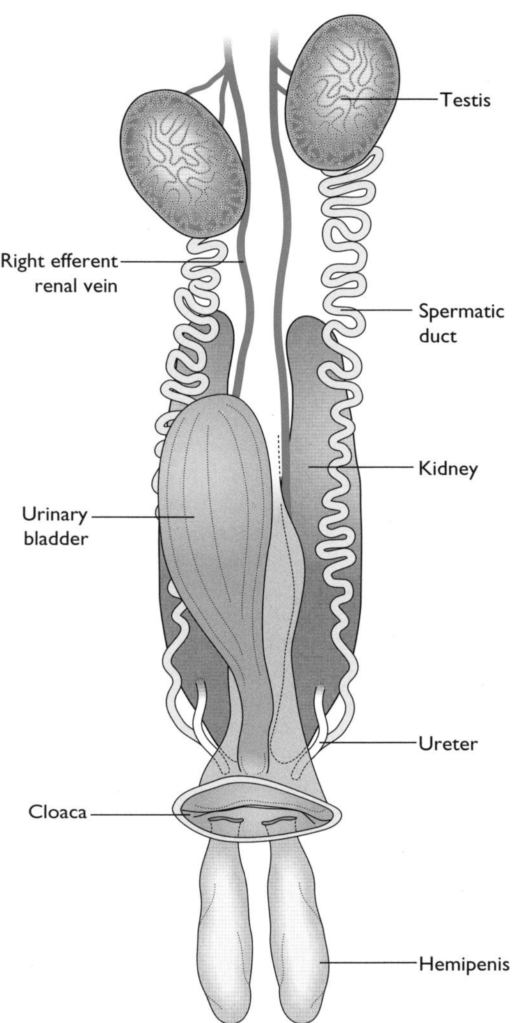

Fig. 15.6 Urogenital system of a male lizard.

Cardiovascular system

Snakes possess the typical reptilian *heart*, and have both *renal* and *hepatic portal* circulations. The heart is generally located at about one third of the length of the body (Fig. 15.11).

Intravenous injection or blood sampling may be carried out by using the ventral venous sinus in the midline of the tail. The jugular vein may also be used but this may require a small incision to visualise it.

Respiratory system

In most snakes the *left lung* is greatly reduced in size or even absent (Fig. 15.11). Only the anterior part of the lung is functional for gaseous exchange. The posterior part is avascular and functions as an air sac that may act as a reserve during periods of apnoea.

Digestive system

Snakes are totally carnivorous and possess six rows of undifferentiated *teeth*, which are replaced continuously (Fig. 15.10). Some

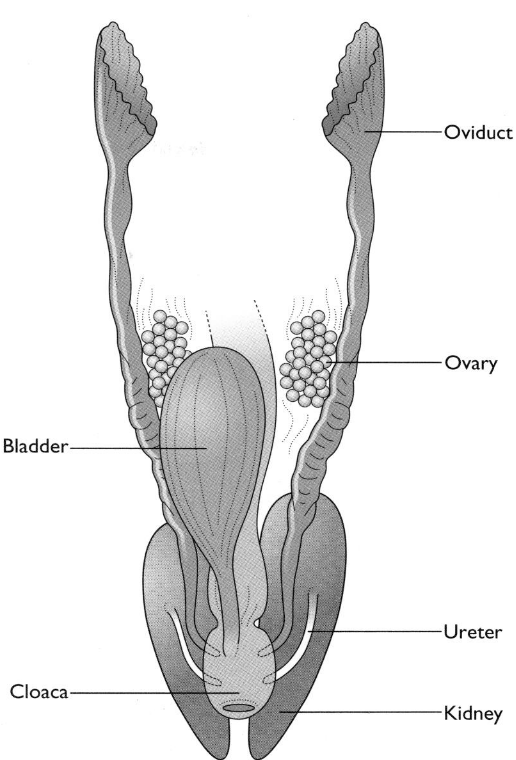

Fig. 15.7 Urogenital system of a female lizard.

species may have modified *fangs* and some are able to produce *venom* from special glands that lie above the oral cavity. The venom is delivered to the prey by the fangs. The *tongue* is thin, forked and mobile and is able to protrude some distance out of the mouth. It is used for olfaction – the snake 'tastes' the environment and the tongue is then brought into contact with *Jacobsen's organ* in the roof of the mouth and information is conveyed by a branch of the olfactory nerve to the brain. Because the body of the snake is long and thin the organs are arranged along its length rather than across the body (Fig. 15.11). The *stomach* is elongated but the *intestines* are relatively short, reflecting the carnivorous diet.

Urogenital system

There is no urinary bladder in snakes and the ureters empty into the *urodeum* section of the *cloaca*. Male snakes possess invaginated *hemipenes* that lie in the base of the tail just caudal to the vent. The hemipenis evaginates into the cloaca of the female to transmit sperm during copulation. Females of very slender species of snake have only one oviduct and ovary.

Sexual differentiation

The method used to determine the sex of a snake depends on its species.

- *Sexual dimorphism*: In some species it is possible to differentiate between the sexes by looking at the colour and the markings.
- *Tail length*: The tail is measured from the vent (the exit of the cloaca) to the tip of the tail. The male usually has a longer tail

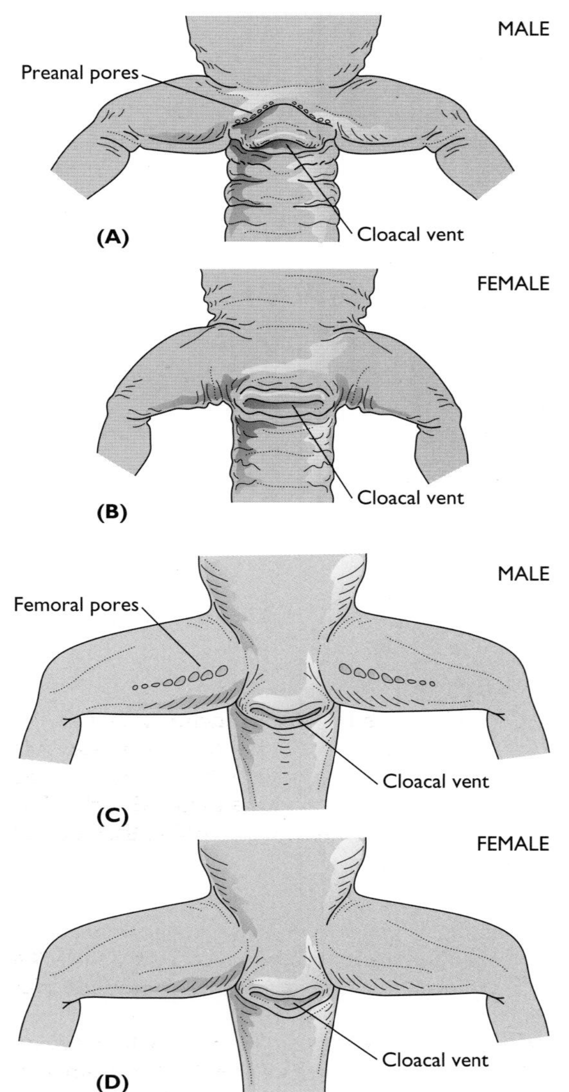

Fig. 15.8 Sexual differentiation in lizards. **(A, B)** Geckos: males have anal or preanal pores in the inguinal region. **(C, D)** Agamas: males have femoral pores.

than the female and the area around the vent may be noticeably swollen. This area houses the hemipenes.

- *Size*: In some species the female is larger than the male.
- *Use of a probe*: This requires experience and great care. A well-lubricated blunt-ended rod is carefully introduced into the cloaca pointing towards the tail. In the male, the probe will travel a longer distance down the cloaca than it does in the female.

Fish

Fish are *ectothermic* vertebrates that live and breathe in water and move with the aid of fins. There are over 30,000 species of fish, which makes them the most numerous of vertebrates. They range in size from the tiny Philippine Island goby, which measures less than 1 cm, to the whale shark, which measures up to 16 m. There are two groups of jawed fish: the *cartilaginous fish* (sharks and rays) and the *bony fish*, which includes all the ornamental fish likely to be kept in captivity. Within the bony fish is the group known as the *Teleosts*, which comprises 20,000 species divided into the *lower Teleosts*, such as carp, salmon and catfish, and the *higher Teleosts*, such as perch, sticklebacks and mackerel. They are found in a wide range of habitats all over the world. Many groups of fish kept in captivity have been selectively bred (e.g., goldfish), which has led to the development of an enormous range of fins, eyes, colour, tails and size. All teleosts have a similar general structure.

General anatomy

Musculoskeletal system

The *fusiform* shape of a fish makes it streamlined for swimming. Locomotion is facilitated by muscle blocks or *myomeres* arranged on either side of the axial skeleton (Fig. 15.12). This enables the body to bend laterally and generate the propulsive force to move forward. The *cranium* is rigid and articulates with the bones of the jaws and opercula apparatus. The number of *vertebrae* varies; ribs in the thoracic region articulate with the vertebrae and support the lateral walls of the body cavity.

Fish possess *fins*, which are responsible for the fish's ability to manoeuvre and remain stable in the water. The fins consist of tissue stretched between rays, which may be stiff and unjointed or soft with many articulations (Fig. 15.13). The fins are attached to small muscles, which fold or extend the fins to produce rapid precise movements. The shape of the *caudal fin* or *tail* provides an indication of the swimming habits of the fish; for example, a forked tail enables the fish to swim at continuous high speeds, while a truncated tail is seen in slow-moving species but allows them to make fast dashes.

Buoyancy in the water is achieved by a gas-filled *swim bladder* in the body of the fish, below the vertebral column (Fig. 15.14). The specific gravity of the Teleosts is greater than that of the surrounding water so there is a tendency to sink if they remain stationary. By altering the volume of air in the swim bladder the fish can rise and remain in one place – they achieve neutral buoyancy despite pressure changes in the water. The swim bladder has evolved from the primitive lung of the lower Teleosts and is a thin-walled diverticulum of the foregut. The structure varies depending on the species:

- *Lower Teleosts*: The swim bladder is linked via a pneumatic duct to the foregut and is described as being *physostomous*. This type occurs mainly in shallow freshwater species. The swim bladder is refilled by rising to the surface and taking a mouthful of air. In bottom-living species the swim bladder may be reduced, enabling them to feed on the river bed.
- *Higher Teleosts*: There is no connection between the foregut and the swim bladder and the bladder is said to be *physoclistous*. The swim bladder is filled during larval development, when there may be a temporary connection with the gut, or it may be filled by a gas gland within the cells of the sac. The gas, which consists mainly of carbon dioxide, is retained in the sac for life by its impermeable walls.

Swim bladder problems are relatively common in aquarium fish. They present as an inability to float upright, to manoeuvre or to swim below the surface. Unfortunately there is very little treatment for the condition.

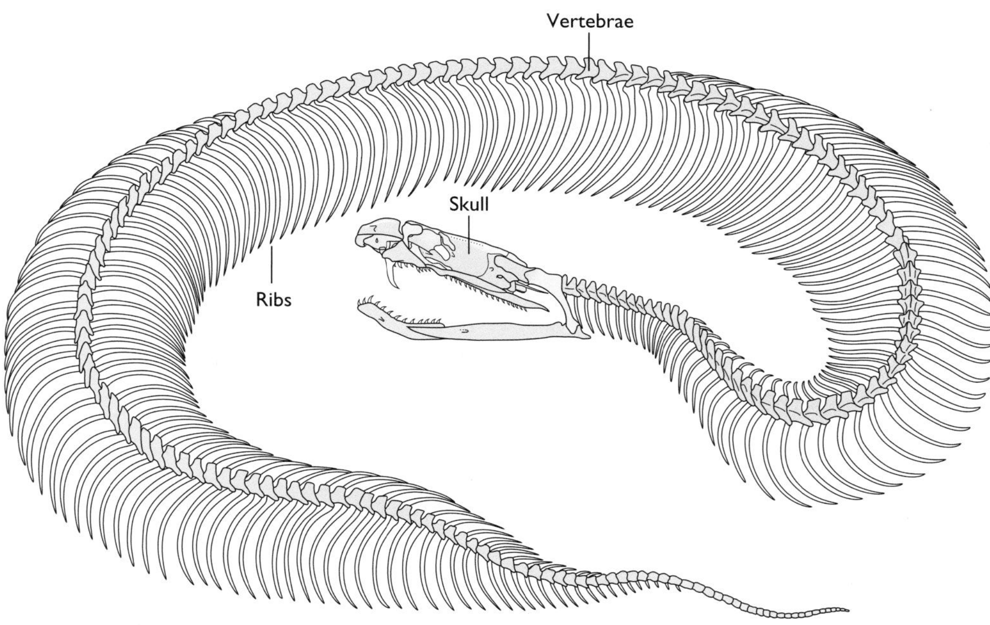

Fig. 15.9 Skeleton of a typical snake.

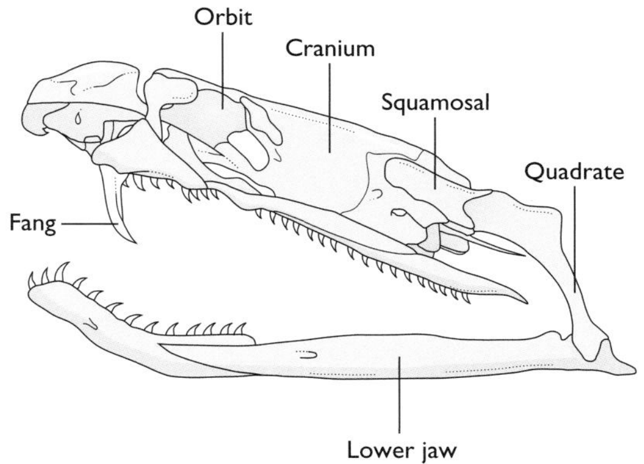

Fig. 15.10 The bones of a snake skull.

Integument

Fish have a scaly skin covered by a layer of *mucus*, which has a fungicidal and bacteriocidal function. Damage to the mucus covering can lead to skin infections and to the formation of ulcers. This layer is referred to as the cuticle or *glycocalyx* and it improves movement through the water by reducing frictional drag. The scales are flexible bony plates on the skin and are arranged like overlapping roof tiles.

Special senses

Teleost fish have the same special senses as mammals: vision, smell, taste, hearing and balance. They also have a *lateral line system* (Fig. 15.13). This consists of a series of shallow channels running over the surface of the body along the lateral midline. At intervals along the line are small clumps of hair cells with tips that are embedded in a gelatinous cup or cupula. If these hair cells are moved by outside vibrations they transmit the information to the brain of the fish, which brings about the appropriate response. The function of the lateral line is to detect disturbance or vibrations in the water caused by objects such as other fish; the lateral line therefore provides a 'touch at a distance' sense. This aids the fish in both the detection of prey in the water and in the avoidance of predators and is thought to be involved in the ability of large shoals to move simultaneously so that they almost behave as one large organism.

Respiratory system

One of the most noteable features of fish is their ability to breathe in water; this is achieved using a specialised system of *gills* (Fig. 15.15).

The gill system involves five lateral *gill slits* on each side of the pharyngeal wall. Each gill consists of a skeletal *gill arch* supporting highly vascularised *gill filaments*. Projecting from these are fine secondary filaments or *lamellae*. At the point where the gill slits open into the pharynx are stiff elongated projections from the gill arch known as *gill rakers*. These act as a screen to protect the delicate gills from particles that could damage them. The gills are covered by protective flaps called the *opercula* (sing. *operculum*). Water is taken in through the mouth and passes over the gills, where gaseous exchange takes place and oxygen passes into the blood. Carbon dioxide passes in the opposite direction and water is forced out through the opercula.

Circulatory system

The heart is a long, folded organ consisting of an atrium and a ventricle. The circulation is described as being *single* (the mammalian circulation is double) because the blood passes through the heart once per circulation. Blood leaves the ventricle and is pumped through the arteries to the gills, where it picks up oxygen. It continues around the body through the other organs, where it picks up nutrients from the digestive system and then delivers oxygen and nutrients to the tissues. In return it collects carbon dioxide and carries this to the gills where it is eliminated. Waste products are also collected and excreted via the kidneys. The blood then flows to the atrium of the heart in the veins.

Fig. 15.11 Internal anatomy of a snake.

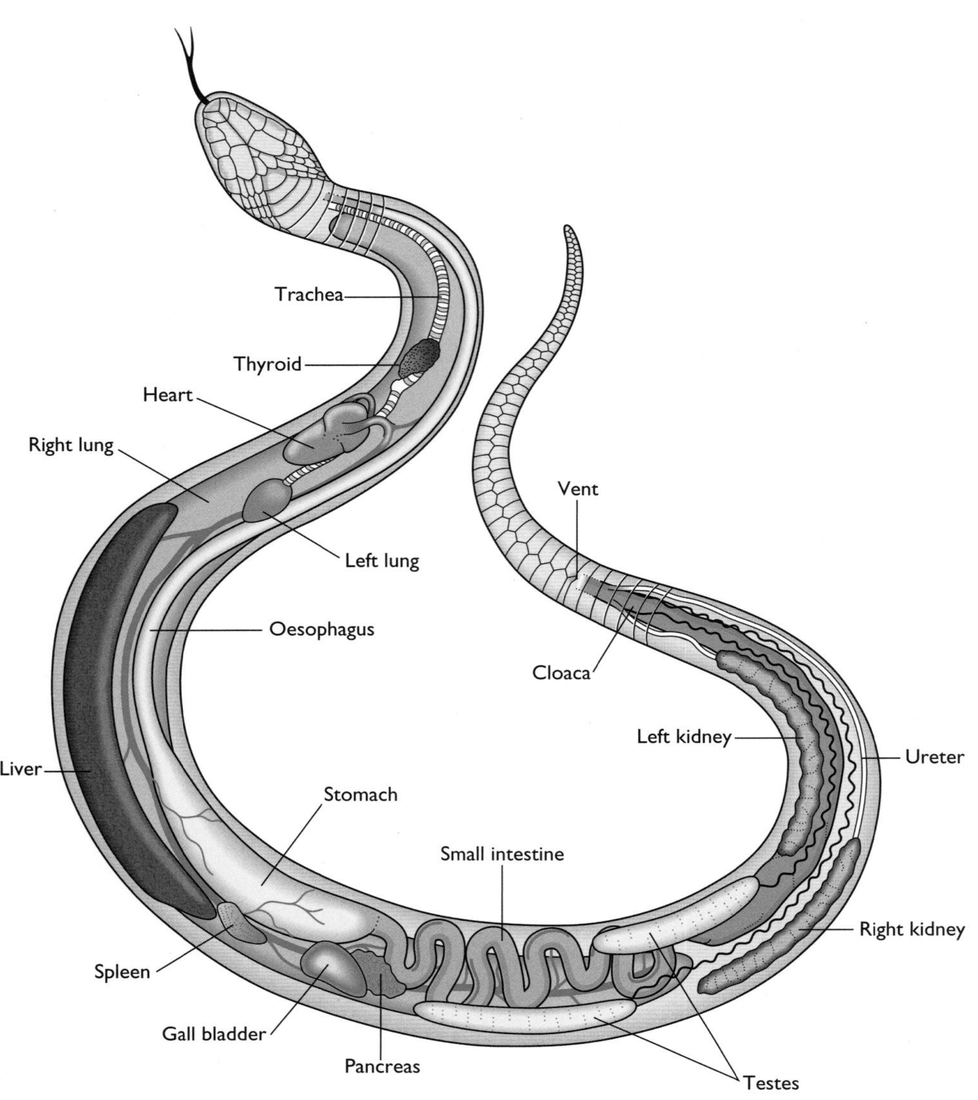

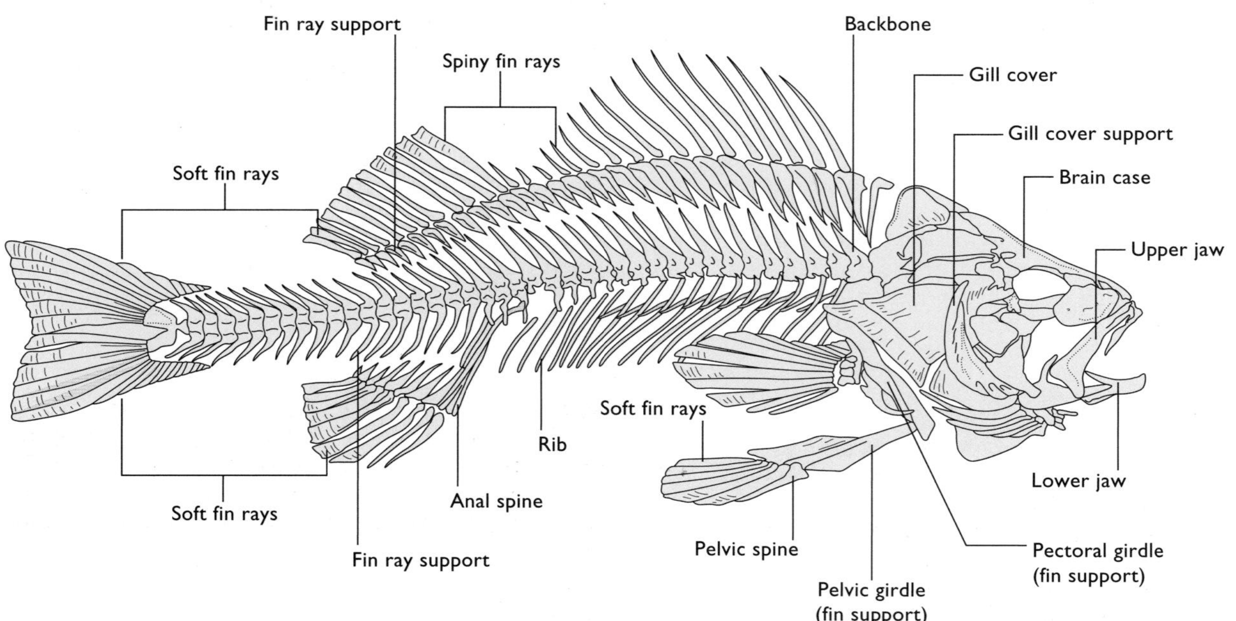

Fig. 15.12 Skeletal structure of a fish.

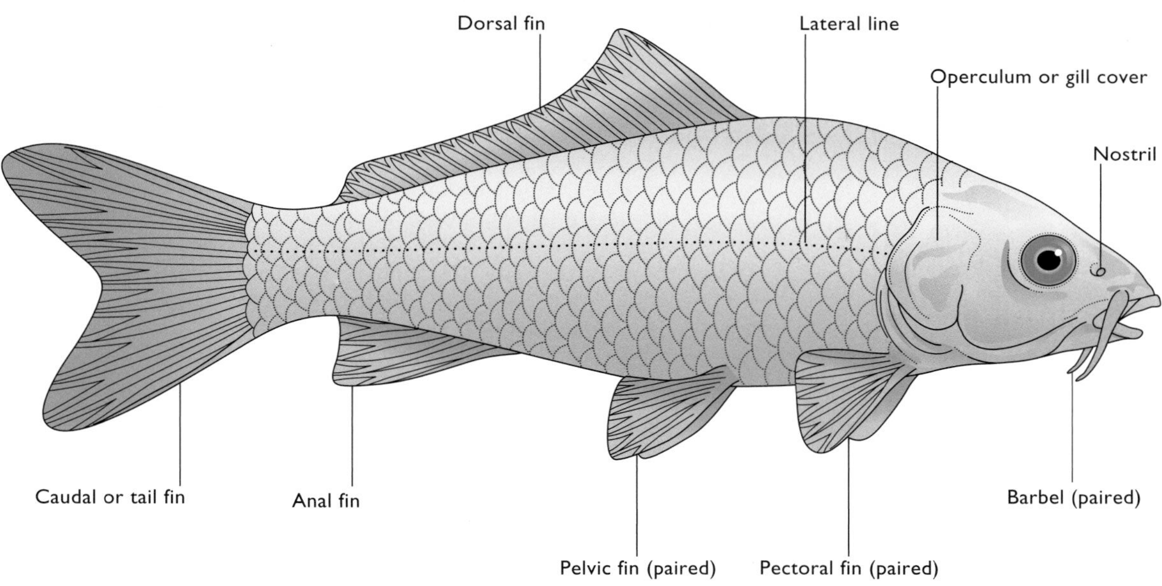

Fig. 15.13 External anatomy of a bony fish.

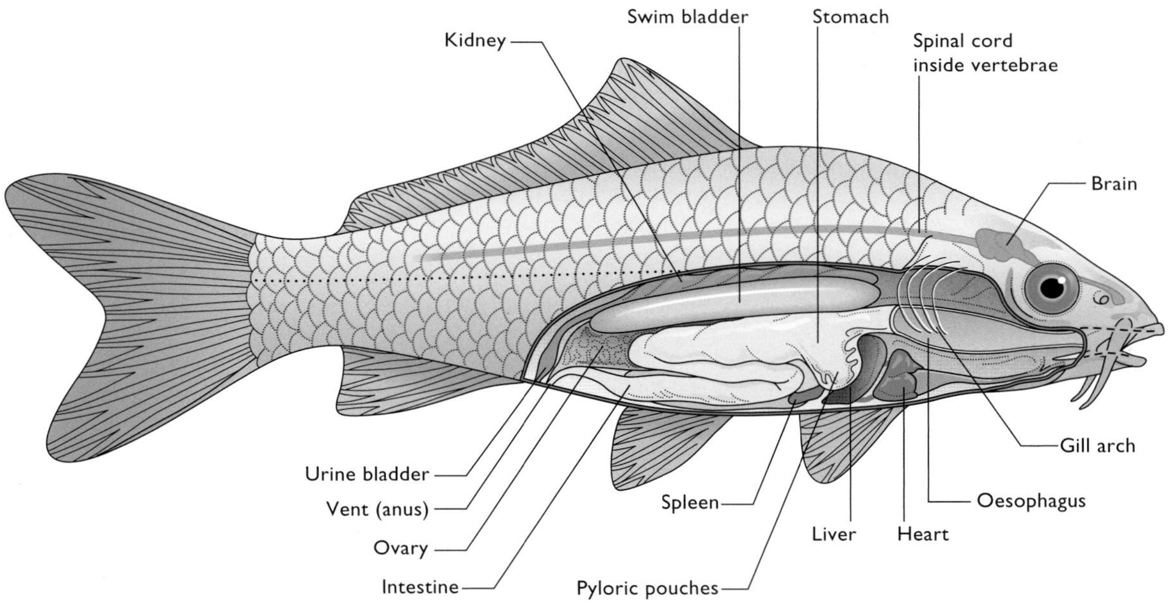

Fig. 15.14 Internal anatomy of a bony fish.

Digestive system

The digestive system of Teleost fish varies according to the type of diet (Fig. 15.14). The method of ingestion depends largely upon suction facilitated by protrusion of the jaws. However, predatory fish have *teeth* on the front of their jaws and the roof of the mouth and also throat teeth just in front of the oesophagus. These are used for catching and holding their prey, which is usually swallowed whole and head first. The *gill rakers* on the inner surface of the gills prevent the food from exiting the mouth through the opercula. Food passes into the *stomach*, which is tube-like, and then into the *intestine*, which is a simple tube of a uniform diameter. The length and structure of the digestive tract varies greatly according to whether the species is a herbivore or carnivore: the gut is longer in herbivorous species than in carnivorous species. Waste materials are evacuated from the *rectum* and *anus*.

Urinary system

The *kidneys* lie ventral to the spine and in some species they may sit like a saddle on the swim bladder (Fig. 15.14). They have a

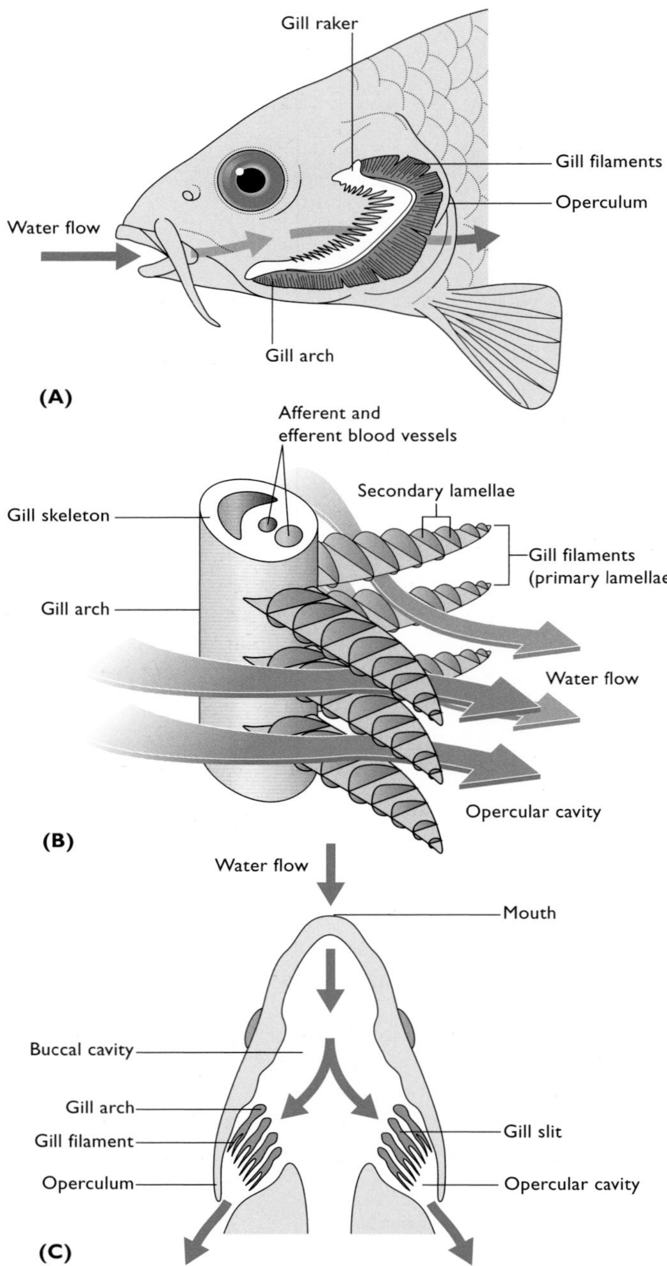

Fig. 15.15 The gill system of a fish. **(A)** Head with the operculum removed. **(B)** Structure of a single gill. **(C)** Horizontal section to show direction of water flow through the buccal cavity.

number of functions including excretion, haemopoiesis and the secretion of hormones.

Osmoregulation varies between freshwater and marine fish. In freshwater, the surrounding water is *hypotonic* so water passes into the body fluids through the gills. The kidney compensates for this and prevents the fish from 'bursting' by excreting large volumes of dilute urine. In the marine environment, the situation is reversed: the surrounding water is *hypertonic*, so water is lost from the body by passive diffusion through the gills. To conserve normal amounts of water within the body the kidney excretes small volumes of concentrated urine.

Nitrogenous waste is excreted by fish in the form of *ammonia*. This is extremely toxic and is only produced in animals that live in a watery environment, which dilutes it. The most important site of nitrogenous excretion in fish is the gills and not the kidneys as in mammals.

Fish kept in a captive environment in the form of a tank must be cleaned out regularly to prevent the ammonia excreted by the kidneys building up and damaging the fish's skin and fins and eventually killing all the tank's inhabitants.

Reproductive system

The majority of Teleosts have separate sexes; however, there is wide diversity in the reproductive patterns and some species may even exhibit parthenogenesis and hermaphroditism. Fertilisation may be:

- *External*: The female lays her eggs in the water and they are fertilised by the male sperm or *milt*; this ritual is known as *spawning*. Very large numbers of eggs are produced because so many are lost to predators and in the moving water. The eggs may be scattered, deposited in nests or buried in the mud at the bottom. Mouth brooders collect the fertilised eggs in their mouth until they hatch, after which the young may use the open mouth as a refuge.
- *Internal*: This is seen in live-bearing species such as guppies, platies and swordtails. The male possesses a *copulatory organ*, usually a modified anal fin, to introduce his sperm into the female, which retains the fertilised eggs in her body. The modified fin is known as a *gonopodium* and is a means of identifying the male. The female stores the milt in her oviduct for several months and several broods can be produced from a single mating. The young may be nourished within her body (*viviparous*) or the eggs may hatch and the live young are then expelled (*oviviparous*).

CHAPTER 16

The horse

Catherine Phillips

The horse appeared in its earliest form 55 million years ago as *Eohippus*, a small, multitoed mammal about 30 cm high. It had four toes on the forelimb and three on the hind limb and a weight-bearing pad under the central toe on each foot. Its teeth were capable of chewing succulent leaves. During its evolution over a period of many millions of years the number of toes reduced and the central third toe became encased in a simple hoof. This species was sequentially replaced by several others with similar skeletal structures and increasingly efficient teeth suitable for eating grass.

During the Lower Pliocene period 10 million years ago, *Pliohippus*, a fully hoofed animal three times the size of the original *Eohippus*, emerged and, by the time *Homo sapiens* had evolved, it had become *Equus*, a recognisable horse. *Equus* appears to have originally come from North America, then migrated southwards and then spread into Asia, Africa and Europe. It became extinct in the Americas 8000 years ago and the different species of *Equus* developed in Asia, Africa and Europe as a result of the different climates and terrains.

The domestic horse *Equus caballus* is a sociable herd-living animal, which – because its wild ancestors might have fallen prey to many different carnivorous species – still retains its primitive instinct to run. The horse has the ability to move very fast, an aspect that has been further developed by selective breeding. Much of its musculoskeletal system is adapted to speed: the single-hoofed central digit where weight is borne on the toe, the well-developed muscles high up on the hindquarters and the sequences in which the feet are lifted from the ground to bring about the different speeds of locomotion. Because a herd of horses must always be prepared for sudden flight they are reluctant to lie down to sleep, and this has led to the evolution of the suspensory and stay apparatus.

Horses evolved to roam large areas in search of food. This was mainly poor-quality grass, which was eaten constantly (grazed) and digested slowly. The flattened table teeth, which grind the grass into boluses that can be easily swallowed, the long length of intestine providing room for the slow digestive progress of tough fibrous ingesta and the large caecum and colon designed to provide a chamber for the microbial breakdown of cellulose in the plant cell walls all enabled the horse to colonise and survive in its ecological niche.

Much of the anatomy and physiology is similar to that of the dog and this chapter is designed to highlight the differences between these two species, not to describe every aspect in repetitious detail.

The skeletal system

The equine skeleton (Fig. 16.1) consists of two separate sections:

- The axial skeleton comprises the skull, vertebral column, ribs and sternum.
- The appendicular skeleton comprises the bones that form the limbs and include the pelvis, which attaches the hind limb, and the scapula, which attaches the forelimb to the body.

The function of the skeleton is to provide a rigid framework for support, protection and movement. It also provides a storage facility for minerals, principally calcium and phosphorus.

The skull

The equine skull (Fig. 16.2) is made up of approximately 37 fused bones, providing a rigid structure with minimal movement; the only moving part is the temporomandibular joint, which is essential for chewing. The major components of the skull are:

- *Mandible*: forms the lower jaw
- *Maxilla*: forms the upper jaw
- *Incisive bone* or *pre-maxilla*: houses the incisor teeth of the upper jaw
- *Orbit*: the eye socket, formed by contributions from several bones
- *Frontal bone*: forms the forehead
- *Nasal bones*: form the nasal cavity.

The functions of the skull are:

1. To protect the more delicate organs of the head (i.e., brain, eye and inner ear)
2. To provide attachment for the hyoid apparatus, which suspends the tongue and the larynx
3. To provide support for the dentition
4. To provide attachment for the muscles of facial expression
5. To form an opening for the entry of air and food

The vertebral column

The vertebral column extends from the base of the skull to the tip of the tail and consists of approximately 54 individual vertebrae (Fig. 16.1).

The function of the vertebral column is:

1. To form a stiff but flexible rod to support the body
2. To house and protect the spinal cord
3. To provide sites of insertion for muscles
4. To provide a means of attachment for the pelvis and ribs

The vertebrae in the horse (Fig. 16.3) are grouped into regions as they are in the cat and the dog, although the numbers of each vertebra may be different.

Vertebral formula for the dog and cat: C7, T13, L7, S3, Cd 20–23.
Vertebral formula for the horse: C7, T18, L6, S5, Cd15–20.

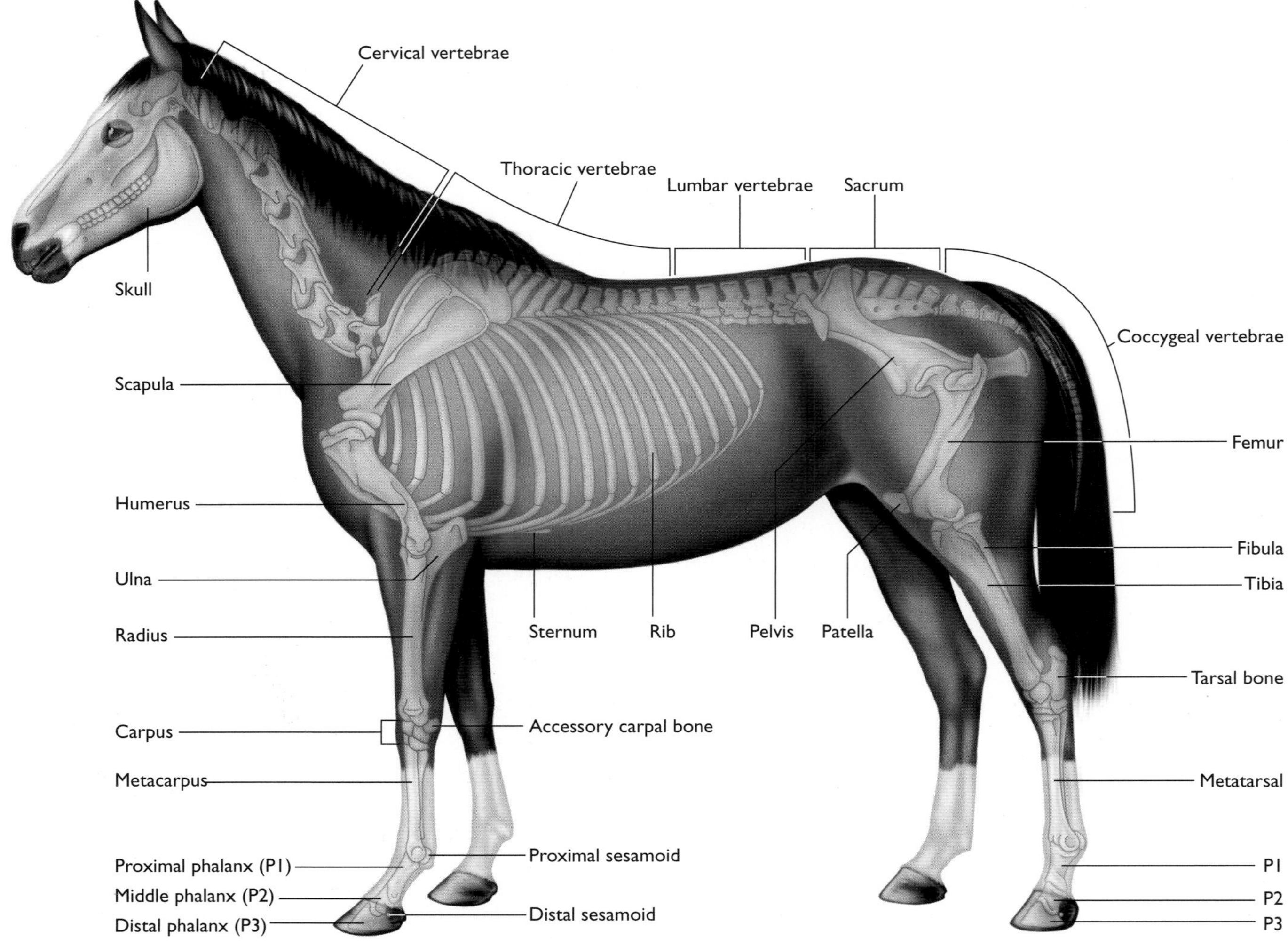

Fig. 16.1 The skeleton of the horse. (With permission from V Aspinall, 2006. The complete textbook of veterinary nursing. London: Butterworth-Heinemann, p. 134.)

The vertebrae (Fig. 16.3) in each region vary in size and shape, which relates to their movement and function.

- *Cervical vertebrae* (7) are found in the neck. The first two are the atlas (C1), distinguished by its large, wing-shaped processes, and the axis (C2), distinguished by a prominent cranial process known as the *dens*. These vertebrae have a large range of motion because they are not inhibited by spinous or transverse processes. The remaining vertebrae (C3–C7) all follow a similar basic pattern (see Chapter 3).

Wobbler syndrome is a developmental condition of the vertebra in the neck presenting commonly as ataxia and/or hind limb paresis and in some cases a tendency to knuckle over in the fetlocks, particularly of the back legs. It is particularly seen in young large horses and may be associated with a rapid growth rate. Treatment may include addressing the animal's nutrition and in some cases cervical surgery may be tried.

- *Thoracic vertebrae* (18) form the dorsal boundary of the thoracic cavity. The first 7–8 vertebrae are covered and protected by the scapula. The thoracic vertebrae have large spinous processes, of which T4–T9 make up the *withers* of the horse. The transverse processes have small accommodating facets allowing for the connection of the ribs. The spinous processes make dorsoventral flexion restricted and lateral flexion minimal. It is the thoracic vertebrae in combination with the muscles that lie beneath that support the rider's weight.
- *Lumbar vertebrae* (5–7; normally 6) are located in the loin area and play a role in the protection of the kidneys. The vertebrae possess large transverse processes, which restrict lateral movement. The spinous processes are much smaller than those of the thoracic vertebrae; however, dorsoventral flexion still remains limited.
- *Sacral vertebrae* (5 fused to form the sacrum) are found in the croup area at the root of the tail. Fusion of the vertebrae in this area means that movement is highly restricted. The pelvis is attached to the sacrum by an interosseous ligament, which forms the sacroiliac joint.
- *Coccygeal or caudal vertebrae* (15–20; average 18) have a basic shape with very small spinous and transverse processes. Towards the end of the tail the vertebrae are little more than rods, which allows great mobility of the tail.

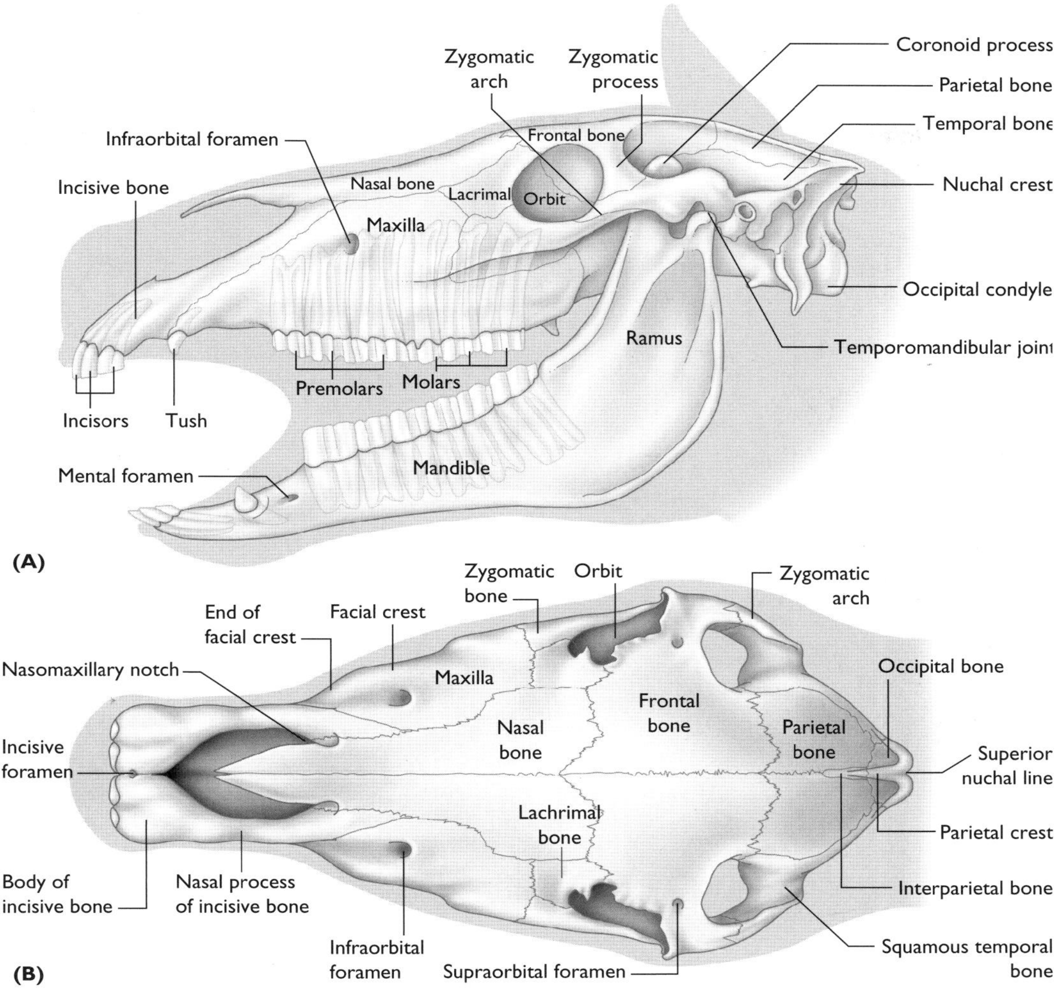

Fig. 16.2 The equine skull. **(A)** Lateral view. **(B)** Dorsal view. (With permission from V Aspinall, 2006. The complete textbook of veterinary nursing. London: Butterworth-Heinemann, p. 135.)

The ribs and sternum

The horse has 18 ribs, although this may vary in some individuals (Fig. 16.1). The ribs play an essential role in housing and protecting the vital internal organs of the thorax. The ribs may be separated into two groups:

- The first eight ribs are the 'true' or 'sternal' ribs (i.e., those that are attached directly to the sternum).
- The final ten ribs are the 'false' or 'asternal' ribs (i.e., those that are attached via cartilage or through one another to the sternum). These form the costal arch.

The appendicular skeleton

The forelimb

Like the dog, the horse has no clavicle or bony connection between the thorax and the forelimbs, which are merely attached by muscular slings, allowing for shock absorption during locomotion.

The bones of the forelimb (Fig. 16.4) are:

- *Scapula* is a large, flat, triangular bone. The scapular spine divides the bone down the middle, each side allowing for the insertion and attachment of the supraspinatus and infraspinatus muscles. A wing of cartilage lies at the proximal end, allowing for further attachment of muscle and connection with the thoracic sling. The scapula meets with the humerus to form the shoulder joint.
- *Humerus* articulates with the scapula and the radius and ulna at the shoulder and elbow joint respectively. The angle at which it lies allows for great shock absorption during movement (Fig. 16.1). The humerus is one of the strongest bones in the equine body.
- *Radius and ulna* are fused in the horse. All equine species bear weight on digit 3, which is the central digit of the primordial pentadactyl limb. The weight is then carried up the strong, single fused bone. The olecranon process at the proximal end of the ulna forms the point of the elbow. The radius, which lies on the medial side of the fused bone, bears most of the weight (Fig. 16.4).
- *Carpus* (Fig. 16.5), known as the *knee*, is made up of eight small bones arranged in two rows. This arrangement further assists in the absorption and distribution of the concussion that travels up the horse's forelimb.

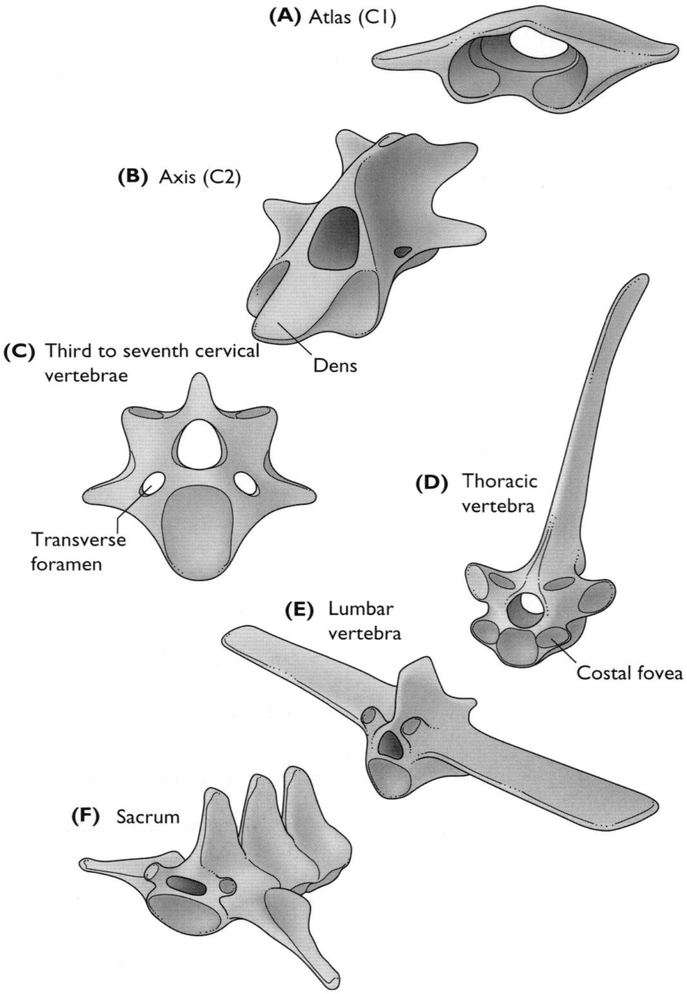

(A) Atlas (C1)
(B) Axis (C2)
(C) Third to seventh cervical vertebrae
Dens
Transverse foramen
(D) Thoracic vertebra
(E) Lumbar vertebra
Costal fovea
(F) Sacrum

Fig. 16.3 The shape of each vertebral type. **(A)** Atlas – CI. **(B)** Axis – C2. **(C)** C3–C7. **(D)** Thoracic vertebra. **(E)** Lumbar vertebra. **(F)** Sacrum.

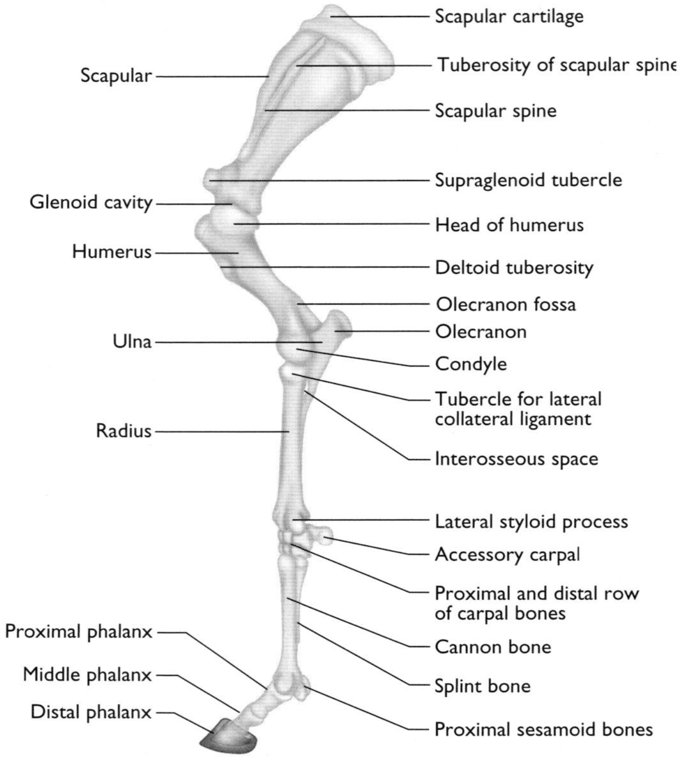

Scapular cartilage
Scapular
Tuberosity of scapular spine
Scapular spine
Supraglenoid tubercle
Glenoid cavity
Head of humerus
Humerus
Deltoid tuberosity
Olecranon fossa
Olecranon
Ulna
Condyle
Tubercle for lateral collateral ligament
Radius
Interosseous space
Lateral styloid process
Accessory carpal
Proximal and distal row of carpal bones
Proximal phalanx
Cannon bone
Middle phalanx
Splint bone
Distal phalanx
Proximal sesamoid bones

Fig. 16.4 The equine forelimb. (With permission from V Aspinall, 2006. The complete textbook of veterinary nursing. London: Butterworth-Heinemann, p. 136.)

Radius
Intermediate carpal bone
Accessory carpal bone
Ulnar carpal bone
III carpal bone
IV carpal bone
III metacarpal bone
IV metacarpal bone
(A)
Radius
Intermediate carpal bone
Radial carpal bone
Ulnar carpal bone
III carpal bone
IV carpal bone
III metacarpal bone (canon)
II metacarpal bone (medial splint)
IV metacarpal bone (lateral splint)
(B)

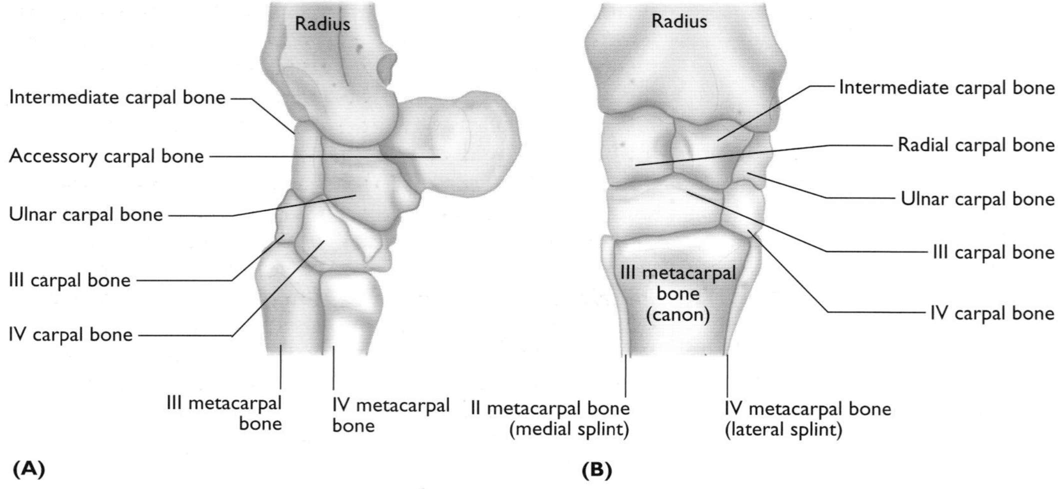

Fig. 16.5 The equine carpus. (With permission from V Aspinall, 2006. The complete textbook of veterinary nursing. London: Butterworth-Heinemann, p. 136.)

The carpus is the equivalent of the human wrist and the bones are arranged as follows:
   - *Upper row*: runs from the medial to lateral surfaces – radial carpal, intermediate, ulnar and accessory carpals. The accessory carpal bone lies behind the ulnar carpal and does not directly bear weight.
   - *Lower row*: These bones simply relate to the metacarpals which lie distal to them and are numbered from II to IV running from medial to lateral.
- *Metacarpals*: There are three metacarpal bones in the horse, which may be numbered 2–4. Of these the third or large metacarpal, also referred to as the *cannon* bone, is fully developed and is the weight-bearer. Metacarpals 2 and 4 are much smaller and lie on either side of the cannon bone. They are referred to as the *splint bones*.
- *Phalanges* (*pasterns* and *pedal bone*): The horse takes its weight on the equivalent of digit 3 (the dog and cat bear weight on digits 2–5 – digit 1 being the dew claw). Three phalanges form the digit. Starting from the proximal end, the first (proximal) phalanx is known as the *long pastern*, the second (medial) phalanx is the *short pastern* and the third (distal) phalanx is the *pedal bone*, which is encased in the hoof. Vital ligaments and tendons run down and around these bones, providing movement and support (see Fig. 16.9).
   - *Fetlock joint* (*metacarpophalangeal joint*) lies between the cannon bone and the long pastern.
   - *Pastern joint* (*proximal interphalangeal joint*) lies between the long and the short pastern.
   - *Coffin joint* (*distal interphalangeal joint*) lies between the short pastern and the pedal bone and incorporates the *navicular* bone.
- *Sesamoids* (*proximal* and *distal*): There are three sesamoid bones in the lower leg. There are two proximal sesamoids located at the back of the metacarpophalangeal or *fetlock joint* and the distal sesamoid or *navicular bone* lies at the back of the pedal bone and is encapsulated within the hoof. The function of these sesamoids is to act as a pulley system for the tendons that pass over, reducing friction and improving efficiency of movement.

The hind limb

The bones of the hind limb (Fig. 16.6) are as follows.

Pelvis

The pelvic girdle (Fig. 16.7) links the spine and the hind limb and is composed of three large flat bones: the *pubis*, the *ischium* and the *ilium*. The pubis forms the floor of the pelvis with the ischium lying caudal to it. The tuber ischii can be felt at the point of buttock. The ilium is the largest bone in the pelvis and is the upper, almost vertical portion. The *wings* or *tubera sacrales* of the ilium can be felt at the croup and the *tuber coxae* forms the points of the hip. All three bones meet to form the acetabulum or hip socket. The *hip joint* is formed by the head of the femur and the acetabulum.

- *Femur* is a large strong bone that provides a large area for the attachment of major muscles of the hind limb. These are largely responsible for generating power and locomotion in the horse.

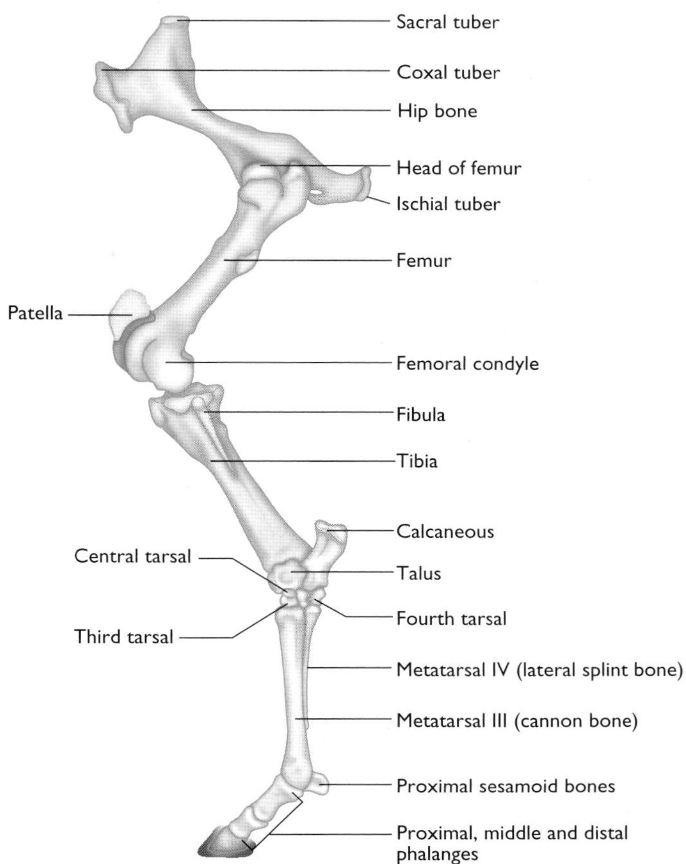

Fig. 16.6 The equine hind limb.

- *Patella* is the equivalent of the human kneecap. It acts as a pulley for the tendons that run over the stifle joint between the femur and the tibia. The *stifle joint* is formed by the distal femur, proximal tibia and patella.
- *Tibia and fibula*: The tibia runs down diagonally from the femur to the hock and is the larger of the two bones allowing for the attachment of the major muscles responsible for the movement of the lower leg. The fibula is much smaller and thinner and lies along the lateral border of the tibia. It tapers to a point at the lower third of the tibia, where it is fused to the tibia.
- *Tarsus* (*hock*) is composed of six small bones, sometimes seven. The bones are arranged in three rows, which are tightly bound by ligaments. The bones of the upper row are the *talus* and the *calcaneus*; the *central tarsus* makes up the middle row; the third row is made up of the first and second tarsal bone, which are fused, and the third tarsal bone. Finally, the fourth tarsal bone is housed in spaces in the middle and lower rows. The body of the calcaneus is extended at its proximal end to form the *tuber calcis* or point of the hock, to which the Achilles tendon is attached.
- *Metacarpals*, *phalanges* and *sesamoids*: The arrangement of the bones distal to the hock follows the same pattern as in the forelimb (Fig. 16.6).

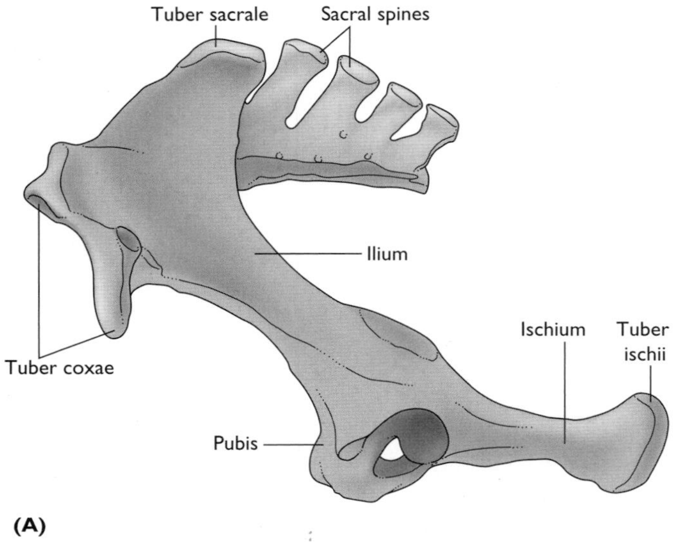

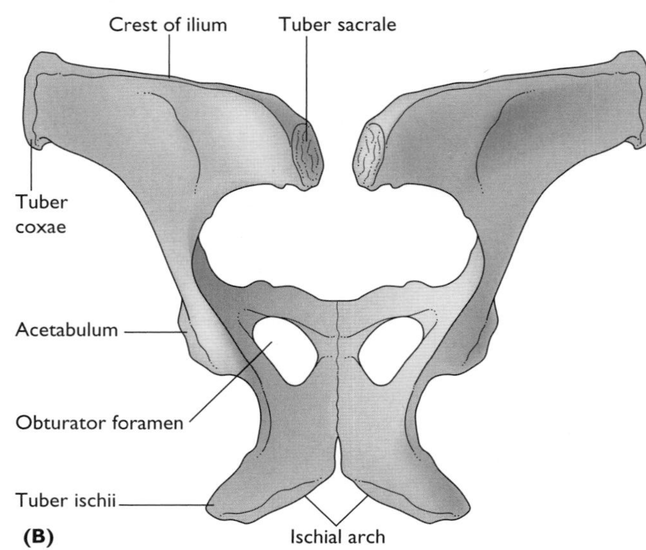

Fig. 16.7 The pelvic girdle of the horse. **(A)** Right lateral view. **(B)** Dorsal view. (After S Sisson, JD Grossman, 1969. Anatomy of the domestic animals, 4th edn. Philadelphia, PA: WB Saunders, pp. 105–106.)

The muscular system

The muscular system is made up of striated muscle that is attached to the skeleton and is under voluntary control. The function of muscle is to bring about movement.

The arrangement of the superficial muscles covering the neck, thorax and abdomen (Fig. 16.8) is similar to that in the dog and cat, with the obvious difference that many are better developed to bring about the rapid locomotion characteristic of the horse.

The limbs of the horse are superbly adapted for speed, although at rest both the fore- and hind limbs support the body. The forelimbs, which should be more or less straight, carry about 60% of the weight and absorb most of the shock during locomotion, especially when landing from a jump. The hind limbs are more angled and provide the main propulsive force. Details of the most significant muscles are shown in Table 16.1.

The hamstring group of muscles – the biceps femoris, semitendinosus and semimembranosus – creates the well-rounded croup area of the body. Their action is to extend the hip and flex the stifle, which provides the main forward thrust and is responsible for the speed of the animal.

Soft tissues of the equine lower leg

The horse is a prey animal and during its evolution it has developed the turn of speed necessary to escape predators. To reduce weight and bulk and improve manoeuvrability, there is little or no muscle below the knee (carpus) and hock (tarsus). The lack of muscle as a protective layer suggests that these structures will be vulnerable to stress and trauma.

The horse has evolved from a three- to four-toed, dog-like animal into the large animal taking its weight on one digit that we recognise today. The central digit is encased in a hoof while the outer toes are reduced to vestigial appendages that no longer reach the ground. This arrangement adds to the horse's ability to run fast.

Ligaments and tendons

Tendons, formed from dense connective tissue, attach muscle to bone. Their function is to harness the pull from muscle contraction that brings about movement. They are less elastic than muscle fibre and have a poor blood supply, which may have an effect on healing.

Important tendons found within the lower leg (Fig. 16.9) include:

- *Deep digital flexor tendon* runs from the deep digital flexor muscle down the back of the limb, over the cannon bone and the proximal and distal sesamoids. It attaches to the third phalanx (P3 or the pedal bone). Its function is to flex the toe.
- *Superficial digital flexor tendon* runs from the superficial digital flexor muscle down the back of the limb, passes over the cannon bone and proximal sesamoids and then splits into two, with one branch attaching to P1 and the other to P2. Its function is to flex the pastern joint.

Rupture of either the deep digital flexor or the superficial digital flexor tendons may be disastrous. The clinical signs include a rising of the toe and a dropping of the fetlock joint.

- *Common digital extensor tendon* runs from the common digital extensor muscle down the front of the limb over the cannon bone and inserts on P1, 2 and 3. Its function is to extend the pastern joint and the toe.
- *Lateral digital extensor tendon* lies on the lateral side of the common digital extensor tendon, running down the limb over the cannon bone and attaching to P1. Its function is to assist in the extension of the pastern joint.

Ligaments attach bone to bone and are similar in structure to tendons. They are relatively less elastic than tendons and, because they also have a poor blood supply, healing may take a long time.

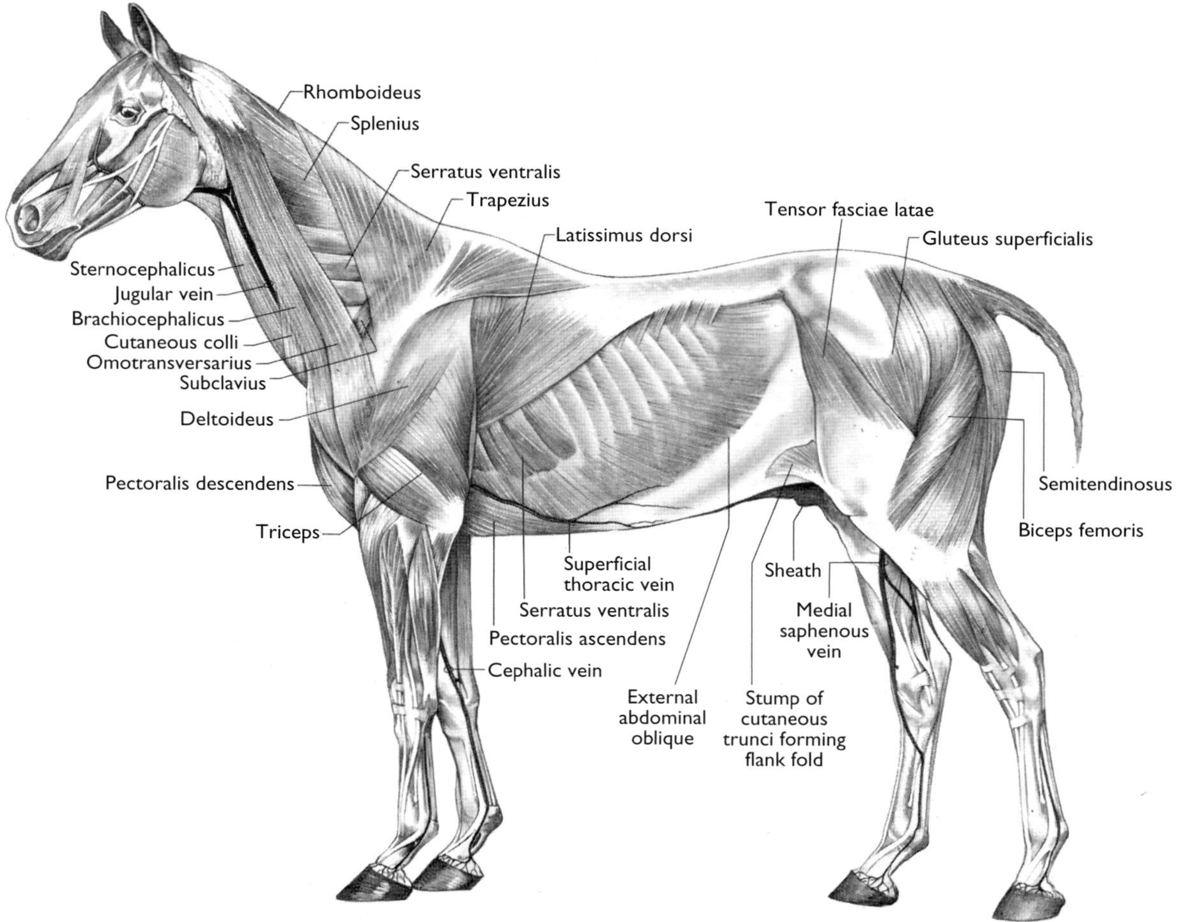

Fig. 16.8 Superficial muscles of the horse. (With permission from KM Dyce, WO Sack, CJG Wensing, 2002. Textbook of veterinary anatomy, 3rd edn. Philadelphia, PA: WB Saunders, p. 570.)

Table 16.1 Important muscles of the horse

Muscle	Action	Origin	Insertion
Brachiocephalicus	Movement of head and neck. Protracts forelimb and extends shoulder	Wing of atlas (first cervical vertebra)	Humerus and shoulder
Sternocephalicus	Movement of head and neck forwards and downwards	Sternum	Mandible
Rhomboideus	Raises shoulder	Nuchal ligament and occipital bone	Scapular (cartilage at proximal end)
Splenius	Elevates and flexes the neck	Behind the poll (at the base of the skull)	Beginning of the trapezius muscle (start of thoracic vertebrae)
Trapezius	Elevates and moves shoulder	Occipital bone, last cervical vertebra (C7) and first 10 thoracic vertebrae (T10)	Spine of the scapula
Longissimus dorsi	Flexes the back and trunk, supports the head and neck (supports the rider's weight)	Ilium, sacrum and thoracic vertebrae	Thoracic vertebrae, last few cervical vertebrae (C4–7), lumbar vertebrae and ribs
Latissimus dorsi	Retracts forelimb and flexes shoulder	Thoracic and lumbar vertebrae	Humerus

Continued

Table 16.1 Important muscles of the horse—cont'd

Muscle	Action	Origin	Insertion
Deltoid	Abducts forelimb, flexes shoulder	Spine of scapula	Proximal humerus
Pectoral	Protracts and retracts forelimb, abducts limb	Sternum	Humerus and scapula
Supraspinatus	Extends forelimb	Scapular spine and cartilage	Proximal humerus, point of shoulder
Infraspinatus	Abducts and rotates forelimb	Scapula, caudal aspect	Humerus
Triceps	Extends elbow	Scapula and humerus	Olecranon process of the ulna
Superficial gluteals	Flexes and extends hip, pulls hind limb towards the body	Tuber coxae of the pelvis	Proximal end of the femur
Biceps femoris	Extends the hip, flexes the stifle and extends the hock	Sacroiliac joint and tuber ischii of the pelvis	Femur, patella and proximal tibia
Semitendinosus	Extends the hip, flexes the stifle and extends the hock	Tuber ischii of the pelvis	Proximal tibia
Semimembranosus	Extends the hip and flexes the stifle	Pelvis	Distal femur and tibia
Gastrocnemius	Flexes the stifle and extends the hock	Femur	Hock

- *Suspensory ligament*, a very important structure, is often referred to as a modified muscle, because it is slightly more elastic than other ligaments and tendons due to the presence of some muscle tissue. The suspensory ligament runs down the back of the limb close to the cannon bone to the level of the proximal sesamoids, where it splits into two. The two branches run either side of the fetlock joint (*metacarpophalangeal joint*) to the front of the limb, connecting with the extensor tendon at the level of P1 (Fig. 16.9). The function of the ligament is to support and suspend the fetlock and prevent over-extension.
- *Medial patella ligaments* originate from the tibial tuberosity and connect to the medial border of the patella. This is a crucial component in the stay apparatus required to lock the equine stifle while resting.

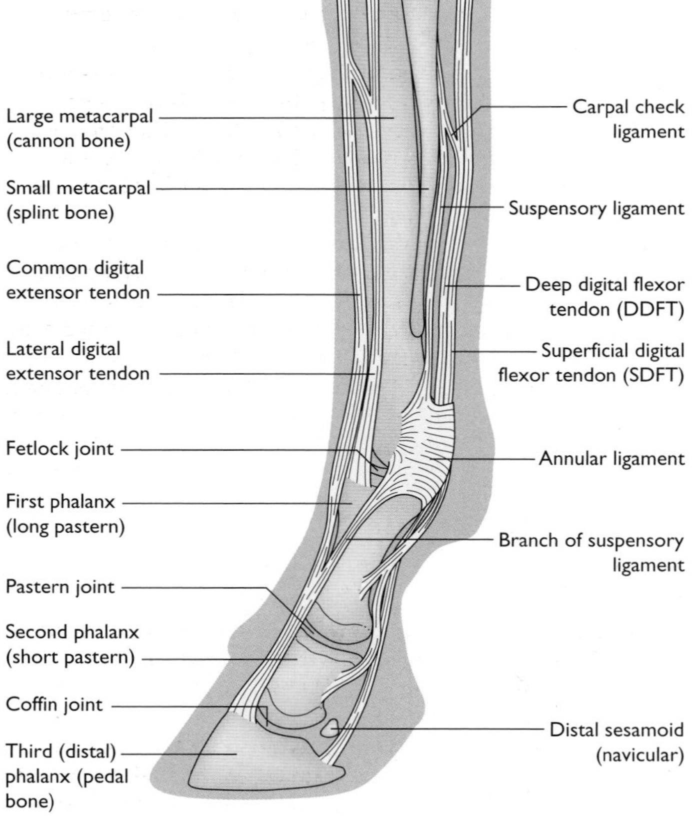

Fig. 16.9 Lateral view of the lower forelimb showing bones, joints, tendons and ligaments.

Upward fixation of the patella is a mechanical condition involving the medial patella ligament. The limb becomes locked in extension and the patient demonstrates lameness in the affected limb.

- *Check ligaments*: There are several in both the fore- and hind limb. They are:
  - Carpal check ligament
  - Radial check ligament
  - Tarsal check ligament

Check ligaments connect ligament to tendon and their function is to prevent strain or over-extension of the joint. The *carpal check ligament* lies just below the carpus and attaches the deep digital flexor tendon to the suspensory ligament, which in turn is attached to the back of the carpus (Fig. 16.9). The *tarsal check ligament* occupies a similar position on the tarsus. The *radial check ligament* lies higher up the forelimb on the back of the distal radius.

The ligaments and tendons in the lower fore- and hind limbs work in conjunction with a variety of muscles to form the *suspensory apparatus* (Fig. 16.10). The function of the suspensory apparatus is to support and suspend the limb and fetlock joint and prevent over-extension and collapse of the limb. It consists of the *suspensory*, *intersesamoidean*, *collateral sesamoidean* and *distal sesamoidean* ligaments, which are attached to the proximal sesamoid bones.

In addition, the suspensory apparatus also contributes to the *stay apparatus*. The stay apparatus involves the coordination

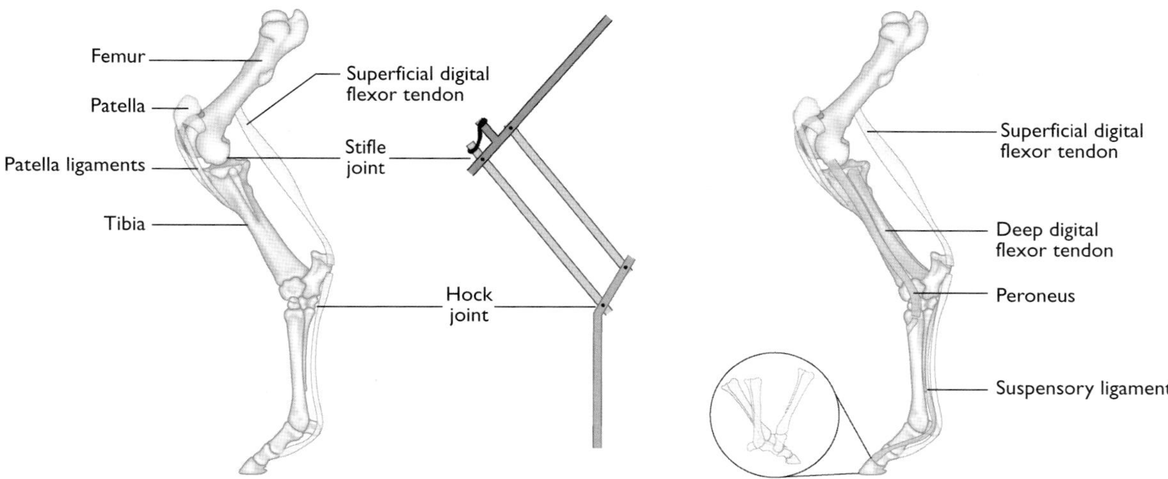

Fig. 16.10 The stay apparatus and suspensory apparatus of the hind limb. (With permission from V Aspinall, 2006. The complete textbook of veterinary nursing. London: Butterworth-Heinemann, p. 141.)

of various muscles, ligaments and tendons in both the fore- and hind limbs, which locks the limbs and joints into position, enabling the horse to rest and sleep in a standing position. The stifle joint of one limb becomes fully locked when most of the body weight is taken by that limb; the other rests on the toe of the hoof. This conserves energy, but every few minutes the horse will shift its weight to the other limb when the muscles begin to tire. This trait is unique to the horse and has evolved because, as a prey animal, the wild horse must be able to make a rapid escape from predators but still must be able to rest. Lying down to sleep would make it more vulnerable to attack.

Structure of the foot and hoof

The equine foot is a complex and important structure. There is a saying within the equine industry: 'No foot no horse', meaning that if the foot is injured the horse will not be able to work and there will be no point in keeping it! Knowledge of the anatomy of the foot and its care is extremely important.

External structures

The internal structures of the foot are surrounded by a protective external capsule called the *hoof* (Fig. 16.11). This is a tough outer covering of epidermal tissue known as *horn*, which is insensitive and overlies the sensitive dermis. The insensitivity of horn enables domesticated horses to have their feet trimmed regularly and to wear shoes held in place by nails knocked into the wall of the hoof. The hoof provides grip, absorbs concussion and promotes circulation.

It consists of the following parts:

- *Frog* is a small, triangular wedge that plays an important role in blood circulation, absorption of concussion and to a certain extent grip.
- *Sole* should be concave in shape and support and protect the structures within the foot. The thickness of the sole varies from horse to horse but generally the horn of the sole is less thick than the horn of the hoof wall and is therefore susceptible to bruising.
- *Bulbs of heel* are located at the back of the foot and work with the frog and sole to assist with circulation and expansion of the foot when it makes contact with the ground.
- *Seat of corn* is the point on the sole where the bars make an angle with the wall of the hoof (Fig. 16.11C).
- *Bars* allow for expansion of the foot and provide strength.
- *Coronet* or *coronary band* is the point from which the horn tissue grows and extends. Horn can take 9–12 months to grow down from the coronet to the tip of the toe on the ground surface. The hoof wall is slightly thicker at the toe than the heel.
- *White line* marks the boundary between the internal and external structures of the foot. The white line is used as a guide by the farrier when nailing shoes onto the hoof. It is sensitive and, if it is penetrated or pinched by an incorrectly positioned nail, the horse will become lame.
- *Periople* forms an outer layer to protect the hoof and maintain moisture levels, which prevent the hoof from becoming dry and brittle.

Internal structures

Inside the hoof are the more sensitive tissues (Fig. 16.11). These consist of:

- *Bones* running from the proximal end to the ground surface are the short pastern or second phalanx, the pedal bone or third phalanx, and the navicular bone or distal sesamoid (Fig. 16.11A).
- *Digital cushion* is a wedge-shaped structure that sits just above the frog and fills the space above the heel of the foot (Fig. 16.11C). It assists with the absorption of concussion and encourages circulation around the tissues of the foot and lower limb every time the foot impacts with the ground.

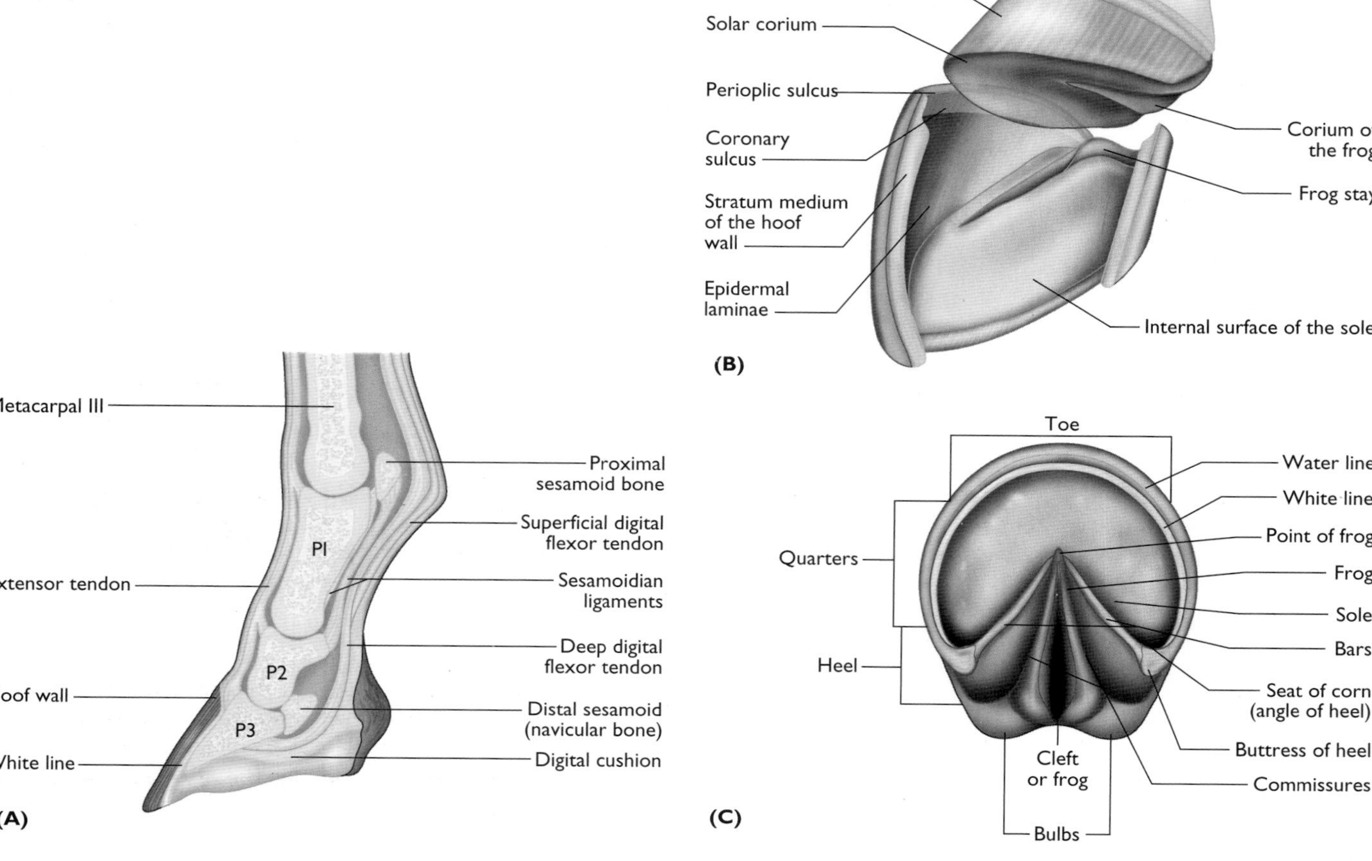

Fig. 16.11 Parts of the equine foot. **(A)** Lateral view of the distal part of the forelimb. **(B)** Dissected view of the relationships of the hoof to the underlying regions of the corium. **(C)** Weight-bearing surface. (With permission from V Aspinall, 2006. The complete textbook of veterinary nursing. London: Butterworth-Heinemann, p. 138.)

- *Lateral cartilages* are two curved discs of cartilage attached to the pedal bone that can be felt just above the coronet band. They work with the digital cushion to assist with the circulation in the foot and to absorb shock. In younger horses the cartilages are highly flexible but as the horse ages they become more fibrous. In cases of extreme trauma and prolonged concussion they may calcify, causing problems with soundness.
- *Corium* is continuous with the skin of the lower leg at the coronet and is the sensitive modified vascular dermis of the foot, which is named according to the insensitive parts of the hoof that it underruns (Fig. 16.11B):
  - *Perioplic corium* supplies the periople with nutrients.
  - *Coronary corium* produces and nourishes the hoof wall.
  - *Laminar corium* consists of the sensitive laminae attached to the periosteum of the pedal bone. These interlock with the insensitive laminae of the hoof wall. It supports the pedal bone and therefore the weight of the horse.

Laminitis is a painful inflammatory condition affecting the laminae of the hoof. It is most commonly associated with overweight ponies but can affect any age or sex or any horse or pony. The patient will be unwilling to move and the affected hooves will feel hot to touch. It is thought to be associated with feeding excess starch such as occurs in lush spring grass or in feeding high levels of grain. Treatment includes altering the diet, reducing the patient's dietary intake by keeping it in a stable during the day (starvation must be avoided because this may lead to hyperlipaemia), the use of analgesics, severely reduced exercise and hosing the hooves with cold running water to ease the pain. In the worst cases the pedal bone may drop or rotate downwards and the hoof may fall off as the attaching laminae break up.

  - *Sole corium* attaches the sole of the pedal bone to the horny sole of the foot.
  - *Frog corium* provides nourishment to the digital cushion and functions with the frog.

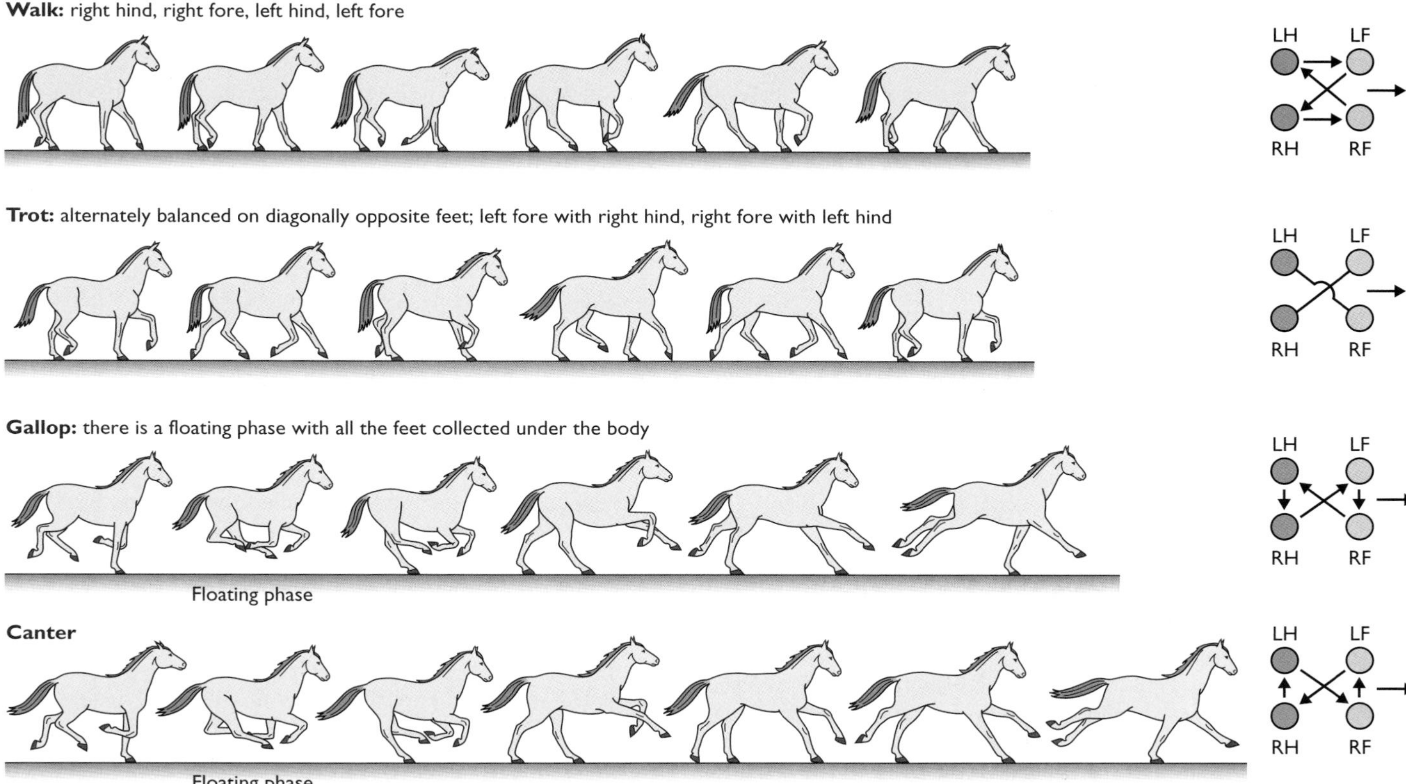

Fig. 16.12 The gaits of the horse. **(A)** Walk. **(B)** Trot. **(C)** Gallop. **(D)** Canter.

Locomotion

The sequence in which a horse lifts its feet from the ground is described as being its *gait*. There are three main types of gait, which define the speed at which the horse moves (Fig. 16.12):

- *Walk* is the slowest gait, during which each foot comes down separately and weight is taken equally on all four feet, which are lifted one at a time.
- *Trot*: The body is alternately balanced on diagonally opposite feet (i.e., left forefoot with right hind foot and right forefoot with left hind foot).
- *Gallop*: During a gallop there is a *floating phase* in which none of the feet are on the ground and they are gathered under the body. When the horse is galloping there are never more than two legs on the ground at the same time. A *canter* is a slower form of the gallop in which both hind feet are still on the ground when the first forefoot returns to the ground.

The nervous system

The nervous system of the horse responds to external and internal stimuli and works closely with the other body systems, particularly the endocrine system, to maintain homoeostasis within the body.

The structure and function of the nervous system, which is largely the same as that in the dog and cat, can be broken down into several component parts:

- *Brain*: housed within the cranium of the skull
- *Spinal cord*: housed within the central canal of the vertebrae
- *Peripheral nerves*: located throughout the body tissues extending to the peripheral and distal anatomy

For further details of nervous system structure and function, see Chapter 5.

The special senses

The horse is an animal of flight, relying heavily on all its senses to survive. The special senses are closely linked to the behavioural responses and it is important to remember that no amount of training can remove the natural flight response, which makes the horse a volatile patient to handle and nurse.

The ear

The ear is an important organ of the body, which enables the animal to hear and provides it with the sensation of balance. The organ is divided into external, middle and inner parts. The external and middle sections are responsible for the collection and transmission of sound waves to the inner ear, which transforms them into nerve impulses to be interpreted by the brain. The middle and inner ear are enclosed within the temporal bone of the skull and only the pinna and the external part of the auditory canal are actually visible. The pinna or ear flap is triangular and rolled distally into a funnel shape. In the horse it is quite mobile and can be turned in the direction of sounds. It also plays an important part in the facial expression of the animal, allowing the veterinary nurse to understand the behavioural and emotional state of the patient and predict any response to external stimuli.

The *guttural pouch* lies within the skull of the horse and is a thin mucosal caudoventral pocket or diverticulum of the Eustachian (auditory) tube that connects the nasopharynx to the middle ear. There is one pouch on each side of the head and each may be found between the base of the skull and the atlas (C1) and the pharynx and the beginning of the oesophagus. There are many important structures that lie very close to the guttural pouch, including the carotid artery and cranial nerves IX, X, XI and XII.

Guttural pouch disease. Regular endoscopy of the guttural pouches is recommended to check their health and that the vital structures lying close to these delicate structures are not being damaged by infection. Conditions of the guttural pouches include empyema (pus-filled), tympany (air-filled and distended), mycosis (fungal infection) and neoplasia such as melanomata. Strangles caused by *Streptococcus equi equi* may also involve the guttural pouches.

The eye

The eye is the organ of sight located within the orbital cavity of the skull and supplied by the optic nerve (II), which carries nerve impulses generated by light rays to the brain. In the horse the eyeball is compressed from front to back and is wider than it is high. It is proportionally larger in relation to its size than the eye of other species. Each eyeball is prominent and sits high up on the side of the head, a position also seen in other prey animals such as the rabbit and the sheep. This gives the horse a wide range of monocular vision and allows it to put its head down to eat while keeping watch for predators (Fig. 16.13). There is only a small area of binocular or 3D vision in front of the head, which allows the horse to judge distances, but this is further reduced by the size and shape of the muzzle.

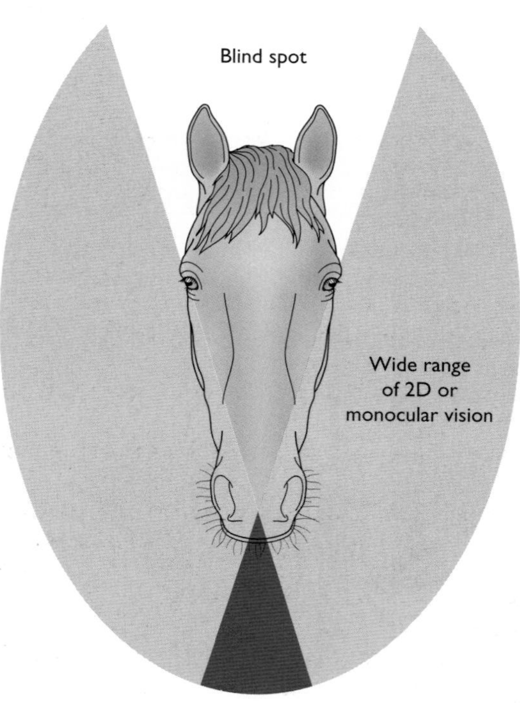

Fig. 16.13 Range of vision seen in the horse.

The basic structure of the eye is similar to that in the dog and cat, with the following differences:

- The cornea is relatively small and oval.
- The choroid contains a tapetum lucidum that lies dorsal to the optic disc and is bluish green in colour.
- The ciliary muscle, which is responsible for altering the shape of the lens to focus images onto the retina, is poorly developed and weak, which means that the equine lens is unable to accommodate as efficiently as those of the dog and the cat.
- The iris is generally dark brown and the pupil within it is a horizontal oval shape but becomes more rounded as it contracts. Newborn foals have a rounded pupil.
- On the margins of the iris, particularly on the upper part, there is a curly, fan-shaped structure called the corpora nigra, which is thought to provide additional shading for the retina to limit the entry of light.
- The retina is often described as being a *ramp retina*. The compressed shape of the eyeball means that all parts of the retina are *not* equidistant from the lens. The upper or dorsal part of the retina is further away and is used for near vision, while the lower or ventral part is closer to the lens and is used for far vision. This makes up for the weakness of the ciliary muscle.

The position of the eyes on the head, the compressed shape of the eyeball and the weakness of the ciliary muscles means that the horse does not locate and focus images on the retina as readily as some predator species. This is not a problem for a prey species that does not need to catch its food; however, when a horse is being ridden and is expected to jump obstacles at speed it must be allowed to see the obstacle from a distance using its binocular facility. As it gets closer to the jump, the jump goes out of focus and it has to remember the details. It then has to adjust the carriage of its head to locate the image on the appropriate part of its retina determined by its distance from the jump. This explains why a horse may move its head up and down as it approaches the jump.

The blood vascular system

As in the dog and cat, the blood vascular system is divided into four main parts:

- *Blood* is very similar in structure and function, although the diagnostic parameters, which are beyond the remit of this text, are different.

Neonatal isoerythrolysis. This is a blood condition affecting neonatal foals. The maternal antibodies transferred via the colostrum attack the foal's erythrocytes and cause anaemia and jaundice. In severe cases this may result in the foal's death. A blood transfusion may be necessary and a gelding may be used as the blood donor.

- The *heart* is an irregular, laterally compressed cone with the larger part lying on the left of centre of the mediastinum and thoracic cavity. The size varies with the size of the horse and its function; the heart of a thoroughbred is larger than that of a draft horse. This is a result partly of inheritance and partly of training, but it may affect the arrangement of the organs around it. The heart usually extends from the second to the sixth intercostal space. Apart from its size there is little to distinguish it from the canine or feline heart.

The most common arrhythmia of the horse is atrial fibrillation, which is characterised by an increased resting heart rate. Horses diagnosed with this condition may be brought back to normal sinus rhythm by the use of quinidine sulphate.

- *Circulation* ensures a continuous flow of blood to all the body cells to deliver nutrients and oxygen and to remove waste products. It comprises many vessels, some of which have more clinical significance for the veterinary nurse than others but all playing an important part in the supply of the animal body.

Normal heart rate in the horse ranges from 25 to 42 beats per minute at rest.

The horse is able to increase the rate to 220–240 beats per minute during extreme exercise.

Pulse rate is measured by applying gentle digital pressure to the *facial artery* as it curves upwards over an area just rostral to the angle of the jaw.

Venepuncture is achieved by using the large *external jugular vein* as it runs down the neck. This can be raised by occluding it in the ventral part of the jugular groove.

- The *lymphatic system* is responsible for returning excess tissue fluid in the form of lymph from the tissues to the circulation. It also monitors the presence of any foreign material in the lymph by passing it through the lymph nodes scattered along the course of the lymphatic vessels. Some superficial lymph nodes can be palpated as a part of a normal health check. The *parotid lymph nodes* are not usually palpable but there are numerous *mandibular nodes* arranged in a forward-pointing V and lying within the intermandibular space. The *retropharyngeal nodes* are arranged in groups within the pharyngeal wall and drain all structures within the upper part of the head. In cases of equine strangles, abscessation of these nodes may lead to infection of the guttural pouches.

The respiratory system

The respiratory system provides the structure and mechanism for oxygen within atmospheric air to be taken into the lungs for effective gaseous exchange and for carbon dioxide produced during cell metabolism to be expelled via the lungs. The parts of the system are similar to those in the dog and cat.

The muzzle of the horse is large but the two *nasal chambers* within are much less spacious than might be expected, as the reserve parts of the cheek teeth and the extensive paranasal sinuses occupy a considerable amount of space. Air passes into the chambers via two large flexible nostrils or *external nares*, which are able to dilate during periods of extreme exercise to increase the volume of inspired air. The *alar fold* forms the ventral margin of each nostril while the dorsal margin leads into a blind-ending pouch called the *false nostril*. Each nasal chamber contains dorsal and ventral *ethmoturbinates or conchae*, which are delicate, coiled bones covered by nasal mucosa. The ethmoturbinates warm, filter and humidify the air before it reaches the trachea and are important in the detection of smell. The right and left nasal chambers extend caudally and communicate with the pharynx. The rostral part of each nasal chamber is divided into three areas called the *dorsal*, *middle* and *ventral meatus*.

Ethmoidal haematomata may develop in the ethmoturbinate region. These lesions affect the performance of the horse and are usually accompanied by a nasal discharge and respiratory noise. They may be removed surgically or by laser ablation via the frontomaxillary opening.

The head of the horse has an extensive system of air-filled *paranasal sinuses*, which communicate with the nasal chambers. Their function is to warm, filter and humidify the inspired air but they also help to reduce the weight of the skull. They consist of:

- *Frontal sinus* lies in the dorsal part of the skull medial to the orbit. There is an opening into the maxillary sinuses via the *frontomaxillary opening* in the floor of the sinus.
- *Two maxillary sinuses* occupy a large proportion of the upper jaw. The caudal cheek teeth are embedded within them. There is a natural slit-like *nasomaxillary opening* into the middle meatus of the nasal chamber.

Sinusitis. The sinus system of the head is susceptible to infection, which may spread from the nasal chambers or from tooth abscesses. Under normal circumstances the sinuses should drain freely into one another and then into the nasal chambers but if infected they may become filled with discharge and drainage and/or irrigation may be necessary. Access to the roots of the teeth may also be gained through the appropriate sinus.

The size of the maxillary sinuses changes as the horse ages. They enlarge considerably after birth as the cheek teeth erupt. This process continues as the teeth migrate forwards and come into wear.

The *pharynx* is divided into three parts:

- *Nasopharynx* is located at the caudal part of the nasal cavity above the soft palate. The openings to the guttural pouches are in the lateral walls.
- *Oropharynx* is located at the caudal part of the oral cavity below the soft palate.
- *Laryngopharynx* extends from the oropharynx to the opening of the oesophagus.

The *larynx* in the horse is an important structure that often fails to function normally (laryngeal hemiplegia) during exercise, necessitating surgical intervention in the performance horse. This structure forms the opening for the trachea. The larynx is comprised of four cartilages, which form a rigid, box-like structure:

- *Epiglottis*: a flap lying on the rostral part of the larynx that covers the glottis and controls the flow of gases into the respiratory tract
- A pair of *arytenoid cartilages*
- *Cricoid cartilage*: forms the ventral floor
- *Thyroid cartilage*

The larynx is suspended from the skull by the *hyoid apparatus*, which allows it to swing backwards and forwards during respiration and swallowing. Within the lumen of the larynx are the *vocal folds*, which are the edges of the mucosal outpouchings known as the lateral ventricles.

Laryngeal hemiplegia. This is usually left-sided and may occur in some larger horses. Affected animals may be referred to as 'roarers', as they produce a strident noise at inspiration. The sound is produced by the passage of air over the passive vocal folds, which results from paralysis of certain muscles. If left untreated, air flow into the respiratory tract is affected, which may affect the performance of the horse. Treatment, as in the dog, is by means of a tie-back. Old-fashioned alternatives included eversion and excision of the affected lateral ventricle by means of an operation known as a Hobday after Sir William Hobday, who pioneered the technique.

The lower respiratory tract, comprising the trachea, bronchi and lung tissue, is similar in structure and function to that in the dog and cat.

The digestive system

The horse is a herbivorous prey species and must be able to take flight at any moment. The wild horse evolved to roam over large areas in search of food, which largely comprised poor-quality fibrous vegetation that would be eaten constantly and digested slowly. The anatomy and physiology of the digestive tract (Fig. 16.14) reflects both these fundamental facts and bears similarity to that of the rabbit. Other herbivorous species include cattle and sheep and their digestive tracts are described in Chapter 17. The parts of the tract are similar to those of the dog and cat; however, the tract is proportionally much longer, because fibre takes longer to break down. The horse is classed as a hindgut fermenter, meaning that the caecum and colon are adapted to provide a chamber in which microbial fermentation of food takes place.

The oral cavity

The muzzle and lips of the horse are highly mobile and sensitive. The whiskers located around the muzzle area are used to feel for and assist in the selection of suitable vegetation. The lips are then used to gather the food into the horse's mouth ready for mastication. The tongue is long and very supple. Its upper surface is covered in a velvet-like layer of delicate papillae. The larger papillae used for detection of taste are fewer in number than in carnivores.

Dentition

The dentition of the horse is clearly adapted to the mechanical breakdown of fibre. The horse has large, flat 'table' teeth and a huge mandible that plays a major role in mastication. The temporomandibular joint has a rotational movement, which allows the teeth to grind the food between them.

Horses have two sets of teeth during their lifetime:

- *Deciduous or milk teeth*: are 24 in total and are gradually discarded over the first five years of life.
- *Permanent teeth* begin to erupt from the age of 2½ years. The full set will be fully erupted and 'in wear' by the age of 6 years (Fig. 16.15). The adult horse has between 36 and 44 teeth; the total number depends on the sex of the individual.

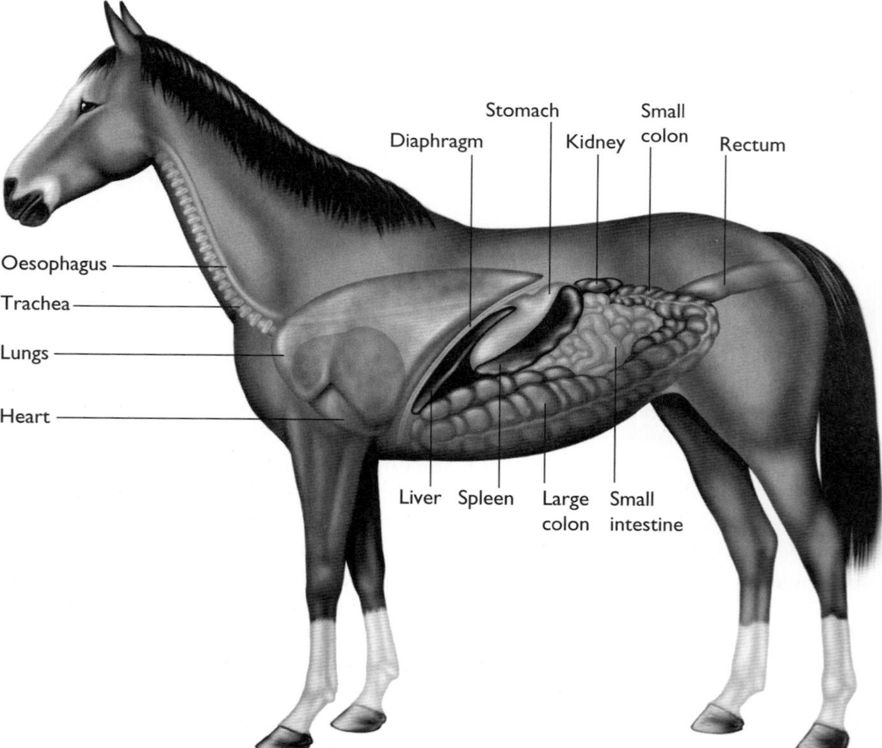

Fig. 16.14 Lateral view of the equine digestive tract. (With permission from V Aspinall, 2006. The complete textbook of veterinary nursing. London: Butterworth-Heinemann, p. 142.)

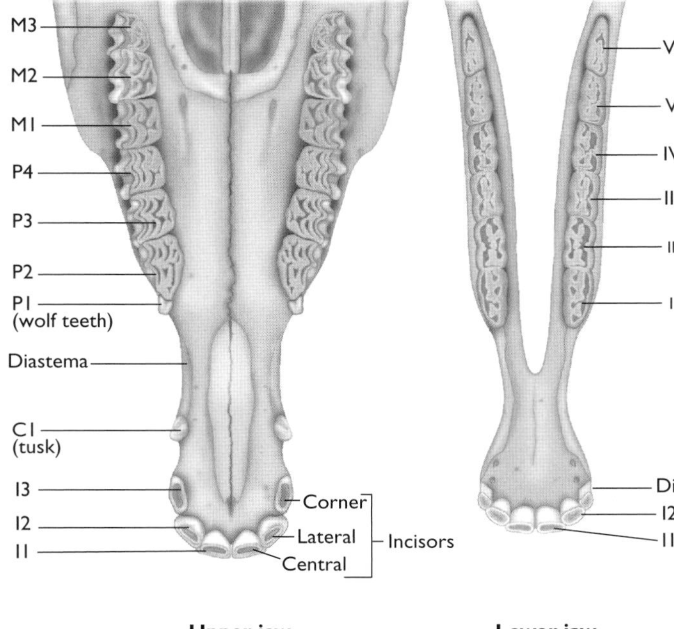

Fig. 16.15 Teeth in the upper and lower jaw of a 4-year-old horse. (With permission from V Aspinall, 2006. The complete textbook of veterinary nursing. London: Butterworth-Heinemann, p. 136.)

Dental formula for the adult male horse (with no wolf teeth):

[**I**3/3, **C**1/1, **PM**3/3, **M**3/3] $\times$ 2 = 40.

Dental formula for the adult female (with no wolf teeth):

[**I**3/3, **C**0/0, **PM**3/3, **M**3/3] $\times$ 2 = 36.

The tooth types are:

- *Incisors* are located at the rostral end of the upper and lower jaw and are responsible for cutting grass as it is taken into the mouth. There are 12 incisors – six in each jaw – which are categorised according to their position as centrals, laterals and corners (Fig. 16.15).
- *Canines* are rudimentary teeth and often fail to erupt in mares, although they may develop in 25%. In stallions these *tushes* develop at around the age of 5 years and cause no problem. They erupt in the space, known as the *diastema*, between the incisors and cheek teeth, closer to the corner incisors than to the premolars (Fig. 16.15).
- *Premolars and molars* (cheek teeth) are flattened teeth primarily used for chewing and grinding up the food into particles small enough to swallow. In each jaw there are six premolars and six molars. In addition, *wolf teeth* (Fig. 16.15) may develop at between 18 months and 5 years of age. These are small, vestigial teeth that develop in front of the premolars, usually in the upper jaw but sometimes in both the upper and lower jaws. They are often removed because they can cause pain and interference with the bit.

Equine teeth are described as being *hypsodontic*: they do not have a layer of enamel over the top or occlusal surface. The enamel casing of the sides is folded, which increases the amount of hard, wearable material. During life the enamel and the softer dentine provide an efficient grinding surface, which wears down as the teeth grow and the animal ages. These changes are described variously as marks, stars and grooves and they can be used to give an indication of the age of an individual horse, although this should never be considered entirely accurate (Fig. 16.16). Each tooth has a huge crown reserve, which enables all the teeth to grow continuously while the occlusal surfaces are worn down by as much as 2–3 mm a year by the mastication process.

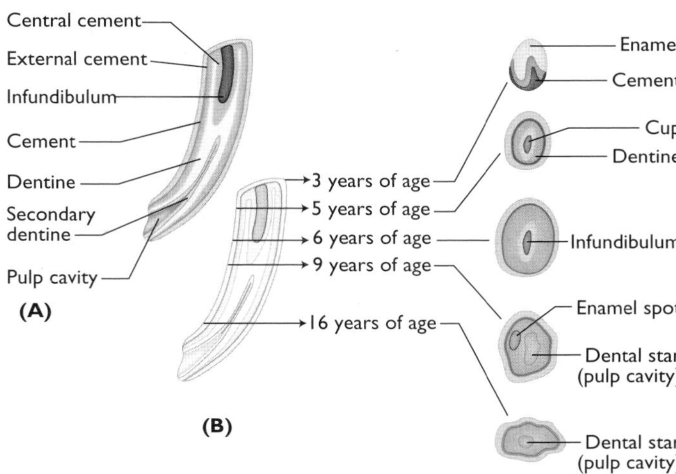

Fig. 16.16 (A) Longitudinal section through an incisor tooth. **(B)** Cross-sections indicate the appearance of the occlusal surface as the tooth wears down. (With permission from V Aspinall, 2006. The complete textbook of veterinary nursing. London: Butterworth-Heinemann, p. 135.)

While in the mouth, the food is mixed with saliva to lubricate and stick the food together to form it into a bolus. The bolus is formed as the food particles are chewed by the molar teeth and movement of the tongue around and against the hard palate. Once sufficiently masticated the bolus is passed to the back of the mouth, towards the throat ready for swallowing. The process of swallowing involves the rising of the soft palate to allow the bolus to travel towards and through the pharynx; the epiglottis then closes over the trachea to prevent any food items from entering the lungs and causing the horse to choke. The bolus then begins its journey to the stomach via the oesophagus.

Oesophagus

The oesophagus is a muscular tube that extends from the throat to the horse's stomach, passing through the thoracic cavity and the diaphragm; its length will vary in relation to the size of the horse, the average being 1.5 m. The bolus is pushed along the oesophagus by a wave of muscular contraction known as peristalsis.

Stomach

The stomach (Fig. 16.17) of the horse is described as being *simple* and is similar to that of the cat, dog and rabbit but very different from the compound stomach of ruminants (e.g., cows and sheep). Digestion, as in the dog and cat, is *monogastric*.

The horse has evolved as a trickle feeder, eating little and often. The stomach is relatively small in comparison to the size of the animal, holding 7–14 l, and is approximately the size of a rugby ball when empty. Food passes from the oesophagus into the stomach via the cardiac sphincter, which prevents food from being regurgitated. Any ingested toxins are difficult to get rid of and often pass through the whole system and they may be responsible for

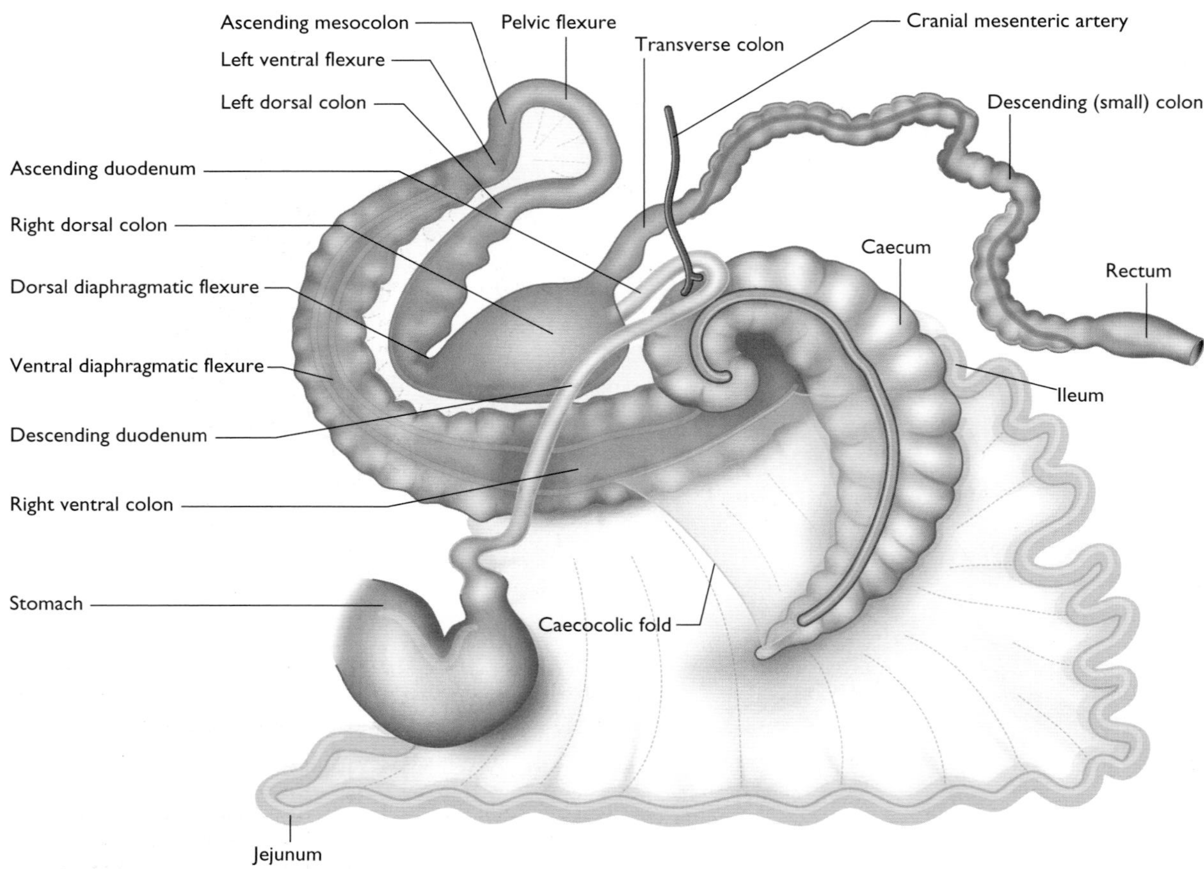

Fig. 16.17 Diagrammatic representation of the equine digestive tract. (With permission from V Aspinall, 2006. The complete textbook of veterinary nursing. London: Butterworth-Heinemann, p. 143.)

inducing colic, which is potentially life-threatening. The stomach empties when it is two-thirds full so food spends a relatively short amount of time here, resulting in minimal digestion. Food passes from the stomach through the pyloric sphincter into the small intestine and is now referred to as chyme.

Small intestine

The small intestine is divided into three sections of varying length, although it is difficult to tell where each one ends and the next begins:

- *Duodenum*: approximately 1 m in length
- *Jejunum*: approximately 20 m in length
- *Ileum*: approximately 1.5 m in length

The total length may range from 20 to 27 m depending upon the size of the horse, and the diameter is just wider than that of an average garden hose. The small intestine ends at the ileocaecal junction. Digestion and absorption of soluble foodstuffs take place within this area.

Large intestine

The large intestine accounts for 65% of the volume of the digestive tract and it is here that microbial digestion of cellulose (complex carbohydrates) takes place (Fig. 16.17). This occurs mainly in the caecum and colon and the process is similar to that seen in rabbits. Mammals are unable to produce the enzymes necessary to break down cellulose found in plant material so they rely on the presence of microorganisms to do it. The microorganisms, consisting mainly of bacteria and protozoa, are specific to the horse's diet and horses are highly sensitive to dietary change, which should always be introduced gradually. Volatile fatty acids resulting from the process are absorbed into the bloodstream and used as energy. In addition, microbial digestion also produces heat, which keeps the animal warm.

The large intestine is divided into three sections:

- *Caecum* is a large, sacculated, blind-ending sac (Fig. 16.17) running along the ventral part of the abdomen. It is approximately 1 m long and can hold up to 35 l of ingesta. The material contains about 90% water but by the time it reaches the colon about 30% has been reabsorbed through the caecal walls.
- *Colon* is where the majority of microbial digestion occurs. The colon can be divided into:
  - *Large colon* is approximately 4 m long and may contain up to 100 l (Fig. 16.17). Food remains here for 36–65 h. In order to allow the organ to sit comfortably within the abdominal cavity it is folded up, giving rise to four distinct but continuous areas. The *right ventral colon* runs from the ileocaecal junction cranially towards the sternum, where it makes a turn at the *sternal flexure* and then becomes the *left ventral colon*. This runs back towards

the pelvis and then makes another turn at the *pelvic flexure*. From here the *left dorsal colon* runs back cranially towards the diaphragm and turns again at the *diaphragmatic flexure* before becoming the *right dorsal colon*, which then travels across the abdomen as the *transverse colon*. These bends can cause impaction of waste food materials, particularly at the pelvic flexure, as at this point the diameter is dramatically reduced from 25 cm to about 5 cm while undergoing a 180° turn.

The structure of the large colon is designed to slow down the passage of food to provide sufficient time for microbial digestion. This works well for horses kept outside and eating grass but stabled horses may be fed on a much drier diet and are unable to move around as freely, which can lead to impactions, particularly at the pelvic flexure, and subsequently colic.

- *Small colon* leads from the transverse colon and is equivalent to the descending colon of the dog. It is narrower but is similar in length. Microbial digestion is of less significance but the passage of ingesta slows and further water is absorbed giving rise to relatively dry faeces.

- *Rectum* continues on from the small colon and is a short storage area for faeces, which accumulate before passing out of the anus. Its length is approximately 30 cm.

Although the microorganisms found within the caecum and colon produce added nutrients such as amino acids, horses, unlike other hindgut fermenters such as the rabbit, do not normally practise coprophagia (eating their own faeces). Foals may eat the faeces of adult horses but this is probably an attempt to colonise their own large intestines with appropriate microorganisms.

The urinary system

The parts of the urinary system of the horse are the same as those in any other mammal and the system carries out the same functions, playing an important role in homeostasis by maintaining water and electrolyte balance.

The kidney

The two kidneys are located in the abdomen, one on either side of the midline close to the diaphragm. The right kidney lies ventral to the last two or three ribs and the first transverse process. The left kidney lies caudal to the right and is located ventral to the last rib and first two or three lumbar transverse processes. In contrast to other species, the kidneys are not the same shape. The right kidney is heart-shaped while the left kidney is more bean-shaped. Both kidneys are smooth in appearance with a deep notch at the renal pelvis. Each kidney weighs approximately 400–600 g, depending upon the size of the horse.

Internally each kidney shows a unipyramidal design: the pyramids of the medulla are fused to form one and their apices are fused to form a common renal crest (Fig. 16.18).

A ureter carries urine from each kidney to the bladder. Each ureter is wide at its origin but narrows further down. The ureters bend caudally as they leave the kidneys and follow a twisting course over the dorsal abdomen to reach the bladder wall close to its neck.

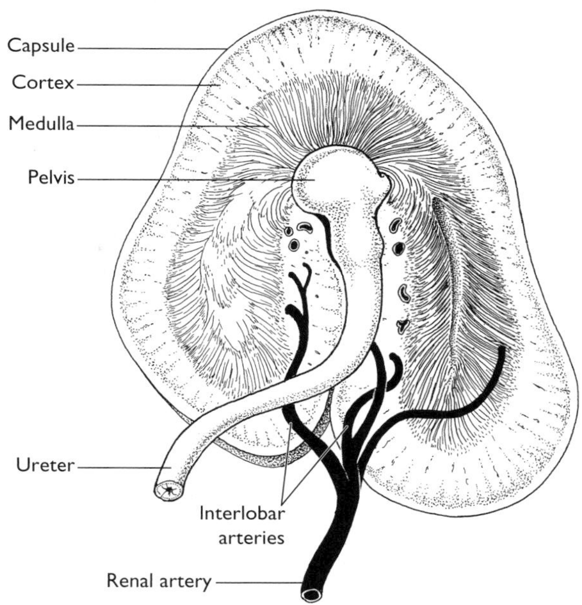

Fig. 16.18 Dorsal section through the equine kidney, semi-schematic. (Redrawn from KM Dyce, WO Sack, CJG Wensing, 2002. Textbook of veterinary anatomy, 3rd edn. Philadelphia, PA: WB Saunders, p. 542.)

Ruptured bladder. During foaling there is a risk of rupturing the bladder of the foal as it is delivered. The affected foal will appear normal after birth but soon afterwards it will cease suckling and fail to produce urine. Within 36 h the abdomen distends and the foal may suffer from respiratory distress. The defect must be repaired surgically.

Urinalysis

Horses produce approximately 20 mL/kg/day of urine. It is usually pale yellow in colour and may be clear or cloudy depending on the amount of calcium carbonate being excreted. The urine is normally alkaline (pH >9) because of the high potassium content of fresh vegetation. Stabled horses may produce urine with a slightly lower pH.

Urinary tract obstruction. This may occur in the horse and is a result of calculi formed from calcium carbonate crystals. Affected individuals may show haematuria after exercise. Diagnosis is confirmed by rectal palpation of the bladder or by ultrasonography. The calculi may be removed surgically or in the mare this may be done manually.

The reproductive system

Male

The parts of the reproductive tract of the male horse or *stallion* (Fig. 16.19) and its associated hormones are similar to those seen in the male dog and cat.

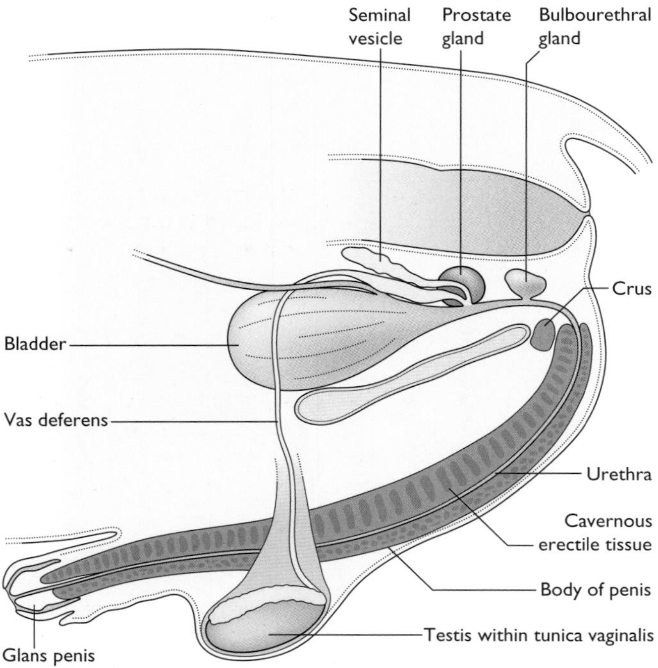

Fig. 16.19 The reproductive organs of the stallion. (Redrawn from KM Dyce, WO Sack, CJG Wensing, 2002. Textbook of veterinary anatomy, 3rd edn. Philadelphia, PA: WB Saunders, p. 561.)

Testis

In the normal stallion there are two testes present within the scrotum, which is located between the hind legs (Fig. 16.19). They are egg-shaped and reach their full size of 8–12 cm at approximately 2 years of age. Once the testes are mature they are responsible for the production of spermatozoa (sperm) and of the male hormone testosterone. Sperm are conducted from the testis up the epididymis and vas deferens during ejaculation and enter the urethra just caudal to the neck of the bladder. They are then deposited in the reproductive tract of the mare by the urethra running within the penis.

The testes of the colt foal may be present in the scrotum at birth or may descend within the first 2 weeks of life.

Accessory glands

The accessory glands are responsible for the production of seminal fluid, whose function is to provide nourishment and an efficient transport medium for the sperm. There are three sets of glands:

- *Prostate* partially surrounds the cranial end of the urethra at its junction with the neck of the bladder. It secretes a clear fluid that cleans the urethra and neutralises the acidity of any remaining urine prior to ejaculation. The prostatic secretions make up the bulk of the seminal fluid.
- *Seminal vesicles or vesicular glands* are a pair of smooth-surfaced, pear-shaped glands located on either side of the bladder. Their fluid is introduced into the ejaculate in the same point at which the vasa deferentia enter the urethra.
- *Bulbourethral glands* are paired glands that lie just dorsal to the urethra as it passes over the ischial arch, leaves the pelvis (Fig. 16.19) and becomes surrounded by erectile tissue.

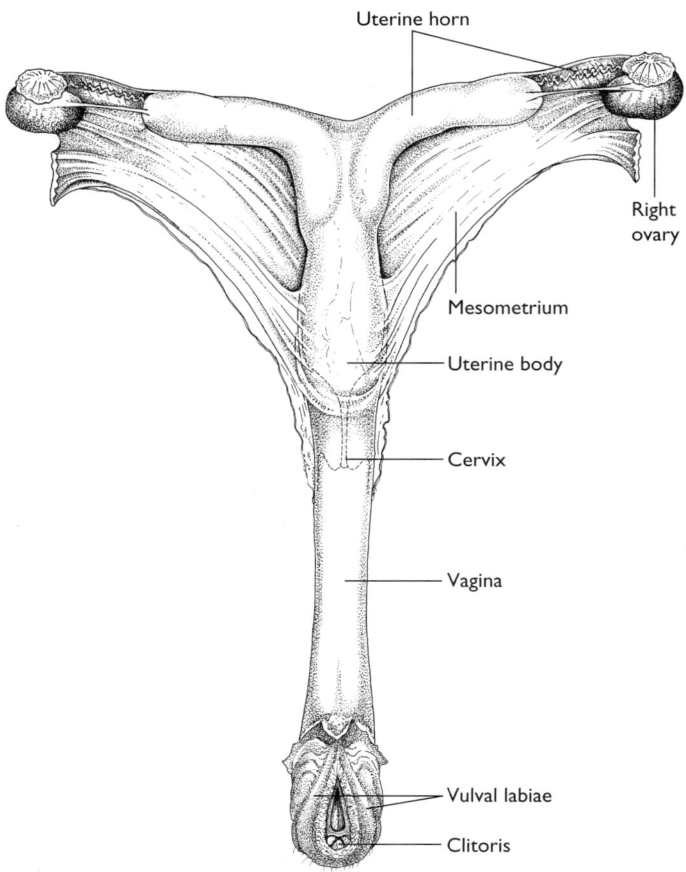

Fig. 16.20 Dorsal view of the reproductive organs of the mare. (Redrawn from KM Dyce, WO Sack, CJG Wensing, 2002 Textbook of veterinary anatomy, 3rd edn. Philadelphia, PA: WB Saunders, p. 555.)

Penis

The penis is the male organ of copulation, which in the stallion lies ventral to the abdominal body wall between the hind legs (Fig. 16.19). It consists of cavernous erectile tissue surrounding the urethra and is supported by a pair of muscular crura that attach it to the ischial arch. The glans penis or the free end has a distinctive mushroom shape. The widest part or corona is some distance from the apex, through which the urethra projects within a central fossa. The body of the penis is long and capable of considerable extension during erection. When not erect the penis is housed within a prepuce for protection. At rest this is thrown into numerous folds, which allows for the erection of the penis. There is no os penis in the stallion.

Female

The parts of the reproductive system of the female horse or *mare* (Fig. 16.20) and their associated hormones are the same as those in the female dog and cat.

Ovary

There are two ovaries, lying one on either side of the midline in the dorsal abdomen and ventral to the area of the fifth lumbar vertebra. In comparison to other species, the ovaries of the mare are quite large – those of a larger mare may be 8–10 cm long. Although they are basically bean-shaped, the free border is deeply indented to form an 'ovulation fossa' from which the mature follicles ovulate. The developing follicles and corpora lutea develop deep within the ovarian tissue and are surrounded by a vascularised layer. This means that they are not particularly prominent and may be difficult to identify by rectal palpation. The ovaries are largely inactive until the mare reaches sexual maturity at around 1–2 years of age.

Granulosa cell tumours are the most common type of ovarian tumour and may affect any age of mare. They are usually benign, slow growing, unilateral and secrete the hormones inhibin and/or testosterone. Clinical signs include irregular or lack of an oestrous cycle, stallion-like behaviour, including aggression and mounting other mares, and development of male characteristics such as a crested neck and increased muscular development.

Uterine tube

This is also referred to as the oviduct or Fallopian tube. There is one leading from each ovary to the uterine horn. Ova, usually one or two at a time, expelled from the ovarian follicles are initially caught by a funnel-shaped *infundibulum* on the end of the uterine tube. They then travel down the tubes, which are about 5 mm in diameter and 10 cm long. Fertilisation occurs within the uterine tubes and only fertilised ova pass through the uterotubular junction into the uterus; unfertilised ova are reabsorbed.

Uterus

The mare is uniparous (naturally gives birth to one foal at a time). This is reflected in the shape of the uterus in that it has a large body and two short, divergent uterine horns (Fig. 16.20). Compare this to the bicornuate uterus exhibited by multiparous or litter-bearing species such as the dog, cat and rabbit (see Fig. 11.6). The embryo will develop in one of the horns and may migrate from one horn to the other up to the time it finally implants in the uterine wall at about 40 days. After this the developing foal will gradually occupy space in the body of the uterus as it grows.

Multiple pregnancies. The shape of the equine uterus means that the mare is not adapted to producing more than one foal at a time. If two ova are fertilised there is insufficient room for them both to grow to full term. If the veterinary surgeon is able to palpate two embryos per rectum, he or she will take steps to abort one of them to avoid the possible death of both foals later on.

Cervix

The cervix forms a tight, muscular seal between the uterus and the vagina that only relaxes during oestrus and parturition. The cervix is 7 cm in length and 4 cm in diameter and when sealed it plays a crucial role in preventing uterine infection. The caudal part of the cervix projects into the vagina and has a lobed appearance that is affected by the changing hormones of the oestrous cycle.

Vagina

The vagina of the mare is an elastic, muscular tube 20–28 cm long and approximately 15 cm in diameter. The distal end is recognised as the vestibule, marked by the urethral opening at the cranial end and the clitoris within the vulva at the caudal end.

Vulva

This is the visual external part of the mare's reproductive tract. The vulval lips situated just below the anus form a final seal to the tract. The clitoris is very prominent in mares in oestrus.

Mammary glands

The two mammary glands or udders of the mare are small and lie on the ventral surface of the caudal abdomen and cranial part of the pelvis. They may be hidden by the hindquarters. Each gland has a single small, cylindrical teat and is covered in sparse hair. The skin is well-supplied with sebaceous and sweat glands.

The oestrous cycle

The onset of sexual maturity in the mare occurs in the spring following her birth so there is a wide range of onset from 12 to 18 months of age. The mare is described as being a *long-day breeder*, meaning that her reproductive cycle is switched on by increasing hours of daylight, which affect the hypothalamus of the brain, which in turn begins to secrete the same controlling hormones that occur in the cat and dog (see Chapter 11). The breeding season runs from early spring to late summer. In the modern breeding industry the mare's oestrous cycle can be manipulated to start breeding much earlier in the year. Within the breeding season the mare will have many periods of oestrus or receptivity to the stallion and is therefore described as being *seasonally polyoestrous*. The mare is also a *spontaneous ovulatory*; she will ovulate without the stimulus of mating and always at approximately the same time of the cycle.

The oestrous cycle lasts 17–21 days, although some mares may have a cycle that lasts as long as 35 days; there is individual variation.

During this period there are two distinct phases:

1. *Oestrus*, often described as being 'in season' or 'on heat', lasts for approximately 3–5 days. The mare is receptive to the stallion and will indicate this by raising her tail, standing with her hind legs apart and squatting, urinating more frequently, and in the presence of a stallion or a 'teaser' she will rhythmically contract her vulva and expose her clitoris, which is known as 'winking'. Ovulation occurs during this phase, usually on the penultimate or last day.
2. *Dioestrus* lasts for 14–16 days and during this phase the mare is non-receptive and behaves normally. Towards the end of dioestrus new follicles start to develop in the ovary and to secrete the hormone oestrogen. When oestrogen in the blood reaches high enough levels to stimulate the behavioural signs of oestrus, the mare progresses into oestrus again.

During the shorter daylight hours of the winter months the oestrous cycles cease and the mare is described as being *anoestrous*.

Acknowledgement

The authors would like to thank Rachel Cook for her contribution to this chapter in previous editions.

CHAPTER 17

Domestic farm animals

For the purposes of this chapter the term 'farm animals' will be taken to mean those species of animal that are kept to provide food or other products such as wool or leather. The term 'domestication' refers to the process in which a species is altered genetically by generations of selective breeding to accentuate characteristics that are of benefit to humans. As a result the species usually becomes dependent on humans and loses its ability to survive in the wild.

The chapter will describe cattle, sheep and pigs and will highlight the important differences in anatomy and physiology from that of the dog or the horse. The domestic fowl or hen, being a bird, is covered in Chapter 13 and the horse in Chapter 16.

Introduction

Of the approximately 15,000 species of mammals and birds, only 30–40 are used as sources of food and fewer than 14 species currently account for 90% of global livestock production. It is thought that the first food animals to have been domesticated were sheep and this probably took place in the Middle East between 9000 and 7000 BC, after the domestication of the dog and long before that of the cat. The evidence for this is the discovery of large numbers of bones of 1-year-old sheep in a settlement in what is now northern Iraq. Goats were domesticated soon afterwards and these two species became the staple food of the nomadic tribes because they are able to move around in search of grass. The domestication of cattle and pigs is associated with the development of more settled communities, which probably occurred soon after 7000 BC. It is thought that the cow was first bred by humans in western Asia and the pig in China.

The cow

The cow (*Bos taurus*) (plural, cattle) is the most common type of domesticated ungulate (hoofed animal). The term 'ox' (plural, oxen) is synonymous with the word 'cow'. The word 'cattle', meaning several cows, is related to the word 'chattels', originally meaning property, indicating that cows were a sign of wealth.

Cattle belong to the order Artiodactyla, even-toed ungulates, and to the family Bovidae and are descended from the extinct Auroch (*Bos primigenius*). It is widely accepted that domestication of the Auroch occurred separately in two areas: in the Near East, giving rise to the humpless *Bos taurus*, and in the Indian subcontinent to the humped *Bos indicus* or Zebu.

The main reason for the domestication of the cow was to provide a regular supply of fresh food. Hunting for food largely depends on luck and if more animals are killed than can be consumed then the surplus will quickly deteriorate. Keeping several cattle means that the 'farmer' has both a living larder and a supply of dairy products. In addition, these animals provide dung to manure the crops and after they are killed they provide leather, horn, bone and fat for tallow candles. The immense strength of the bulls also meant that they could be used to pull wagons and ploughs, which improved crop production.

Musculo-skeletal system

The skeleton

The skeleton of the cow consists of the axial, appendicular and splanchnic skeletons (Fig. 17.1). The bones of the skeleton follow the same basic plan seen in the dog with a few functional differences.

Axial skeleton

The skull The bones forming the skull (Figs. 17.2 and 17.3) are the same as they are in the dog but the relative proportions are different. The nasal and oral parts of the skull are long as they are in the horse. The frontal bones are extensive and form about half of the entire length of the skull (Fig. 17.2) and the entire roof of the cranium. The posterior borders of the bone form the central *frontal eminence*, with the parietal bones (Fig. 17.3) and this is the highest point of the skull. At the junction of the posterior part and the lateral border of the frontal bone on each side is the horn core or *processus cornus*, from which horn material develops. Each horn is elongated, pigmented and conical in shape and the size; curvature and direction of the horns varies among individuals and breeds.

Horn is the tough outer covering of epidermal tissue containing a high proportion of keratin, which makes it both hard and insensitive. Below the epidermal layer is the more sensitive dermis, which is attached to the horn core. Horn grows from the dermis by means of horn tubules in the same way as the horn forming the equine hoof. The horn material at the base of the horn is soft and slightly transparent and is more sensitive than the rest of the horn.

Horns are found in both sexes of cattle but those in the bull are much larger. Unlike the antlers seen in the deer family, horns are not shed and replaced annually. Some breeds of cattle (e.g., Aberdeen Angus and Jerseys) are naturally polled (hornless) but most have horns which are usually removed when the calf is young to make handling easier and safer and to prevent damage to others in the herd.

The nasal cavity is much smaller than you might expect from the size of the skull and is mainly filled with coiled turbinate bones. In the caudal part of the cavity the nasal septum does not reach to the floor, forming a single median channel that leads from the paired nasal chambers into the nasopharynx.

The system of paranasal sinuses within the skull is very complicated and is poorly developed in the young calf; it does not reach its full size for several years. The *maxillary sinus* occupies much of the upper jaw above the cheek teeth. The *frontal sinus* is large and comprises several compartments of which the caudal

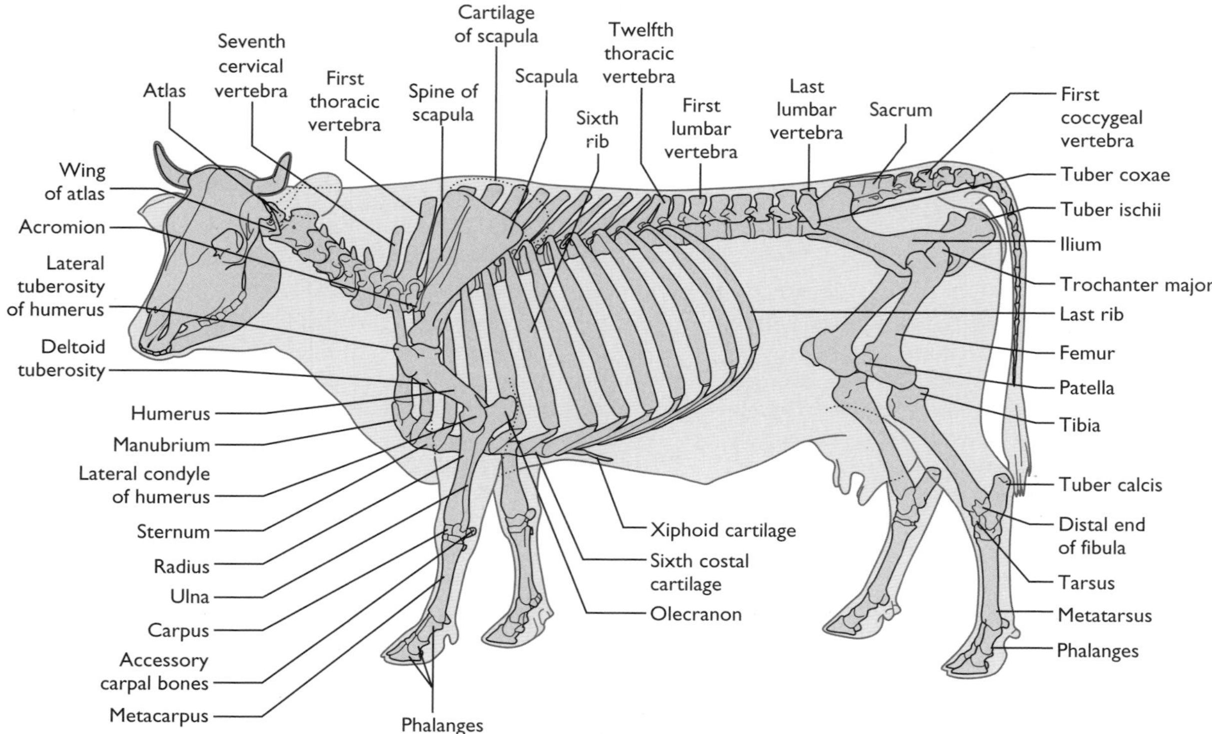

Fig. 17.1 The skeleton of the cow. (After S Sisson, JD Grossman, 1969. Anatomy of the Domestic Animals, 4th edn. Philadelphia and London: WB Saunders, p. 126.)

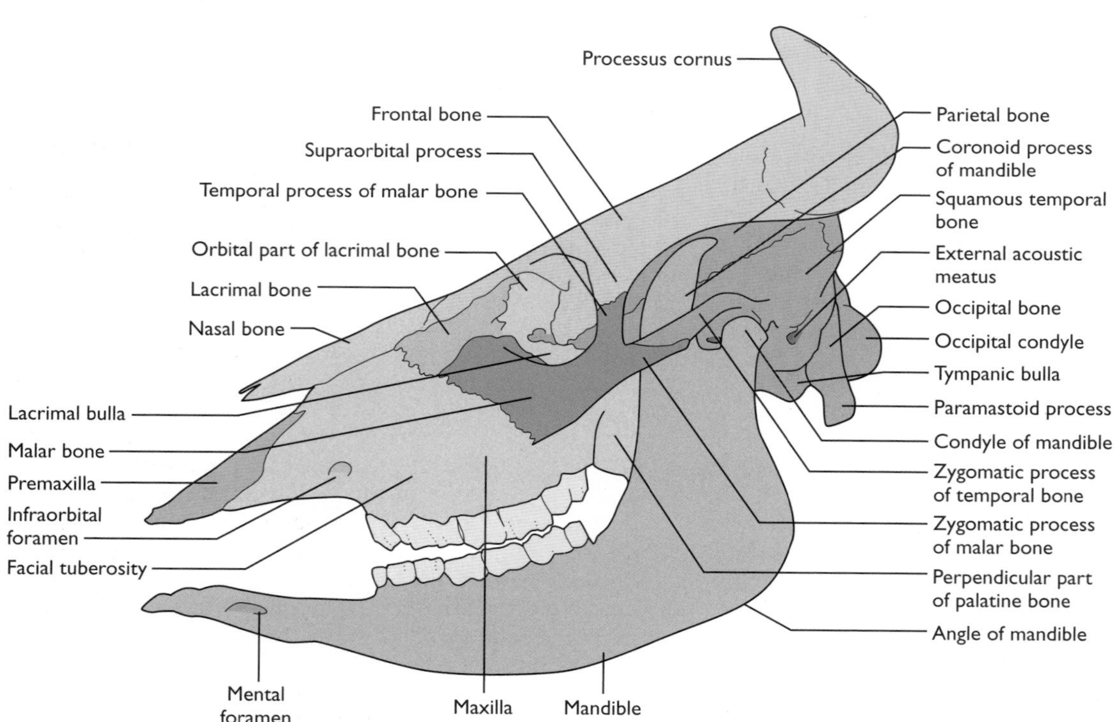

Fig. 17.2 An ox skull: lateral view. The jaws are separated for the sake of clearness. (After S Sisson, JD Grossman, 1969. Anatomy of the Domestic Animals, 4th edn. Philadelphia and London: WB Saunders, p. 132.)

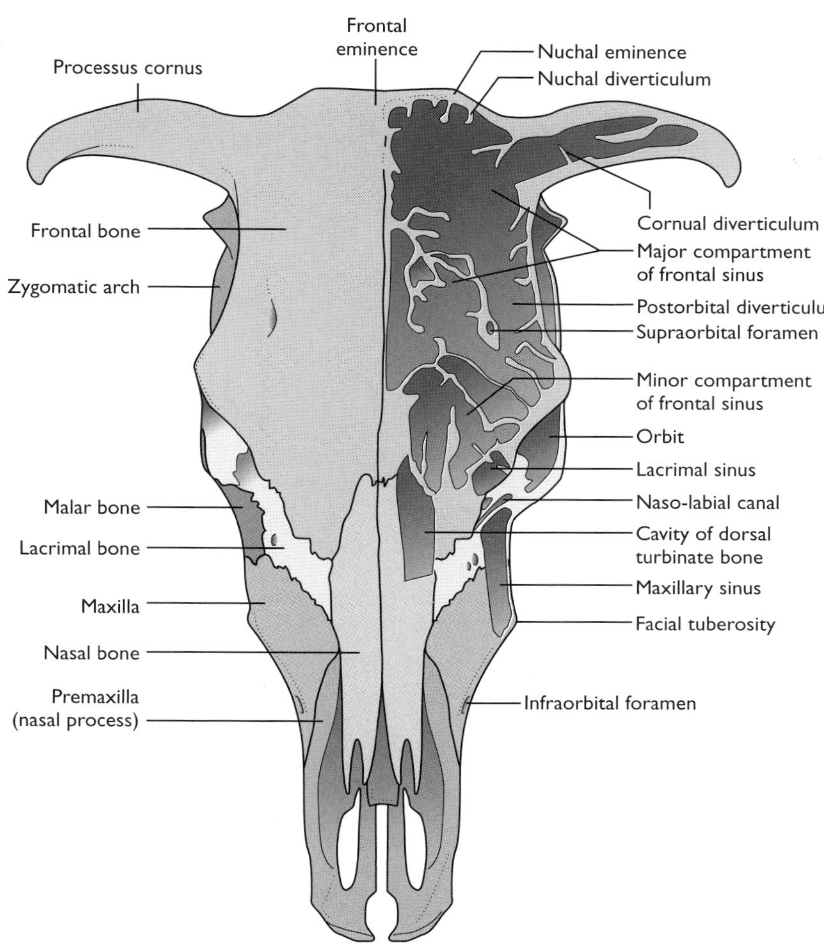

Fig. 17.3 An ox skull: dorsal view, sinuses opened. (After S Sisson, JD Grossman, 1969. Anatomy of the Domestic Animals, 4th edn. Philadelphia and London: WB Saunders, p. 144.)

is the most important. It lies mainly within the frontal bone, covers the dorsal part of the brain case and penetrates into the horn core. When adult cattle are dehorned an opening into the sinus is exposed and this is potentially an area that may be attacked by flies, leading to fly strike. To avoid flies and damage by frosts, adult cattle should be dehorned in the autumn or spring. If the procedure is done on a cold day, it may appear as if 'smoke' is leaving the horn core as the warm air in the sinuses condenses in the cold outside air. The remaining hole soon heals by second intention.

Disbudding means the removal of the horn buds in young calves. It is carried out before the calf is 2 months old and as soon as the horn bud can be seen. It should only be done using a heated iron under local anaesthetic by a trained competent stock-keeper.

Dehorning means the removal of a fully developed horn. It should not be a routine procedure and should only be done for the animal and the herd's welfare. It should be performed by a veterinary surgeon under a local anaesthetic because it involves cutting and sawing sensitive tissues. The sensitive dermis of the horn is supplied by the cornual nerve, which divides into two branches that supply either side of the horn base. The site for the nerve block with local anaesthetic is midway along a line drawn between the top of the eye and the base of the horn.

Humane Slaughter: The anatomy of the frontal sinus is relevant to the technique used in the humane slaughter of cattle. Placement of the captive bolt gun is at the intersection of two diagonal lines running from the lateral canthus of each eye to the base of the opposite horn. The bolt then passes through the shallowest part of the frontal sinus on its route to the brain. The use of any other site may lead to the bolt being lodged in the sinus and not in the brain.

Vertebral column The vertebral formula for the cow is C7 T13 L6 S5 Cd18-20. The shape of each vertebral region conforms to the pattern previously described; however, the cervical vertebrae are shorter than those of the horse, the thoracic vertebrae are larger, the lumbar vertebrae are longer and the sacrum, consisting of five vertebrae, is much more fused than in the horse so it is less easy to distinguish the individual spinous processes. The 18–20 coccygeal vertebrae are longer and better developed than in the horse. The first 5–6 have complete arches and spinous processes and relatively large transverse processes, which is in contrast to the almost tube-like coccygeal vertebrae of the dog and cat.

The curve of the vertebral column is different to that of the horse (Figs. 17.1 and 16.1), giving a much more level outline. This is partly due to the fact that the tips of the spinous processes from the second thoracic vertebra to the middle of the lumbar spine are almost in a straight line. The cervical curve is very slight and the promontory created by the top of the scapula and the spinous processes of the first few thoracic vertebrae is more pronounced. The promontory of the sacrum is also more obvious, especially in individuals where the sacrum is tilted upwards. The neck has a great degree of mobility, which allows the cow to raise and lower its head and to lick its flank with its tongue.

Ribs and sternum The cow has 13 pairs of ribs, of which 8 are sternal and 5 are asternal. They are wider, flatter and less curved than those of the horse. In many individuals there may be a 14th rib, which is usually floating and may correspond to an additional thoracic vertebra or to the first lumbar vertebra. The sternum consists of seven sternebrae and it is wider and flatter than that of the horse.

Appendicular skeleton

As a general rule cattle lead less active lives than horses so knowledge of the detailed musculature and skeletal anatomy of the limbs is less important. However, cattle are prone to infection and trauma of the feet, which is often related to the type of husbandry to which they are subjected. Lameness problems may occupy a significant proportion of the work of a large animal veterinary surgeon particularly on dairy farms.

The forelimb The upper forelimb follows the same pattern as that of other mammals and consists of the *scapula*, the *humerus* and its associated muscles, and the whole is enclosed within the skin of the trunk so that, in most breeds, it fits closely to the thoracic wall. The bony landmarks, such as the prominent spine of the scapula and the point of the shoulder, are relatively easy to palpate as the muscles are less well developed than they are in the horse. The action of the large shoulder joint is mainly flexion and extension. There are synovial bursae associated with the tendon of the triceps as it attaches to the olecranon of the ulna. These may become inflamed and be a cause of lameness.

The original plan of the lower part of the limb of all mammals, birds and reptiles has five digits and is known as the *pentadactyl limb*. Through the process of evolution this plan has modified according to function so that now the dog and cat bear weight on digits 2–5 (see Chapter 3), the horse bears weight on one digit, number 3 (see Chapter 16) and is described as an odd-toed ungulate, while the cow bears weight on two digits, numbers 3 and 4, and is described as an even-toed ungulate. The remaining bones of the lower limb have either disappeared completely or have become merely vestigial, meaning that they are present in a reduced form and have no function. This has an effect on the anatomy of the bones of the lower forelimb, which are also modified to bear weight:

The *radius* is short and relatively broad. This is the main weight bearer. The distal end lies nearer to the medial plane than the proximal end so the bone lies slightly obliquely in the forelimb, causing the forelimb to incline medially and the foot to incline laterally. This produces a 'knock-kneed' appearance, which does not seem to interfere with locomotion.

The *ulna* is slender and fused at its distal end to the radius. (Compare this to the separate radius and ulna seen in the dog and cat.) It projects below the distal radius, forming the styloid process, which aids the stability of the carpal joint.

The *carpus* consists of six short bones arranged in two rows. The proximal row comprises the radial, intermediate, ulnar and accessory carpals and the distal row consists of the fused second and third carpals and a separate fourth carpal. The bones are linked by synovial joints and most of the action, which is flexion and extension, is between the distal radius and ulna and the proximal carpal bones.

Metacarpals comprise a single large cannon bone resulting from fusion of the third and fourth metacarpals and the division is quite visible skeletally. There is also a small metacarpal bone that is about 3–4 cm in length and lies against the proximal lateral border of the larger bone. It does not articulate with the carpus and is the remains of metacarpal 5.

The third and fourth *digits* are separate (Fig. 17.4) and fully functional and each consists of three phalanges and three sesamoid bones. The second and fifth digits are vestigial and consist of one or two small bones lying behind the fetlock joint (metacarpo-phalangeal joint) that do not articulate with any other bone. They do not make contact with the ground and may be referred to as the dew claws.

- *First phalanx* is relatively short and narrow.
- *Second (middle) phalanx* is about two-thirds the length of the first phalanx. The first and second phalanges are enclosed in the same sheath of hairy skin, which extends to the coronets of the hoof covering each toe.
- *Third phalanx* is shaped like the hoof in which it lies and is similar to half of the equine hoof (Fig. 17.5). It has four surfaces: articular, axial (in the cleft between the toes), abaxial and the sole surface that takes the weight.

Within the foot and embedded within the fibro-cartilaginous tissue of the lower limb, there are four *proximal sesamoids* – two associated with each digit on the palmar surface of the fetlock joint (Fig. 17.6). There is also a *distal sesamoid* lying on the palmar surface of each coffin joint; this is the equivalent of the navicular bone of the horse.

The joints within the foot of the cow follow a similar pattern to that in the equine foot and only allow flexion and extension:

- *Fetlock joint* is located between the metacarpus and the first phalanx. This is the first duplicated joint within the lower limb.

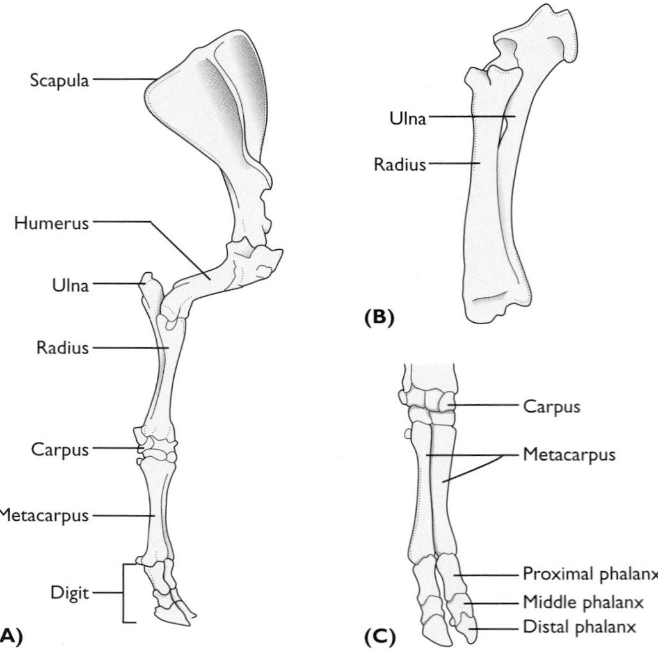

Fig. 17.4 The forelimb of the cow. **(A)** Bones of the forelimb. **(B)** Radius and ulna – note the fused distal end. **(C)** Distal forelimb; weight is taken on digits 3 and 4.

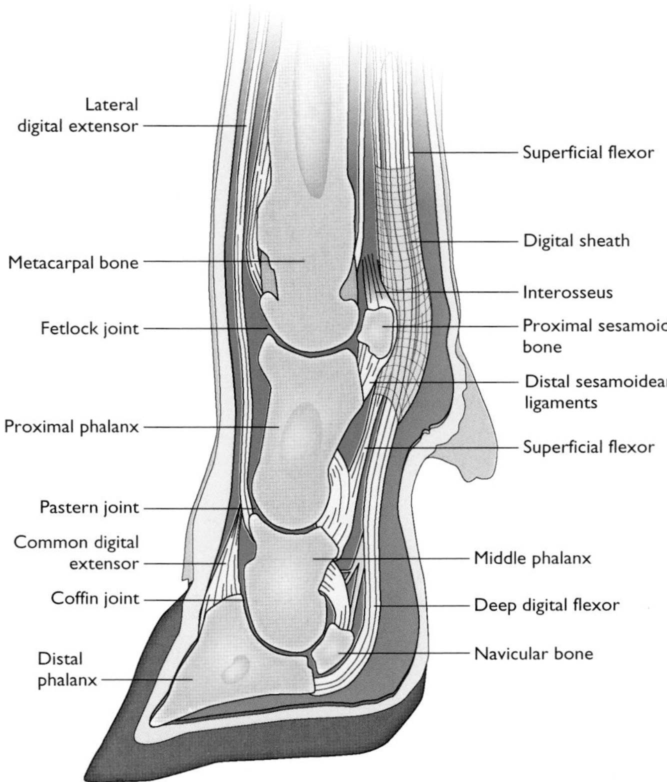

Fig. 17.5 The sagittal section of the bovine foot, splitting the lateral digit. (Reproduced with permission from KM Dyce, WO Sack, CJG Wensing, 2002. Textbook of Veterinary Anatomy, 3rd edn. Philadelphia, PA: WB Saunders, p. 736.)

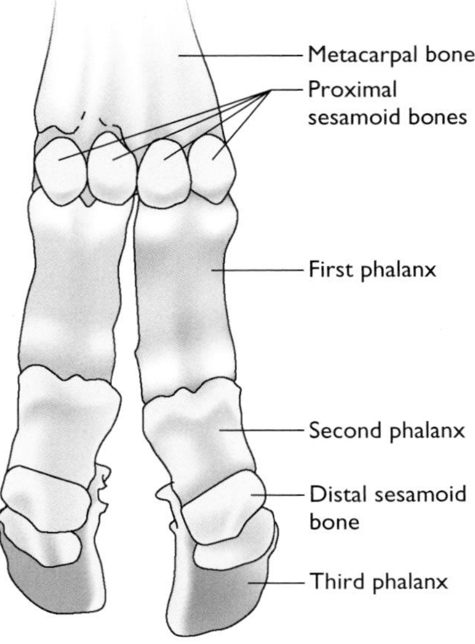

Fig. 17.6 The bones of the distal part of the forelimb of the ox: plantar view. (After S Sisson, JD Grossman, 1969. Anatomy of the Domestic Animals, 4th edn. Philadelphia and London: WB Saunders, p. 150.)

- *Pastern joint* is located between the first and second phalanges.
- *Coffin joint* is located between the second and third phalanges.

The hind limb The *pelvic girdle* of the cow comprises the ilium, ischium and pubis, all of which make a contribution to the acetabulum, which forms the socket of the hip joint. The girdle is robust and angular, resulting in the characteristic bony appearance of the hind end, which is also partly due to the poor development of the muscles around the croup (root of the tail). The 'pin bones' or tuber ischii (Fig. 17.1) are triangular, easily palpated and project well above the vulva on either side of the tail. The sacro-sciatic ligament runs from the dorsal angle of each tuber ischii to attach to the sacrum and forms part of the roof of the pelvic cavity. The 'hook bones' or tuber coxae are very obvious on either side of the sacrum and lumbar spine and the line connecting both tubers is at an angle to the horizontal indicating the slope of the pelvis. This angulation has an effect on the way in which the femur is set in the hip joint, which affects the conformation of the hind limb and a tendency to concussive trauma if abnormally tilted.

The *sacro-sciatic ligament* is not covered by muscle, which makes it easy to palpate when checking for softening prior to calving. Softening results from the changes in hormones around the time of birth. Stretching of the softened ligament facilitates the passage of the calf through the birth canal. The external sign of this is that the cow's tail droops due to reduced support by the ligament.

The head of the relatively short cylindrical *femur* is smaller than that of the horse and it sits in the acetabulum supported by the round ligament to form the *hip joint*. The action of the joint is principally flexion and extension, although there is also a degree of rotation associated with flexion, which makes sure that the stifle joint does not impinge on the abdomen.

The *stifle joint* formed by the distal femur and the proximal tibia is similar to that of the horse. The *patella* is long, narrow and very thick.

The plan of the lower limb reflects the fact that weight is taken on digits 3 and 4.

Tibia is the only weight bearer of the lower limb.

Fibula is much reduced and consists of two parts – a rudimentary proximal end, which is fused with the lateral condyle of the tibia, and at the distal end a separate and palpable lateral malleolus (Fig. 17.7). The proximal surface of this bone articulates with the distal end of the tibia and the distal surface rests on the fibular tarsal bone.

Tarsus – consists of five short bones (Fig. 17.7) arranged in three approximate rows. The largest bones are:

- *Tibial tarsal* (talus): articulates with the fibular tarsal and the fused central and fourth tarsal; part of the proximal row
- *Fibular tarsal* (calcaneous): articulates with the tibial tarsal and bears the tuber calcis; which forms the very obvious point of the hock to which the Achilles tendon attaches; part of the proximal row
- *Central and fourth tarsals*: fused to form a large bone (Fig. 17.7) that extends across the width of the tarsus and articulates with all the bones; forms the middle row
- *First tarsal*: small bone that articulates with the central tarsal and distally with the metatarsus; part of the distal row
- *Second and third tarsals*: fused to form a small bone which articulates distally with the metatarsus; part of the distal row

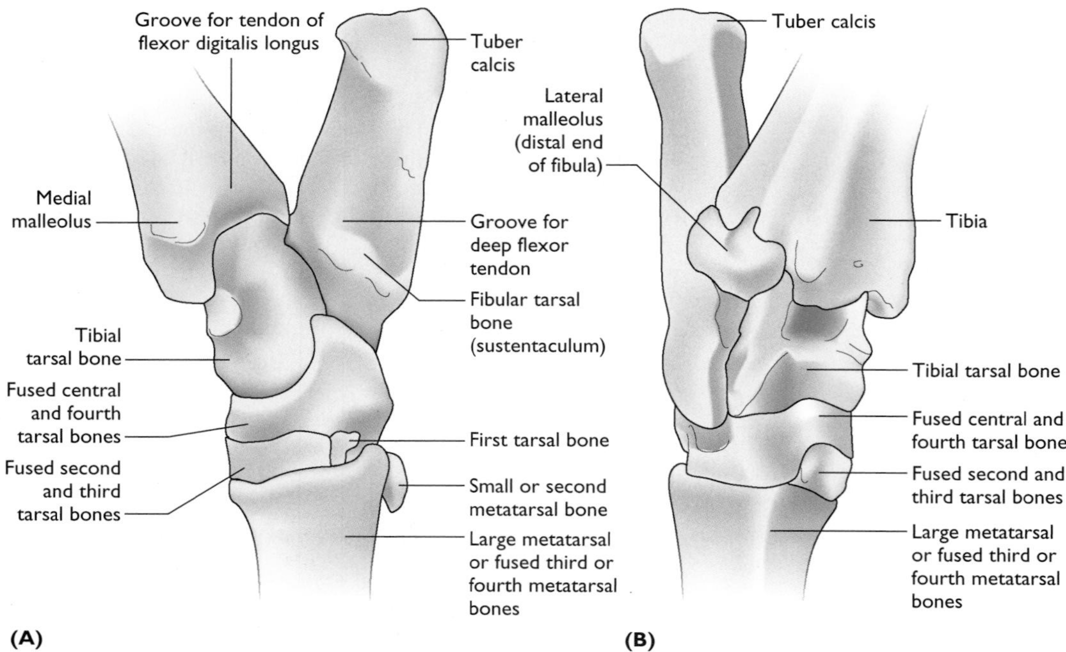

Fig. 17.7 The right tarsus and adjacent bones of the ox. **(A)** Medial view. **(B)** Dorso-lateral view. (After S Sisson, JD Grossman, 1969. Anatomy of the Domestic Animals, 4th edn. Philadelphia and London: WB Saunders, p. 154.)

The bones are linked by synovial joints and the action of the *hock joint* is flexion and extension. The conformation of this joint is significant in animals selected for breeding and the points of the hocks should be vertically below the pin bones when viewed from the back and the side. Abnormal posture may lead to problems in locomotion and may potentially damage the tendons and synovial structures of the digits.

The skeletal anatomy of the hind foot is similar to that described in the forefoot. The single metatarsus is larger than the metacarpus and in cross section is obviously four-sided, which gives the lower hind limb a much more substantial appearance. Research has shown that there is an increased incidence of hind limb problems, which has never been explained.

Splanchnic skeleton

As in the dog and cat the splanchnic skeleton is defined as those bones that are located in soft tissues and are not attached to the skeleton itself. In the cow it is represented by a pair of bones known as the *ossa cordis* within the heart (Fig. 17.8). They lie within the fibrous tissue surrounding the atrioventricular and arterial openings and they consist of islands of fibrocartilage in which there are nodules of bone, which, it is assumed, add extra strength to the tissue.

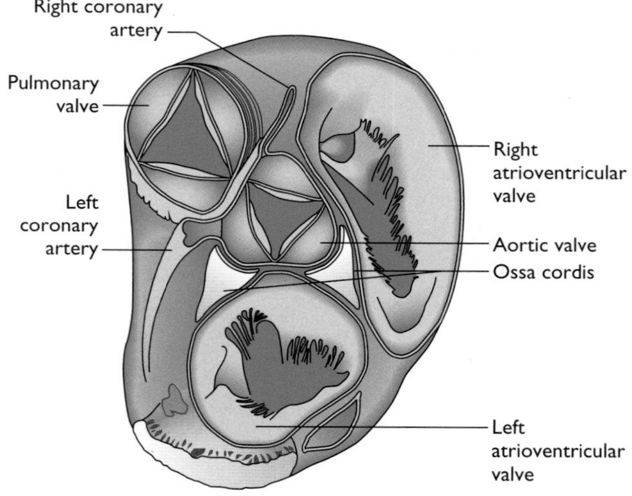

Fig. 17.8 The dorsal view of the base of the bovine heart after removal of the atria. The ossa cordis on both sides of the aortic valve have been exposed. (Reproduced with permission from KM Dyce, WO Sack, CJG Wensing, 2002. Textbook of Veterinary Anatomy, 3rd edn. Philadelphia, PA: WB Saunders, p. 224.)

Muscles and tendons

The function of a muscle and its tendinous attachment to a bone is to bring about locomotion, and in prey species this is primarily to escape predators. Horses rely on speed but as a species *Bos taurus* is not designed for running fast, relying instead on size and the numbers in the herd for protection. Thus the muscles in the horse that are linked to running and jumping are well developed and those in the cow, exactly the same anatomically, are much less developed. However, some breeds of modern cattle (e.g., Hereford, Aberdeen Angus, Charolais and Limousin) are kept for food, which means that as a result of many years of selective breeding the muscles of the lumbar spine and the neck and the proximal parts of the limbs have been developed to produce the choicest cuts of beef. Thus the names and locations of the muscles (Fig. 17.9) are the same but the relative sizes will differ from other species and the degree of development will vary between breeds.

Muscles and tendons of the lower limbs

The muscles of the lower limbs of the cow have a similar arrangement to those in the horse except that the cow has two digits

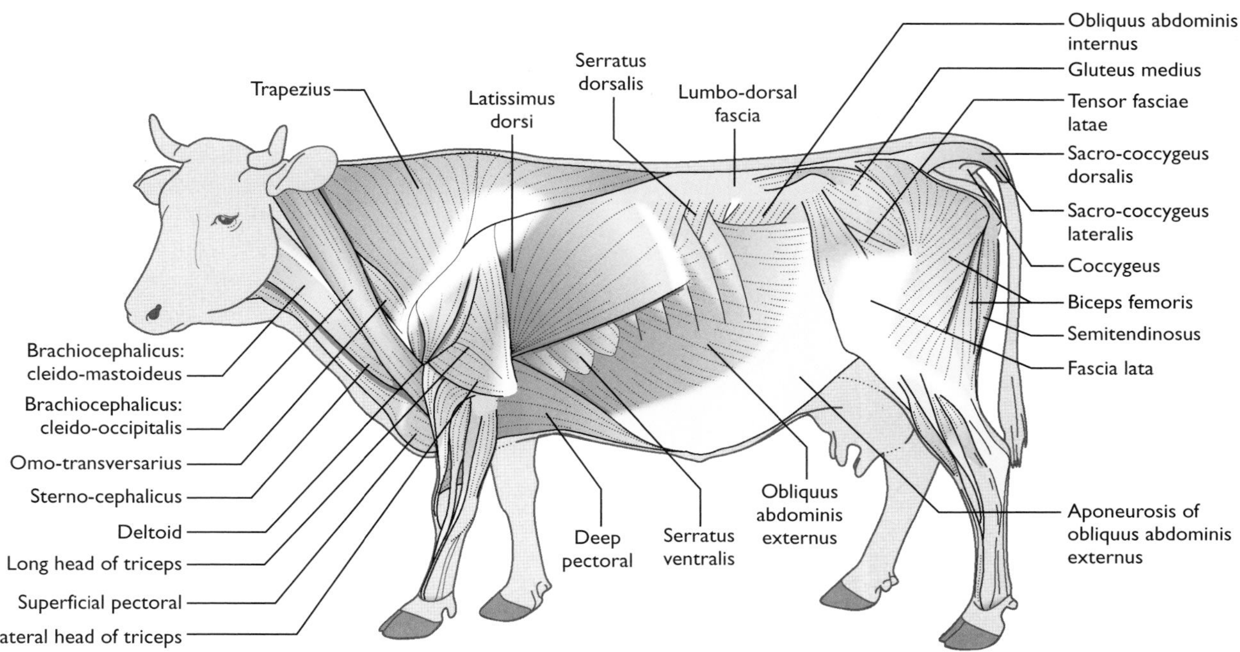

Fig. 17.9 The superficial muscles of the ox, after removal of cutaneous muscle. (After S Sisson, JD Grossman, 1969. Anatomy of the Domestic Animals, 4th edn. Philadelphia and London: WB Saunders, p. 350.)

whereas the horse only has one, which alters the way in which tendons of the digital flexor and extensor muscles insert on the bones (Table 17.1). Figure 17.10 illustrates the arrangement of the tendons as they pass down the limb and then split up to attach to the digits.

As in the dog and the horse, the bellies of the muscles supplying the lower limbs attach on the upper parts of the limbs and their action is brought about by means of long tendons that attach to the appropriate bones lower down the limb. These tendons are relatively superficial but are protected from traumatic damage by the overlying skin and by *synovial sheaths* wrapped around them or by *bursae*, which provide a more discrete cushioning. When the muscle contracts and the tendon moves the synovial fluid lubricates and prevents friction (Fig. 17.11).

Inflammation of a bursa, or bursitis, or of a tendon sheath or tenosynovitis is quite common and it is important to know the anatomy of the area in order to diagnose which structure is affected. Inflammation of these structures presents as swelling, pain, heat and a reduction or loss of function of the joint or muscle.

Interdigital ligaments prevent the two toes from splaying apart as weight is taken on them. The fibres of these structures pass between the two digits at the level of the proximal phalanges and then lower down towards the distal phalanges.

Interosseous muscle is located on the palmar and plantar surfaces of the lower limbs lying along the length of the metacarpus or metatarsus (Fig. 17.12). This flat muscle is fleshy in the young animal but eventually becomes a completely tendinous band running from the carpal joint distally around the structures of the foot. Its five principal branches link with the three extensor tendons (Figs. 17.10 and 17.12) and terminate on the proximal sesamoid bones. This structure forms a 'sling', which is tensed when the fetlock is overextended and the foot takes weight. The superficial digital flexor muscle assists the interosseus in preventing overextension of the fetlock joint.

The hooves

As a member of the order Artiodactyla, the cow bears weight on two toes (digits 3 and 4) and each digit is enclosed in a horny case or hoof that protects the sensitive internal structures. (NB: Horn is the insensitive keratinised epithelium from which hooves, claws and horns are made.) There are four hooves on each limb: the two dewclaws, which consist only of a wall and a bulb and are of no significance, and the two chief digits, which conform to the shape of the distal phalanges (Fig. 17.13).

Each hoof or claw may be considered to have three surfaces:

- Abaxial or outer surface, which is convex from side to side and is ridged which may indicate uneven horn production
- Axial or interdigital surface, which is concave and also ridged
- Ground surface, which consists of a slightly concave sole pointed at the front and a wider softer bulb at the back, which is continuous with the skin

The two claws curve towards each other at both ends, touching each other at the bulbs and sometimes at the apices (Fig. 17.13). The lateral claw is usually larger and it takes the majority of the cow's weight – it may vary in the hind foot.

The structure of each claw is similar to that of the horse and consists of:

Periople is part of the dermis or corium that forms the horn tissue of the wall and lies in a 10 mm flat coronary band above the coronary border of the hoof. It is partly covered with hairy skin and is intermediate in consistency between the soft epidermis and the hard horn. At the back of the foot it is wider and merges with the bulbs of the hoof. The corium itself continues under the

Table 17.1 Muscles of the lower limbs

Muscle	Origin	Insertion	Action
Fore limb			
Extensor group			
Extensor carpi radialis	Lateral condyle of the humerus	Metacarpal tuberosity	Extends and fixes the carpal joint
Extensor carpi obliquus	Lateral border and dorsal surface of the radius	Head of the medial metacarpal bone	Extends the carpus
Common digital extensor	Lateral condyle of the humerus and from the ulna	Third phalanx	Extends the digits. Adducts the digits
Medial digital extensor	Lateral condyle of the humerus	Second and third phalanges of the medial digit	Extends the digits. Abducts the digits
Lateral digital extensor	Lateral ligament of the elbow joint, lateral tuberosity of the radius, and the ulna	Second and third phalanges of the medial digit	Extends the digits. Abducts the digits
Flexor group			
Flexor carpi radialis	Medial condyle of the humerus	Proximal end of the medial metacarpus	Flexes the carpus and extends the elbow
Flexor carpi ulnaris	Medial condyle of the humerus and medial surface of the olecranon	Proximal edge of the accessory carpal bone	Flexes the carpus and extends the elbow
Ulnaris lateralis	Lateral condyle of the humerus	Lateral surface and proximal border of the accessory carpal and the large metacarpal bone	Flexes the carpus and extends the elbow
Superficial digital flexor	Medial condyle of the humerus and a ridge on the posterior surface of the radius	Proximal extremity of the second phalanx and the distal extremity of the first phalanx	Flexes the digits and the carpus and extends the elbow
Deep digital flexor	Medial condyle of the humerus, medial surface of the olecranon, posterior surface of the proximal radius	Cartilage of the third phalanx	Flexes the digits and the carpus and extends the elbow
Hind limb			
Extensor group			
Long digital extensor	Caudal surface of the distal femur; shares its origin with the peroneus tertius	Tendon starts as it passes over the hock and is bound by two annular ligaments. It inserts on the third phalanx.	Extends the digits, flexes the hock and assists in fixing the stifle joint
Medial digital extensor	Caudal surface of the distal femur. Shares its origin with the peroneus tertius	Tendon starts as it passes over the hock and is bound by two annular ligaments. It inserts on the second phalanx of the medial digit.	Extends the digits, flexes the hock and assists in fixing the stifle joint
Lateral digital extensor	Lateral ligament of the stifle joint and lateral condyle of the tibia	Passes over the lateral surface of the hock and inserts on the dorsal surface of the second phalanx of the lateral digit	Extends the digits and flexes the hock
Short digital extensor	Caudal surface of the femur	On the tendon of the long digital extensor	Assists the long digital extensor
Flexor group			
Peroneus longus	Lateral condyle of the tibia and on the fibrous band that represents the shaft of the fibula	First tarsal bone and on the proximal end of the large metatarsal bone	Inwardly rotates the hock joint
Peroneus tertius	Caudal surface of the distal femur with the long and medial digital extensors	Proximal end of the large metatarsal and the fused second and third tarsal bones	Flexes the hock
Anterior tibialis	Lateral surface of the tibial tuberosity and crest	Medial aspect of the hock inserting on the metatarsal bone and the fused second and third tarsal bones	Flexes the hock
Superficial digital flexor	Dorsal surface of the mid-shaft of the femur	Proximal extremity of the second phalanx and the distal extremity of the first phalanx	Flexes the digits and extends the hock; part of the Achilles tendon
Deep digital flexor	Lateral condyle of the tibia	Cartilage of the third phalanx	Flexes the digits and extends the hock

Remember – extensor tendons to the digits run on the dorsal surface of the limb; flexor tendons to the digits run on the palmar or plantar surface of the limb.

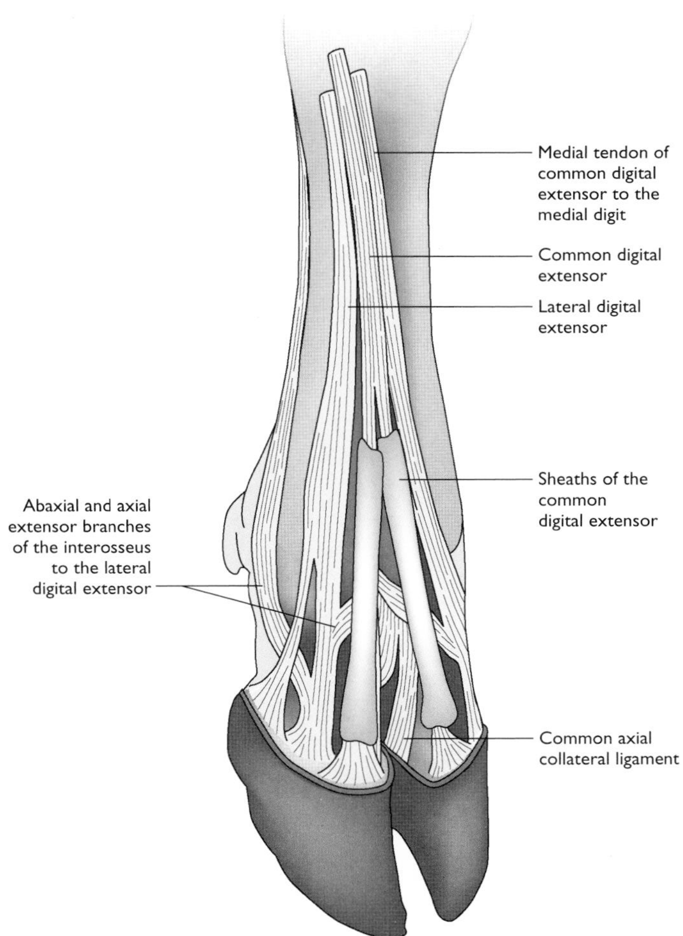

Fig. 17.10 The dorsal view of the bovine right forefoot. (Reproduced with permission from KM Dyce, WO Sack, CJG Wensing, 2002. Textbook of Veterinary Anatomy, 3rd edn. Philadelphia, PA: WB Saunders, p. 738.)

overlying horn material as the sensitive coronary corium, which supplies the horn tissue with nutrients allowing it to grow. It is less well developed than in the horse, which results in a weaker union between the outer horn and the corium, which may be the reason why the cow has evolved a greater weight-bearing surface than in the horse.

Wall forms the greater part of the abaxial and axial surfaces. The distal border makes contact with the ground along the whole length of the abaxial surface but, because the axial surface is slightly concave, only the toe of this part of the wall touches the ground. The wall thins out as it becomes the bulbs of the heel.

Sole is a relatively smooth area within the angle between the abaxial and axial parts of the wall (Fig. 17.13). It is separated from the wall by the *white line*, which is generally lighter in colour. This area is sensitive and is an area of weakness, so infection, penetration or bruising by objects such as stones may result in lameness. Infection may track up into the corium and break out at the coronary band. The lateral hind claw is more commonly affected. The sole gradually merges into the bulb in the centre of the foot – the exact location of the junction depends on the extent of the *digital cushion*, which lies beneath the bulb (Fig. 17.13).

Bulb is the main weight-bearing part of each hoof and it takes up the greater part of the ground surface. It is relatively soft but the greater thickness of the epidermal tissue increases its protectiveness. The tendon of the deep digital flexor is separated from the corium of the bulbs by a digital cushion, which is a mass of fatty elastic tissue designed to absorb concussion during locomotion.

In an adult cow, horn tissue grows at the rate of approximately 5 mm/month from the coronary band and this is balanced by wear from the ground surface. The angle that the wall makes with the ground should be approximately 45–50°. Overgrowth of the tissue may occur at the toe, which shifts weight onto the bulbs of the heel. This changes the angle with the ground and overgrowth is exacerbated because wear is reduced, resulting in twisted and deformed toes. Overgrowth of the sole is most often seen in the hind feet, usually on the lateral claw. Routine assessment of cattle feet and corrective trimming to return the foot to normal size and shape must be carried out regularly by the veterinary surgeon or a qualified foot trimmer.

Digestive system

The cow is a herbivore: it is adapted to eat plant material. The cell walls of plants consist of complex carbohydrates such as cellulose and, because no mammal produces an enzyme capable of breaking these down, initial digestion relies on the action of micro organisms living within a fermentation chamber adapted from part of the gut. The stomach of the cow, in the cranial part of the digestive system, is described as being compound and has evolved to form two chambers, known as the rumen and the reticulum, or the rumenoreticulum, giving rise to the terms 'ruminant' and 'cranial fermenter'. The rumenoreticulum contains an enormous population of micro organisms. There are about 25–50 billion bacteria and 200–500 thousand protozoa in a millilitre of ruminal fluid. Table 17.2 compares digestive systems of other types of herbivorous species. Examples of caudal fermenters are described in Chapters 14 and 16.

Oral cavity

The size of the oral cavity is shorter and wider than in the horse. The *lips* are thick and fairly immobile. The central part of the upper lip and the area between the nostrils form the *muzzle* or planum nasolabiale, which is hairless, often pigmented (depending on breed), smooth, cool and damp due to the secretions of the nasolabial glands. The lower lip is also hairless but the remainder of the area surrounding the mouth is covered in normal hairy skin and tactile hairs used as sensing probes.

The *tongue* may be pigmented with a wide root and body and a narrow mobile tip, which aids prehension and the formation of a food bolus. The posterior part of the back of the tongue forms an elliptical prominence, which is made obvious by a transverse depression in front of it. In front of this prominence the surface is covered in numerous tough backward-pointing papillae. These are extremely rough to the touch, which also aids in prehension. On the surface of the prominence are a variety of different shapes of papillae, some of which have taste buds at their base.

The *hard palate* is wide and usually pigmented. The incisive bone is covered in a thick layer of dense connective tissue

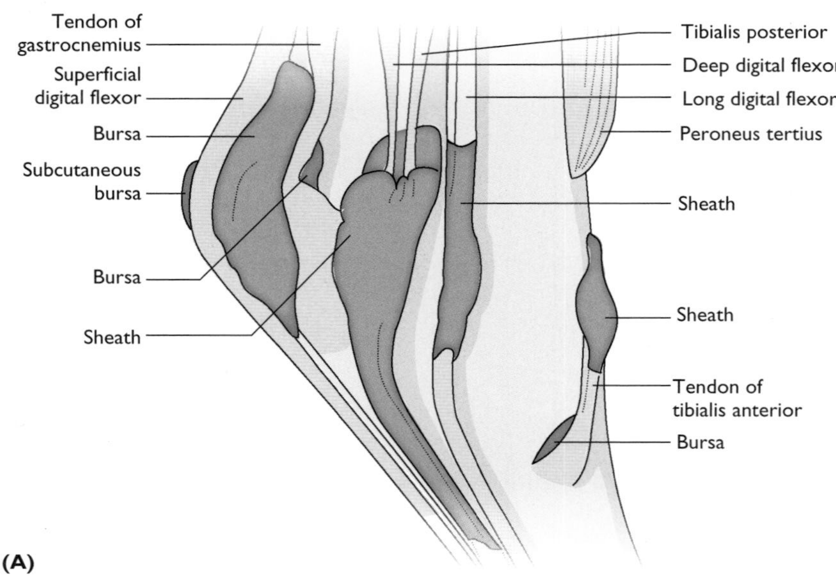

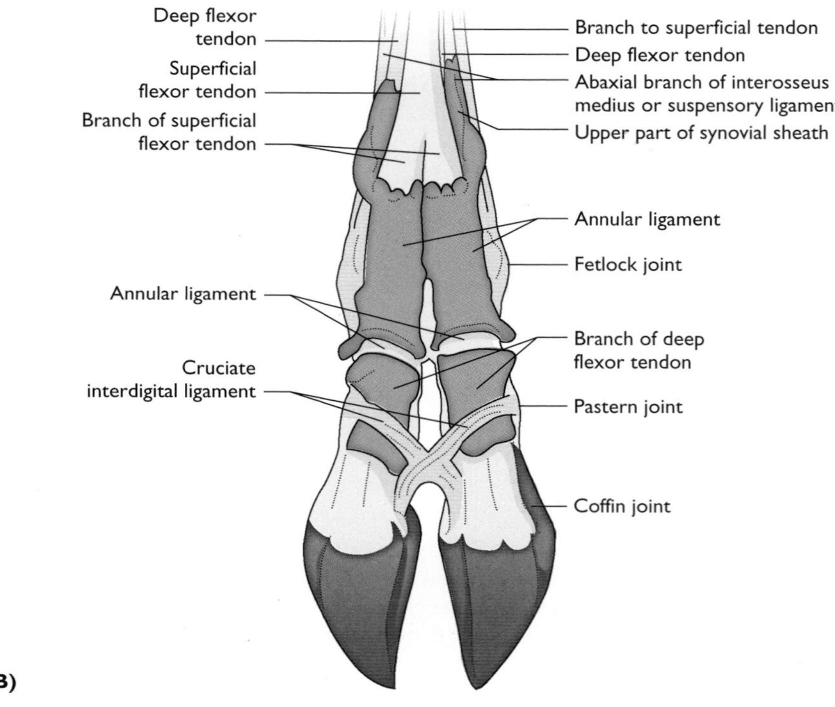

Fig. 17.11 **(A)** The left tarsus of the ox with synovial sheaths and bursae injected: medial view. **(B)** The distal part of the limb of the ox with synovial sheaths injected: plantar view. (After S Sisson, JD Grossman, 1969. Anatomy of the Domestic Animals, 4th edn. Philadelphia and London: WB Saunders, p. 360.)

covered in horny epithelium and forming the *dental pad*. This takes the place of the upper incisors and is used to break off plant material before it is chewed and swallowed. Towards the junction with the soft palate, the hard palate is covered in a series of serrated ridges and at the back of the cavity the covering of the palate becomes smooth.

The *salivary glands*, consisting of the parotid, mandibular and sublingual glands, secrete a fluid that consists mainly of mucus and water. In the cow there is no amylase and the main function of saliva is to lubricate the food, form a bolus, neutralise the acid formed by ruminal micro organisms and it may prevent excessive frothing in the rumen.

Teeth

The dental formula of the permanent teeth is:

$(I0/4, C0/0, PM3/3, M3/3) \times 2 = 32.$

There are no incisors or canines in the upper jaw and there are eight incisors in the lower jaw (Fig. 17.14). These are arranged in a continuous fan-like arcade that is opposed to the dental pad. In most mammals there are six incisors but in the cow the canine tooth on either side may be considered to have become the extra incisors. There is a wide gap or *diastema* between the incisors and the cheek teeth, the premolars and molars, of which there are three of each type on either side in

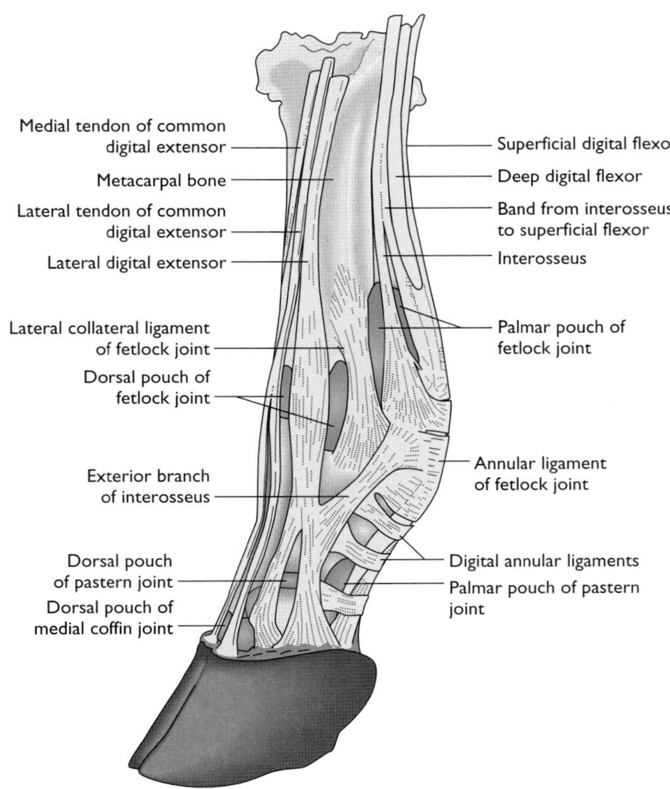

Fig. 17.12 The bovine left forefoot: lateral view. (Reproduced with permission from KM Dyce, WO Sack, CJG Wensing, 2002. Textbook of Veterinary Anatomy, 3rd edn. Philadelphia, PA: WB Saunders, p. 739.)

both jaws. These increase in size from front to back and are arranged in such a way that one tooth is opposed to two teeth in the opposite jaw. The enamel of each tooth is arranged in prominent crescent-shaped ridges and the flattened or 'table' surfaces slope from side to side. These uneven surfaces, coupled with the circular action of the bovine temporomandibular joint, result in an efficient grinding mechanism that turns the plant material into a pulp.

The teeth are described as being hypsodontic as they are in the horse (cf. brachydontic teeth of the dog, cat and pig). This means that they sit tall above the gum, do not have a layer of enamel over the top and the enamel over the sides is folded, which increases the area of hard material used for grinding. As the animal ages the crowns of the teeth wear down, which is compensated for by the continuous growth of the teeth and when growth eventually stops the roots are exposed. The crowns only wear away completely in very old animals.

Abdominal cavity

Cranial digestive tract

The *oesophagus*, which is wider and more dilatable than that of the horse, leads from the pharynx and enters the rumen via the *cardia*. The stomach is described as being compound (cf. the stomachs of the dog, cat. horse and pig which are described as being simple) and consists of four chambers. The largest are the *rumen and reticulum*, which form the fermentation chamber in which a population of micro organisms begin the breakdown of complex carbohydrates such as cellulose. The rumen extends from the eighth rib to the pelvic inlet (Fig. 17.15), occupying the greater part of the left side of the animal. The reticulum is much smaller and lies cranial to the rumen under the cover of the sixth to eighth rib. It is closely opposed to the diaphragm, on the other side of which is the heart. It lies above the xiphoid process of the sternum; applying pressure to this area with your knee may elicit a pain response if the organ is diseased.

Traumatic reticulitis, or 'wire' is a condition in which a cow ingests a penetrating foreign body such as a piece of wire or other metal debris. The weight of the wire and the normal contractions of the rumen and reticulum cause the foreign body to fall to the bottom of the reticulum, where it may penetrate the reticular wall, resulting in grunting with the ruminal movements. The foreign body may further penetrate the diaphragm, causing reticuloperitonitis, and even the pericardium surrounding the nearby heart, leading to reticulopericarditis. The treatment is to open the rumen (rumenotomy) and manually retrieve the foreign body from the depths of the reticulum.

The two chambers are divided by a series of pillars that encircle and project into the lumen but in fact the two may almost be considered to one organ – the *rumenoreticulum*. These pillars create folds that are visible externally (Fig. 17.16), producing a sac-like appearance. The cardia, at the end of the oesophagus, opens into both the rumen and the reticulum and leading from this is a thick-walled gutter known as the *reticular groove*, which eventually opens into the third chamber, the omasum. This groove is important in unweaned calves. During suckling the groove forms a complete tube that channels milk directly from the oesophagus into an omasal canal and then into the abomasum, thus avoiding the processes in the rumenoreticulum. It is the act of suckling that causes the tube to form, and incorrect presentation of the milk (e.g., in some bucket-fed systems) may cause milk to spill over into the rumenoreticulum where it may become sour, resulting in digestive upsets. As the animal matures use of the reticular groove decreases, although some soluble nutrients dissolved in saliva during mastication may still bypass the rumenoreticulum.

The third chamber of the compound stomach is the *omasum*, which lies within the abdomen to the right of the midline (Figs. 17.15 and 17.16) under the cover of ribs 8–11. Within the lumen there is an *omasal canal*, which connects at one end with the reticular groove via a *reticulo-omasal opening* and at the other end with the abomasum via a large oval *omaso-abomasal opening*. This allows the passage of more liquid ingesta straight into abomasum bypassing the omasum.

The fourth chamber is the *abomasum*, which lies flexed on the floor of the abdomen (Figs. 17.15 and 17.16) and the lower pole of the omasum sits within its angle. It is divided into the fundus and body, which connects with the omasum and the pyloric part, which connects with the duodenum. Within the pylorus is a large swelling, the *torus pyloricus*, which narrows the passage through the pylorus but its true function is unknown. The abomasum is attached externally to the rumen and reticulum so it moves when they contract. It is in the abomasum that enzymic digestion occurs as it would in the simple stomach of other species.

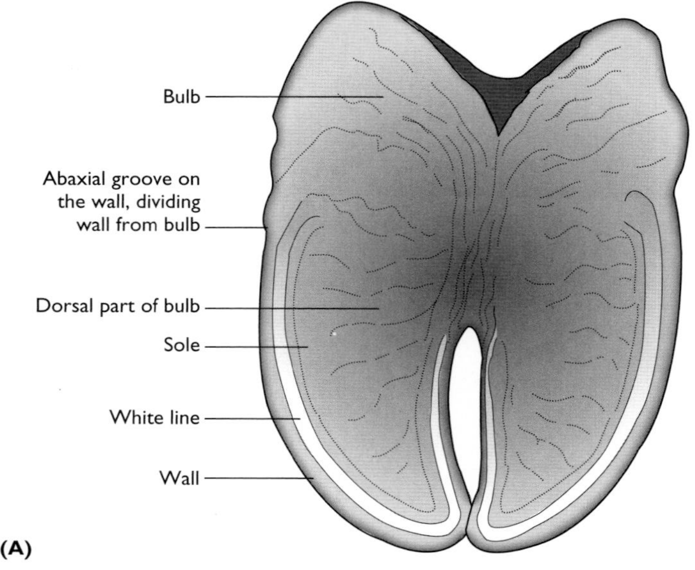

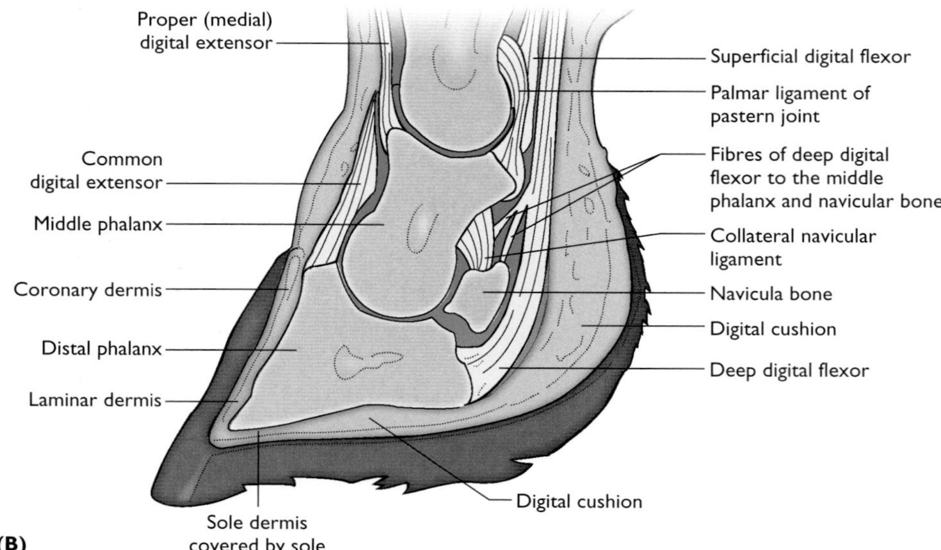

Fig. 17.13 **(A)** The ground surface of the hooves of the bovine forefoot. **(B)** The sagittal section of the medial digit of the bovine forefoot. (Reproduced with permission from KM Dyce, WO Sack, CJG Wensing, 2002. Textbook of Veterinary Anatomy, 3rd edn, Philadelphia. PA: WB Saunders, p. 740/741.)

Displaced abomasum may occur to the right or to the left and both conditions are associated with intensively fed and high-yielding dairy cows, although it can occur spontaneously in other cows. The abomasum becomes atonic, fills with gas and liquid ingesta and the organ rises out of its normal position into the dorsal abdomen. Percussion of the dorsal anterior abdomen either on the left or the right may be diagnosed by a pinging sound when the last rib is flicked with a finger. The condition is painful and may be life threatening. A displaced abomasum may be further complicated by spontaneous torsion and apart from the obvious differences, it relates to gastric torsion in the dog. Treatment includes deflation of the organ through the abdominal wall, followed by an abomasoplexy (fixing the deflated organ to the abdominal wall to prevent recurrence). In some cases placing the cow on its back and gently rolling it from side to side may be enough to free the abomasum so that it returns to its normal position. The patient may be given spasmolytics, analgesics and a high-fibre diet to encourage gut motility.

Epithelial linings: Each chamber of the compound stomach is lined with *keratinised stratified squamous epithelium* and has a characteristic appearance according to its location and function:

- *Reticulum* is arranged into folds about 1 cm high enclosing four-, five- or six-sided spaces, creating a honeycomb or reticulated effect. The spaces are subdivided into smaller cells and the floors are covered in horny papillae. Towards the junction with the rumen the pattern modifies and merges with the pattern of the ruminal epithelium.
- *Rumen* consists of numerous papillae that vary in prominence, depending on age and diet of the individual cow and the area of the rumen. The shapes of the papillae vary from rounded to conical or leaf-shaped.

The abrasive nature of the epithelial lining was originally thought to assist in the maceration and breakdown of the fibrous food material but it is now known that the upper keratinised layer protects against damage by tough plant material whilst

Table 17.2 Types of digestive system found within the herbivores

Species	Latin name	Cranial fermenter – fermentation takes place within an adaptation of the stomach (i.e., foregut)	Caudal fermenter – fermentation takes place within the caecum and/or colon (i.e., hindgut)
Cow	*Bos taurus*	✓	
Sheep	*Ovies aries*	✓	
Goat	*Capra hircus*	✓	
Deer	(generic term)	✓	
Horse	*Equus caballus*		✓
Rabbit	*Oryctolagus cuniculus*		✓
Chinchilla	*Chinchilla lanigera*		✓
Guinea pig	*Cavia porcellus*		✓
Camelids (i.e., llamas and alpacas)	*Lama glama and Lama pacas*	✓	
African elephant	*Loxodonta africana*		✓
Antelope	(generic term)	✓	

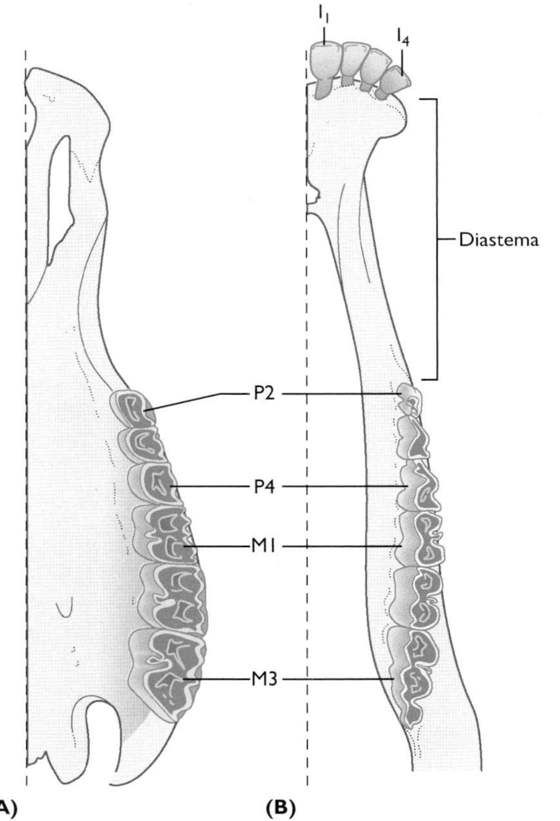

Fig. 17.14 (A) The left half of the upper and **(B)** the right half of the lower jaw of cattle. Note the different shapes of the upper and lower cheek teeth and the large diastema. (Reproduced with permission from KM Dyce, WO Sack, CJG Wensing, 2002. Textbook of Veterinary Anatomy, 3rd edn. Philadelphia, PA: WB Saunders, p. 638.)

the deeper layers absorb volatile fatty acids (VFAs) resulting from microbial fermentation within the chambers.

Omasum: The cavity of the chamber is almost completely filled with about a hundred longitudinal folds or laminae, which hang from the greater curvature and the sides, thus resembling a book. There are about a dozen particularly long ones with shorter ones interspersed between them and even shorter ones between those. The area around the reticulo-omasal and omaso-abomasal openings are free of these folds.

Tripe. This is the term applied to the lining and underlying muscular tissue of the rumen and reticulum when it is removed from the carcass of a cow. In life it is a greeny-brown colour, resulting from staining with plant material, but when washed it becomes white or pale grey. Tripe is considered to be a great delicacy in parts of the UK, when washed tripe may be served cooked with onions and white sauce. Unwashed tripe still has plant material sticking to it and this provides a better level of nutrition when it is fed to dogs.

- *Abomasum* is divided into two parts: the *piriform sac*, which consists of the fundus and the body and is analogous with the simple stomach of other species, and the *pyloric* part, which leads into the duodenum. The whole organ is lined with a pinkish slimy glandular mucosa. At the omaso-abomasal junction the epithelium becomes columnar with occasional goblet cells. The mucosa of the fundus and body contains true peptic glands and its function relates to that of the simple stomach, while the mucosa of the pyloric part secretes only mucus. The internal surface area is increased by the presence of large folds that spiral over the walls of the fundus and body. These folds reduce in the flexed area of the abomasum and terminate in a form of plug that prevents the reflux of ingesta into the omasum. The lining of the pyloric part has a few lower folds. At the exit of the pylorus is a torus or swelling that is capable of enlargement but its function is unknown.

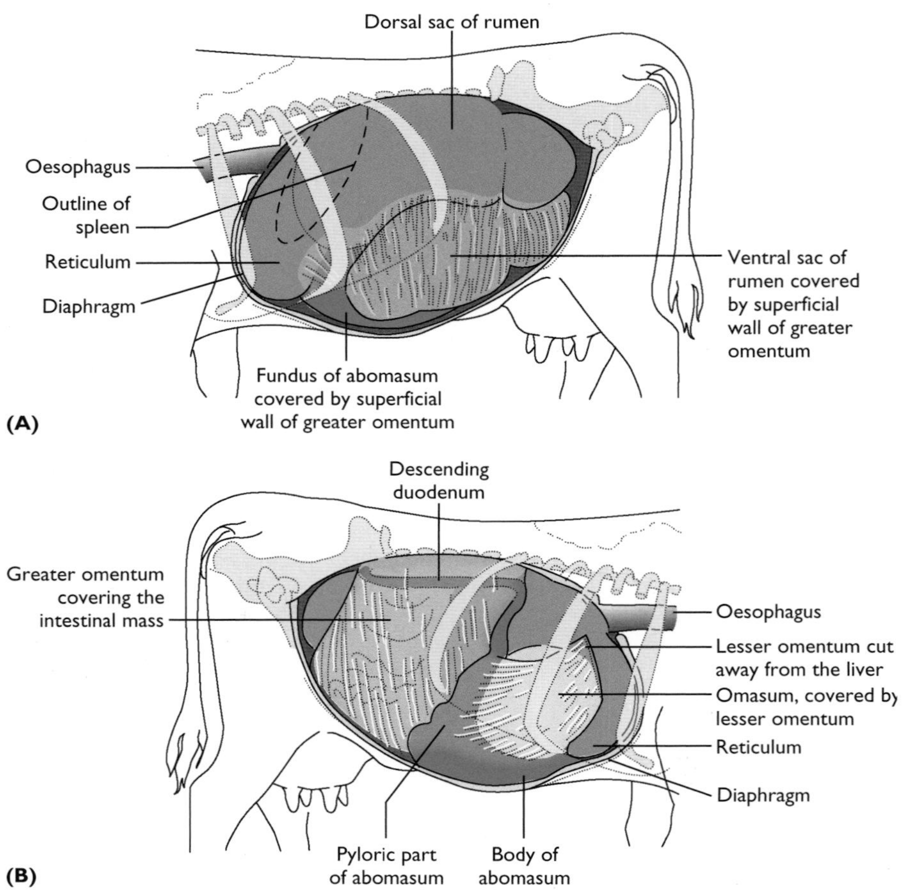

Fig. 17.15 The topography of the abdominal viscera. **(A)** The relationship of the abdominal viscera to the left abdominal wall. **(B)** Relationship of the abdominal viscera to the right abdominal wall: the liver has been removed. (Reproduced with permission from KM Dyce, WO Sack, CJG Wensing, 2002. Textbook of Veterinary Anatomy, 3rd edn. Philadelphia, PA: WB Saunders, p. 670.)

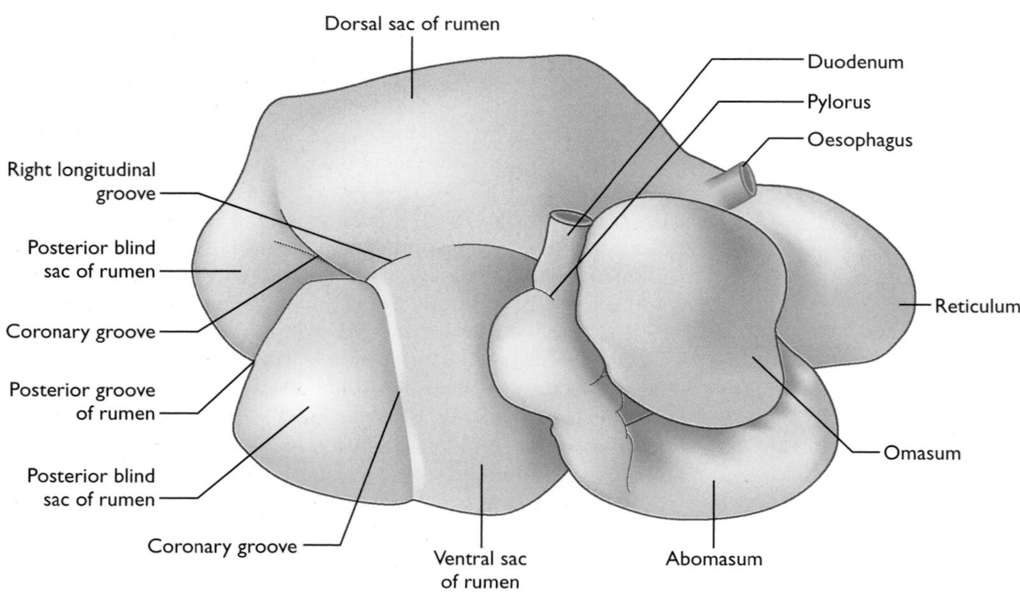

Fig. 17.16 The stomach of the ox: right view. (After S Sisson, JD Grossman, 1969. Anatomy of the Domestic Animals, 4th edn. Philadelphia and London: WB Saunders p. 458.)

Function The cow ingests plant material by using a combination of the tongue and lips, which tear the fibrous stems and leaves from the plant then pinch it off between the incisors and the dental pad. The food is masticated using the tongue, the flattened abrasive surfaces of the table teeth and the circular motion of the temporomandibular joint. The food is ground into a fibrous pulp and the tongue, cheeks and lips help to form a bolus which is swallowed.

The bolus travels along the oesophagus by peristalsis and enters the rumenoreticulum. The walls of the compound stomach contain bundles of smooth muscle that run in both longitudinal and circular directions. These initiate a regular sequence of rhythmic contractions that mix and redistribute the food backwards and forwards through both the rumen and reticulum. These contractions are repeated several times per minute passing between the two chambers and are interspersed with periods of regurgitation during which food passes back up the oesophagus and into the oral cavity by antiperistalsis. Here the food is remasticated and reinsalivated – a process known as *chewing the cud* – and it is then reswallowed and, because it is heavy with saliva, it tends to drop through the cardia into the reticulum. Food within the rumenoreticulum tends to be layered; the food that is well chewed and impregnated with saliva is heavy and falls to the bottom, while the food that is less well chewed and not as wet is lighter and lies above it. The uppermost layer consists of a mixture of carbon dioxide and methane produced by microbial fermentation. It is the food in the middle layers that is most likely to be regurgitated for further mastication.

Rumination is a process that enables the cow to search for food, ingest it quickly and then chew it at a later time. It involves the processes of regurgitation, remastication, reinsalivation and reswallowing. Remastication is a slower, more relaxed activity than the initial chewing and the regurgitated material consists mainly of roughage and fluid and very little concentrate. Cattle spend an average of eight hours a day ruminating with periods of activity scattered throughout the day. The process appears to be mainly reflex and the main stimulus appears to be the presence of roughage in the reticulum or near to the cardia.

Eructation, or more colloquially, belching, allows the cow to expel via the mouth and nostrils methane and carbon dioxide produced by the microbial fermentation process. This occurs at a rate of 1–3 eructations per minute and a large proportion of the methane is inspired and recycled by absorption in the lungs. Both eructation and regurgitation cause a temporary small dilation of the oesophagus running up towards the mouth, which may be observed when a cow is sitting down and quietly ruminating.

After spending some time within the rumen and reticulum, food that is sufficiently soaked and macerated reaches the reticulo-omasal orifice and may either pass directly into the abomasum or, if requiring further processing, will pass into the omasum. Here contractions squeeze fluid out of the ingesta, further grind the more solid material and then pass it into the abomasum. Peristaltic contractions within the abomasum are similar to those within the simple stomach. There is maximum activity within the pyloric region and least within the fundus.

Microbial activity within the rumenoreticulum converts plant material into VFAs, carbon dioxide, methane, ammonia and microbial cells. These are utilised by the cow as sources of energy, high-quality protein and many water-soluble vitamins. Acetic acid is an example of a VFA produced within the rumen. It is absorbed through the rumen wall and is used as an energy source by both the muscles and the mammary glands. The microbes are able to use non-protein nitrogen sources such as urea and ammonia and convert it into their own body protein. In this way the association between the host cow and its microbial flora is an example of a symbiotic or a mutualistic relationship. The digestive process within the abomasum relies on the secretion of enzymes and is similar to that in a simple stomach. It is mainly aimed at the digestion of protein by the action of pepsin.

Neonatal development: At the time of birth the abomasum of the calf occupies about 60% of its final adult size while the rumen and reticulum are very small and appear to be collapsed. The omasum is also small and forms a linking bridge between the rumen and the abomasum. The lining of the abomasum is immature and only begins to change after a few days. This may be linked to its ability to absorb colostral antibodies unchanged within the first few days of life.

As the calf grows there are few observable changes in the structure of the forestomach until the calf starts to show an interest in solid food, which is generally from about 2 to 3 weeks of age, and the availability of suitable forage will affect normal development. Exposure to a plant diet must continue for some time for development to continue and a return to a milk diet will stop the process. After this the abomasum grows steadily while the rumen and reticulum develop extremely rapidly. Opinions differ as to when the compound stomach reaches its final adult proportions but it is sometime between 3 and 12 months of age.

Caudal digestive tract

The parts of the small and large intestine are similar to those in the dog and there are no specific adaptations to a herbivorous diet. They mainly lie to the right of the midline and in the cranial abdomen, partly under the ribs (Fig. 17.15). The total length and capacity is relatively small – about 50 m – which indicates the efficiency of digestion in the compound stomach.

Anatomically the most obvious difference is in the colon. This is divided into ascending, transverse and descending parts but the ascending part is wound into an elaborate double spiral (Fig. 17.17) known as the *ansa spiralis*. The first part spirals towards the centre of the coil while the second part spirals outwards and eventually leads into the transverse colon.

Function The food material that leaves the abomasum includes undigested fibre, some micro organisms and proteins and some sugars produced by the micro organisms. There may also be proteins, fats and carbohydrates that are not able to be digested in the rumenoreticulum but will be digested in the small intestine. Enzymic digestion continues in the small intestine with the aid of pancreatic enzymes and bile from the liver and gall bladder but its major function is in the absorption of the majority of the digested nutrients. Water and VFAs are absorbed by the large intestine and the VFAs are used as a source of energy by the body tissues. The faeces excreted by the cow consist of some undigested food, water and metabolic waste and its consistency is an indicator of the health of the individual. Normal manure is a dark greenish brown and of a dropping consistency. It should not be runny or overly solid but it will vary according to the type of diet; for example, cows on lush spring grass may produce profuse watery green diarrhoea.

Urinary system

The arrangement of the urinary system is the same as for other mammalian species: a pair of kidneys are each drained by a

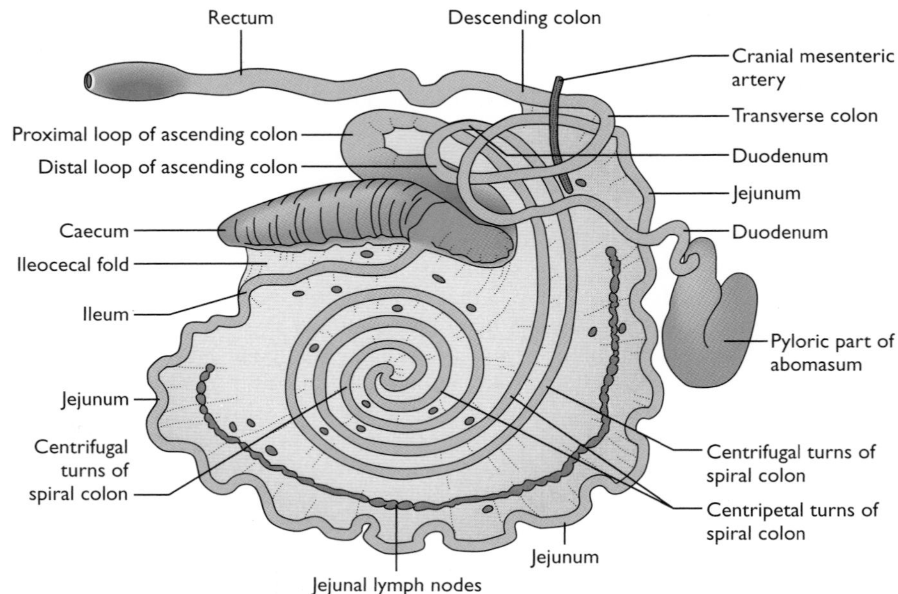

Fig. 17.17 The right lateral view of the bovine intestinal tract: schematic. (Reproduced with permission from KM Dyce, WO Sack, CJG Wensing, 2002. Textbook of Veterinary Anatomy, 3rd edn. Philadelphia, PA: WB Saunders, p. 684.)

ureter, which conducts urine into the urinary bladder. This, in turn is drained by a single urethra, which conveys urine out of the body. However, the position and the external appearance of the bovine kidney is different from that of the canine, feline or equine kidneys.

Position

- *Right kidney* is ellipsoidal in shape, is slightly flattened (Fig. 17.18) and lies in the expected position in the right dorso-lumbar area of the abdomen below the last rib and the transverse processes of L2-3. This is close to the liver, pancreas, duodenum and colon but the position varies with the respiratory phase of the living animal. The hilus is wide and lies on the ventromedial surface of the kidney. The ureter runs from the hilus following a retroperitoneal route across the dorsal abdominal wall and into the pelvic cavity.
- *Left kidney* is flattened at its cranial pole and is thicker at its caudal pole (Fig. 17.18) and it lies behind and ventral to the right kidney under L2-4 almost in the midline, which is a result of the postnatal growth of the rumen. It hangs in a long fold of mesentery and rests on the adjacent mass of intestine and is flattened by the rumen. Its ureter crosses the dorsal surface of the kidney to reach the left side of the abdomen and then it runs in a similar fashion to the right ureter. In a starved animal, when the rumen may be much less distended, the kidney may come to lie much closer to the left side. The position of the kidney in life moves with the animal's respiration.

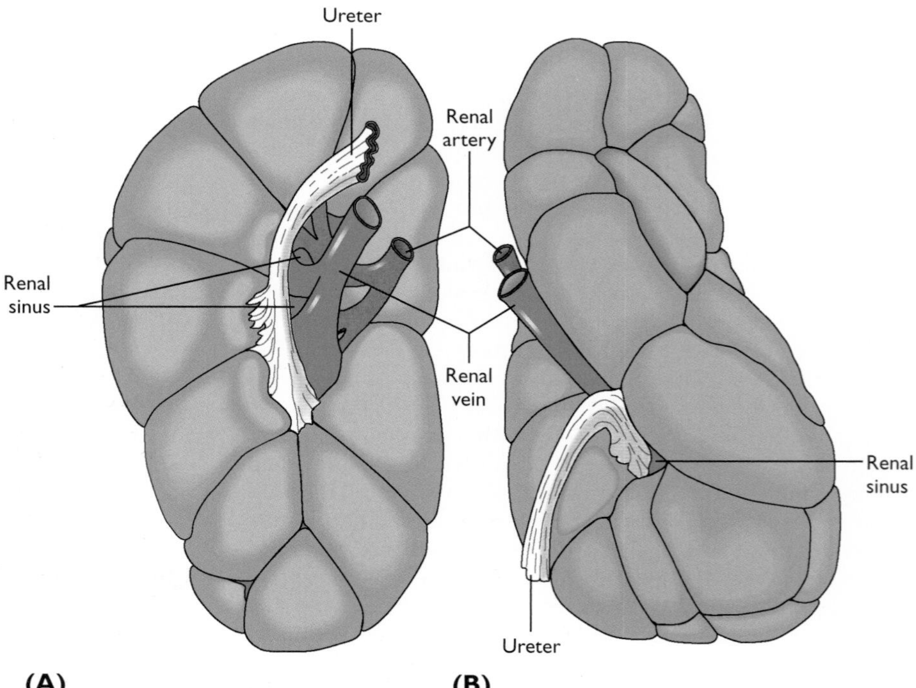

Fig. 17.18 Ventral views of **(A)** the right kidney and **(B)** the left kidney. (Reproduced with permission from KM Dyce, WO Sack, CJG Wensing, 2002. Textbook of Veterinary Anatomy, 3rd edn. Philadelphia, PA: WB Saunders, p. 687.)

External appearance

The kidney of the cow is lobated, being divided into at least 12 lobes by deep fissures (Fig. 17.18). The kidney is multipyramidal: each lobe contains a separate medullary pyramid, which is capped by a continuous cortex, although it may appear that this is also lobed. The apex of each pyramid drains into a cup or calyx derived from the ureter. These calyces join together to form two larger cups draining the cranial and caudal poles of the kidney and they combine to form the single ureter that leaves via the hilus. There is no renal pelvis corresponding to that in the canine or feline kidney.

The whole kidney is covered in a tough capsule, which in a healthy kidney may be easily stripped away except in the hilar region. In a normal animal each kidney is surrounded by a large amount of fat, which provides additional protection.

Suet. The slightly granular fat traditionally used for making dumplings and suet puddings is taken from the lumbar area of the bovine carcass around the outside of each renal capsule.

Normal bovine urine is pale to medium yellow in colour and should be clear. The normal pH is about 8 and therefore slightly alkaline, which is characteristic of a herbivorous diet. The specific gravity should be 1.015–1.030.

Reproductive system

Female

The female of the species *Bos taurus* is known as a cow; the young cow, up to the time that she has her first calf, is known as a heifer.

Reproductive tract

The parts of the tract are the same as in other mammals but the shape of the tract (Fig. 17.19) differs from other species:

- *Ovary*: The adult ovaries lie in the caudal abdomen, close to the pelvic inlet. Each is attached to the body wall and the uterus by means of the *broad ligament* and, except in advanced pregnancy when the ovaries are pulled down by the weight of the gravid uterus, they do not move much further forward. Each ovary is oval and is surprisingly small for such a large animal, being not much longer than 4 cm. Both the follicles and the mature corpora lutea project from the ovarian tissue and are manually palpable per rectum, providing evidence of the reproductive phase of the individual cow.
- *Uterine tube*: Long and tortuous (Fig. 17.19). The *infundibulum* opens over the lateral part of the ovary and lies within the mesosalpinx. There is a gradual transition from the tube to the uterine horn.
- *Uterus*: In the adult, the uterus lies almost entirely within the abdominal cavity. On external examination it appears to consist of a long *body* (apparently about 15 cm long) and two divergent *uterine horns*, which curve ventrally; however, internally, the body is very short (about 3 cm long) and the caudal parts of the long horns, which lie side by side, are incompletely fused except for a connection by the superficial (Fig. 17.19) dorsal and ventral *intercornual ligaments*. These form a small pocket that opens cranially and provides a useful means of fixing the tract digitally during a rectal examination. The consistency of the uterine wall varies

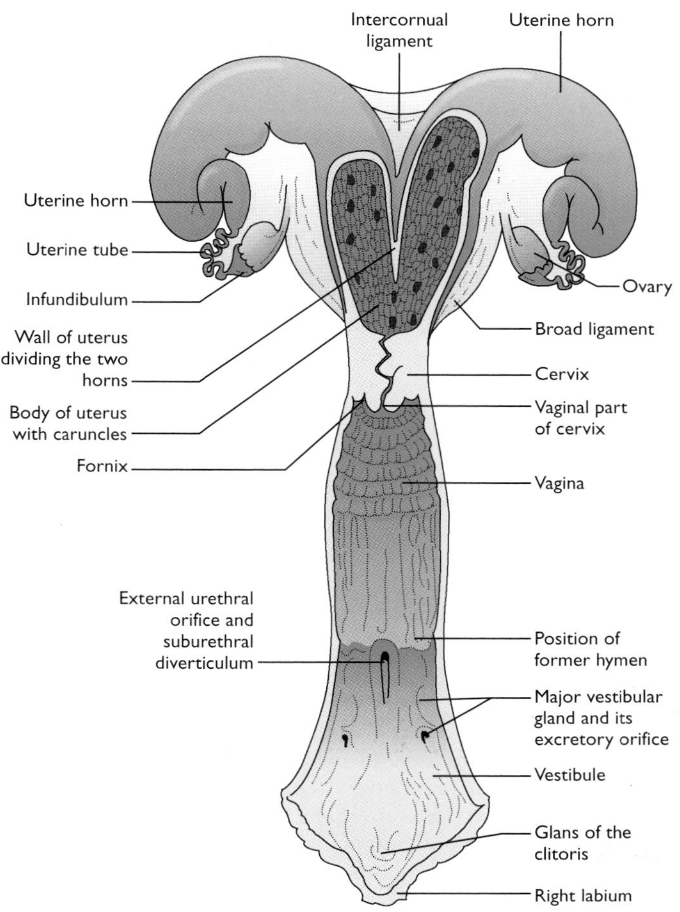

Fig. 17.19 The bovine reproductive organs: dorsal view. The uterus, cervix, vagina and vestibule have been opened. (Reproduced with permission from KM Dyce, WO Sack, CJG Wensing, 2002. Textbook of Veterinary Anatomy, 3rd edn. Philadelphia, PA: WB Saunders, p. 699.)

and stimulation of the uterine muscle during rectal examination causes it to contract and become much firmer; this is most obvious during oestrus.

Internally the *endometrium* varies in both colour and thickness according to the phase of the oestrous cycle. Distributed over the surface are noticeable *caruncles*, which, in the mature but non-pregnant cow, may be 15 mm long and project above the endometrial surface. There are about 40 caruncles arranged in four more or less regular rows in the wider parts of each horn. During pregnancy the surface of the caruncles become enlarged, pitted and invaded by villi from the allanto-chorion to form *cotyledons*. The cotyledonary placenta (cf. zonary placenta of the dog and cat) is a characteristic of ruminants and it is through these cotyledons that exchange of nutrients and gases between the dam and the foetus takes place (Fig. 17.30). The mucosa of the uterine body is much smoother and leads into the cervix through the narrowing of the internal cervical orifice.

- *Cervix*: About 10 cm long with a dense muscular wall that may be as much as 2–3 cm thick. The *cervical canal* forms a spiral and is usually tightly closed. During pregnancy it is sealed by a mucous plug secreted by the cervical mucosa. There is a very obvious delineation between the uterus and the cervix and then the cervix and the vagina, which makes passage of a catheter difficult except when the cow is in oestrus or pregnant.

- *Vagina*: A featureless organ divided in a ratio of 3:1 between the vagina and the *vestibule*. The boundary between the two is marked by the *external urethral orifice*, which is the entrance to the urethra and bladder lying on the floor of the vagina and within about 10 cm of the ventral junction of the two labia. The vagina is able to markedly expand during parturition, which is brought about by the presence of low longitudinal folds seen only when the organ is collapsed. The vestibule slopes ventrally to open between the two *vulval labia*, which are flaccid, wrinkled and joined dorsally and ventrally; the ventral junction bears a number of long hairs. Lying between the two labia is the clitoris, which may be about 10 cm in length and the tip may be visible at the ventral labial junction.

The mammary glands

The cow has four mammary glands or quarters, which are collectively known as the *udder* and are much larger than those seen in the horse. Each gland bears one principal *teat*, which averages about 6–7 cm in length, and each teat has one teat *orifice*. Accessory or supernumerary teats are not uncommon, particularly on the two hind quarters. These may be associated with glandular tissue but are considered to be an undesirable characteristic because the extra teats interfere with the design of the milking cluster and they are sometimes removed from young calves destined to be replacement heifers.

The appearance of the udder varies greatly between individuals, breed and the degree of maturity. Young heifers will have small underdeveloped udders while a dairy cow in full milk may have an extremely large udder that may weigh as much as 60 kg. An obvious *intermammary groove* divides the udder into right and left but the boundary between the fore- and hindquarters is less distinct. The skin of the udder is thin, supple and freely moveable and is covered with fine soft hairs, while the skin of the teats is more firmly attached and is hairless.

The dorsal surface of the udder fits snuggly against the abdominal wall but the part below the pelvis is narrower and is pressed between the thighs. The udder is suspended from the abdominal wall by a well-developed *suspensory apparatus* that runs caudally and is attached to the pubic symphysis by a strong tendon.

An average dairy cow will produce about 7000 l of milk in a single lactation, which is far more than is needed by her calf. Research has shown that it takes 500 l of blood flowing through the udder to produce 1 l of milk, so it follows that the blood supply to the tissue is of high volume and is very important and very complicated. The main arteries to the udder are derived from the *external pudendal* and the *perineal arteries*. The external pudendal artery, which may be as much as 1.5 cm in diameter, passes within the abdominal cavity along the ventral abdominal wall and then through the inguinal canal into the udder, where it divides into cranial and caudal branches supplying the fore- and hindquarters on the same side. The veins draining the udder form a venous circle at its base from which the blood is carried away by three large veins, linked by various tributaries, back into the venous circulation. This arrangement guarantees a choice of drainage routes even if the animal is sitting down. The tissue of the udder is well supplied with supramammary lymph nodes and numerous lymphatic vessels.

Dry cows. The lactation period of the dairy cow is artificially prolonged by milking. The milking period begins a few days after calving, which allows the calf to ingest colostrum from its dam, and continues until about 2 months before the next calf is due – a period of about 10 months. The dairy cow is usually inseminated about 60 days after calving and is therefore pregnant for much of the lactation. At the end of the lactation the cow is 'dried off' and the mammary tissue undergoes partial involution, which is quickly reversed as the next calf is born.

Mastitis, This is inflammation of the mammary glands and is of particular significance in high-yielding dairy cows. Causative pathogens may be spread from cow to cow (e.g., *Staphylococcus aureus*) or be contracted from the environment (e.g., *Esherichia coli* or *Streptococcus uberis*). Clinical signs, depending on cause, may include a hot swollen and tender quarter, production of thin discoloured milk often containing clots and in severe cases the cow may show signs of systemic illness such as pyrexia and anorexia. In the worst cases the cow may lose the quarter and may even die.

Oestrous cycle of the cow

Most dairy cows are produced by artificial insemination (AI) and lactation cannot occur without the cow giving birth to a calf. The bull calves produced may be reared for beef and the females may be kept to become replacement heifers for the herd. Beef breeds may be mated naturally by running with a bull but however the next generation of cattle is produced, it is important to be able to recognise the signs of a cow in oestrus.

- Sexual maturity in the cow occurs at 8–12 months of age. Smaller breeds of cow mature earlier than large breeds (e.g., Jerseys about 8 months old; Friesians about 11 months old) and it seems to coincide with the animal reaching about two-thirds of its final body size. The first oestrus may be affected by time of year and nutritional level.
- The cow is a spontaneous ovulator (she ovulates without the stimulus of mating).
- The average length of the oestrous cycle is 21–22 days. It may be only 20 days in heifers.
- The oestrus period, which is defined as the time when the cow will allow herself to be mounted, is 12–24 h. The average time is 18 h and it may be shorter in heifers.
- Ovulation usually occurs 10–15 h after the end of oestrus.
- Insemination, either by natural mating or by AI, is usually done about 12 h after the start of oestrus.
- Signs of oestrus, which is described as 'bulling', include:
  - The cow will stand rather than lie down, with her tail raised and her ears pricked.
  - She may bellow and may arch her back frequently or stretch.
  - She may be generally restless.
  - She will allow other cows or a bull to mount her: this is the most reliable sign.
  - She may also have a clear mucoid vaginal discharge and sometimes the vulva is swollen.
  - She may also mount other cows.
- In some cows, particularly heifers, there may be bleeding from the vulva. This occurs within 1–3 days of the end of oestrus and is described as metoestrous bleeding. Mating at this time seldom results in conception.

Table 17.3 Gestation periods of farm animals

Species	Length of gestation period in days	Length of gestation period in weeks
Cow	280	40
Sheep	147	21
Goat	154	22
Pig	114	16

The gestation period of the cow is shown in Table 17.3.

Male

The male of the species *Bos taurus* is known as a bull; a young castrated male is known as a bullock and these are usually reared to supply beef. Castration increases the rate of growth and prevents/reduces the development of male secondary sexual characteristics such as aggression. Some breeds of bull (e.g., Friesian and Jersey) are difficult to handle and are therefore rarely kept. Cows of these breeds are usually impregnated by AI.

Castration can be done without the use of a local anaesthetic before the calf has reached 2 months of age and may be performed by the stockkeeper. Bloodless castration (e.g., by means of a rubber ring) may only be done in the first week of life. If the calf is older than 2 months, then a veterinary surgeon must perform the operation and a local anaesthetic must be used.

Reproductive tract

The parts of the male tract bear the same names as those in other mammals but, in particular, the shape and type of accessory glands are different (Fig. 17.20):

Scrotum: The scrotum is pendulous and is suspended between the hind legs, further forward than in the horse. The skin, which closely follows the outline of the testes, is usually flesh coloured and covered with fine hairs. There is an obvious division between the two testes and a constricted neck at the junction of the scrotum with the body wall. In many individuals, particularly in bullocks, there is a large pad of 'cod fat' around the inguinal part of the cord. Just in front of the scrotum there are 2 or 4 small rudimentary teats. These are functionless but notice is taken of their number and spacing in dairy bulls, as this characteristic may be passed on to their female offspring.

Testis: These are elongated, oval and are larger than those in the stallion measuring 10–12 cm in length. A healthy testis is freely moveable within the scrotum and the external surface feels smooth except for a winding pattern of intracapsular blood vessels. The *cauda epididymis* or tail forms a conspicuous conical swelling from the ventral surface and usually feels firm but is softer for a short time after ejaculation. The *deferent duct* goes up towards the inguinal canal on the medial surface of the testis and lies in the caudal part of the *spermatic cord*. The cord, consisting of the deferent duct and the testicular vessels wrapped in the tunica vaginalis, must be identified when using the Burdizzo method of castration. The deferent ducts from either side pass over the dorsal surface of the bladder, through the tissue of the prostate and, at the point where each enters the urethra, the tubes form a swollen *ampulla* and then become surrounded by the *seminal vesicles* (Fig. 17.20).

Accessory glands: These secrete the seminal fluid in which spermatozoa are propelled into the female tract during ejaculation. They (Fig. 17.20) consist of the following:

- The *seminal vesicles* are large lobulated irregular glands lying lateral to the ampullae of the deferent ducts. The glands are flexed back on themselves and provide the bulk of the seminal fluid.

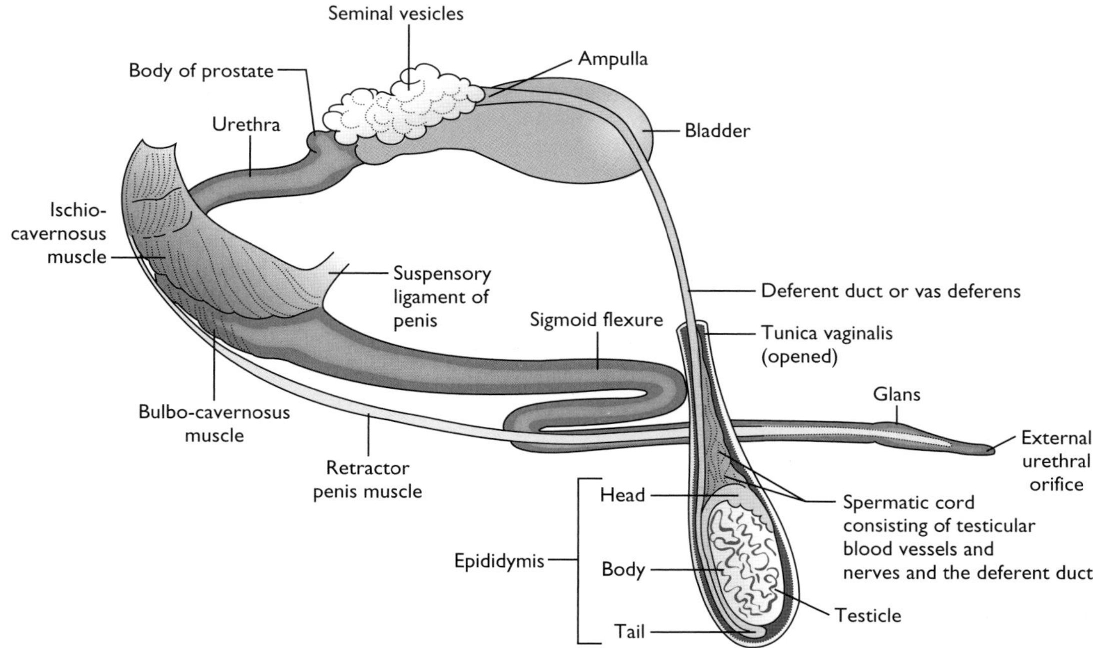

Fig. 17.20 General view of the genital organs of the bull. (After S Sisson, JD Grossman, 1969. Anatomy of the Domestic Animals, 4th edn. Philadelphia and London: WB Saunders, p. 597.)

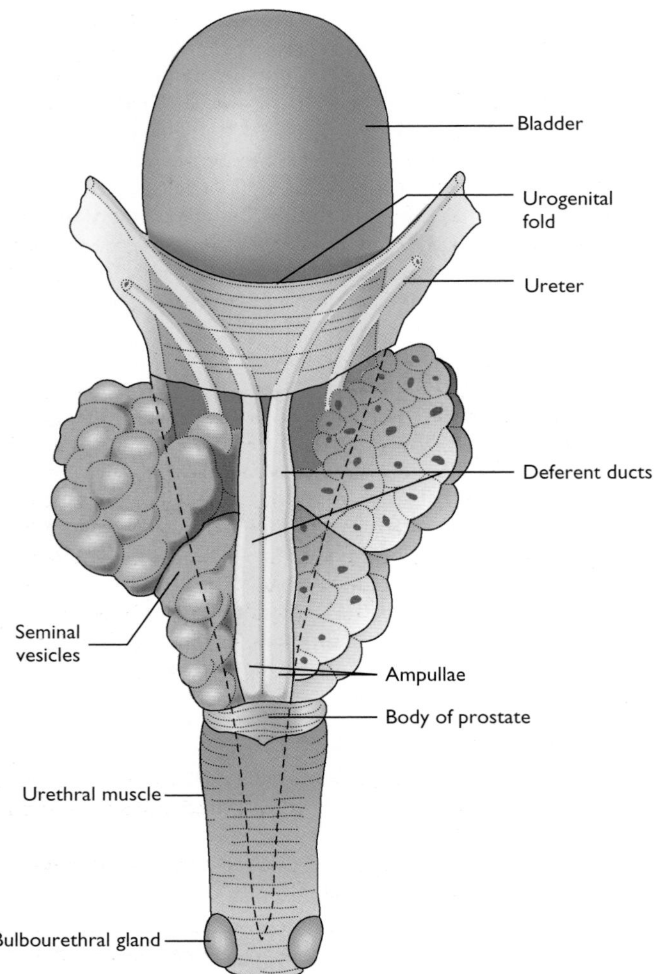

Fig. 17.21 The internal genital organs of the bull: dorsal view. The right vesicle is sectioned frontally. The dotted line indicates the backward extension of the peritoneum. (After S Sisson, JD Grossman, 1969. Anatomy of the Domestic Animals, 4th edn. Philadelphia and London: WB Saunders, p. 598.)

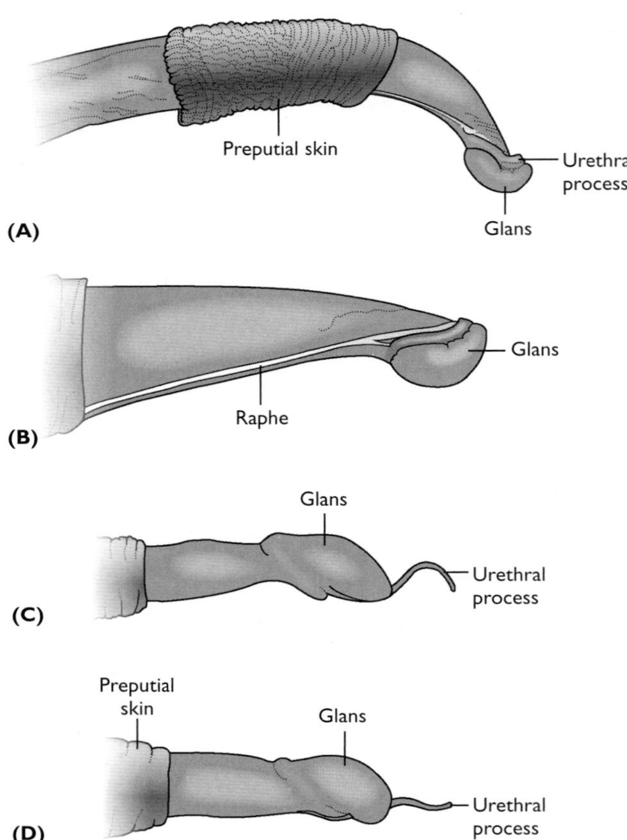

Fig. 17.22 Right lateral view of the distal end of the bull's penis, **(A)** flaccid and **(B)** erect; and the distal end of **(C)** the ram's and **(D)** the buck's penis. (Reproduced with permission from KM Dyce, WO Sack, CJG Wensing, 2002. Textbook of Veterinary Anatomy, 3rd edn. Philadelphia, PA: WB Saunders, p. 718.)

- The *prostate* is pale yellow in colour and consists of two parts – the body which stretches across the dorsal surface of the neck of the bladder and a second part which surrounds the pelvic part of the urethra and is hidden by the urethral muscle.
- The *bulbourethral glands* are smaller than those in the stallion; they lie dorsal to the urethra at the level of the ischial arch (Fig. 17.21), mainly covered by erectile tissue. Their watery secretions are produced before the main ejaculate to flush the penile urethra before the arrival of the sperm.

Penis: This is about 1 m long and is made of fibro-elastic tissue, which makes it relatively rigid even before erection (Fig. 17.20). Just behind the scrotum it forms an S-shaped curve known as the *sigmoid flexure*. About 30 cm is folded up when the penis is fully retracted but this straightens out during erection. The *glans penis* is about 8 cm long and is flattened dorsoventrally with a tip, known as the *urethral process* that is pointed and twisted (Fig. 17.22). The external urethral orifice opens within the groove formed by the twist. During the latter stages of erection the urethral process spirals around to the left as intromission is completed.

The *root* of the penis is attached to the ischial arch by two rod-like crura, which are surrounded by powerful ischiocavernosus muscles (Fig. 17.20) containing well-developed cavernous spaces. The *body* is cylindrical and comprises the two crura and the spongy part of the urethra all wrapped in the tunica albuginea. The amount of cavernous erectile tissue around the body is small so the penis only slightly increases in length and diameter during erection, merely becoming more rigid, and the process may be very rapid. After ejaculation, the sigmoid flexure is reinstated by the *retractor penis muscle* running from the flexure to the root (Fig. 17.20).

Prepuce: Long and narrow, this opens about 5 cm caudal to the umbilicus. The opening is small and surrounded by long hairs. The lining membrane is folded longitudinally and coiled tubular glands lie within the covering of stratified squamous epithelium.

The sheep

The domestic sheep (*Ovis aries*) belongs to the order Artiodactyla and the family Bovidae, as do cows, goats and deer. It is descended from the Asiatic mouflon (*Ovis orientalis*), although European breeds may also be derived from the Urial (*Ovis vignei*); both species are in danger of extinction in the wild. In the UK there are about 70 recognised sheep breeds and 12 recognised crosses, representing a huge range of coat type and colour, size, horns and use. Meat breeds include the Border Leicester, Charollais, Hampshire and Suffolk; wool breeds include Dorset, Cotswold, Ryeland and Herdwick, although most breeds will cross over between uses and there is a tendency to produce cross breeds, particularly for fattening. Many of the pure 'old-fashioned' breeds are in danger of dying out and are classed as rare breeds (e.g., Ronaldsay and Soay according to the Rare Breeds Survival Trust).

The sheep may be described as a multipurpose animal because it provides wool, meat and milk and for thousands of years it has been an important agricultural species. The sheep was one of the first species to be domesticated by prehistoric humans in the Middle East around 9000 years ago. They may have originally been hunted for their meat, then rounded up by dogs and later have been managed and shepherded as flocks. The main reason for keeping sheep at this time would be to guarantee a source of fresh meat; however, the advantages of their coat were soon discovered. The wild sheep had a coat that had both hair and wool fibres, which provides warmth, insulation and weather resistance and which was moulted in the spring. This discarded fibre would have been gathered, spun and woven into cloth, leading to the development of a textile industry around 10,000–8000 BC. Over the centuries the sheep has also been used to provide milk for its lambs and then later for humans. Nowadays in many parts of the world the sheep is still milked and the milk is used to provide a drink and for making butter and cheese.

Over the centuries desirable qualities in both the conformation of the animal, producing better-quality meat, and in the quality of the fleece, have been selected, resulting in breeds that are good for one quality or the other. Wool production reached its peak in the Middle Ages and for hundreds of years the principal industry in western Europe was wool. Parts of England (e.g., Norfolk and the Cotswolds) still bear the legacy of the wool industry, shown by the size of their churches and their textile mills.

Musculo-skeletal system

The skeleton

Axial skeleton

Skull: The dorsal profile of the skull is domed over the cranium and slopes caudally towards the neck. This gives a different shape from that of the cow but it may be hidden by the location and the size of the horns. In some breeds (e.g., Border Leicester), the standards require a Roman nose.

Many breeds are naturally polled but when horns do occur they are present in both ewes and rams. In a few breeds (e.g., Jacobs), multiple horns may develop and this is described as being polycerate. This condition is often linked with problems in closure of the cranial sutures and defects in the eyelids. The horns arise from the frontal bone but some curve around so far that their final position is related to the parietal bone of the skull in contrast to the temporal bone of the cow. The frontal sinus penetrates the base of the horn but does not reach as far up as it does in cattle. The horns, which are often extremely curled, depending on breed, and ridged, are triangular in cross section and sometimes grow so close to the skin of the face that there is a risk of pressure necrosis. Treatment of this may necessitate removing part of the horn.

Vertebral formula: C7 T13 L6-7 S4 Cd16-18. With the exception of the cervical vertebrae, variation in number is quite common in the sheep and there may be 14 thoracic vertebrae or 7 lumbar vertebrae or even an indeterminate extra vertebra between the two regions.

Sacrum usually consists of four fused vertebrae but the most caudal may be entirely separate or only partially fused.

Coccygeal vertebrae: In short-tailed sheep there may be only 3 vertebrae and in breeds with long tails there may be as many as 24.

Ribs and sternum: The 13th rib is often a floating rib, as is the 14th rib if it is present.

Docking: It is usual to dock the tails of lambs, especially of those breeds that are turned out to roam freely on the moors and uplands of the UK during the summer months. Faeces may become trapped under the tail, resulting in scalded skin and a smell that will attract flies, leading to fly strike, which may be fatal in a sheep that is not regularly checked. Docking and castrating may be done by the shepherd using a rubber ring in the first week of life. The tail must be left long enough to cover the vulva of the female or the anus of the male. If docking and castrating are performed over the age of 3 months it must be done under local anaesthetic by a veterinary surgeon.

Appendicular skeleton

The sheep is an even-toed ungulate that bears weight on digits 3 and 4, so the basic layout of the fore- and hind limbs is very similar to that seen in cattle.

The foot: Each distal phalanx is housed within a hoof whose structure is the same as in cattle.

Footrot, which presents as lifting of the horn of the hoof and erosion of the sole and heels, leading to pain, is the single most important cause of lameness in the national flock, particularly in breeding ewes. It is the result of a chronic infection caused by the bacteria *Dichelobacter nodosus*. Badly infected animals should be culled, while less severe cases may be treated with long-acting parenteral tetracyclines. Steps should be taken to prevent the spread between individuals and between flocks. More importantly, the condition should be prevented by vaccination, the use of zinc sulphate or formalin footbaths and by biannual foot checking and foot trimming. The trimmings may harbour infection and should be disposed of appropriately.

Splanchnic skeleton

There is no representative of the splanchnic skeleton in the sheep because it does not possess the ossa cordis, found in the heart of cattle, or the os penis, found in the penis of dogs and cats

Digestive system

As shown in Table 17.2, the sheep is a herbivorous cranial fermenter, meaning that the foregut has evolved to form the rumen in which fermentation of plant material takes place.

Oral cavity

Lips are thin and mobile and the upper lip is divided by a deep *philtrum*, which allows the sheep to nibble grass, leaving it very short. Generations of grazing by sheep (and also by rabbits which have a similar deep philtrum; see Chapter 14) have resulted in the development of the classic downland turf, which is short, dense and springy.

Hard palate: The dental pad lies on the more rostral part and the remainder is covered in irregular ridges with smooth edges. It may also be partially pigmented.

Tongue: Similar to that of the cow but the tip is smooth and the whole structure is covered in short, blunt papillae. The raised prominence, seen in cattle, is not nearly so obvious in the sheep and the root of the tongue is quite smooth. These differences reflect the differences in prehension between cattle and sheep: sheep nibble grass using their incisors and dental pad, while cattle tear off blades of grass using their prehensile tongues.

Teeth: The dental formula of the permanent teeth is:

$$(I0/4, C0/0, PM3/3, M3/3) \times 2 = 32 \quad \text{(i.e., the same as the cow)}.$$

The incisor teeth form a strongly curved arch, which has a sharp edge needed for cropping the grass. The cheek teeth have a thinner overlying layer of cement than those of cattle and it is often blackened by food deposits.

Abdominal cavity

The general arrangement of the stomach of the sheep is similar to that of the cow and its average capacity is about 15 l, compared to an average medium-sized cow, whose capacity may be 135–180 l. The reticulum is relatively larger than it is in the cow, the omasum is much smaller and the abomasum is larger and longer.

The parts, the arrangement and the function of the intestines are the same as in the cow.

Urinary system

The kidneys of the sheep are quite different to those of the cow and more closely resemble those of the dog in both their external and internal structure. They are regular in shape and, as they are enclosed in large amounts of fat, they are less likely to be distorted by pressure from other organs. The left kidney is less likely to be displaced by the rumen.

Reproductive system

Female

The female of the species *Ovis aries* is known as a ewe.

Reproductive tract

The tract is similar to that of the cow with the following differences:

- *Ovary*: These are almond shaped and about 1 cm in length. During the breeding season the outline of the ovary is more likely to be irregular because it is broken up by the formation of several ova and their subsequent change into corpora lutea. This reflects the wide occurrence of twin or even multiple births.
- *Uterine tube*: This is relatively long and there is no clear boundary between the uterine tube and the horn. The tube itself is very convoluted in the area close to the infundibulum.
- *Uterus*: This is similar to that of the cow. The two horns are 10–12 cm long and are coiled in a spiral. The caudal parts are joined by the intercornual ligament, making the body, which is actually less than 2.5 cm long, seem longer than it actually is. Internally the caruncles are relatively small, with a concave depression on each free surface.
- *Cervix*: A large number of irregular circular folds project into the cervical canal, fitting closely together and making catheterization of the uterus very difficult.
- *Vulva*: This is about 2.5 cm in length with thick labia. The ventral commissure points downwards. The clitoris is short.
- *Mammary glands*: There are two glands situated in the inguinal region of the abdomen. These are relatively small and hemispherical in shape. In breeds used for cheese production the glands may be larger. The teats are cylindrical and not always hairless. Closure of the teat canal is achieved without the presence of a sphincter muscle.

Oestrous cycle of the sheep

Most lambs are conceived naturally because rams are relatively easy to keep on a farm, although some breeds and some individuals, particularly those that are horned, may be aggressive and deserve respect. Detection of the signs of oestrus is also quite difficult and breeding may be more successful if a ram, running with the ewe flock, is allowed to detect the receptive ewes without the help of the stockman. The majority of sheep breeds will lamb once a year, although some breeds have been selectively improved to lamb twice a year (e.g., Dorset Horn). Mating or tupping usually takes place between August and October and lambing between December and April, when there is sufficient new grass to allow the ewes to produce milk and to feed the newborn lambs as they are weaned.

The ewe is described as being *seasonally polyoestrous*: the non-pregnant ewe has many periods of oestrus (defined as the time when she will accept the ram) during a defined breeding season. The ewe is a *short-day breeder*: she will begin to cycle in response to the declining hours of daylight seen in the autumn. After the season is over there is a long period of anoestrus.

- Sexual maturity in the ewe occurs at 6–7 months of age.
- The length of the breeding season is said to vary with the breed. Those breeds that were developed in parts of the world with a severe winter climate have short breeding seasons; those developed in milder climates have a longer breeding season.
- The average breeding season runs from August to December.
- The sheep is a spontaneous ovulator: she ovulates without the stimulus of mating.
- The average length of the oestrous cycle is 16 days.
- The oestrous period lasts for about 30 h.
- Ovulation occurs towards the end of the oestrous period; two or three ova will be produced at the same time.
- The optimal time for mating is from the middle of the oestrous period to the end but because the ram is usually running with the ewe, he will attempt to mate and she will only allow it when the cycle of hormones is correct.
- Signs of oestrous, which are often very subtle and difficult to detect, include:
  - Tendency to seek out the ram and stand beside him
  - Slight swelling of the vulva
  - Shaking of the tail, which helps to spread her scent

The average length of the gestation period in the ewe is 147 days (Table 17.3). The placenta of the ewe is cotyledonary, as seen in the cow (Fig. 17.30).

Synchronisation of oestrus. This is done to make certain that many ewes come into season together, ensuring a tight lambing season. The technique may also be used to bring the ewes into season earlier than normal so that lambing time is advanced. It may involve the use of a teaser or vasectomised ram, whose presence will stimulate the ewes to cycle, or the use of intravaginal sponges soaked in pregnant mare serum gonadotrophin. The sponge is left in place for 12 days and when it is withdrawn the ewe comes into oestrus and mating takes place. It is recommended to use one ram for 12 ewes.

Use of a raddle. A raddle, consisting of a harness and a marker attached to the brisket of the ram, is used to identify which ewes have been mated. When the ram mounts the ewe he makes a coloured mark on her rump. The colour of the raddle is changed every 9 days. If a ewe fails to conceive she will come into season within the next 3 weeks and be mated again and a different coloured mark will be left on her rump. By noting the colour of the raddle marks, the farmer can group ewes according to their date of mating and thus lambing date and take note of any ewes who have not conceived; these are the ones with several different coloured marks on their rumps.

Male

The male of the species *Ovis aries* is called a ram.

Castration. Ram lambs are usually castrated within a few days of birth and this may be carried out by the shepherd without an anaesthetic. The most common way of doing this is by the use of a rubber band placed externally around the spermatic cord and it is done at the same time as the tails are docked. Castration after 3 months of age must be done by a veterinary surgeon and under a local anaesthetic.

Reproductive tract

The parts of the tract are similar to those seen in the bull with the following differences:

Scrotum: This is sometimes hidden by wool, which may affect fertility because it affects the ability to dissipate heat. Rudimentary teats are common in rams.

Accessory glands: These consist of the seminal vesicles, prostate and bulbourethral glands and their function is to secrete seminal fluid to wash the spermatozoa into the female tract.

Penis: This is similar to that of the bull but the free end is distinctive (Fig. 17.22). The *urethral process* extends beyond the glans penis for approximately 4 cm and is long and twisted. The urethra opens at the tip. In the past this vermiform appendage was snipped off to reduce the fertility of a ram.

Pregnancy diagnosis. This is commonly done by ultrasound scanning between 50 and 90 days of pregnancy. Skilled technicians can distinguish the approximate age and number of the fetuses, which provides the shepherd with sufficient information to decide the correct nutritional level for each ewe and to organise the lambing process for the whole flock. Underfeeding a ewe who is carrying two or more lambs may cause a condition called Twin Lamb Disease, which is due to hypoglycaemia. This may result in the death of both the ewe and the lambs.

The pig

The domestic pig (*Sus scrofa domesticus or Sus domesticus*) is a member of the order Artiodactyla and the family Suidae and is considered to be a subspecies of the wild boar (*Sus scrofa*). The pig is thought to have been first domesticated around 7000 BC and at a similar time to when other animal species such as cattle and sheep and plant species such as wheat and barley were also being domesticated. Around the world there are thought to have been at least seven sites of pig domestication, mainly in Asia and the Middle East, but the first site is thought to have been in Turkey. Archaeological evidence shows that pigs were abundant in temperate to hot regions of the world. One of the reasons for the large numbers of sites is that pigs are very adaptable and as omnivores, they are able to consume a wide range of different foods, making them easy to domesticate. In some parts of the world, such as New Zealand and Australia, pigs have escaped to become feral and have caused substantial environmental damage. In parts of the UK the wild boar has returned, whether as a planned reintroduction or as an escape from wild boar farms, and is also causing damage and a threat to walkers in the countryside.

The domestic pig is mainly used to provide pork and other foods such as ham, sausages and bacon and in spite of various religious restrictions, pork is the most widely consumed meat worldwide. There are now hundreds of breeds of pig of all different sizes but the original native pig in the UK was a large rangy animal with floppy ears that was kept in orchards and then later in the backyards of cottages. In the late eighteenth century a small, fat, prick-eared breed of pig was imported from Asia and crossing these two breeds formed the basis for all breeds until the 1950s. In 1955 the government recommended that British farming should focus on three main breeds, the Large White, Landrace and Welsh, which would mainly provide bacon. This led to the near extinction of many native breeds but the more recent revival of interest in rare breeds such as the Gloucester Old Spot and the Tamworth has led to an increase in their numbers and an increased interest in the range of foods and tastes that they can provide.

Nowadays pigs may be intensively farmed in multi-pig units or extensively in open fields with individual huts providing protection from the weather, both heat and cold. More recently they have become popular pets with an increase in numbers of breeds such as the American mini pig, Kune Kune and the Vietnamese potbellied pig. Because there are some structural and nutritional similarities between the pig and human, pigs are now commonly used in biomedical research, particularly for surgical procedures used in human medicine.

External features

The overall shape of the pig is a cylinder that tapers slightly towards the hind end. The head and neck form a cone that merges with the rest of the body at the level of the forelimbs. The upper surface of the head is usually concave depending on the breed; those with long skulls such as the Tamworth have a less obvious concavity than those with short skulls such as the Gloucester Old Spot or the Berkshire. The caudal part of the skull is high and then the outline gradually slopes towards the shoulders. The neck is short, although as in all mammals there are still seven cervical vertebrae, which means that the angle of the mandible lies relatively close to the shoulder joint, restricting the animal's ability to turn its head from side to side.

One of the most obvious features of the pig is its strong snout or rostrum, formed by a disc-shaped moveable tip to the muzzle, which incorporates the upper lip. The snout is supported by the *rostral bone* (Fig. 17.23), which is not seen in other animals and lies at the rostral end of the nasal septum. The levator labii superioris muscle, which is the main mover of the snout, attaches to this bone. The snout enables the pig to perform its characteristic 'rooting' behaviour in search of food and this is further helped by the sloping 'cutaway' profile of its lower mandible.

Rooting behaviour may be discouraged by the application of a nose ring to the dorsal border of the snout. Nose ringing is not recommended for animals kept entirely indoors and because it is considered to be a mutilation, it should not be done on outdoor animals unless it is really necessary. Nose ringing should only be carried out by someone who is trained and is competent to perform the procedure.

The lips are firm and the upper lip is deeply notched on either side to allow the upper canine or tusk to project outside it. The eyes are small, set deeply in the orbit and fringed in light eyelashes. Pigs have no tapetum lucidum so their night vision is poor. The oval ears have a wide base and attach to the high caudal part of the head. They have a pointed tip and in many breeds the ear flap falls forward over the eyes (lop-eared; e.g., Gloucester Old Spot, Duroc and Landrace) while in a few others the ear is pricked upright (e.g., Tamworth, Large White and Wild Boar).

The skin is thick and overlies a thick layer of subcutaneous fat, which makes the pig difficult to palpate and to listen to the heart. The pig has fewer sebaceous glands than other species and they are generally smaller; however, the sweat glands are much larger and in some cases are visible to the naked eye. They are found in various areas of the body and around the lower limbs, digits and the prepuce. The skin is sparsely covered in coarse bristles; the more highly developed the breed, the fewer the hairs; wild boar are covered in hair. The bristles are usually arranged in groups of three and are more numerous on the neck and back. Those around the snout and chin are sinus hairs.

The skeleton

Axial skeleton

The skull The bones making up the skull bear the same names as those of other mammals (Figs. 17.23 and 17.24) but their shape varies. The skull of primitive wild pigs is almost pyramidal but selective breeding to produce more modern breeds has resulted in a greater height above the brain. Above and caudal to the quite small orbit is an obvious *temporal line* (Fig. 17.23), which runs into the zygomatic process of the temporal bone. The zygomatic arch is very strong and deep with a wide articular surface for the temporomandibular joint, which allows the pig a forceful bite.

The size of the cranial cavity, and the brain within it, is small compared to the size of the cranium due to the enormous development of the *frontal sinuses*. In the young pig these are quite small and are confined to the anterior part of the frontal bone, but as the pig grows they extend laterally and caudally, almost as far as the occipital condyles, and are subdivided into at least six compartments. The brain is well protected by the double layer of bone and the frontal sinus and this may have evolved as result of the pig's habit of rooting and the tendency to fight using sharp upward thrusts of the tusks.

The external nares of the pig are round and lead into the nasal cavities, which are long and narrow and extend beyond the level of the orbits. They are filled with the conchae covered in the nasal mucosa, which contains the receptors responsible for the sense of

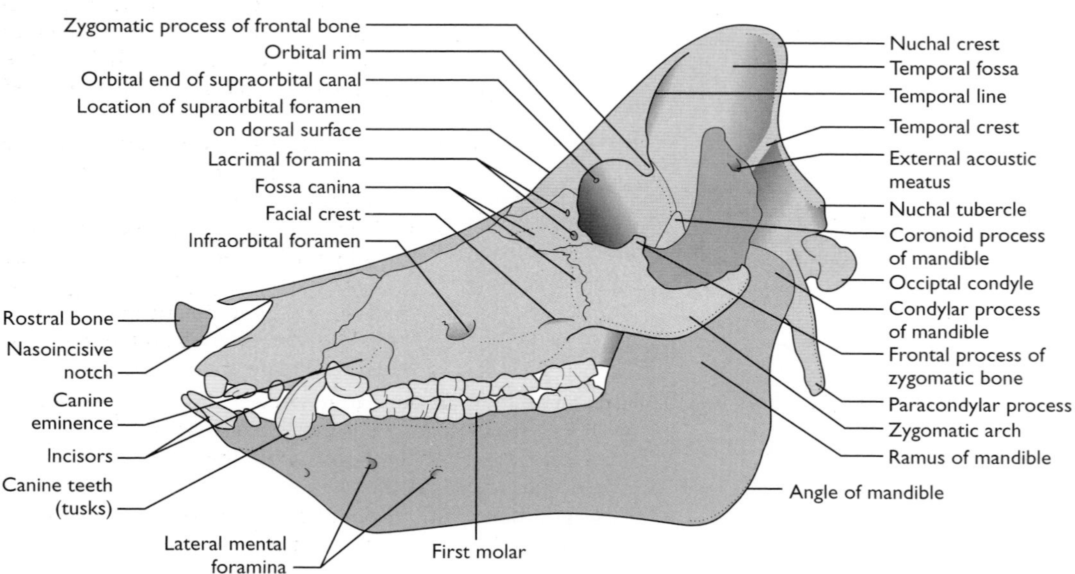

Fig. 17.23 The skull of the boar. (Reproduced with permission from KM Dyce, WO Sack, CJG Wensing, 2002. Textbook of Veterinary Anatomy, 3rd edn. Philadelphia, PA: WB Saunders, p. 763.)

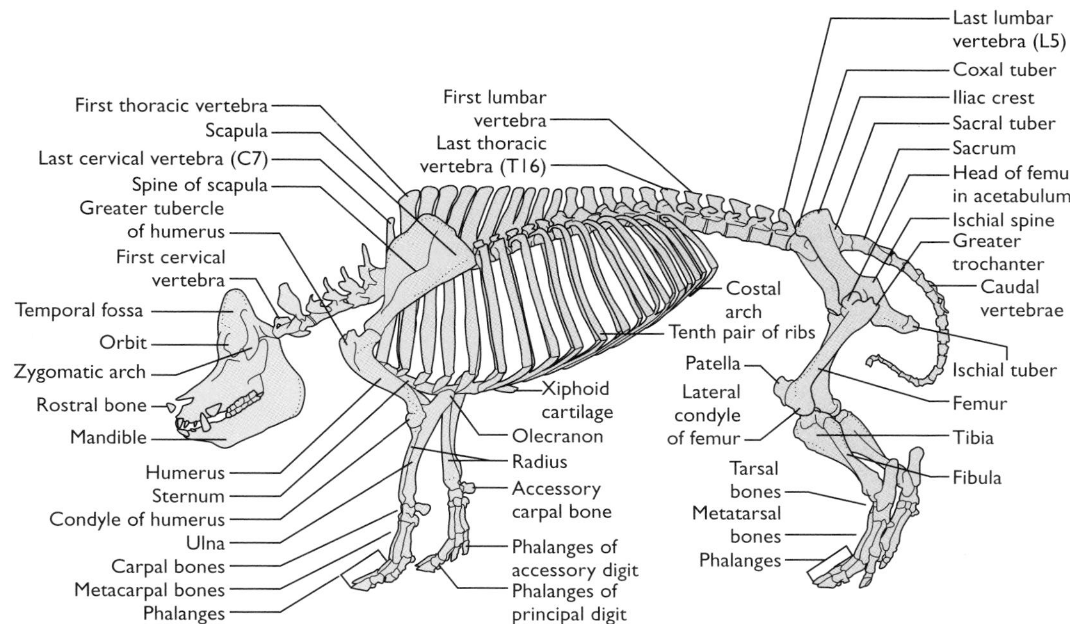

Fig. 17.24 The skeleton of the boar. (Reproduced with permission from KM Dyce, WO Sack, CJG Wensing, 2002. Textbook of Veterinary Anatomy, 3rd edn. Philadelphia, PA: WB Saunders, p. 762.)

smell. This is particularly acute in the pig, a fact that is used to locate truffles in France.

Vertebral column The vertebral formula (Fig. 17.24) is C7 T14-15 L6-7 S4 Cd20-23.

The bodies of the *cervical vertebrae* are elliptical and the vertebral arches are transversely wide and there is quite a gap between adjacent arches. The last cervical vertebra (C7) has a spinous process, which is in the region of 10 cm in length. There are 14–15 *thoracic vertebrae*, although 16 or 17 have been recorded, and there are 6–7 *lumbar vertebrae*. Selective breeding has resulted in the production of pigs with longer backs because this is the most valuable part of the carcass, providing more bacon, chops and hams. The *sacrum* consists of four vertebrae that fuse as the animal ages but this is never as complete as it is in other animals. The first four or five *coccygeal vertebrae* have well-developed articular processes and the vertebral arches are complete but in the remainder the anatomical features gradually diminish. In many cases the first coccygeal vertebra unites with the sacrum. The last 15 vertebrae form the curly part of the tail.

Tail docking. This is not considered to be a routine procedure and should only be done as a last resort, if there is evidence of injury. In addition, the management system and the environmental conditions should be examined and altered if necessary. Docking must be done before the seventh day of life and should only be performed by a trained, competent operator.

Ribs and sternum There are 14–15 pairs of ribs, of which 7 are sternal and 7 or 8 are asternal. They are quite strongly curved except towards the costal arch. On the last five or six ribs the tubercle fuses with the head. If a 15th rib is present it is usually floating and is only about 2–3 cm in length but in some cases it is fully developed and its costal cartilage forms part of the costal arch. The sternum consists of six sternebrae. The thoracic cavity is much more barrel-shaped than that of the cow or the horse, which results from the stronger curve of the ribs and the fact that they vary less in their relative lengths.

Appendicular skeleton

The pig is an even-toed ungulate that bears weight on digits 3 and 4, as do cattle and sheep; however, there are a pair of accessory digits or dewclaws, which are much more obvious than in the other species. These digits have a full set of phalanges (Fig. 17.25), unlike the dew claws of cattle. The whole foot is referred to as the pig's trotters, which in many parts of the world are treated as culinary delicacies.

Foot problems in pigs are rare unless they are kept on a very hard or sharp substrate. Running on concrete helps to keep the hooves worn down so that trimming is rarely necessary. Joint problems are more common and this may be most likely to occur in breeds bred for rapid weight gain. Immature skeletons cannot support the weight of a fully fattened young pig, leading to the breakdown of articular cartilage and bone deformities.

The forelimb The pattern of both the forelimb and hind limb is reflected in the fact that weight is borne on two digits:

- *Scapula* is very wide with an obvious triangular spine that may be palpable. The spine curves backwards over the infraspinous fossa and bears a large tuberosity (Fig. 17.24). The neck is well defined.
- *Humerus* is short and strong with a marked slope so that it resembles an italic letter '*f*'. The musculo-spiral groove is shallow.
- *Radius/ulna* are separate bones, although they are held closely together by the *interosseus ligament* with little or no *interosseus space*. The *radius* is short, narrow and thick and the shaft

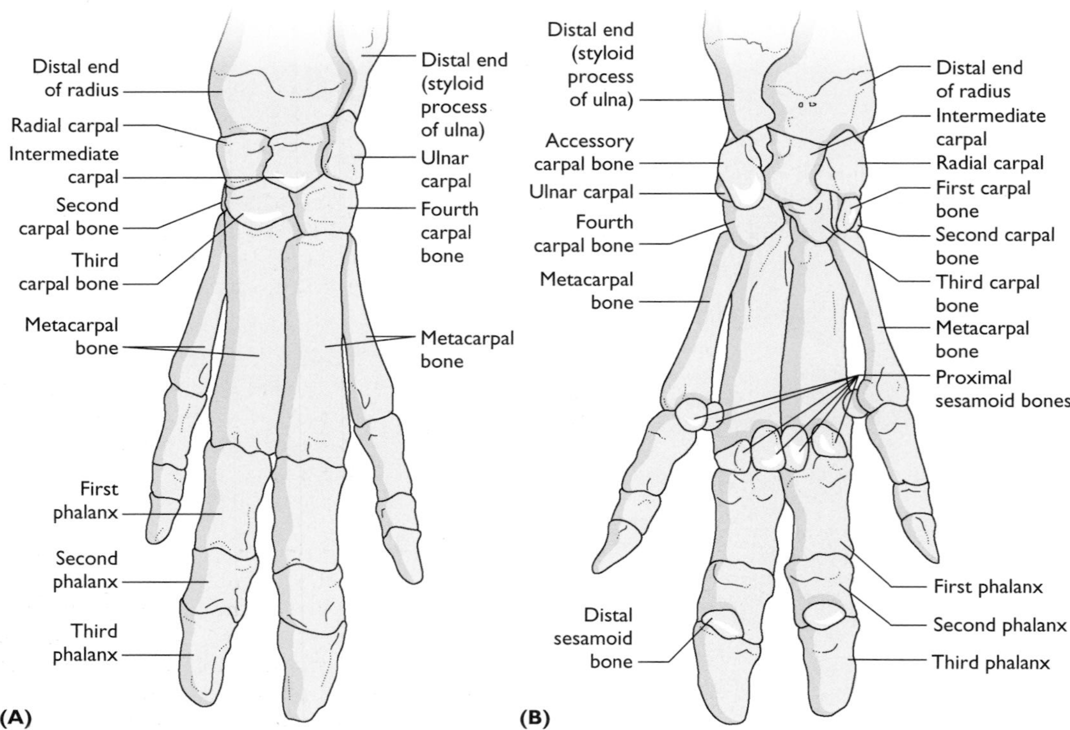

Fig. 17.25 The skeleton of the distal part of the left thoracic limb of the pig. **(A)** Dorsal view. **(B)** Plantar view. (After S Sisson, JD Grossman, 1969. Anatomy of the Domestic Animals, 4th edn. Philadelphia and London: WB Saunders, p. 180.)

increases in width towards the distal end, where it articulates with the radial and intermediate carpal bones. The *ulna* is weight bearing and is therefore much larger, longer and heavier than the radius and the shaft is curved. The proximal end is large and bent medially, while the distal end is relatively small and articulates with the ulnar and accessory carpal bones.

- *Carpus* consists of eight bones, four in each row. The proximal row is similar to that seen in the cow; in the distal row the *fourth carpal* is the largest bone and articulates with the *intermediate* and *ulnar carpals* above it and the fourth and fifth metacarpals below it (Fig. 17.25). The *carpal joint* is very moveable and will allow flexion of almost 180°.

On the caudomedial aspect of the carpus are the so-called *carpal glands*. These lie just below the skin and open through several visible ducts. They are thought to be associated with territorial scent marking.

- *Metacarpals*: There are four long bones. The first is absent; the third and fourth are the largest and bear weight; the second and fifth are much smaller and they bear the accessory digits. The proximal ends of the second and fifth bones lie a little behind the other two and the fifth is much thicker than the second metacarpals.
- *Digits*: Each digit consists of three phalanges and three sesamoids (Fig. 17.25). The bones of digits 3 and 4 resemble those of the cow, while those of the accessory digits, which do not normally touch the ground, are similar but much smaller.

The hind limb

- *Pelvic girdle* consists of the ilium, ischium and pubis and is a long narrow structure. The ilium and ischium lie almost in a line with each other. The pubic symphysis is thick and the two pubic bones lie almost in a horizontal plane. The symphysis does not usually undergo complete ossification. The pelvic inlet is elliptical and oblique and the floor of the pelvis, particularly in the sow, is wide and flattened; in the boar the floor is concave. The acetabulum lies a little further back than in the cow.
- *Femur* has a wide strong shaft. The head is strongly curved and there is a distinct neck. On the articular surface there is a large fovea, marking the attachment of the round ligament.
- *Tibia/fibula* are two distinct bones with a wide interosseus space between them. The *tibia* is much the larger and its shaft curves medially. The proximal part of the tibial crest is very prominent and curves outwards. The *fibula* bears weight and is a similar length to that of the tibia with a wide flattened proximal end and a narrower but thicker distal end. The proximal end articulates with the lateral condyle of the tibia, while the distal end forms the lateral malleolus.
- *Tarsus* consists of seven bones. The tibial and fibular tarsal are similar to that in the cow and the fibular tarsal bears the tuber calcis, to which the Achilles tendon attaches. The third bone in this 'row' is the central tarsal. The distal row comprises four tarsal bones, of which the fourth is the largest.

- *Metatarsals/digits* follow a similar pattern to those seen in the forelimb but the bones are larger. The proximal and medial phalanges of each digit are a little longer and narrower than they are in the forelimb.

Covering the end of each distal phalanx, in both the fore- and hind limbs, is a *hoof*, which is similar in structure to that seen in cattle but they are straight (i.e., do not curve inwards) and have a soft digital pad or bulb, which is set away from the sole and wall. The hooves covering the accessory digits are similar in structure but bear no weight except on soft ground.

Digestive system

The pig is an omnivore: it is adapted to eat all types of food and this may be one contributing factor to its successful domestication in many parts of the world.

Oral cavity

The *lips* extend quite far back on the face but the mouth does not open as wide as the mouth of the dog, for example. The upper lip is short and merges with the snout and the lower lip is small and pointed. The *hard palate* is long and narrow and there is no dental pad. In the centre is a furrow and on either side there are a series of prominent palatine ridges. These stop abruptly as the hard palate becomes the *soft palate*. At this point there are two patches, which are the *tonsils* of the soft palate; these are the only tonsils seen in the pig, which is different to the tonsils in the wall of the oropharynx in other species. The soft palate is thick and extends to the middle of the epiglottis. In many cases there is a small extension hanging down into the oropharynx; this is the *uvula*, which is also seen in humans.

The *tongue* is long and narrow with a pointed apex. The entire oral cavity, including the cheeks, is covered in a smooth mucous membrane.

Teeth

The dental formula of the permanent teeth is:

$(I3/3, C1/1, PM4/4, M3/3) \times 2 = 44.$

Pigs have the largest number of teeth of all the domestic animals. The upper *incisors* are small and curved and are separated from each other by spaces. The lower incisors lie close together and are straight, projecting forwards to meet the upper teeth in a grasping action. The *canine teeth or tusks* are small in the sow and only their tips project from the mouth, while the tusks of the boar are large and project from the mouth. These are used as weapons by fighting boars and some stockmen remove them to prevent injury to themselves and to other pigs. The upper canine may be 8–10 cm long, while the lower canine may reach up to 20 cm in length. The pulp cavity remains open for up to 2 years, after which a proper root develops and the tooth stops growing. The *premolars and molars* increase in width and length from front to back and the number of roots increases with the size of the tooth. These teeth are very large and are much more like the cheek teeth of the dog than the grinding teeth of herbivores. The surface of the crown is covered in irregular cusps, which is ideal for crushing food.

Piglets are born with eight teeth – incisors and canines – and these are often known as 'needle' teeth because they are so sharp. There is a risk that they may injure the teats of the sow during suckling or littermates as they fight for the teats. Some stockmen may clip the teeth within hours of birth.

Teeth clipping or grinding in piglets. This should not be done as a routine and only after there is evidence of injury to the sow or to the littermates. The management system or the environmental conditions should be checked and altered if necessary. The procedure involves reducing the points of the corner or canine teeth either by using a grinder, which is less likely to split the tooth, or by using sharp clippers. It should not be done later than the seventh day and should be performed by a trained and competent operator.

Clipping the tusks of boars. This is permissible if there is risk of damage to other pigs or to handlers but it is not considered to be a routine procedure. The tusks are reduced in size under anaesthesia because the tooth pulp is sensitive.

Food passes from the oral cavity into the pharynx, which has a particular feature not seen in other animals. Arising from the pharyngeal wall and dorsal to the entrance of the oesophagus is a *pharyngeal diverticulum*. This is about 1 cm long in piglets and 3–4 cm long in adult pigs. Externally this diverticulum lies at approximately the level of the base of the ear and its only significance is that during oral dosing there is a risk of penetration by the nozzle of the doser. Medication should be deposited in the oropharynx, which externally lies about 2.5 cm higher, level with the lateral canthus of the eye.

Abdominal cavity

Food material, having been masticated in the mouth and swallowed, passes down the short straight oesophagus into the stomach. The digestive tract of the pig within the abdominal cavity resembles that of the dog, although it is important to remember that they are not related. The following differences should be noted:

Stomach: This is a simple stomach as seen in the horse and the dog. It is divided into a large rounded left part and a small right part ending in the *pylorus*. It has a large capacity and when full the pyloric part may touch the floor of the abdomen by the right costal arch. The oesophagus enters obliquely through a slit-like cardia and is bounded above and to the left by a muscular fold leading into a *diverticulum* (Fig. 17.26), which is not seen in other species. The stomach is lined with a soft glandular mucosa divided into different areas (Fig. 17.26), which are easily distinguishable by their different colours. Within the pylorus is a prominence, the *torus pyloricus*, consisting of muscle and fat. This is similar to that seen in ruminants but its function is unknown.

Small intestine is similar to that of the dog. The *bile duct* enters the duodenum about 3 cm from the pylorus and the single *pancreatic duct* enters about 12 cm from the pylorus. The entrance papillae are visible to the naked eye in slaughtered specimens.

Large intestine: Most of this is wider than the small intestine. The ileum joins the caecum obliquely and projects into it. The *caecum* itself is blind-ending and is about 20–30 cm long (Fig. 17.27). The colon is as wide as the caecum to begin with and then gradually narrows. It can be thought of as the familiar ascending, transverse and descending parts. Most of the *ascending colon* is

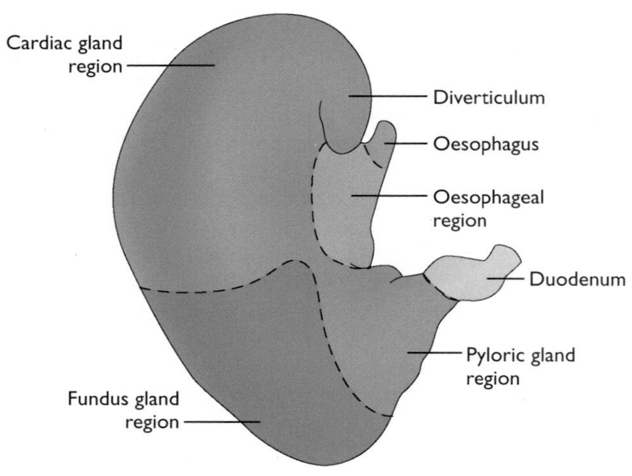

Fig. 17.26 Diagram of the mucous membrane of the stomach of the pig. (After S Sisson, JD Grossman, 1969. Anatomy of the Domestic Animals, 4th edn. Philadelphia and London: WB Saunders, p. 491.)

arranged in three close double spiral coils held by the mesentery (Fig. 17.27). As the ascending part comes out of the spiral, it travels forwards towards the sublumbar region, turns left across the abdomen as the *transverse colon* and then passes backwards as the *descending colon*, as it does in the dog. The transverse and descending parts of the colon are held in place by a short mesentery. The colon then passes through the pelvic cavity as the *rectum* and terminates at the anus.

Atresia ani, or congenital absence of an anus. This occurs relatively frequently in piglets and is something that should always be checked in the newborn litter. The condition may be inherited and may be traceable to a particular boar. Affected piglets are unable to defecate and untreated piglets may survive for up to 4 weeks. If the rectum terminates close to the exterior skin, an opening may be surgically created by the veterinary surgeon but the piglet will be incontinent because it will have no anal sphincter.

Urinary system

The parts of the urinary system are the same as those in other mammalian species. The two kidneys are positioned more or less symmetrically and the right kidney does not touch the liver – both facts are different to the anatomy seen in other species.

The pig kidney is longer and thinner than in other species (Fig. 17.28). The renal pelvis consists of a central cavity with a large recess, or major calyx, at either end which drains into the pelvis. Urine formed by the renal nephrons drips into the renal papillae, each formed by fusion of several pyramids, and then drains into one of the ten minor calyces and so into the pelvis. Urine is conveyed from the kidney via the ureter to the bladder. The bladder lies entirely within the abdominal cavity and is entirely covered in peritoneum. When full it may reach as far forward as the umbilicus.

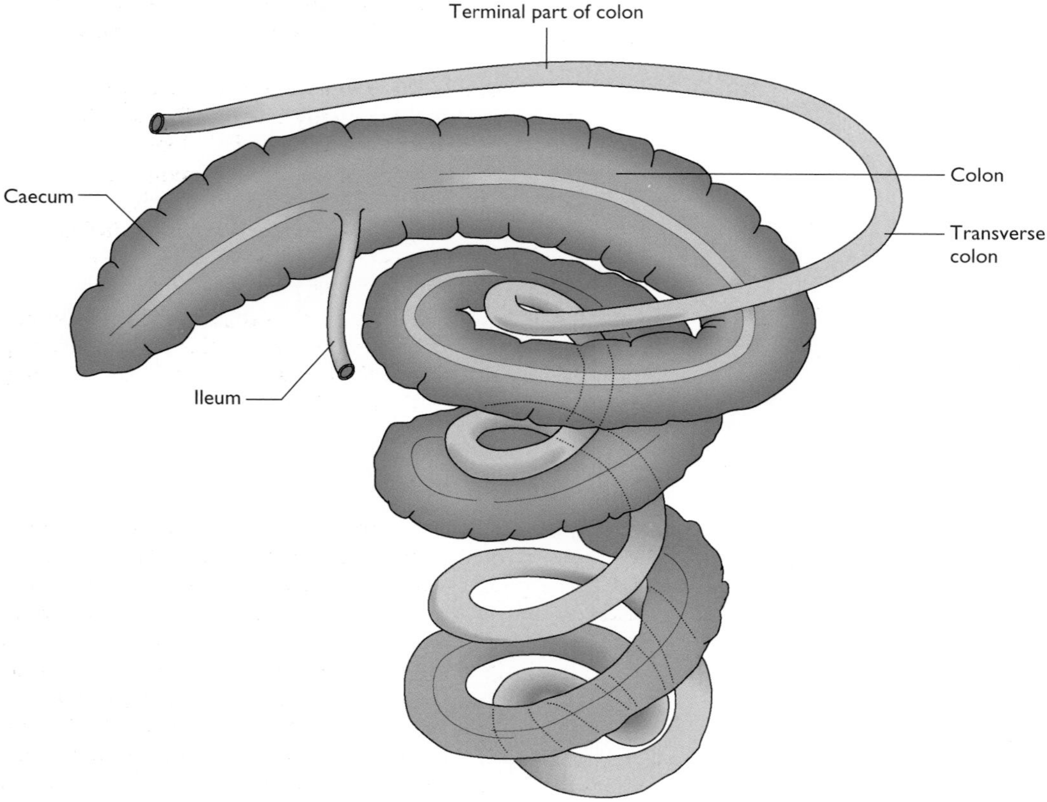

Fig. 17.27 Diagram of the caecum and colon of the pig. Coils of colon have been pulled apart. Anatomy of the Domestic Animals. (After S Sisson, JD Grossman, 1969. Anatomy of the Domestic Animals, 4th edn. Philadelphia and London: WB Saunders, p. 493.)

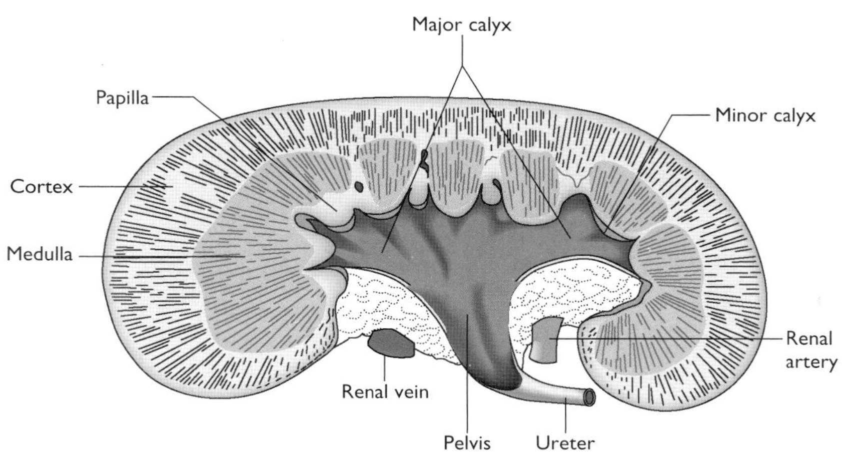

Fig. 17.28 Pig's kidney sectioned through poles and hilus. (Reproduced with permission from KM Dyce, WO Sack, CJG Wensing, 2002. Textbook of Veterinary Anatomy, 3rd edn. Philadelphia, PA: WB Saunders, p. 783.)

Reproductive system

Female

The female of the species *Sus scrofa domesticus* is known as a sow; the young pig up to the time she has her first litter is known as a gilt. Parturition in the pig is known as farrowing.

Reproductive tract

The parts of the tract are the same as those in other mammals. The pig is a multiparous species (i.e., litter bearing) and the uterus (Fig. 17.29) is described as being bicornuate, with long uterine horns designed to support the development of many piglets.

- *Ovary*: About 5 cm in length with an irregular lobulated appearance caused by the presence of many follicles or corpora lutea which protrude from the surface. Each ovary is hidden inside the *ovarian bursa* and suspended by a long *mesovarium*, which means that the position of the ovary is variable; both ovaries may lie close to one flank a few centimetres from the pelvic inlet but within the abdominal cavity.
- *Uterine tube*: The *infundibulum* opens within the ovarian bursa and the tube then continues within the mesosalpinx and opens into the uterine horn without a noticeable constriction.
- *Uterus*: The *uterine horns* are long and convoluted (Fig. 17.29). In the non-pregnant state they may be as long as 1 m and in the pregnant state they may be up to 2 m long. This provides sufficient space for the development of a large litter of piglets. They are suspended by an extensive broad ligament or mesometrium, which allows the horns to be very mobile. They lie somewhere between the roof and floor of the abdomen cranial to the pelvic inlet. During pregnancy the broad ligament enlarges considerably and allows the gravid horns to fall to the abdominal floor. At full term the uterus almost fills the ventral half of the abdomen, pushing the intestines out of the way and reaching to the stomach and liver.

  The *uterine body* is short and at the junction of the horns with the body the deeper layers of circular smooth muscle form a complex sphincter, which functions during farrowing. It allows one piglet at a time to pass from one or other of the horns into the body and out of the birth canal, thus preventing a collision that might occur if both horns contracted at the same time, possibly resulting in dystocia. The sphincter does not work in early pregnancy when transuterine migration occurs. This process allow embryos to travel from one horn, across the uterine body, into the opposite horn so that equal numbers of embryos implant in each horn, making optimal use of the available space for development. There is no implantation within the uterine body.
- *Cervix* is much longer than in other species; half of it lies within the abdominal cavity and half within the pelvic cavity. The beginning and end are ill defined as it merges with the uterus and the vagina (Fig. 17.29). The mucosal lining of the cervical canal forms a series of prominences within the lumen, which interlock and close the canal. During oestrus and just before farrowing, the cervix becomes enlarged and swollen and the prominences become soft and indistinct.
- *Vagina and vestibule*: The urethra enters the floor of the reproductive tract more cranially than in other species, making the vagina short and the vestibule long.
- *Vulva* is conical and slopes so that the opening faces dorsocaudally. The clitoris lies between the vulval labia and is about 6 cm long in the mature sow but is difficult to see. Very large clitorises may be associated with a pseudohermaphrodite or intersex condition.
- *Mammary glands*: Most sows have seven pairs of glands, which are suspended from the ventral body wall of the thoracic and abdominal cavities, as in the dog and cat. The teats are long and perforated by two teat orifices.

Oestrous cycle of the sow

Most piglets are conceived by AI rather than by natural mating because boars are difficult to keep and manage. They are large, sometimes aggressive and in order to maintain fertility, a boar should not be overused. A boar should only be expected to serve one sow a day and in a natural mating system you would need one boar for 10–20 sows; these would not all be in season at the same time. In a system using AI, an ejaculate from one boar can inseminate 100–200 sows. It is important to understand and manage the oestrous cycle of the sow because failure to detect the signs and to inseminate the sow at the correct time is one of the biggest causes of low conception rates and consequently low pig production.

- Sexual maturity in the sow occurs around 6 months of age. This may be delayed if a sow is kept on her own. In gilts

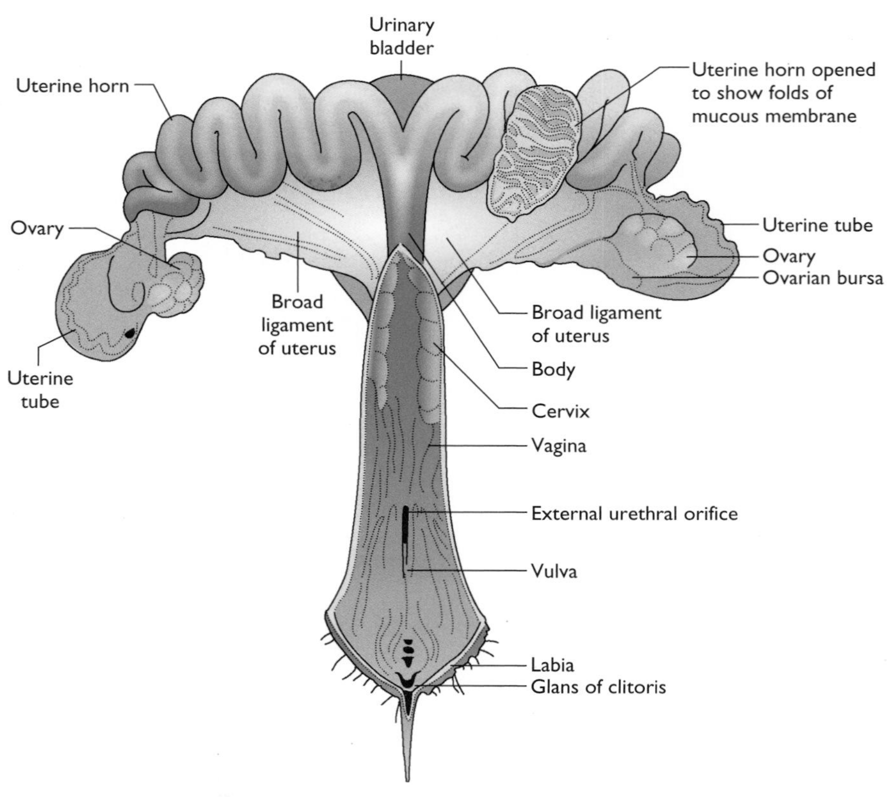

Fig. 17.29 The genital organs of the sow: dorsal view. The vulva, vagina and cervix are slit open. (After S Sisson, JD Grossman, 1969. Anatomy of the Domestic Animals, 4th edn. Philadelphia and London: WB Saunders, p. 622.)

kept in groups, sexual maturity may occur before 6 months of age.

- The sow is described as being *polyoestrous* with a period of *lactational anoestrus*, which lasts until the piglets are weaned. Cycling will restart 4–7 days after weaning.
- The reproductive hormones of the sow do not respond to the changing seasons, so the sow continues to cycle throughout the year.
- The sow is a spontaneous ovulator.
- The average oestrous cycle lasts for 21 days.
- The oestrous period lasts for 2–3 days, averaging 48–60 h (i.e., the time when the sow will allow mating, sometimes called 'standing heat').
- Ovulation occurs during the last third of oestrus, 36–42 h after the start of the oestrous period. Many ova will be produced.
- Signs of oestrus include:
  - Sow will stand still and allow the boar to mount.
  - She will assume a rigid stance, often with her ears pricked and quivering, when pressure is applied to her back; this is the back pressure test.
  - Vulval lips are red and swollen with a thin mucoid discharge.
  - A group-housed sow will actively seek out the boar.
  - She may also show reduced appetite, restlessness, grunting, chomping jaws and increased alertness.
  - In the absence of a boar, a sow may respond to sound recordings of a boar or sprays containing boar pheromones.

The average length of gestation is 114 days (Table 17.3). The foetuses are attached to the endometrium of the uterus by a *diffuse placenta*, which is similar to that seen in the mare (Fig. 17.30). The structure of the placenta may explain the lack of transplacental antibody transfer, which means that it is vital that the neonatal piglet receives its colostrum.

Male

The male of the species *Sus scrofa domesticus* is known as a boar. A castrated pig is sometimes referred to as a hog.

Reproductive tract

The parts of the boar's reproductive tract are the same as in other species but there are a few differences.

Scrotum lies a short distance from the anus (Fig. 17.31) and is not as well-defined as in other male animals.

Testis is large and oval in outline. The epididymis is closely attached to the testis and its very large tail forms a blunt projection at the posterior part, which is at the uppermost point of the scrotum (Fig. 17.31), just below the anus. The ductus deferens is long and convoluted and lies within the long spermatic cord. The cremaster muscle, which pulls the testis closer to the body, is also well developed.

Accessory glands

- *Seminal vesicles*: The pair are pale pink in colour, lobed, very large and extend into the abdominal cavity (Fig. 17.31). They cover the posterior part of the bladder, ductus

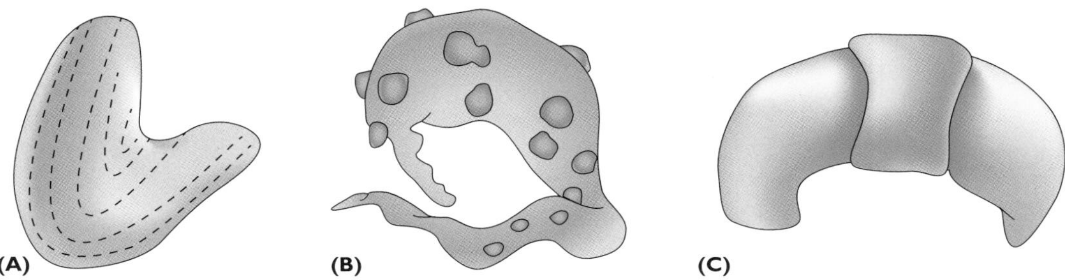

Fig. 17.30 Placental types according to the distribution of chorionic projections (villi) on the endometrium. **(A)** Diffuse placenta in the mare. **(B)** Cotyledonary placenta (cow, goat, sheep). **(C)** Zonary placenta (dog, cat). (Reproduced with permission from WO Reece, 2009. Functional Anatomy and Physiology of Domestic Animals. Philadelphia, PA: Wiley-Blackwell, p. 486.)

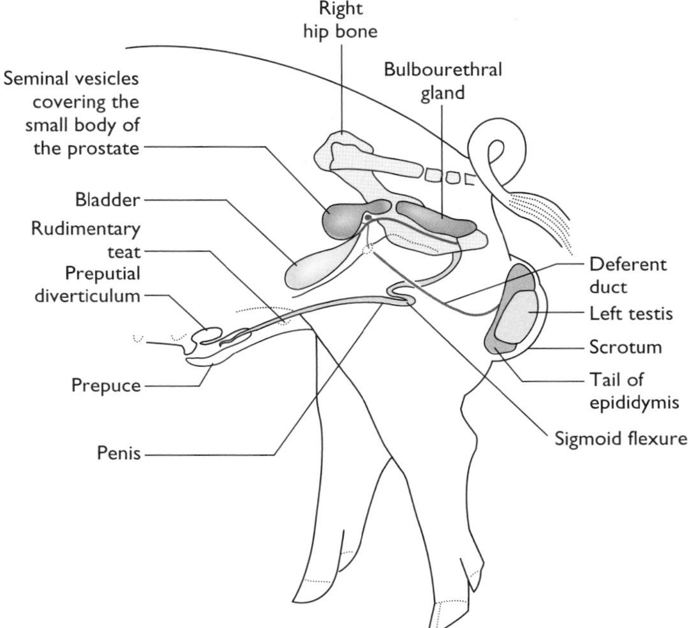

Fig. 17.31 Diagram showing the reproductive organs of the boar *in situ.* (Reproduced with permission from KM Dyce, WO Sack, CJG Wensing, 2002. Textbook of Veterinary Anatomy, 3rd edn. Philadelphia, PA: WB Saunders, p. 790.)

deferentia, as they enter the urethra, the body of the prostate, the anterior part of the urethra and the bulbourethral glands. Their secretion is thick, cloudy and slightly acid.

- *Prostate*: This is much smaller and consists of the body, which lies over the neck of the bladder and underneath the seminal vesicles, and a less distinct part, which surrounds the pelvic urethra. Fluid is discharged into the urethra through several small ducts.
- *Bulbourethrals*: Large, dense and almost cylindrical. They lie on either side and on the posterior side of the pelvic urethra. Each gland has a large duct, which enters the urethra at the level of the ischial arch.

These accessory glands are poorly developed in male piglets that are castrated early. During ejaculation the boar may produce as much as 200–500 ml of seminal fluid. The bulk of the fluid is secreted by the prostate and the bulbourethral glands. The sperm-rich fraction is only about 2–5% of the ejaculate.

Castration. This is routinely performed to increase weight gain and to reduce 'boar taint' – the smell associated with meat from male animals. It should only be done if it is really necessary and may be performed by a trained competent stockman before the age of 7 days. If older animals are to be castrated then it must be done by a veterinary surgeon.

Penis: Similar structure to the penis of the bull. The penis is about half a metre in length and has a sigmoid flexure (Fig. 17.31), which lies in front of the scrotum. The shaft is twisted counterclockwise for one complete turn. The anterior end has no glans penis and is also spirally twisted, similar to a corkscrew, especially during erection. The external urethral orifice is slit-like and lies ventrally, close to the end.

During erection, increasing blood pressure in the cavernous erectile tissue straightens the sigmoid flexure and the penis increases in length by 25%. The diameter of the shaft increases and both the longitudinal twist and the corkscrew spiral become more pronounced. During mating, which takes about 30 min, the end of the penis passes through the cervix and enters the uterus.

Prepuce: This is relatively long with a narrow opening surrounded by a few stiff hairs. It houses the free end of the penis. In the dorsal wall of the cranial part, which is wider, there is a *preputial diverticulum* which varies in size between individuals. It contains a foul-smelling liquid, which consists of cell debris soaked in urine. This produces the characteristic smell of a boar and contains the pheromone that encourages a sow to stand immobile during mating. This is also found in the saliva and breath of a boar.

References and recommended sources of further information

References

Adams, D. R. (1986). *Canine anatomy*. Ames, IA: Iowa State University Press.

Arthur, G. H. (1964). *Wright's veterinary obstetrics* (3rd ed.). London: Baillière Tindall.

Aspinall, V. (2001). *Anatomy and physiology for veterinary nurses*. Stroud, Gloucestershire: Keyskills Co. Ltd.

Aspinall, V. (2006). *The complete textbook of veterinary nursing*. London: Butterworth-Heinemann.

Aspinall, V. (2014a). *Clinical procedures in veterinary nursing* (3rd ed.). London: Butterworth-Heinemann.

Beaver, B. V. (1992). *Feline behaviour*. Philadelphia, PA: W.B. Saunders.

Beynon, P. (Ed.), (1996). *BSAVA manual of psittacine birds*. Cheltenham, Gloucestershire: British Small Animal Veterinary Association.

Beynon, P., & Cooper, J. E. (Eds.), (1992). *Manual of exotic pets*. Cheltenham, Gloucestershire: British Small Animal Veterinary Association.

Beynon, P., Lawton, M. P. C., & Cooper, J. E. (1992). *BSAVA manual of reptiles*. Cheltenham, Gloucestershire: British Small Animal Veterinary Association.

Bowden, C., & Masters, J. (Eds.), (2001). *Pre-veterinary nursing textbook*. Oxford: Butterworth-Heinemann.

Boyd, J. S. (2001a). *Colour atlas of clinical anatomy of the dog and cat* (2nd ed.). London: Mosby.

Budras, K. -D., Sack, W. O., & Röck, S. (2003). *Anatomy of the horse* (4th ed.). Hanover: Schlutersche.

Butcher, R. L. (Ed.), (1992). *Manual of ornamental fish*. Cheltenham, Gloucestershire: British Small Animal Veterinary Association.

Colville, T., & Bassett, J. M. (2002a). *Clinical anatomy and physiology for veterinary technicians*. St Louis, MO: Mosby.

Cooper, J. E. (2002). *Birds of prey – Health and disease*. Oxford: Blackwell Science.

Coumbe, K. (2001). *The equine veterinary nursing manual*. Oxford: Blackwell Science.

Dyce, K. M., Sack, W. O., & Wensing, C. J. G. (1996a). *Textbook of veterinary anatomy* (2nd ed.). Philadelphia, PA: W.B. Saunders.

Ekarius, C. (2008). *Storey's illustrated breed guide to sheep, goats, cattle and pigs*. North Adams, MA: Storey Publishing.

Evans, H. E. (1993). *Miller's anatomy of the dog* (3rd ed.). Philadelphia, PA: W.B. Saunders.

Evans, J. M., & White, K. (1988). *The book of the bitch*. Guildford: Henston.

Flecknell, P. (Ed.), (2000). *BSAVA manual of rabbit medicine and surgery*. Quedgeley, Gloucestershire: British Small Animal Veterinary Association.

Frandson, R. D., & Spurgeon, T. L. (1992). *Anatomy and physiology of farm animals*. Philadelphia, PA: Lea & Febiger.

Freeman, W. H., & Bracegirdle, B. (1966). *Atlas of histology*. London: Heinemann.

Fullick, A. (2000). *Biology*. Oxford: Heinemann.

Harvey Pough, F., Heiser, J. B., & McFarland, W. N. (1993). *Vertebrate life* (3rd ed.). Basingstoke: Macmillan.

Hillyer, E. V., & Quesenberry, K. E. (1997). *Ferrets, rabbits and rodents – Clinical medicine and surgery*. Philadelphia, PA: W.B. Saunders.

King, A. S., & McClelland, J. (1984). *Birds – Their structure and function*. London: Baillière Tindall.

Laber-Laird, K., Swindle, M. M., & Flecknell, P. (Eds.), (1996). *Handbook of rodent and rabbit medicine*. Oxford: Pergamon.

Lane, D. R. (1991). *Jones' animal nursing* (5th ed.). Oxford: Pergamon.

Lane, D. R., & Cooper, B. (Eds.), (1999). *Veterinary nursing*. (2nd ed.). Oxford: Butterworth-Heinemann.

Long, S. (2006). *Veterinary genetics and reproductive physiology*. Oxford: Butterworth-Heinemann.

Mader, D. R. (1996). *Reptile medicine and surgery*. Philadelphia, PA: W.B. Saunders.

McArthur, S. (1996). *Veterinary management of tortoises and turtles*. Oxford: Blackwell Science.

Meredith, A., & Redrobe, S. (Eds.), (2002). *Manual of exotic pets* (4th ed.). Quedgeley, Gloucestershire: British Small Animal Veterinary Association.

Michell, A. R., & Watkins, P. E. (1989). *An introduction to veterinary anatomy and physiology*. Cheltenham, Gloucestershire: British Small Animal Veterinary Association.

Okerman, L. (1994). *Diseases of domestic rabbits*. Oxford: Blackwell Science.

Phillips, W. D., & Chilton, T. J. (1989). *A-level biology*. Oxford: Oxford University Press.

Pickering, W. R. (1996). *Advanced human biology*. Oxford: Oxford University Press.

Reece, W. O. (1991). *Physiology of domestic animals*. Philadelphia, PA: Lea & Febiger.

Roberts, M. B. V. (1986). *Biology – A functional approach* (4th ed.). Walton-on-Thames, Surrey: Nelson.

Roberts, R. J. (Ed.), (2001). *Fish pathology* (3rd ed.). Philadelphia, PA: W.B. Saunders.

Roberts, V., & Scott-Park, F. (2008). *BSAVA manual of farm pets*. Gloucester: BSAVA.

Ruckebusch, Y., Phaneuf, L. -P., & Dunlop, R. (1991). *Physiology of small and large animals*. Philadelphia, PA: B.C. Decker.

Samuelson, D. A. (2007). *Textbook of veterinary histology*. St Louis, MO: Saunders-Elsevier.

Shively, M. J., & Beaver, B. G. (1985). *Dissection of the dog and cat*. Ames, IA: Iowa State University Press.

Silver, C. (1990). *Guide to the horses of the world*. London: Treasure Press.

Sisson, S., & Grossman, J. D. (1969). *Anatomy of the domestic animals* (4th ed.). Philadelphia, PA: W.B. Saunders.

Smith, B. J. (1999a). *Canine anatomy*. Philadelphia, PA: Lippincott Williams & Wilkins.

Sturkie, P. D. (Ed.), (1976). *Avian physiology*. New York: Springer Verlag.

Turner, T. (1994). *Veterinary notes for dog owners*. London: Popular Dogs.

Upton, J., & Soden, D. (1996). *An introduction to keeping sheep* (2nd ed.). Ipswich: Farming Press.

Warren Dean, M. (1995). *Small animal care and management*. New York: Delmar Publishers.

Web references

Abbott, K. A., & Lewis, C. J. (2005). Current approaches to the management of ovine footrot. *The Veterinary Journal*, *169*(1), 28–41, http://www.sciencedirect.com/science/article/pii/S1090023304001303. Accessed December 2013.

Aurochs. http://en.wikipedia.org/wiki/Aurochs. Accessed August 2013.

Boars. http://cal.vet.upenn.edu/projects/swine/bio/fem/conc/boar.html. Accessed January 2014.

Cattle. http://en.wikipedia.org/wiki/Cattle. Accessed August 2013.

Domestication. http://en.wikipedia.org/wiki/domestication. Accessed August 2013.

Domestic pig. http://en.wikipedia.org/wiki/domestic_pig. Accessed December 2013.

Estrus in swine. http://cal.vet.upenn.edu/projects/swine/bio/fem/estr.html. Accessed January 2014.

Hall, J. B., & Silver, S. Nutrition and feeding of the cow-calf herd: Digestive system of the cow. www.ext.vt.edu. Accessed November 2013.

HistoryWorld. History of the domestication of animals. http://www.historyworld.net/wrldhis/PlainTextHistories.asp?historyid=ab57. Accessed August 2013.

Pigs. https://www.rbst.org.uk/pigs-information. Accessed December 2013.

Further information

Aspinall, V. (2011). *The complete textbook of veterinary nursing.* London: Butterworth-Heinemann.

Aspinall, V. (2014b). *Clinical procedures in veterinary nursing.* London: Butterworth-Heinemann.

Boyd, J. S. (2001b). *Colour atlas of clinical anatomy of the dog and cat* (2nd ed.). London: Mosby.

Colville, T., & Bassett, J. M. (2002b). *Clinical anatomy and physiology for veterinary technicians.* St Louis, MO: Mosby.

Dyce, K. M., Sack, W. O., & Wensing, C. J. G. (1996b). *Textbook of veterinary anatomy* (2nd ed.). Philadelphia, PA: W.B. Saunders.

Lane, D. R., & Cooper, B. (Eds.), (2007). *Veterinary nursing* (4th ed.). Oxford: Butterworth-Heinemann.

Smith, B. J. (1999b). *Canine anatomy.* Philadelphia, PA: Lippincott Williams & Wilkins.

Introduction to anatomical terminology

Many of the words used in anatomy and physiology will be unfamiliar to you and may often appear rather daunting. However, if you become aware of the concept of breaking down a word into its component parts, then the word can be 'dissected' to discover its meaning. This technique is useful when trying to understand the veterinary 'jargon' used by vets, as well as within the broader context of anatomy and physiology.

A *prefix* is found at the beginning of a word, such as *peri* in pericardium. The prefix itself has a general meaning (e.g., *peri* means 'around'), but when combined with another word it gives a specific meaning: pericardium meaning literally 'around the heart'. Prefixes are given in Table A.1.

A *suffix* is found at the end of a word, such as *cyte* in osteocyte. Suffixes also have a general meaning – *cyte* means 'cell' – but when added to a word it becomes specific: osteocyte means 'bone cell'. Suffixes are given in Table A.2.

The *root* of a word is the essence of its meaning (e.g., *pericardium*). The root often refers to the organ, structure or disease in question; the root *cardium* relates to the heart. It can be considered as the 'word element', which is often derived from a Latin or Greek word. Roots are given in Table A.3.

Other words simply have a meaning that can be used within a word; for example, *genesis* means 'creation' or 'origination'. Thus, *carcinogenic* means that something 'creates' cancer; similarly, *pathogenic* means 'causing disease'.

Table A.1 Common prefixes

Prefix	Meaning	Examples
A-	Without; not	*Avascular* – without a blood supply
Anti-	Working against; counteracting	*Antibody* – neutralises antigens; *antiseptic* – inhibits growth of bacteria; *antihistamine* – inhibits the effects of histamine
Ante- (also Pre-)	Before	*Anterior* – structures at the front of the body; *antenatal* – before parturition; *prepubic* – in front of the pubis
Brady-	Slow	*Bradycardia* – slow heart rate; *bradypnoea* – slower than normal breathing
Cyto-	A cell	*Cytotoxic* – something that has a damaging effect on cells (e.g., cytotoxic drugs)
Dys-	Difficult; impaired	*Dyspnoea* – difficulty in breathing; *dysplasia* – an abnormality of development
Endo-	Within	*Endometrium* – the inner lining of the uterus; *endothelium* – the layer of epithelial cells that lines the inside of the heart and blood vessels
Epi-	Upon; outside of	*Epidermis* – the outermost layer of the skin; *epiglottis* – cartilaginous structure that guards the entrance to the larynx
Eryth(ro)-	Red	*Erythrocyte* – red blood cell; *erythema* – redness of the skin
Hyper-	Excessive; increased	*Hypertensive* – high blood pressure; *hypertrophy* – increase in the size of a tissue or organ
Hypo-	Decreased; deficient; beneath	*Hypothermia* – low body temperature; *hypodermis* – the subcutis that lies beneath the skin
Peri-	Around; in the region of	*Periosteum* – the connective tissue that surrounds a bone; *perianal* – around the anus
Poly-	Many; much	*Polyoestrous* – having more than one oestrous cycle a year; *polyarthritis* – inflammation of several joints; *polypeptide* – a compound containing three or more linked amino acids
Post-	After; behind	*Postmortem* – after death; *postoperative* – after a surgical operation; *posterior* – towards the rear
Pyo-	Pus	*Pyometra* – presence of pus in the uterus; *pyoderma* – bacterial infection of the skin
Tachy-	Rapid	*Tachycardia* – elevated heart rate

Table A.2 Common suffixes

Suffix	Meaning	Examples
-aemia	Relates to the blood	*Ischaemia* – reduced or deficient blood supply; *viraemia* – the presence of virus particles in the bloodstream
-cyte (cyto- is the prefix used)	A cell	*Erythrocyte* – red blood cell; *chondrocyte* – cartilage cell; *hepatocyte* – liver cell
-ectomy	Surgical removal of	*Thyroidectomy* – removal of the thyroid gland
-genic	Giving rise to; causing	*Pathogenic* – causing disease; *carcinogenic* – causing neoplasia or cancer
-ia/-iasis	Condition or state	*Hypoplasia* – incomplete development of an organ or tissue; *distichiasis* – presence of a double row of eyelashes
-itis	Inflammation	*Arthritis* – inflammation of a joint; *hepatitis* – inflammation of the liver; *conjunctivitis* – inflammation of the conjunctiva of the eye
-oma	Tumour, neoplasm	*Sarcoma* – malignant tumour; *lipoma* – benign tumour of adipose tissue
-osis	Disease order or state	*Osteochondrosis* – a developmental disease of articular cartilage
-ostomy	Surgical opening	*Tracheostomy* – opening into the trachea; *colostomy* – opening into the colon

Table A.3 Common roots of words

Root word	Meaning	Examples
Arthr(o)	Joint; articulation	*Arthrodesis* – surgical fusion of a joint; *arthritis* – inflammation of a joint
Cardi(o)	Heart	*Cardiology* – the study of the heart and its function; *myocardium* – muscle layer of the heart
Chondr(o)	Cartilage	*Chondrocyte* – cartilage cell; *perichondrium* – membrane that covers cartilage
Cyst(o)	Bladder	*Cystotomy* – incision into the bladder; *cystitis* – inflammation of the urinary bladder
Derm(ato)	Skin	*Dermatitis* – inflammation of the skin
Gloss(o) (also lingual)	Tongue	*Hypoglossal* – situated below the tongue (also *sublingual*)
Haem(ato/o)	Blood	*Haematemesis* – vomiting blood; *haemorrhage* – the escape of blood from a ruptured vessel
Hepat(o)	Liver	*Hepatocyte* – liver cell; *hepatic artery* – artery that supplies blood to the liver
Hist(io/o)	Tissue	*Histology* – the study of tissues
Mamm(o) (also mast(o))	Breast; mammary gland	*Mammogram* – radiograph of a mammary gland; *mastectomy* – surgical removal of mammary gland
Metr(a/o)	Uterus	*Endometrium* – lining of the uterus; *metritis* – inflammation of the uterus
My(o)	Muscle	*Myositis* – inflammation of a voluntary muscle
Neur(o)	Nerve	*Neuralgia* – pain in a nerve; *neuron* – nerve cell
Ophthalm(o)	Eye	*Ophthalmoscope* – instrument used to examine the interior of the eye
Orchi(d)	Testis (testicle)	*Orchitis* – inflammation of a testis; *cryptorchid* – having an undescended testicle
Oste(o)	Bone	*Osteomyelitis* – inflammation of bone
Pneum(o)	Air or gas; lung	*Pneumonia* – inflammation of the lung tissue; *pneumothorax* – the presence of free air in the thorax
-pnoea	Respiration; breathing	*Apnoea* – temporary cessation in breathing
Ren-	Kidney	*Renal artery* – the artery that supplies the kidney with blood
Rhin(o)	Nose	*Rhinitis* – inflammation of the mucous membrane of the nose
Trich(o)	Hair	*Trichosis* – any disease of, or abnormal growth of hair
Vas(o)	Vessel; duct	*Vascular* – pertaining to blood vessels; *vasoconstriction* – decrease in the diameter of a blood vessel; *vasectomy* – excision of the vas deferens (deferent duct)

APPENDIX 2

Multiple choice questions and answers

These multiple choice questions are based on the facts in the book, so why not test your understanding of what you have read? There is one correct answer to each question. The answers can be found on page 258.

Section 1 The dog and cat

1. Principles of cell biology

1.1 The cell membrane is mainly composed of:
a. a single layer of protein molecules
b. a protein bilayer
c. a phospholipid bilayer
d. a polysaccharide bilayer

1.2 Which of the following is *not* found in the nucleus of the cell?
a. centrioles
b. chromosomes
c. DNA
d. nucleoli

1.3 Which organelle is the site for ATP production?
a. nucleolus
b. mitochondrion
c. Golgi complex
d. ribosome

1.4 What is the function of the rough endoplasmic reticulum in the mammalian cell?
a. storage of lysosomal enzymes
b. synthesis and transport of proteins
c. synthesis of glucose
d. production of ATP

1.5 During which stage of mitosis do the chromosomes line up in the middle of the cell?
a. prophase
b. anaphase
c. metaphase
d. telophase

1.6 When does 'crossing-over' take place during meiosis?
a. metaphase
b. prophase
c. anaphase
d. telophase

1.7 Fluid that has a lower osmotic pressure than that of plasma is said to be:
a. hypotonic
b. isotonic
c. hypertonic
d. isometric

1.8 Which of the following cations is in a relatively higher concentration in the intracellular fluid than in the extracellular fluid?
a. potassium
b. iodine
c. sodium
d. chloride

1.9 Which of the following is *not* an example of a structural protein?
a. collagen
b. enzymes
c. elastin
d. keratin

1.10 Which of the following statements is the least accurate?
a. an acidic solution has a pH of below 7
b. the pH scale is a measure of a solution's hydrogen ion content
c. an alkaline substance releases hydrogen ions when dissolved in a solution
d. the pH of body fluids is 7.35

2. The tissues and body cavities

2.1 Which of the following is *not* a connective tissue?
a. bone
b. cartilage
c. muscle
d. blood

2.2 Which type of tissue covers the external and internal surfaces of the body?
a. connective
b. skin
c. areolar
d. epithelial

2.3 Where would you find simple cuboidal epithelium?
a. lining the bladder
b. lining the upper respiratory tract
c. lining the renal nephron
d. in the epidermis

2.4 What type of epithelium lines the ureters?
a. simple squamous
b. ciliated columnar
c. transitional
d. stratified squamous

2.5 Which of the following is an example of a simple coiled gland?
a. salivary
b. sweat
c. duodenal
d. sebaceous

2.6 Which type of cartilage is found in the epiglottis?
a. hyaline
b. fibrous
c. elastic
d. globular

2.7 Which type of bone tissue is found in the cortices of all types of bone?
a. spongy
b. cancellous
c. hyaline
d. compact

2.8 The contractile protein that makes up the thin filaments of a muscle fibre is:
a. actin
b. elastin
c. collagen
d. myosin

2.9 What is the name given to the serous endothelium that lines the inside of the thoracic cavity?
a. parietal peritoneum
b. parietal pleura
c. visceral peritoneum
d. mediastinum

2.10 What is found within the peritoneal cavity?
a. pleural fluid
b. the pericardium
c. peritoneal fluid
d. the mediastinum

3. The skeletal system

3.1 Which of the following is a splanchnic bone?
a. tuber calcis
b. patella
c. os penis
d. calcaneus

3.2 Where do the primary centres of ossification appear in a long bone?
a. the diaphysis
b. the ends
c. the epiphyses
d. the epiphyseal plate

3.3 Which bone of the skull lies at the base of the orbit and is the region through which the tears drain into the nose?
a. sphenoid
b. ethmoid
c. occipital
d. lacrimal

3.4 Which of the following joints is an example of an amphiarthrosis?
a. the temporomandibular
b. sutures of the skull
c. between the bodies of the vertebrae
d. between the skull and the atlas

3.5 Which part of the mandible articulates with the temporal region of the skull?
a. masseteric fossa
b. condylar process
c. coronoid process
d. occipital condyle

3.6 Which part of a thoracic vertebra articulates with the tubercle of a rib?
a. the spinous process
b. the costal fovea
c. the transverse fovea
d. the neural arch

3.7 How many sternebrae is the sternum made up of?
a. 7
b. 13
c. 3
d. 8

3.8 The olecranon fossa receives which part of the ulna during extension of the elbow?
a. olecranon
b. anconeal process
c. coronoid process
d. styloid process

3.9 On which bone would you find the medial malleolus?
a. tibia
b. fibula
c. femur
d. radius

3.10 How many short bones are found in the tarsus?
- **a.** 5
- **b.** 7
- **c.** 3
- **d.** 2

4. The muscular system

4.1 What is the unit of contraction in a muscle called?
- **a.** motor unit
- **b.** sarcomere
- **c.** origin
- **d.** insertion

4.2 Which of the following muscles protracts the forelimb and bends the neck laterally?
- **a.** brachialis
- **b.** biceps brachii
- **c.** brachiocephalicus
- **d.** biceps femoris

4.3 Which muscle inserts on the coronoid process of the mandible?
- **a.** temporalis
- **b.** masseter
- **c.** digastricus
- **d.** pterygoid

4.4 Where do the extraocular muscles insert?
- **a.** linea alba
- **b.** optic foramen
- **c.** the orbit
- **d.** the sclera

4.5 Through which of the openings in the diaphragm does the thoracic duct pass?
- **a.** oesophageal hiatus
- **b.** aortic hiatus
- **c.** inguinal ring
- **d.** caval foramen

4.6 Which of the following muscles does *not* insert on the linea alba?
- **a.** external abdominal oblique
- **b.** transversus abdominis
- **c.** rectus abdominis
- **d.** internal abdominal oblique

4.7 Which muscle inserts on the spine of the scapula?
- **a.** trapezius
- **b.** infraspinatus
- **c.** pectoralis
- **d.** latissimus dorsi

4.8 The patella is found in the tendon of insertion of which muscle?
- **a.** biceps femoris
- **b.** gastrocnemius
- **c.** semitendinosus
- **d.** quadriceps femoris

4.9 Which muscle flexes the hock?
- **a.** gastrocnemius
- **b.** biceps femoris
- **c.** anterior tibialis
- **d.** pectineus

4.10 Which of the following muscles is *not* a component of the Achilles tendon?
- **a.** semimembranosus
- **b.** biceps femoris
- **c.** semitendinosus
- **d.** superficial digital flexor

5. The nervous system and special senses

5.1 Which of the following structures is *not* part of the peripheral nervous system?
- **a.** cranial nerve V
- **b.** spinal nerves supplying the intercostal muscles
- **c.** hypothalamus
- **d.** a neuromuscular junction

5.2 Which of the following carry nerve impulses towards the cell body of a neuron?
- **a.** axons
- **b.** nodes of Ranvier
- **c.** myelin
- **d.** dendrons

5.3 Which of the following statements is *false?*
- **a.** Sensory nerve fibres carry information towards the central nervous system.
- **b.** Most nerve fibres within the grey matter of the brain are myelinated.
- **c.** A ganglion is a collection of nerve cell bodies.
- **d.** The autonomic nervous system consists mainly of visceral motor nerves.

5.4 The pons, medulla and cerebellum together form the –
- **a.** forebrain
- **b.** midbrain
- **c.** hindbrain
- **d.** cerebral hemispheres

5.5 Working from the outer surface of the brain to the inside, the meningeal layers are:
- **a.** pia mater, arachnoid mater, dura mater
- **b.** dura mater, arachnoid mater, pia mater
- **c.** arachnoid mater, dura mater, pia mater
- **d.** dura mater, pia mater, arachnoid mater

5.6 The aqueduct of Silvius lies within which part of the central nervous system?
- **a.** midbrain
- **b.** hindbrain
- **c.** spinal cord
- **d.** forebrain

5.7 Which of the cranial nerves is responsible for gustation?
- **a.** olfactory
- **b.** glossopharyngeal
- **c.** optic
- **d.** trochlear

5.8 Which of the following statements is *true?*
- **a.** The photoreceptor cells within the back of the eye and known as rods are responsible for colour vision.
- **b.** The pupil of the cat is rounded.
- **c.** Aqueous humour lies within the posterior chamber of the eye.
- **d.** The cells of the tapetum lucidum reflect light back to the photoreceptor cells of the retina.

5.9 Which of the following reflexes is routinely used to test for the level of anaesthesia?
- **a.** palpebral
- **b.** panniculus
- **c.** anal
- **d.** patellar

5.10 Which structure is used to monitor balance?
- **a.** organ of Corti
- **b.** tympanic membrane
- **c.** malleus
- **d.** utricle and saccule

6. The endocrine system

6.1 The chemical messengers sent out by the organs of the endocrine system are:
- **a.** glucose
- **b.** enzymes
- **c.** hormones
- **d.** nerve impulses

6.2 Which of the following statements about endocrine glands is *false?*
- **a.** They may be controlled by levels of chemicals or other hormones in the blood.
- **b.** They secrete hormones directly into their target organs by means of a duct.
- **c.** They secrete hormones that are designed to specifically affect the target organ and no other.
- **d.** They secrete hormones directly into the bloodstream.

6.3 Which of the following are classed as endocrine glands?
- **a.** ovary
- **b.** pancreas
- **c.** thyroid gland
- **d.** all of the above

6.4 Which of the following hormones is secreted by the posterior pituitary?
- **a.** ACTH
- **b.** TSH
- **c.** ADH
- **d.** FSH

6.5 Which of the following hormones has an effect on the kidney?
- **a.** ADH
- **b.** oxytocin
- **c.** TSH
- **d.** calcitonin

6.6 Which of the following is *not* secreted by the adrenal cortex?
- **a.** aldosterone
- **b.** cortisol
- **c.** oestrogen
- **d.** adrenaline

6.7 When an animal is very frightened and likely to attack you, which of the following is happening inside the animal?
- **a.** Salivary secretion increases so the animal dribbles.
- **b.** Blood glucose levels rise.
- **c.** Respiratory rate slows down.
- **d.** Levels of cortisol and corticosterone in the blood decrease.

6.8 Polydipsia, polyuria, polyphagia and bilateral symmetrical alopecia are symptoms of:
- **a.** diabetes mellitus
- **b.** diabetes insipidus
- **c.** Addison's disease
- **d.** Cushing's disease

6.9 Testosterone is secreted by which cells?
- **a.** islets of Langerhans
- **b.** Sertoli cells
- **c.** Brunner's glands
- **d.** cells of Leydig

6.10 Hypoglycaemia or lowered blood glucose will stimulate the secretion of which pancreatic hormone?
- **a.** glucagon
- **b.** insulin
- **c.** antidiuretic hormone
- **d.** somatostatin

7. The blood vascular system

7.1 Which of the following statements is *true?*
- **a.** Blood entering the right atrium is well oxygenated.
- **b.** The right ventricle pumps blood into the systemic circulation via the pulmonary vein.
- **c.** Blood returning to the heart enters the left atrium via the cranial and caudal venae cavae.
- **d.** The right ventricle pumps blood into the pulmonary circulation via the pulmonary artery.

7.2 Which branch of the aorta transports oxygenated blood to the kidneys?
a. renal vein
b. hepatic artery
c. renal artery
d. hepatic portal vein

7.3 The fibrous threads that attach the mitral valve to the papillary muscle of the ventricular wall are known as:
a. Purkinje fibres
b. chordae tendineae
c. bundle of His
d. collateral ligaments

7.4 Which granulocyte produces histamine?
a. basophil
b. eosinophil
c. neutrophil
d. macrophage

7.5 Which of the following are essential to the blood clotting mechanism?
a. potassium and vitamin D
b. calcium and vitamin K
c. sodium and vitamin C
d. iron and vitamin B

7.6 The area of modified cardiac muscle cells in the wall of the right atrium that initiates the heartbeat is referred to as the:
a. atrioventricular node
b. Purkinje fibres
c. bundle of His
d. sinoatrial node

7.7 In the fetal circulation, the shunt that connects the pulmonary artery and aorta is called the:
a. ductus venosus
b. foramen ovale
c. ductus arteriosus
d. falciform ligament

7.8 What is the name of the main lymphatic duct that arises in the abdomen?
a. tracheal duct
b. cisterna chyli
c. right lymphatic duct
d. cisterna magna

7.9 Which of the following is *not* a function of the spleen?
a. production of thrombocytes
b. storage of blood
c. destruction of worn out red blood cells
d. production of lymphocytes

7.10 Which of the following cells is involved in the humoral immune response?
a. macrophage
b. B lymphocyte
c. neutrophil
d. T lymphocyte

8. The respiratory system

8.1 What prevents food from entering the nasal chamber when an animal swallows?
a. nasal septum
b. soft palate
c. epiglottis
d. nasal conchae

8.2 Which part of the respiratory system is also responsible for the production of sound?
a. hyoid apparatus
b. eustachian tube
c. pharynx
d. larynx

8.3 Which type of epithelium lines the trachea?
a. ciliated columnar
b. simple squamous
c. stratified squamous
d. transitional

8.4 Which of the following is *true?* The route taken by the inspired air from the pharynx into the lungs is:
a. trachea, larynx, bronchi, bronchioles, alveolar ducts, alveolar sacs
b. larynx, bronchi, trachea, bronchioles, alveolar sacs, alveolar ducts
c. larynx, trachea, bronchioles, bronchi, alveolar sacs, alveolar ducts
d. larynx, trachea, bronchi, bronchioles, alveolar ducts, alveolar sacs

8.5 Where does gaseous exchange take place in the respiratory system?
a. bronchioles, alveolar ducts and alveoli
b. alveoli only
c. respiratory bronchioles only
d. alveolar ducts and alveoli

8.6 What is the fourth lobe of the right lung of a dog called?
a. apical lobe
b. cardiac lobe
c. the right lung does not have a fourth lobe
d. accessory lobe

8.7 Which muscle is responsible for increasing the volume of the thoracic cavity during inspiration?
a. diaphragm
b. hypaxial
c. external oblique
d. epaxial

8.8 Which reflex prevents over-inflation of the lungs?
a. Howell–Jolly
b. Hering–Breuer
c. cough
d. Flehman's

8.9 The chemoreceptors that monitor oxygen levels and the pH of the blood are located in the:
a. bronchi and bronchioles
b. alveoli
c. aortic and carotid bodies
d. jugular vein

8.10 The air left in the airways and lungs after a forced expiration is referred to as:
a. residual volume
b. dead space
c. vital capacity
d. tidal volume

9. The digestive system

9.1 The process of breaking food down into small, soluble units is known as:
a. ingestion
b. digestion
c. absorption
d. excretion

9.2 The cleft in the upper lip is known as the:
a. soft palate
b. carnassial
c. philtrum
d. tubercle

9.3 The formula for the deciduous dentition in the cat is:
a. [**I**3/3, **C**1/1, **PM** 3/2] × 2 = 26
b. [**I**3/3, **C**1/1, **PM** 3/3] × 2 = 28
c. [**I**3/3, **C**1/1, **PM** 4/4, **M** 2/3] × 2 = 42
d. [**I**3/3, **C**1/1, **PM** 3/2, **M** 1/1] × 2 = 30

9.4 Which of the following is *not* part of the small intestine?
a. stomach
b. duodenum
c. jejunum
d. ileum

9.5 Food passes through the parts of the large intestine in which order?
a. ascending colon, descending colon, transverse colon, caecum, rectum
b. descending colon, transverse colon, ascending colon, rectum, caecum
c. caecum, ascending colon, descending colon, transverse colon, rectum
d. caecum, ascending colon, transverse colon, descending colon, rectum

9.6 The chief cells in the gastric mucosa produce which part of the gastric juices?
a. pepsin
b. pepsinogen
c. hydrochloric acid
d. mucus

9.7 Which salivary gland lies within the orbit of the skull?
a. parotid
b. sublingual
c. mandibular
d. zygomatic

9.8 Food resulting from digestion in the stomach is:
a. chyme with an acid pH
b. chyle with a neutral pH
c. chyme with an alkaline pH
d. bile with a neutral pH

9.9 Which of the following is *not* a function of the liver?
a. production of plasma proteins
b. storage of iron
c. regulation of fluid volume in the fluid compartments
d. formation of red blood cells in the fetus

9.10 Amino acids resulting from the digestion of protein are carried to the liver by the:
a. lacteals
b. hepatic portal vein
c. hepatic vein
d. hepatic artery

10. The urinary system

10.1 Which of the following statements is *false*?
a. The position of the kidney in the abdomen is described as being retroperitoneal.
b. The right kidney is caudal to the left kidney.
c. The kidneys lie in the cranial abdomen closely attached to the lumbar hypaxial muscles.
d. The ovaries and the adrenal glands lie close to the cranial pole of each kidney.

10.2 The basin-shaped structure in the centre of the kidney is called the:
a. cortex
b. hilus
c. pelvis
d. medulla

10.3 The loop of Henle of each nephron:
a. lies within the medulla and is lined with simple squamous epithelium
b. lies in the cortex and is lined with cuboidal epithelium
c. lies in the medulla and is lined with columnar epithelium
d. lies in the kidney pyramids and collects urine from several nephrons

10.4 Which of the following does *not* occur in the proximal convoluted tubule?
a. secretion of penicillin
b. reabsorption of glucose
c. control of acid–base balance
d. reabsorption of water

10.5 Which of the following statements is *false?*
a. Aldosterone is secreted by the anterior pituitary gland at the base of the brain.
b. Aldosterone acts mainly on the distal convoluted tubules and controls the reabsorption of sodium.
c. ADH is secreted when an animal is dehydrated.
d. The release of aldosterone is stimulated by angiotensin.

10.6 Which of the following hormones does *not* have an effect on the kidney?
a. renin
b. aldosterone
c. antidiuretic hormone
d. erythropoietin

10.7 If an animal is over-hydrated, which of the following will happen?
a. Blood pressure will fall and will be detected by baroreceptors in the blood vessel walls.
b. Osmotic pressure will rise and the osmoreceptors will stimulate the thirst centre.
c. Secretion of ADH will decrease and a large volume of dilute urine will be excreted.
d. Water will be resorbed into the capillaries of the medulla from the loops of Henle.

10.8 If an animal is fed on a high-salt diet, which of the following will *not* happen?
a. The osmotic pressure of the blood will increase.
b. Water will be drawn into the circulation by osmosis, increasing the circulating blood volume.
c. The animal will become hypertensive.
d. Aldosterone secretion will rise and sodium will be resorbed from the distal convoluted tubules.

10.9 The bladder is lined by which type of epithelium?
a. squamous
b. ciliated columnar
c. transitional
d. cuboidal

10.10 Normal urine contains:
a. glucose, water and urea
b. water, salts and urea
c. protein, amino acids and water
d. urea, crystals and glucose

11. The reproductive system

11.1 Which of the following is *not* a function of the male reproductive tract?
a. secretion of hormones to produce the secondary sexual characteristics
b. transportation of urine from the bladder to the outside of the body
c. production of fluids to wash the sperm into the female tract
d. production of sperm to fertilise the ova of the female

11.2 At what age would you expect to find the testes in the scrotum of the dog?
a. 12 weeks post-partum
b. 35 weeks of gestation
c. just prior to parturition
d. 6 months post-partum

11.3 Which of the following are seen in the cat and *not* in the dog?
a. bulbourethral glands
b. preprostatic urethra
c. barbed glans penis
d. all of the above

11.4 The os penis of the dog lies:
a. ventral to the urethra
b. dorsal to the urethra
c. caudal to the prostate
d. in the centre of the urethra

11.5 Spermatozoa are produced:
a. by mitosis and contain the diploid number of chromosomes
b. by meiosis and contain the haploid number of chromosomes
c. by binary fission and contain the haploid number of chromosomes
d. by meiosis and contain the diploid number of chromosomes

11.6 The bitch and the queen are described as:
a. primigravid
b. uniparous
c. multigravid
d. multiparous

11.7 Pseudocyesis is better known as:
a. pregnancy
b. fertilisation
c. false pregnancy
d. ovulation

11.8 The fold of peritoneum supporting the uterus within the peritoneal cavity is the:
a. broad ligament
b. mesosalpinx
c. mesovarium
d. mesocolon

11.9 The queen is described as being:
a. a spontaneous ovulator and seasonally polyoestrous
b. an induced ovulator and monoestrous
c. an induced ovulator and seasonally polyoestrous
d. a spontaneous ovulator and monoestrous

11.10 Within the inner cell mass of the developing embryo the ectoderm forms:
- **a.** the lining of the digestive tract
- **b.** the trophoblast
- **c.** the skin and nervous system
- **d.** the musculoskeletal system

12. The common integument

12.1 In which layer of the epidermis are new cells manufactured?
- **a.** stratum granulosum
- **b.** stratum germinativum
- **c.** stratum lucidum
- **d.** stratum corneum

12.2 In which layer of the skin are the sensory nerve endings found?
- **a.** hypodermis
- **b.** epidermis
- **c.** dermis
- **d.** subcutis

12.3 Where do the ducts of the sebaceous glands open into?
- **a.** the surface layer of the epithelium
- **b.** the hair follicle
- **c.** the sweat glands
- **d.** the hypodermis

12.4 Where are ceruminous glands found?
- **a.** opening onto the eyelids
- **b.** around the circumference of the anus
- **c.** associated with each hair follicle
- **d.** in the external ear canal

12.5 Which of the following statements is the most accurate?
- **a.** Each hair follicle contains one guard hair and several wool hairs.
- **b.** Each hair follicle contains a wool hair only.
- **c.** Each hair follicle contains one wool hair and several guard hairs.
- **d.** Each hair follicle contains several guard hairs and many wool hairs.

12.6 How many pads are found on the hind paw of the dog?
- **a.** 7
- **b.** 4
- **c.** 5
- **d.** 6

12.7 Which muscle unsheathes the claws of a cat?
- **a.** digital extensor muscle
- **b.** digital flexor muscle
- **c.** carpal flexor muscle
- **d.** carpal extensor muscle

12.8 Which part of the distal phalanx is covered by the claw?
- **a.** anconeal process
- **b.** sole
- **c.** ungual process
- **d.** claw fold

12.9 Where are sudoriferous glands found in the dog?
- **a.** at the base of the tail
- **b.** on the nose and foot pads
- **c.** associated with each hair follicle
- **d.** in the ear canal

12.10 Which of the following is *not* a function of the integument?
- **a.** secretion of pheromones
- **b.** production of vitamin E
- **c.** protection from invasion by bacteria
- **d.** thermoregulation

Section 2 Comparative Anatomy and Physiology

13. Birds

13.1 Which of the following characteristics is possessed only by the class Aves?
- **a.** ability to fly
- **b.** feathers
- **c.** ability to lay eggs
- **d.** warm blood

13.2 The sternum of the bird is extended into a flattened:
- **a.** coracoid
- **b.** quadrate
- **c.** keel
- **d.** pygostyle

13.3 Which of the following statements is *false?*
- **a.** Some of the bones of the skeleton are filled with sacs full of air to reduce the weight.
- **b.** There are always seven cervical vertebrae in the neck no matter how long the neck.
- **c.** At the base of the tail is a preen gland whose secretions are vital for the health of the feathers.
- **d.** There is no diaphragm to divide the body cavity into thorax and abdomen.

13.4 The feathers attached to the ulna of the wing are the:
- **a.** contour feathers
- **b.** filoplume
- **c.** primaries
- **d.** secondaries

13.5 Which is the most developed special sense in the bird?
- **a.** sight
- **b.** touch
- **c.** smell
- **d.** taste

13.6 Which of the following statements is *false?*
- **a.** Air passes through the lungs twice; the second passage is the most efficient.
- **b.** Many thin-walled air sacs lead out of the lungs and occupy most of the body cavity.
- **c.** The lungs are large, flexible and spongy and lie close to the ventral body wall.
- **d.** There is no diaphragm separating the thorax from the abdomen.

13.7 The passage of food down the digestive tract is:
- **a.** crop, proventriculus, gizzard, duodenum, jejunum
- **b.** oesophagus, stomach, duodenum, jejunum
- **c.** gizzard, proventriculus, crop, duodenum, ileum
- **d.** oesophagus, crop, gizzard, proventriculus

13.8 In the bird, the principal excretory product is:
- **a.** urea
- **b.** ammonia
- **c.** urates
- **d.** bile

13.9 Which part of the female reproductive tract is responsible for the addition of albumen to the bird's egg?
- **a.** magnum
- **b.** isthmus
- **c.** shell gland
- **d.** vagina

13.10 By which method could you identify the sex of a budgerigar?
- **a.** DNA testing
- **b.** surgical sexing
- **c.** sexual dimorphism
- **d.** by listening to the birdsong

14. Small mammals

14.1 Members of the order Lagomorpha can be distinguished from members of the order Rodentia by examination of:
- **a.** ears
- **b.** genitalia
- **c.** teeth
- **d.** cheek muscles

14.2 The digestive tract of the rabbit and the herbivorous rodent has an enlarged:
- **a.** stomach
- **b.** spleen
- **c.** jejunum
- **d.** caecum

14.3 The dental formula of the rabbit is:
- **a.** [**I**1/1, **C**0/0, **PM**0/0, **M** 3/3] × 2 = 16
- **b.** [**I**2/1, **C**0/0, **PM**3/2, **M** 3/3] × 2 = 28
- **c.** [**I**1/1, **C**0/0, **PM**1/1, **M** 3/3] × 2 = 20
- **d.** [**I**3/3, **C**1/1, **PM**3/3, **M** 1/2] × 2 = 34

14.4 The space between the incisors and the cheek teeth of rabbits and rodents is known as the:
- **a.** diastema
- **b.** philtrum
- **c.** dewlap
- **d.** acromion

14.5 Young that are born blind, deaf, hairless and totally dependent on the mother are described as being:
- **a.** precocial
- **b.** nidicolous
- **c.** altricial
- **d.** nidifugous

14.6 Which of the following species gives birth to precocial young?
- **a.** *Mustela putorius furo*
- **b.** *Oryctolagus cuniculus*
- **c.** *Mus musculus*
- **d.** *Chinchilla lanigera*

14.7 Which of the following species is an induced ovulator?
- **a.** the ferret
- **b.** the mouse
- **c.** the guinea pig
- **d.** the chipmunk

14.8 Which of the following statements is *false?*
- **a.** Jill ferrets can suffer from a fatal anaemia if not allowed to breed at regular intervals.
- **b.** The jill is a spontaneous ovulator and ovulation occurs on the tenth day of the season.
- **c.** Ferrets are true carnivores and belong to the family Mustelidae.
- **d.** The male ferret has a J-shaped os penis that lies in the caudal portion of the penis.

14.9 The males of which of the following species have teats on the ventral body wall?
- **a.** *Rattus norvegicus*
- **b.** *Tamias sibiricus*
- **c.** *Cavia porcellus*
- **d.** *Mesocricetus auratus*

14.10 The gestation period of the chinchilla is:
- **a.** 111 days
- **b.** 9 weeks
- **c.** 28–32 days
- **d.** 15–18 days

15. Reptiles and fish

15.1 Tortoises and terrapins belong to the order:
- **a.** Rhynchocephalia
- **b.** Crocodilia
- **c.** Chelonia
- **d.** Squamata

15.2 Which of the following statements is *false?*
- **a.** The body cavity of the reptile is not divided into two by a diaphragm.
- **b.** In the peripheral circulation of the reptile a renal portal system transports blood from the hind limbs and tail directly to the kidney.
- **c.** Reptiles do not possess a bladder for the storage of urine.
- **d.** Reptiles may be oviparous (egg layers) or ovoviviparous (live bearers).

15.3 The sex of a tortoise can be determined by examining:
- **a.** the tail length: males have longer tails
- **b.** the plastron: that of the female is convex and of the male is concave
- **c.** the caudal scute: in the female it may curve upwards
- **d.** all of the above

15.4 The ability of some species of lizard to shed the tail and grow a new one is known as:
- **a.** ecdysis
- **b.** autotomy
- **c.** caecotrophy
- **d.** mutation

15.5 Jacobsen's organ, located in the mouth of some reptiles, is associated with which sense?
- **a.** smell
- **b.** sight
- **c.** hearing
- **d.** touch

15.6 Which one of the following statements is *false?*
- **a.** Snakes do not have eyelids but have a transparent spectacle over the eye.
- **b.** Some snakes show evidence of vestigial legs.
- **c.** All species of snake have external ears, which they use to detect their prey.
- **d.** Some snakes lay eggs while others bear live young.

15.7 Which body system does not open into the cloaca of the snake?
- **a.** digestive
- **b.** urinary
- **c.** reproductive
- **d.** circulatory

15.8 In fish a physostomous swim bladder is refilled with air by:
- **a.** a gas gland lying in the wall of the bladder
- **b.** swimming to the surface and taking a mouthful of air
- **c.** excretory gases formed by the gut
- **d.** descending to the bottom and increasing the air pressure

15.9 The ability of shoals of fish to move simultaneously is thought to be linked to the presence of:
- **a.** the lateral line
- **b.** chromatophores in the skin that change colour
- **c.** the presence of the glycocalyx, which reduces friction
- **d.** coordinated movements of the tail fins

15.10 The function of the gill rakers projecting from the gill arches is to:
- **a.** extract oxygen from the water passing over them
- **b.** prevent damage to the gills by food particles taken into the mouth cavity
- **c.** prevent damage to the gills from objects in the water
- **d.** support the gill arches

16. The horse

16.1 The horse has evolved to take weight on which digit of the pentadactyl limb?
- **a.** 1
- **b.** 2
- **c.** 3
- **d.** 4

16.2 The vertebral formula of the horse is:
- **a.** C7 T18 L6 S5 Cd15-20
- **b.** C7 T12-13 L7 S4 Cd16
- **c.** C7 T13 L7 S3 Cd20-23
- **d.** C7 T15 L5-6 S3 Cd18

16.3 The joint between the short pastern bone and the pedal bone is known as the:
- **a.** pastern
- **b.** knee
- **c.** fetlock
- **d.** coffin

16.4 The full set of permanent teeth is present in the jaw and is in wear by what age?
- **a.** 4 years
- **b.** 5 years
- **c.** 6 years
- **d.** 7 years

16.5 The sesamoid bone housed within the hoof is known as the:
- **a.** navicular
- **b.** pedal
- **c.** coffin
- **d.** fabella

16.6 Which statement best describes the function of the splenius muscle?
- **a.** It abducts the forelimb and flexes the shoulder.
- **b.** It extends the hip, flexes the stifle and extends the hock.
- **c.** It elevates and flexes the neck.
- **d.** It protracts the forelimb and extends the shoulder.

16.7 From which point on a horse's foot does horn grow?
- **a.** the sole
- **b.** the coronet
- **c.** the periople
- **d.** the frog

16.8 The normal resting heart rate of the horse is:
- **a.** 120–180 beats per minute
- **b.** 80–120 beats per minute
- **c.** 25–42 beats per minute
- **d.** 130–325 beats per minute

16.9 Food passes through the large colon in the following order:
- **a.** right dorsal colon, left dorsal colon, left ventral colon, right ventral colon
- **b.** right dorsal colon, right ventral colon, left dorsal colon, left ventral colon
- **c.** left ventral colon, right ventral colon, right dorsal colon, left dorsal colon
- **d.** right ventral colon, left ventral colon, left dorsal colon, right dorsal colon

16.10 Which of the following most accurately describes the reproductive pattern of the mare?
- **a.** The mare is a short-day breeder, seasonally polyoestrous and an induced ovulator.
- **b.** The mare is a long-day breeder, seasonally polyoestrous and a spontaneous ovulator.
- **c.** The mare is a long-day breeder, monoestrous and an induced ovulator.
- **d.** The mare is a short-day breeder, monoestrous and a spontaneous ovulator.

17. Farm animals

17.1 Which of the following species is *not* part of the order Artiodactyla?
- **a.** *Bos taurus*
- **b.** *Equus caballus*
- **c.** *Capra hircus*
- **d.** *Sus scrofa domesticus*

17.2 The descriptive term meaning an animal is 'many horned' is:
- **a.** polled
- **b.** multiparous
- **c.** polycerate
- **d.** vestigial

17.3 Which of the following statements concerning the anatomy of the cow is *false*?
- **a.** The peroneus longus muscle originates on the lateral condyle of the tibia and inserts on the first tarsal bone and the proximal end of the large metatarsal bone and its function is to bring about inward rotation of the hock.
- **b.** The interdigital ligaments run between the two toes on each foot and prevent the digits from splaying apart when weight is taken.
- **c.** The ulna and radius of the cow are separate bones, as they are in the dog and the horse.
- **d.** The phalanges of the 2nd and 5th digits are vestigial and are known as the dew claws.

17.4 Which of the following best describes the epithelial lining of the omasum of a ruminant?
- **a.** pinkish in colour with openings of digestive glands distributed over the majority of the mucosa
- **b.** arranged in deep longitudinal folds with shorter folds between them
- **c.** covered in numerous rounded and conical-shaped papillae
- **d.** arranged in low folds encompassing 4-, 5- or 6-sided spaces to create a honeycomb effect

17.5 The ansa spiralis of the ruminant digestive tract is part of which organ?
- **a.** oesophagus
- **b.** rumen
- **c.** transverse colon
- **d.** ascending colon

17.6 With reference to the oestrous cycle, the ewe is described as:
- **a.** spontaneous ovulator, seasonally polyoestrous and a short day breeder
- **b.** induced ovulator, seasonally polyoestrous and a long day breeder
- **c.** spontaneous ovulator, monoestrous and a short day breeder
- **d.** induced ovulator, monoestrous and a long day breeder

17.7 The vertebral formula of the pig is:
- **a.** C7 T13 L6-7 S4 Cd16-18
- **b.** C7 T13 L6 S5 Cd18-20
- **c.** C7 T18 L6 S5 Cd15-20
- **d.** C7 T14-15 L6-7 S4 Cd20-23

17.8 The type of placenta described as being diffuse is seen in which species?
- **a.** dog and cat
- **b.** pig and horse
- **c.** dog and sheep
- **d.** cow and pig

17.9 Which of the following male animals has a pair of large seminal vesicles, a corkscrew-shaped penis and a preputial diverticulum?
- **a.** ram
- **b.** stallion
- **c.** boar
- **d.** bull

17.10 The gestation period of the ewe is:
- **a.** 114 days
- **b.** 21 weeks
- **c.** 154 days
- **d.** 40 weeks

Multiple choice answers

1

1.1	c
1.2	a
1.3	b
1.4	b
1.5	c
1.6	b
1.7	a
1.8	a
1.9	b
1.10	c

2

2.1	c
2.2	d
2.3	c
2.4	c
2.5	b
2.6	c
2.7	d
2.8	a
2.9	b
2.10	c

3

3.1	c
3.2	a
3.3	d
3.4	c
3.5	b
3.6	c
3.7	d
3.8	b
3.9	a
3.10	b

4

4.1	b
4.2	c
4.3	a
4.4	d
4.5	b
4.6	c
4.7	a
4.8	d
4.9	c
4.10	a

5

5.1	c
5.2	d
5.3	b
5.4	c
5.5	b
5.6	a
5.7	b
5.8	d
5.9	a
5.10	d

6

6.1	c
6.2	b
6.3	d
6.4	c
6.5	a
6.6	d
6.7	b
6.8	d
6.9	d
6.10	a

7

7.1	d
7.2	c
7.3	b
7.4	a
7.5	b
7.6	d
7.7	c
7.8	b
7.9	a
7.10	b

8

8.1	b
8.2	d
8.3	a
8.4	d
8.5	b
8.6	d
8.7	a
8.8	b
8.9	c
8.10	a

9

9.1	b
9.2	c
9.3	a
9.4	a
9.5	d
9.6	b
9.7	d
9.8	a
9.9	c
9.10	b

10

10.1	b
10.2	c
10.3	a
10.4	c
10.5	a
10.6	d
10.7	c
10.8	d
10.9	c
10.10	b

11

11.1	b
11.2	a
11.3	d
11.4	b
11.5	b
11.6	d
11.7	c
11.8	a
11.9	c
11.10	c

12

12.1	b
12.2	c
12.3	b
12.4	d
12.5	a
12.6	c
12.7	b
12.8	c
12.9	b
12.10	b

13

13.1	b
13.2	c
13.3	b
13.4	d
13.5	a
13.6	c
13.7	a
13.8	c
13.9	a
13.10	c

14

14.1	c
14.2	d
14.3	b
14.4	a
14.5	c
14.6	d
14.7	a
14.8	b
14.9	c
14.10	a

15

15.1	c
15.2	c
15.3	d
15.4	b
15.5	a
15.6	c
15.7	d
15.8	b
15.9	a
15.10	b

16

16.1	c
16.2	a
16.3	d
16.4	c
16.5	a
16.6	c
16.7	b
16.8	c
16.9	d
16.10	b

17

17.1	b
17.2	c
17.3	c
17.4	b
17.5	d
17.6	a
17. 7	d
17.8	b
17.9	c
17.10	b

Index

Note: Page numbers followed by *f* indicate figures, *b* indicate boxes and *t* indicate tables.

C

F

G

H

N

O

P

S

V

W

X

Y

Z